Bright Futures

FOURTH EDITION

Guidelines for Health Supervision of Infants, Children, and Adolescents

EDITORS

Joseph F. Hagan, Jr, MD, FAAP

Judith S. Shaw, EdD, MPH, RN, FAAP

Paula M. Duncan, MD, FAAP

SUPPORTED, IN PART, BY

US Department of Health and Human Services

Health Resources and Services Administration

Maternal and Child Health Bureau

PUBLISHED BY

American Academy of Pediatrics

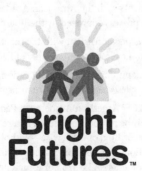

prevention and health
promotion for infants,
children, adolescents,
and their families™

American Academy of Pediatrics

DEDICATED TO THE HEALTH OF ALL CHILDREN®

D1379348

This publication has been produced by the American Academy of Pediatrics. Supported, in part, under its cooperative agreement (U04MC07853) with the US Department of Health and Human Services, Health Resources and Services Administration (HRSA), Maternal and Child Health Bureau (MCHB).

Suggested citation: Hagan JF, Shaw JS, Duncan PM, eds. *Bright Futures: Guidelines for Health Supervision of Infants, Children, and Adolescents.* 4th ed. Elk Grove Village, IL: American Academy of Pediatrics; 2017

American Academy of Pediatrics Bright Futures National Center Staff

Chief Medical Officer
Senior Vice President, Child Health and Wellness
American Academy of Pediatrics: *V. Fan Tait, MD*

Director, Division of Developmental Pediatrics and Preventive Services: *Darcy Steinberg-Hastings, MPH*

Manager, Bright Futures National Center: *Jane Bassewitz, MA*

Manager, Bright Futures Implementation: *Kathryn Janies*

American Academy of Pediatrics Publishing Staff

Director, Department of Publishing: *Mark Grimes*

Senior Editor, Professional/Clinical Publishing: *Eileen Glasstetter, MS*

Production Manager, Clinical/Professional Publications: *Theresa Wiener*

Editorial Specialist: *Amanda Helmholz*

Manager, Art Direction and Production: *Linda Diamond*

Manager, Art Direction and Production: *Peg Mulcahy*

Senior Vice President, Membership Engagement and Marketing and Sales: *Mary Lou White*

Marketing Manager, Practice Publications: *Mary Jo Reynolds*

Printed in the United States of America

3-333/0217

3 4 5 6 7 8 9 10

BF0043

ISBN: 978-1-61002-022-0
eBook: 978-1-61002-023-7
Library of Congress Control Number: 2016940985

Dedication

This work honors our coeditor, Paula Duncan, MD, FAAP, without whose energy, insight, and spirit these *Guidelines* would not have achieved relevance for current pediatric practice.

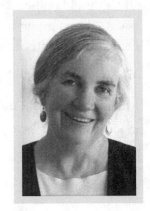

A graduate of Manhattanville College, Dr Duncan received her medical degree from Women's Medical College in Philadelphia and completed her pediatric residency at Albany Medical Center and at Stanford University Medical Center, where she was also a Clinical Scholar in Adolescent Medicine.

In her early career in adolescent medicine, Dr Duncan committed to the primary and community-based care that she recognized as essential to her patients' healthy growth and development. She identified a mid-career opportunity to improve child and adolescent health in her community and left practice to serve as Medical Director of the Burlington (Vermont) School Department, where she was an early leader in the design of school-based health services. In addition, she created an innovative and nationally recognized curriculum for HIV/AIDS education for grades 4 through 12. From 1987–2001, she facilitated the Vermont public-private partnership of health care delivery at Vermont Department of Health, and served as state Maternal and Child Health Director from 1993–1998. Dr Duncan later became Youth Project Director for the Vermont Child Health Improvement Program at The Robert Larner, M.D. College of Medicine at the University of Vermont, where she is Clinical Professor in Pediatrics.

Dr Duncan's career has also been one of service in her community and on the national level. She was vice president of the American Academy of Pediatrics (AAP) Vermont Chapter (1990–1994) and later president of the Vermont Medical Society (2009). Her national work with the AAP includes serving as coeditor of the AAP's *Bright Futures Guidelines,* 3rd and 4th editions (2008 and 2017) and the *Bright Futures Tool and Resource Kit* (2009) as well as chairing the AAP Bright Futures Steering Committee.

Her contributions have been honored in national and AAP awards, including the Executive Committee Clifford Grulee Award, which recognizes long-term accomplishments and outstanding service to the AAP. She also received the AAP Section on Pediatric Dentistry Oral Health Services Award, and the AAP Council on Community Pediatrics Job Lewis Smith Award, which recognizes lifelong outstanding career achievement in community pediatrics.

The US Department of Health and Human Services, Health Resources and Service Administration (HRSA) Maternal Child Health Bureau (MCHB) Director's Award was presented to Dr Duncan in 2007 "in recognition of contributions made to the health of infants, mothers, children, adolescents, and children with special health needs in the Nation." In 2011, Dr Duncan was recipient of the Abraham Jacobi Award, which is presented to a pediatrician who is a member of both the AAP and the American Medical Association. This award recognizes long-term, notable national contributions to pediatrics in teaching, patient care, and/or clinical research.

Dr Duncan reminds us that "the heart of Bright Futures is establishing trust to build a therapeutic relationship." She has championed and devoted her career to the use of strength-based approaches. And this is who she is. Dr Duncan's warmth, joyfulness, and ability to see the best in people enable her to behold the innate strengths of families. It is her passion to teach all of us how to see families as she does and serve them better. This focus on strengths and protective factors in the clinical encounter of preventive services is her essential contribution to our *Bright Futures Guidelines*, 4th Edition.

We are in Paula's debt for her collegiality and great wisdom. And we cherish her friendship.

Joe Hagan

Judy Shaw

Mission Statement, Core Values, and Vision of the American Academy of Pediatrics

Mission

The mission of the American Academy of Pediatrics (AAP) is to attain optimal physical, mental, and social health and well-being for all infants, children, adolescents, and young adults. To accomplish this mission, the AAP shall support the professional needs of its members.

Core Values

We believe

- In the inherent worth of all children; they are our most enduring and vulnerable legacy.
- Children deserve optimal health and the highest quality health care.
- Pediatricians, Pediatric Subspecialists, and Pediatric Surgical Specialists are the best qualified to provide child health care.
- Multidisciplinary teams including patients and families are integral to delivering the highest quality health care.

The AAP is the organization to advance child health and well-being and the profession of pediatrics.

Vision

Children have optimal health and well-being and are valued by society. Academy members practice the highest quality health care and experience professional satisfaction and personal well-being.

Bright Futures Mission Statement

The mission of Bright Futures is to promote and improve the health, education, and well-being of infants, children, adolescents, families, and communities.

Contents

Bright Futures Health Promotion Themes

CONTENTS

Bright Futures Health Supervision Visits

Bright Futures: A Comprehensive Approach to Health Supervision

Bright Futures: Guidelines for Health Supervision of Infants, Children, and Adolescents describes a system of care that is unique in its attention to health promotion activities and psychosocial factors of health and its focus on youth and family strengths. It also is unique in recognizing that effective health promotion and disease prevention require coordinated efforts among medical and nonmedical professionals and agencies, including public health, social services, mental health, educational services, home health, parents, caregivers, families, and many other members of the broader community. The *Guidelines* address the care needs of **all** children and adolescents, including children and youth with special health care needs and children from families from diverse cultural and ethnic backgrounds.

Since 2001, the Maternal and Child Health Bureau (MCHB) of the US Department of Health and Human Services' Health Resources and Services Administration has awarded cooperative agreements to the American Academy of Pediatrics (AAP) to lead the Bright Futures initiative. With the encouragement and strong support of the MCHB, the AAP and its many collaborating partners developed the third and fourth editions of the *Bright Futures Guidelines.*

An Evolving Understanding of Health Supervision for Children

When the Bright Futures Project Advisory Committee convened for the third edition, the members began with key questions: What is Bright Futures? How can a new edition improve upon existing guidelines? Most important, how can a new edition improve the desired outcome of

guidelines, which is child health? We turned to the previous editions of *Bright Futures Guidelines* for insight and direction.

The first edition of the *Bright Futures Guidelines,* published in 1994, emphasized the psychosocial aspects of health. Although other guidelines at the time, notably the AAP *Guidelines for Health Supervision,* considered psychosocial factors, Bright Futures emphasized the critical importance of child and family social and emotional functioning as a core component of the health supervision encounter. In the introduction to the first edition, Morris Green, MD, and his colleagues demonstrated this commitment by writing that Bright Futures represents "…'a new health supervision' [that] is urgently needed to confront the 'new morbidities' that challenge today's children and families."[1] This edition continues this emphasis.

The second edition of the *Bright Futures Guidelines,* published in 2000, further emphasized that care for children could be defined and taught to both health care professionals and families. In collaboration with Judith S. Palfrey, MD, and an expert advisory group, Dr Green retooled the initial description of Bright Futures to encompass this new dimension: "Bright Futures is a vision, a philosophy, a set of expert guidelines, and a practical developmental approach to providing health supervision to children of all ages from birth to adolescence."[2]

For the third edition of the *Bright Futures Guidelines,* the AAP's cooperative agreement with the MCHB created multidisciplinary Bright Futures expert panels working through the Bright Futures Education Center.[3] The panels, which first met in September 2003, further adapted the

Guidelines to clinical primary care by enumerating appropriate universal and selective screening and developing anticipatory guidance recommendations for each health supervision visit. Evidence was sought to ground these recommendations in science and a process was established to encourage needed study and to accumulate new evidence as it became available. The third edition expanded the definition of Bright Futures to be "a set of principles, strategies, and tools that are theory based, evidence driven, and systems oriented that can be used to improve the health and well-being of all children through culturally appropriate interventions that address their current and emerging health promotion needs at the family, clinical practice, community, health system, and policy levels."

Following publication in 2008, the Bright Futures Implementation Project demonstrated to practices that health supervision could be improved by using the *Bright Futures Guidelines.* Subsequent study demonstrated that practices and clinics could successfully implement the screening and guidance recommended.[4]

Developing the Fourth Edition

From its earliest conception and planning, the experts who have contributed to Bright Futures have viewed primary care health supervision as a service intended to promote health. Like our predecessors, we view health as not simply the absence of disease, but rather the presence of mental, physical, family, and social wellness. This wellness in infants, children, adolescents, and young adults is intended to prevent disease and promote health. It has always been the Bright Futures vision that the strength of families and communities is essential to child health.

We assert that health, broadly considered, requires a healthy family and a healthy community, and we now have the science to support our belief. New knowledge of early brain development and the importance of nurturance to avoid or lessen

trauma and stress on the developing brain not only tells us that our long-held beliefs regarding health promotion might actually be true but also guides our contemporary work in this endeavor. The new science of epigenetics brings parents and caregivers to our care domain. If we cannot address the environmental and social determinants of health for parents—and alter their epigenetics—we will not change the developmental trajectory of their children or their grandchildren. In this fourth edition, clinicians will find emphasis on this uniquely pediatric endeavor. A new team of experts was convened to develop a new health promotion theme: *Promoting Lifelong Health for Families and Communities.* It provides a current review of the science of development and insight for how this science might be applied in our practices and clinics.

Since the last edition, new evidence has been developed regarding health supervision activities. We have actively sought this evidence since the previous edition and with MCHB support of young investigators, many contributions to this work have been made. Clinicians are directed to the *Evidence and Rationale chapter* so that they might understand how to apply this evidence to their work.

As was done for the previous edition, 4 multidisciplinary expert panels were convened for the age stages of infancy, early childhood, middle childhood, and adolescence. Each panel was cochaired by a pediatrician content expert and a panel member who represented family members or another health profession. The 39 members of the expert panels were individuals who represented a wide range of disciplines and areas of expertise. These representatives included mental health experts, nutritionists, oral health practitioners, family medicine providers, nurse practitioners, family and school representatives, and members of AAP national committees with relevant expertise (eg, AAP Committee on Psychosocial Aspects of Child and Family Health, AAP Committee on

Practice and Ambulatory Medicine, and AAP Committee on Adolescence).

Also, as was done with the previous edition, the *Bright Futures Guidelines* were posted for public review before publication. External reviewers who represented AAP committees, councils, and sections; professional organizations; institutions; and individuals with expertise and interest in this project provided more than 3,500 comments and endorsements that were essential to the final revisions of the *Guidelines*.

Building on Strengths, Moving in New Directions

Recognizing that the science of health care for children continues to expand, the *Bright Futures Guidelines* developers have been consistently encouraged to consider which Bright Futures concepts from earlier editions could be used and further developed to drive positive change and improve clinical practice. As a result, the third edition, and now the fourth edition, build on the strengths of previous editions while also moving in new directions. The *Bright Futures Guidelines* serve as the recommended preventive services to be delivered to infants, children, adolescents, and their families.

An Emphasis on the Evidence Base

An ongoing theme in the evolution of Bright Futures involves exploration of the science of prevention and health promotion to document effectiveness, measure outcomes, and promote additional research and evidence-based practice. An evidence panel for the third edition composed of members of AAP Section on Epidemiology (known as SOEp) was convened to conduct systematic research on the Bright Futures recommendations. The Panel drew from expert sources, such as the Cochrane Collaboration,[5] the US Preventive Services Task Force,[6] the Centers for Disease Control and Prevention Community Guide,[7]

professional organizations' policy and committee work, the National Guideline Clearinghouse,[8] and *Healthy People 2010*.[9]

In this fourth edition, evidence expert Alex Kemper, MD, FAAP, advised the Bright Futures Steering Committee and editors. Dr Kemper was especially helpful in areas where research and practice are changing rapidly or are investigational. Available evidence continues to guide our work. Our process of evidence discernment is discussed in the *Evidence and Rationale chapter* and new evidence is highlighted.

A Recognition that Health Supervision Must Keep Pace With Changes in Family, Community, and Society

In any health care arrangement, successful practices create a team composed of families, health care professionals, and community experts to learn about and obtain helpful resources. In so doing, they also identify gaps in services and supports for families. The team shares responsibility with, and provides support and training to, families and other caregivers, while also identifying and collaborating with community resources that can help meet family needs. New evidence, new community influences, and emerging societal changes dictate the form and content of necessary health care for children.[10] Bright Futures places special emphasis on several areas of vital importance to caring for children and families, including social determinants of health, care for children and youth with special health care needs, and cultural competence. Discussion of these issues is woven throughout the Bright Futures Health Promotion Themes and Bright Futures Health Supervision Visits.

A Pledge to Work Collaboratively With Families and Communities

Health supervision care is carried out in a variety of settings in collaboration with health care professionals from many disciplines and in concert with families, parents, and communities. Bright Futures health supervision involves families and parents in family-centered medical homes, recognizes the strengths that families and parents bring to the practice of health care for children, and identifies resources and educational materials specific for individual families. All of us who care for children are challenged to construct new methodologies and systems for excellent care that embody this vision for health care that optimizes the health and well-being of all infants, children, adolescents, and young adults.

References

1. Green M, ed. *Bright Futures: Guidelines for Health Supervision of Infants, Children, and Adolescents.* Arlington, VA: National Center for Education in Maternal and Child Health; 1994

2. Green M, Palfrey JS, eds. *Bright Futures: Guidelines for Health Supervision of Infants, Children, and Adolescents.* 2nd ed. Arlington, VA: National Center for Education in Maternal and Child Health; 2000

3. Hagan JF, Shaw JS, Duncan PM, eds. *Bright Futures: Guidelines for Health Supervision of Infants, Children, and Adolescents.* 3rd ed. Elk Grove Village, IL: American Academy of Pediatrics; 2008

4. Duncan PM, Pirretti A, Earls MF, et al. Improving delivery of Bright Futures preventive services at the 9- and 24-month well child visit. *Pediatrics.* 2015;135(1):e178-e186

5. The Cochrane Collaboration: The Reliable Source of Evidence in Health Care. http://www.cochrane.org. Accessed July 7, 2006

6. *The Guide to Clinical Preventive Services: Report of the United States Preventive Services Task Force.* 3rd ed. Washington, DC: International Medical Publishing; 2002

7. Centers for Disease Control and Prevention. The Community Guide. https://www.thecommunityguide.org. Accessed December 30, 2016

8. US Department of Health and Human Services, National Guideline Clearinghouse. http://www.guideline.gov. Accessed December 30, 2016

9. US Department of Health and Human Services. *Healthy People 2010: Understanding and Improving Health.* 2nd ed. Washington, DC: Government Printing Office; 2000

10. Schor EL. Rethinking well-child care. *Pediatrics.* 2004;114(1): 210-216

BRIGHT FUTURES: A COMPREHENSIVE APPROACH TO HEALTH SUEPRVISION

Contributors

Bright Futures Expert Panels

Infancy

Deborah Campbell, MD (Cochairperson)

Barbara Deloian, PhD, RN, CPNP (Cochairperson)

Melissa Clark Vickers, MEd

George J. Cohen, MD (retired)

Tumaini R. Coker, MD, MBA

Dipesh Navsaria, MD, MPH, MSLIS

Beth Potter, MD

Penelope Knapp, MD

Rocio Quinonez, DMD, MS, MPH, FRCDC

Karyl Rickard, PhD, RDN

Elizabeth P. Elliott, MS, PA-C

Early Childhood

Cynthia S. Minkovitz, MD, MPP (Cochairperson)

Donald B. Middleton, MD (Cochairperson)

Joseph M. Carrillo, MD

Peter A. Gorski, MD, MPA

Christopher A. Kus, MD, MPH

Nan Gaylord, PhD, RN, CPNP-PC

Francisco Ramos-Gomez, DDS, MS, MPH

Madeleine Sigman-Grant, PhD, RD

Manuel E. Jimenez, MD, MS

Middle Childhood

Edward Goldson, MD (Cochairperson)

Bonnie A. Spear, PhD, RDN (Cochairperson)

Scott W. Cashion, DDS, MS

Paula L. Coates, DDS, MS

Anne Turner-Henson, PhD, RN

Arthur Lavin, MD

Robert C. Lee, DO, MS

Beth A. MacDonald

Eve Spratt, MD, MS

Jane A. Weida, MD

Adolescence

Martin M. Fisher, MD (Cochairperson)

Frances E. Biagioli, MD (Cochairperson)

Pamela Burke, PhD, RN, FNP, PNP

Shakeeb Chinoy, MD

Arthur B. Elster, MD

Katrina Holt, MPH, MS, RD

M. Susan Jay, MD

Jaime Martinez, MD

Vaughn Rickert, PsyD[†]

Scott D. Smith, DDS, MS

Bright Futures Evidence Expert

Alex Kemper, MD

Promoting Lifelong Health for Families and Communities Theme

Frances E. Biagioli, MD

Deborah Campbell, MD

Joseph Carrillo, MD

Shakeeb Chinoy, MD

James Duffee, MD, MPH

Arthur B. Elster, MD

Andrew Garner, MD, PhD

Nan Gaylord, PhD, RN, CPNP

Penelope Knapp, MD

Colleen Kraft, MD

Robert C. Lee, DO, MS

Anne Turner-Henson, PhD, RN

Melissa Clark Vickers, MEd

American Academy of Pediatrics

Board of Directors Reviewers
David I. Bromberg, MD, FAAP

Pamela K. Shaw, MD, FAAP

Staff
Vera Frances "Fan" Tait, MD
Principal Investigator

Roger F. Suchyta, MD
Senior Medical Advisor

Darcy Steinberg-Hastings, MPH
Coprincipal Investigator

Jane B. Bassewitz, MA
Project Director, Bright Futures National Center

Kathryn M. Janies
Manager, Bright Futures Implementation

Jonathan Faletti
Manager, Chapter Programs

Bonnie Kozial
Manager, Injury, Violence, and Poison Prevention

Stephanie Mucha, MPH
Manager, Children With Special Needs Initiatives

Linda Paul, MPH
Manager, Committees and Sections

Elizabeth Sobczyk, MPH, MSW
Manager, Immunization Initiatives

JBS International, Inc.
Deborah S. Mullen, Project Director

Anne Brown Rodgers, Senior Science Writer
and Editor

Nancy L. Keene, Senior Science Writer

Reference Librarian
Jae N. Vick, MLS

Other Contributors
Paul H. Lipkin, MD
AAP Council on Children With Disabilities

Michelle M. Macias, MD
AAP Section on Developmental and Behavioral
Pediatrics

Jamie Meringer, MD
The Robert Larner, M.D. College of Medicine at
the University of Vermont

Amy E. Pirretti, MS

Organizations and Agencies That Participated in the Bright Futures Project Advisory Committees

Bright Futures Steering Committee
The Bright Futures Steering Committee oversees
the Bright Futures National Center (BFNC) efforts.
The steering committee provides advice on activities and consultation to chairpersons and staff of
the BFNC and the center's Project Implementation
Advisory Committee (PIAC).

Paula M. Duncan, MD (Chairperson), American
Academy of Pediatrics

Leslie Carroll, MUP, Family Voices

Edward S. Curry, MD, American Academy
of Pediatrics

Joseph F. Hagan, Jr, MD, American Academy
of Pediatrics

Mary Margaret Gottesman, PhD, RN, CPNP,
National Association of Pediatric Nurse
Practitioners

Judith S. Shaw, EdD, MPH, RN, Academic
Pediatric Association

Jack T. Swanson, MD, American Academy
of Pediatrics

Elizabeth Edgerton, MD, MPH (Federal Liaison),
Health Resources and Services Administration,
Maternal and Child Health Bureau

Erin Reiney, MPH, CHES (Federal Liaison), Health
Resources and Services Administration, Maternal
and Child Health Bureau

CONTRIBUTORS

Bright Futures Project Implementation Advisory Committee

The BFNC PIAC provides guidance on activities and consultation to chairpersons and staff of the BFNC on implementation of Bright Futures across disciplines. The PIAC members serve as representatives on the center's PIAC, reporting on Bright Futures activities to constituents and eliciting organizational interest and support. Members promote Bright Futures content and philosophy to other national, state, and local organizations; assist in increasing collaborative efforts among organizations; and promote center activities by offering presentations, and trainings, to colleagues within constituent organizations.

Paula M. Duncan, MD (Chairperson)
American Academy of Pediatrics

Christopher M. Barry, PA-C, MMSc
American Academy of Physician Assistants

Martha Dewey Bergren, DNS, RN, NCSN
National Association of School Nurses

Gregory S. Blaschke, MD, MPH
Oregon Health & Science University
Doernbecher Children's Hospital

Laura Brey, MS
National Association of School-Based
Health Centers

Paul Casamassimo, DDS
American Academy of Pediatric Dentistry

James J. Crall, DDS, ScD
American Academy of Pediatric Dentistry

Michael Fraser, PhD, CAE
Association of Maternal and Child
Health Programs

Sandra G. Hassink, MD
Thomas Jefferson University
Nemours/Alfred I. duPont Hospital for Children

Seiji Hayashi, MD, MPH
Health Resources and Services Administration,
Bureau of Primary Health Care

Stephen Holve, MD
Indian Health Service

Christopher A. Kus, MD, MPH
Association of Maternal and Child
Health Programs

Sharon Moffatt, RN, BSN, MS
Association of State and Territorial Health Officials

Ruth Perou, PhD
Centers for Disease Control and Prevention

Richard E. Rainey, MD
Blue Cross Blue Shield Association

Beth Rezet, MD
Association of Pediatric Program Directors

Judith S. Shaw, EdD, MPH, RN
Academic Pediatric Association

Bonnie A. Spear, PhD, RDN
American Dietetic Association

David Stevens, MD
National Association of Community
Health Centers

Myrtis Sullivan, MD, MPH
National Medical Association

Felicia K. Taylor, MBA
National Association of Pediatric
Nurse Practitioners

Modena Wilson, MD, MPH
American Medical Association

Bright Futures Project Implementation Advisory Committee Federal Liaisons

Elizabeth Edgerton, MD, MPH
Health Resources and Services Administration,
Maternal and Child Health Bureau

Seiji Hayashi, MD, MPH
Health Resources and Services Administration,
Bureau of Primary Health Care

Stephen Holve, MD
Indian Health Service

Ruth Perou, PhD
Centers for Disease Control and Prevention

Erin Reiney, MPH, CHES
Health Resources and Services Administration,
Maternal and Child Health Bureau

Acknowledgments

The fourth edition of *Bright Futures: Guidelines for Health Supervision of Infants, Children, and Adolescents* could not have been created without the leadership, wise counsel, and unwavering efforts of many people. We are grateful for the valuable help we received from a wide variety of multidisciplinary organizations and individuals.

Under the leadership of Michael C. Lu, MD, MS, MPH, associate administrator for Maternal and Child Health (MCH), Health Resources and Services Administration, the project has benefited from the dedication and guidance of many MCH Bureau staff, especially Elizabeth Edgerton, MD, MPH, director for the Division of Child, Adolescent and Family, and Erin Reiney, MPH, CHES, the Bright Futures project officer. We also acknowledge the contributions of Chris DeGraw, MD, MPH, former Bright Futures project officer. His commitment to and guidance of the Bright Futures initiative were invaluable.

We are grateful to the American Academy of Pediatrics, in particular Fan Tait, MD; Darcy Steinberg-Hastings, MPH; and Jane Bassewitz, MA, for their vision, creativity, support, and leadership as we drafted the fourth edition. We also thank Alex Kemper, MD, for his leadership in guiding the evidence review process. We are thankful to Anne Rodgers, our excellent science writer, who was so effective in helping us to say clearly what we wished to communicate.

We appreciate Leslie Carroll, MUP; Edward S. Curry, MD; Mary Margaret Gottesman, PhD, RN, CPNP; Jack T. Swanson, MD; Frances E. Biagioli, MD; Deborah Campbell, MD; Barbara Deloian, PhD, RN, CPNP; Martin M. Fisher, MD; Edward Goldson, MD; Donald B. Middleton, MD; Cynthia S. Minkovitz, MD, MPP; and Bonnie A. Spear, PhD, RDN, who were always available to us as our core consultants. Their continual review helped ensure that our recommendations would be relevant to practice and applicable to the community setting.

We are extremely grateful to the 4 multidisciplinary expert panels for their tremendous commitment and contributions in developing the fourth edition of the *Guidelines,* as well as to the expert group that worked to develop the new *Promoting Lifelong Health for Families and Communities theme.*

We also acknowledge the help and expertise of Paul H. Lipkin, MD, and Michelle M. Macias, MD, who updated and revised the infancy and early childhood developmental milestones; Jamie Meringer, MD, who assisted in developing content on e-cigarettes; and Claire McCarthy, MD; Jenny Radesky, MD; and Megan A. Moreno, MD, MSEd, MPH, who assisted in developing content related to social media.

We also wish to acknowledge the significant contributions of American Academy of Pediatrics staff, especially Kathryn Janies, Jonathan Faletti, and Bonnie Kozial, who have worked diligently to ensure the success of Bright Futures.

Throughout the process of developing and revising this edition of the *Guidelines,* we relied on numerous experts who reviewed sections of the document, often multiple times. Their careful review and thoughtful suggestions improved the *Guidelines* immeasurably. In summer 2015, the entire document was posted on the Bright Futures Web site for external review. During this time, we received more than 3,500 comments from across all disciplines (ie, health care, public health professionals, child care professionals, educators), parents, and other child health advocates throughout the United States. We are most grateful to those who took the time to ensure that the *Guidelines* are as complete and scientifically sound as possible.

The passion and commitment of all of these individuals and partners have significantly advanced the field of health care for all infants, children, and adolescents.

—*Joseph F. Hagan, Jr, MD, FAAP; Judith S. Shaw, EdD, MPH, RN, FAAP; and Paula M. Duncan, MD, FAAP, editors*

ACKNOWLEDGMENTS

In Memoriam

The Bright Futures experts, consultants, staff, and editors wish to acknowledge the loss of dear friends and colleagues since the publication of the last edition. We are forever grateful for their contributions to children and their families.

Morris Green, MD, FAAP, a leader in the field of child behavior and emotional health and an early proponent of family-centered care, was editor of the *Bright Futures Guidelines,* 1st Edition, and coeditor of the second edition. Dr Green practiced pediatrics in Indiana for more than 45 years; for 20 years he was physician-in-chief of the James Whitcomb Riley Hospital for Children and chairman of the Indiana University School of Medicine Department of Pediatrics. He died in August of 2013 at the age of 91. Morris was an important consultant and role model in the development of the third edition.

Polly Arango was a cofounder of Family Voices, a national family organization dedicated to family-centered care for children and youth with special health care needs or disabilities, and of Parents Reaching Out, an organization educating and advocating for New Mexico parents of disabled children. She died in June of 2010 at the age of 68. Polly Arango served on the expert panels for the *Bright Futures Guidelines,* 3rd and 4th editions. We are indebted to Polly for centering our work on the families in which children grow and develop.

Thomas Tonniges, MD, FAAP, served as director of community pediatrics at the American Academy of Pediatrics (AAP) and helped to bring the Bright Futures projects to the AAP. He died in October of 2015 at the age of 66. While in private practice before coming to the AAP, Dr Tonniges was instrumental in developing the national model for the medical home. Tom's leadership in the Bright Futures Pediatric Implementation Project has fostered an improving standard for pediatric and adolescent health supervision care.

Vaughn Rickert, PsyD, was a scholar and professor of adolescent medicine and was a past president of the Society for Adolescent Medicine. Dr Rickert was professor of pediatrics and the Donald P. Orr Chair in Adolescent Medicine at Indiana University School of Medicine and Riley Hospital for Children where he was the director of the Section of Adolescent Medicine. He died in June of 2015 at the age of 62. Vaughn's contributions to the Bright Futures Adolescent Expert Panel were essential to the behavioral care components of health supervision care.

May they rest in peace.

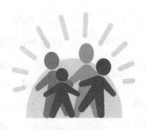

What Is Bright Futures?

AN INTRODUCTION TO THE FOURTH EDITION OF

Bright Futures: Guidelines for Health Supervision of Infants, Children, and Adolescents

Bright Futures is a set of principles, strategies, and tools that are theory based, evidence driven, and systems oriented that can be used to improve the health and well-being of all children through culturally appropriate interventions that address their current and emerging health promotion needs at the family, clinical practice, community, health system, and policy levels.

Bright Futures is . . .

. . . a set of principles, strategies, and tools . . .

The Bright Futures principles acknowledge the value of each child, the importance of family, the connection to community, and that children and youth with special health care needs are children first. These principles assist the health care professional in delivering, and the practice in supporting, the highest quality health care for children and their families.

Strategies drive practices and health care professionals to succeed in achieving professional excellence. Bright Futures can assist pediatric health care professionals in raising the bar of quality health care for all of our children, through a

thoughtfully derived process that will allow them to do their jobs well.

This book is the core of the Bright Futures tools for practice. It is not intended to be a textbook, but a compendium of guidelines, expert opinion, and recommendations for health supervision visits. Other available Bright Futures resources can be found at **https://brightfutures.aap.org.** The *Bright Futures Tool and Resource Kit* that accompanies this book is designed to assist health care professionals in planning and carrying out health supervision visits. It contains numerous charts, forms, screening instruments, and other tools that increase practice efficiency and efficacy.

. . . that are theory based, evidence driven . . .

The rationale for a clinical decision can balance evidence from research, clinical practice guidelines, professional recommendations, or decision support systems with expert opinion, experience, habit, intuition, preferences, or values. Clinical or counseling decisions and recommendations also can be based on legislation (eg, seat belts), common sense not likely to be studied experimentally (eg, sunburn prevention), or relational evidence (eg, television watching and violent behavior). Most important, clinical and counseling decisions are responsive to family needs and desires expressed in the context of patient-centered decision making. It follows that much of the content of a health supervision visit is the theoretical application of scientific principles in the service of child and family health.

Strong evidence for the effectiveness of a clinical intervention is one of the most persuasive arguments for making it a part of child health supervision. On the other hand, if careful studies have shown an intervention to be ineffective or even harmful, few would argue for its inclusion. Identifying and assessing evidence for effectiveness was a central element of the work involved in developing this edition's health supervision recommendations. The multifaceted approach we used is described in greater detail in the *Evidence and Rationale chapter*.

... and systems oriented ...

In the footsteps of Green and Palfrey[1] (the developers of earlier editions of the *Bright Futures Guidelines*), we created principles, strategies, and tools as part of a Bright Futures system of care. That system goes beyond the schema of individual health supervision visits and encompasses an approach that includes continuous improvements in the delivery system that result in better outcomes for children and families. Experience since the release of the third edition demonstrates the ability of practices to effect these changes.[2] Knowing what to do is important; knowing how to do it is essential.

A systems-oriented approach in a Bright Futures practice means moving beyond the status quo to become a practice where redesign and positive change are embodied every day. Methods for disseminating and applying Bright Futures knowledge in the practice environment must be accomplished with an understanding of the health care system and environment.

... that can be used to improve the health and well-being of all children ...

The care described by Bright Futures contributes to positive health outcomes through health promotion and anticipatory guidance, disease prevention, and early detection of disease. Preventive services address these child health outcomes and provide guidance to parents and children, including children and youth with special health care needs.

These health outcomes,[3] which represent physical and emotional well-being and optimal functioning at home, in school, and in the community, include

- Attaining a healthy weight and body mass index, and normal blood pressure, vision, and hearing
- Pursuing healthy behaviors related to nutrition, physical activity, safety, sexuality, and substance use
- Accomplishing the developmental tasks of childhood and adolescence related to social connections, competence, autonomy, empathy, and coping skills
- Having a loving, responsible family who is supported by a safe community
- For children with special health care needs or chronic health problems, achieving self-management skills and the freedom from real or perceived barriers to reaching their potential

... through culturally appropriate interventions ...

Culture is a system of shared values and beliefs and learned patterns of behavior that are not defined simply by ethnicity or race. A culture may form around sexual orientation, religion, language, gender, disability, or socioeconomic status. Cultural values are beliefs, behaviors, and ideas that a group of people share and expect to be observed in their dealings with others. These values inform interpersonal interactions and communication, influencing such critical aspects of the provider-patient relationship as body language, touch, communication style and eye contact, modesty, responses to pain, and a willingness to disclose mental or emotional distress.

Cultural competence (knowledge and awareness of values, behaviors, attitudes, and practices within a system, organization, and program or among individuals that enables them to work effectively cross-culturally) is intricately linked to the concept and practice of family-centered care. Family-centered care in Bright Futures honors the strengths, cultures, traditions, and expertise that everyone brings to a respectful family-professional partnership. With this approach to care, families feel they can make decisions, with providers at different levels, in the care of their own children and as advocates for systems and policies that support children and youth with special health care needs. Cultural competence requires building relationships with community cultural brokers who can provide an understanding of community norms and links to other families and organizations, such as churches or social clubs.

● ● ● that address their current and emerging health promotion needs ● ● ●

The third edition identified 2 health issues in current child health practice, as major concerns for families, health care professionals, health planners, and the community—promoting healthy weight and promoting mental health. They were highlighted as "Significant Challenges to Child and Adolescent Health" throughout that edition of the *Bright Futures Guidelines* and the *Bright Futures Tool and Resource Kit.* These remain important issues of focus in child and youth health supervision care.

Lifestyle choices strongly influence weight status and effective interventions are family based and begin in infancy. The choice to breastfeed, the appropriate introduction of solid foods, and family meal planning and participation lay the ground-work for a child's lifelong healthy eating habits. Parents also influence lifelong habits of physical

activity and physical inactivity. Through Bright Futures' guidance on careful monitoring, interventions, and anticipatory guidance about nutrition, activity level, and other family lifestyle choices, health care professionals can play an important role in promoting healthy weight for all children and adolescents.

A 1999 surgeon general's report described mental health in childhood and adolescence as the achievement of expected developmental, cognitive, social, and emotional milestones and of secure attachments, satisfying social relationships, and effective coping skills.[4] This remains an appropriate definition and its achievement is a goal of health supervision. As many as 1 in 5 children and adolescents has diagnosable mental or addictive disorder that is associated with at least minimum impairment.

This edition broadens our attention to health and mental health in addressing the new sciences of early brain development and epigenetics and the impact of social determinants of health on child and family health and well-being. *(For more on this issue, see the Promoting Lifelong Health for Families and Communities theme.)* Child health care professionals champion a strength-based approach, helping families identify their assets that enhance their ability to care for their child and guide their child's development. Bright Futures provides multiple opportunities for promoting lifelong health in the health supervision visits.

● ● ● at the family level ● ● ●

The composition and context of the typical or traditional family have changed significantly over the past 3 decades. Fewer children now reside in a household with their biological mother and father and with only one parent working outside the home. Today, the term *family* is used to describe a unit that may comprise a married nuclear family; cohabiting family; single-parent, blended, or stepfamily; grandparent-headed household; single-gender parents; commuter or long-distance family; foster family; or a larger community family with several

Bright Futures Guidelines for Health Supervision of Infants, Children, and Adolescents

WHAT IS BRIGHT FUTURES?

individuals who share the caregiving and parenting responsibilities. Each of these family constellations presents unique challenges to child-rearing for parents as well as children.

Families are critical partners in the care of children. A successful system of care for children is family centered and embraces the medical home and the dental home concepts. In a Bright Futures partnership, health care professionals expect that families come to the partnership with strengths. They acknowledge and reinforce those strengths and help build others. They also recognize that all (health care professionals, families, and children) grow, learn, and develop over time and with experience, information, training, and support. This approach also includes encouraging opportunities for children and youth that have been demonstrated to correlate with positive health behavior choices. For some families, these assets are strongly ingrained and reinforced by cultural or faith-based beliefs. They are equally important in all socioeconomic groups. Most families can maximize these assets if they are aware of their importance. *(For more on this issue, see the Promoting Family Support theme.)*

Collaboration with families in a clinical practice is a series of communications, agreements, and negotiations to ensure the best possible health care for the child. In the Bright Futures vision of family-centered care, families must be empowered as care participants. Their unique ability to choose what is best for their children must be recognized.

...the clinical practice level...

To further define the diversity of practice in the care of children, it is important to consider the community of care that is available to the family. The clinical practice is central to providing health supervision. Practices may be small or large, private or public sector, or affiliated with a hospital. A rural solo practice, suburban private practice of one or several physicians and nurse practitioners,

children's service within a multidisciplinary clinic, school-based health center, dental office, community health center, and public health clinic are all examples of practices that provide preventive services to children. Each model consists of health care professionals with committed and experienced office or clinic staff to provide care for children and their families.

To adequately address the health needs, including oral health and emotional and social needs, of a child and family, child health care professionals always will serve as care coordinators. Health care professionals, working closely with the family, will develop a centralized patient care plan and seek consultations from medical, nursing, or dental colleagues, mental health professionals, nutritionists, and others in the community, on behalf of their patients, and will facilitate appropriate referrals when necessary. Care coordination also involves a knowledge of community services and support systems that might be recommended to families. At the heart of the Bright Futures approach to practice is the notion that every child deserves a medical and dental home.

A medical home is defined as primary care that is accessible, continuous, comprehensive, family centered, coordinated, compassionate, and culturally effective.[5] In a medical home, a child health care professional works in partnership with the family and patient to ensure that all the medical and non-medical needs of the patient are met. Through this partnership, the child health care professional can help the family and patient access and coordinate specialty care, educational services, out-of-home care, family support, and other public and private community services that are important to the overall health of the child and family.

Nowhere is the medical home concept more important than in the care of children and youth with special health care needs. For families and

4

health care professionals alike, the implications of caring for a child or youth with special health care needs can be profound. *(For more on this issue, see the Promoting Health for Children and Youth With Special Health Care Needs theme.)*

The dental home[6] provides risk assessment and an individualized preventive dental health program, anticipatory guidance, a plan for emergency dental trauma, comprehensive dental care, and referrals to other specialists. *(For more on this issue, see the Promoting Oral Health theme.)*

... and the community, health system, and policy levels.

One of the unique and core values of Bright Futures is the commitment to advocacy and action in promoting health and preventing disease, not only within the medical home but also in partnership with other health and education professionals and others in the community. This core value rests on a clear understanding of the important role that the community plays in influencing children's health, both positively and negatively. Communities in which children, youth, and families feel safe and valued, and have access to positive activities and relationships, provide the essential base on which the health care professional can build to support healthy behaviors for families at the health supervision visits. Understanding the community in which the practice or clinic is located can help the health care professional learn the strengths of that community and use and build on those strengths. Data on community threats and assets provide an important tool that providers can use to prioritize action on specific health concerns.

The Bright Futures comprehensive approach to health care also encompasses continuous improvements in the overall health care delivery system that result in enhanced prevention services, improved outcomes for children and families, and the potential for cost savings.

Bright Futures embodies the concept of synergy between health care professionals, who provide health promotion and preventive services to individual children and families, and public health care professionals, who develop policies and implement programs to address the health of populations of children at the community, state, and national levels. Bright Futures has the opportunity to serve as a critical link between the health of individual children and families and public policy health goals. *Healthy People 2020*,[7] for example, is a comprehensive set of disease prevention and health promotion objectives for the nation over the current decade of this century. Its major goals are to increase the quality and number of years of healthy life and to eliminate health disparities. In its leading health indicators, *Healthy People 2020* enumerates the 12 most important health issues for the nation.

- Access to health services
- Clinical preventive services
- Environmental quality
- Injury and violence
- Maternal, infant, and child health
- Mental health
- Nutrition, physical activity, and obesity
- Oral health
- Reproductive and sexual health
- Social determinants
- Substance abuse
- Tobacco

Many of the themes for the Bright Futures Health Supervision Visits were chosen from these leading health indicators to synchronize the efforts of office-based or clinic-based health supervision and public health efforts. This partnership role is explicitly mentioned in the American Academy of Pediatrics (AAP) policy statement on the pediatrician's role in community pediatrics, which recommends that pediatricians "…should work collaboratively with public health departments and colleagues in related professions to identify and mitigate hindrances to the health and well-being of children in the communities they serve. In many cases, vitally needed services already exist in the community.

Pediatricians can play an extremely important role in coordinating and focusing services to realize maximum benefit for all children."[8] This is true for all health care professionals who provide clinical primary care for infants, children, and adolescents. The *Bright Futures Tool and Resource Kit* includes templates and Web sites to aid these efforts.

Who Can Use Bright Futures?

The themes and visits described in Bright Futures are designed to be readily applied to the work of child health care professionals and practice staff who directly provide primary care, and the parents and children who participate in these visits. One of the greatest strengths of Bright Futures is that its content and approach resonate with, and are found useful by, a wide variety of professionals and families who work to promote child health. Evaluations of Bright Futures have found that although the *Guidelines* themselves are written in a format to be particularly useful for health care professionals who work in clinical settings, they have been adopted and adapted by public health care professionals as the basis for population-based programs and policies, by policy makers as a standard for child health care, by parent groups, and by educators who train the next generation of health care professionals in a variety of fields.[9]

The health care of well or sick children is practiced by a broad range of professionals who take responsibility for a child's health care in a clinical encounter. These health care professionals can be family medicine physicians, pediatric and family nurse practitioners, pediatricians, dentists, nutritionists, nurses, physical and occupational therapists, social workers, mental health professionals, physician assistants, and others. Bright Futures does not stop there, however. These principles and recommendations have been designed with many partners in mind because these professionals do not practice in a vacuum. They work collaboratively with other health care professionals and support personnel as part of the overall health care system.

A review of the key themes that provide cross-cutting perspectives on all the content of Bright Futures will reveal how collaborative work contributes to the goals. The discussions for each age group will be helpful to all health care professionals and families who support and care for children and youth. The *Bright Futures Tool and Resource Kit* has materials and strategies to enhance the ability of the medical home and community agencies to efficiently identify mutual resources, communicate well with families and each other, and partner in designing service delivery systems.

How Is Bright Futures Organized?

The richness of this fourth edition of the *Bright Futures Guidelines* reflects the combined wisdom of the child and adolescent health care professionals and families on the Bright Futures infancy, early childhood, middle childhood, and adolescence expert panels. Each panel and many expert reviewers carefully considered the health supervision needs of an age group and developmental stage. Their work is represented in several formats in the *Guidelines*.

- The first major part of the *Guidelines* is the **health promotion themes.** These thematic discussions highlight issues that are important to families and health care professionals across all the developmental stages. The health promotion themes are designed for the practitioner or student who desires an in-depth, state-of-the-art discussion of a certain child health topic with evidence regarding effectiveness. These comprehensive discussions also can help families understand the context of their child's health and support their child's and family's health. Information from the 4 expert panels about these themes as they relate to specific developmental stages from birth to early adulthood was blended into each health promotion theme discussion.

■ The second major part of the *Guidelines* is the **visits.** In this part, practitioners will find the core of child health supervision activities, described as Bright Futures Visits (Box 1).

Bright Futures Visits, from the Prenatal Visit to the Late Adolescent Visit, are presented in accordance with the *Bright Futures/AAP Recommendations for Preventive Pediatric Health Care (Periodicity Schedule),*[10] which is the standard for preventive care for infants, children, and adolescents and is used by professional organizations, federal programs, and third party payers.

Each visit within the 4 ages and stages of development begins with an introductory section that highlights key concepts of each age. This information is followed by detailed, evidence-based guidance for conducting the visit.

The visits sections are designed to be implemented as state-of-the-art practice in the care of children and youth. The visits describe the essential content of the child and family visit and interaction with the provider of pediatric health care and the health care system in which the service is provided.

This clinical approach and content can be readily adapted for use in other situations where the health and development of children at various ages and stages is addressed. This might include home visiting programs or helping the parents of children in Head Start or other child care or early education programs understand their children's health and developmental needs. Colleagues in public health or health policy will find the community- and family-based approach embedded in the child and adolescent health supervision guidance. Educators and students of medicine, nursing, dentistry, public health, and others will find the *Bright Futures Guidelines* and the supporting sample questions, anticipatory guidance, and *Bright Futures Tool and Resource Kit* materials especially useful in understanding the complexity and context of health supervision visits and in appreciating the warmth of the patient contact that the Bright Futures approach ensures.

Box 1

A Bright Futures Health Supervision Visit

A Bright Futures Visit is an age-specific health supervision visit that uses techniques described in this edition of the *Bright Futures: Guidelines for Health Supervision of Infants, Children, and Adolescents,* although modifications to fit the specific needs and circumstances of communities and practices are encouraged. The Bright Futures Visit is family driven and is designed for practitioners to improve their desired standard of care. This family-centered emphasis is demonstrated through several features.

- Solicitation of parental and child concerns.
- Surveillance and screening.
- Assessment of strengths.
- Discussion of certain visit priorities for improved child and adolescent health and family function over time. Sample questions and anticipatory guidance for each priority are provided as starting points for discussion. These questions and anticipatory guidance points can be modified or enhanced by each health care professional using Bright Futures.
- Use of the *Bright Futures Tool and Resource Kit* content and processes.

Implementing Bright Futures

Carrying out Bright Futures means making full use of all the Bright Futures materials. For child health care professionals who wish to improve their skills, Bright Futures has developed a range of resources and materials that complement the *Guidelines,* and can be found on the Bright Futures Web site.

Finally, the *Bright Futures Tool and Resource Kit* allows health care professionals who wish to improve their practice or services to efficiently and comprehensively carry out new practices and practice change strategies. The Bright Futures tools also are compatible with suggested templates for the electronic health record (EHR), although using the *Bright Futures Tool and Resource Kit* does not require an EHR. These tools include

- A **Bright Futures Previsit Questionnaire,** which a parent or patient completes before the practitioner begins the visit. Clinicians who had experience with the American Medical Association's *Guidelines for Adolescent Preventive Services* (known as *GAPS)* approach will note that this questionnaire functions similarly to the Trigger Questionnaire in the "gathering information" phase. When the questionnaire is completed, the family's agenda, and many of the child's strengths, screening requirements, and intervention needs, is highlighted. The questionnaire helps parents understand the goals for the visit, introduces topics that will be covered, and encourages parents to list the questions and concerns that they wish to discuss. It also helps the health care professional sort the many appropriate clinical topics for the day's visit into topics that are essential to the child and family at this visit. It includes interval history (ie, changes that have occurred to the child and family since the last visit) and history

that is necessary for the disease detection, disease prevention, and health promotion activities of the visit. It also is a useful tool for surveillance, as it helps bring the health care professional up-to-date with the child's health.

- **Screening tools,** such as standardized developmental assessment tests and screening questionnaires that allow health care professionals to screen children and youth for certain conditions at specific visits.
- The **Bright Futures Visit Chart Documentation Form,** which corresponds to the *Bright Futures Guidelines* tasks for that visit and the information that is gleaned from the parent questionnaire. It reduces repetitive charting and frees the clinician for more face-to-face time with the child or youth. This form allows for replication of significant positive findings from the parent questionnaire without duplication of charting. Topics are organized so that positive findings detected in the parent questionnaire easily flow to the chart instrument to document how the health care professional has addressed the need that has been identified. The chart visit documentation form also records the physical examination findings, the assessments, and the interventions that are agreed upon with the family.
- The **Bright Futures Preventive Services Prompting Sheet,** which affords an at-a-glance compilation of work that is done over multiple visits to ensure completeness and increase efficiency.
- **Parent/Child Anticipatory Guidance Materials,** which reinforce and supplement the information discussed at the visit. These materials guide the health care professional in that they contain general principles and instructions for how the health care professional can communicate information with families.

Bright Futures Tool and Resource Kit elements improve the health care professional's efficiency in identifying the correct interventions and ensure that the valuable visit time will be sufficient to address the family's questions and agenda, the child's needs, and the prioritized anticipatory guidance recommended by the Bright Futures expert panels.

Using Bright Futures to Improve the Quality of Care

The *Bright Futures Guidelines* present an expanded implementation approach that builds on change strategies for office systems. This approach allows child health care professionals who deliver care consistent with Bright Futures to engage their office staff, families, public health colleagues, and even community agencies in quality improvement activities that will result in better care.

In an effort to examine the feasibility of implementing the *Bright Futures Guidelines,* the AAP supported a 9-month learning collaborative that examined implementation strategies for health supervision visits for children at the 9 Month and 2 Year Visits.[2] Twenty-one practices from across the country improved their health care processes to support the new *Bright Futures Guidelines.* To accomplish this, practices made measurable changes in the following areas:

- Delivery of preventive services
- Use of structured developmental screening
- Use of strength-based approaches and a mechanism to elicit and address parental concerns
- Establishment of community linkages that facilitate effective referrals and access to needed community services for families and collaboration with other child advocates

- Use of a recall and reminder system
- Use of a practice mechanism to identify children with special health care needs and ensure that they receive preventive services

The study found that using the Bright Futures approach involved all the office staff in improvements that were important to patient care and demonstrable on chart audit. Many of the changes did not involve additional work but rather a more coordinated approach. Practices learned actionable changes from one other as they progressed.

In addition to the focus on systematic improvement, using Bright Futures has other potential benefits as well. Health care professionals may use the data they gather to satisfy future recertification requirements. Many of the public health national performance measures will be met through implementing of Bright Futures, such as safe sleep position, developmental screening, and adolescent well-child visit.[11,12] In addition, as health insurers link reimbursement to documentation of the delivery of quality preventive services, child health care professionals will have ready access to the data that demonstrate the high caliber of their work.

References

1. Green M, Palfrey JS, eds. *Bright Futures: Guidelines for Health Supervision of Infants, Children, and Adolescents.* 2nd ed. Arlington, VA: National Center for Education in Maternal and Child Health; 2002

2. Duncan PM, Pirretti A, Earls MF, et al. Improving delivery of Bright Futures preventive services at the 9- and 24-month well child visit. *Pediatrics.* 2015;135(1):e178-e186

3. Schor EL. Personal communication; 2006

4. US Department of Health and Human Services. *Mental Health: A Report of the Surgeon General.* Rockville, MD: US Department of Health and Human Services, Substance Abuse and Mental Health Services Administration, Center for Mental Health Services, National Institutes of Health, National Institute of Mental Health; 1999

5. American Academy of Pediatrics Medical Home Initiatives for Children With Special Health Care Needs Project Advisory Committee. The medical home. *Pediatrics.* 2002;110(1 pt 1): 184-186

6. Hale KJ. Oral health risk assessment timing and establishment of the dental home. *Pediatrics.* 2003;111(5 pt 1):1113-1116

7. US Department of Health and Human Services. *Healthy People 2020.* http://www.healthypeople.gov. Accessed October 21, 2016

8. Rushton FE Jr; American Academy of Pediatrics Committee on Community Health Services. The pediatrician's role in community pediatrics. *Pediatrics.* 2005;115(4):1092-1094

9. Zimmerman B, Gallagher J, Botsko C, Ledsky R, Gwinner V. *Assessing the Bright Futures for Infants, Children and Adolescents Initiative: Findings from a National Process Evaluation.* Washington, DC: Health Systems Research Inc; 2005

10. American Academy of Pediatrics Committee on Practice and Ambulatory Medicine Bright Futures Periodicity Schedule Workgroup. Recommendations for preventive pediatric health care. *Pediatrics.* 2016;137(1):e20153908

11. Lu MC, Lauver CB, Dykton C, et al. Transformation of the Title V Maternal and Child Health Services Block Grant. *Matern Child Health J.* 2015;19(5):927-931

12. Kogan MD, Dykton C, Hirai A, et al. A new performance measurement system for maternal and child health in the United States. *Matern Child Health J.* 2015;19(5):945-957

WHAT IS BRIGHT FUTURES?

Bright Futures Health Promotion Themes

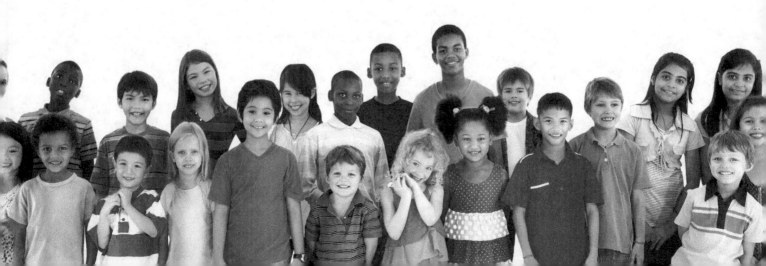

An Introduction to the Bright Futures Health Promotion Themes

Understanding certain key topics of importance to families and health care professionals is essential to promoting the health and well-being of children, from birth through adolescence and young adulthood. The *Bright Futures: Guidelines for Health Supervision of Infants, Children, and Adolescents* provide an in-depth, state-of-the-art discussion of these Bright Futures Health Promotion Themes, with evidence regarding effectiveness of health promotion interventions at specific developmental stages, from birth to early adulthood. These discussions are designed for the health care professional or student who desires detailed discussion of these child health topics. In addition, health care professionals can use these comprehensive discussions to help families understand the context of their child's health and support their child's and family's development.

Most of the health promotion themes contained in the third edition have been updated and carried over to the fourth edition, though several changes of note were made.

- Information on caring for *children and youth with special health care needs* was extracted from a number of themes and consolidated into one theme devoted to this issue.
- In light of the growing appreciation of the critical role that *social determinants of health* and *social media* play in the health and well-being of children, youth, and families, this edition of *Bright Futures Guidelines* has 2 new themes devoted to these topics.

- Information in the third edition's *Promoting Community Relationships and Resources theme* was incorporated into the other themes.

The 12 health promotion themes in this edition are

- Promoting Lifelong Health for Families and Communities
- Promoting Family Support
- Promoting Health for Children and Youth With Special Health Care Needs
- Promoting Healthy Development
- Promoting Mental Health
- Promoting Healthy Weight
- Promoting Healthy Nutrition
- Promoting Physical Activity
- Promoting Oral Health
- Promoting Healthy Sexual Development and Sexuality
- Promoting the Healthy and Safe Use of Social Media
- Promoting Safety and Injury Prevention

Promoting Lifelong Health for Families and Communities

Every child deserves a bright future, growing in a nurturing family and living in a supportive community. From the moment of conception, individuals grow in physical and relational environments that evolve and influence each other over time and that shape their biological and behavioral systems for life. Dramatic advances in a wide range of biological, behavioral, and social sciences have shown that each child's future depends on genetic predispositions (the biology) and early environmental influences (the ecology), which affect later abilities to play, learn, work, and be physically, mentally, and emotionally healthy. Box 1 provides definitions for several key terms related to the lifelong health of children, families, and communities.

Box 1

Definitions of Key Terms Related to Lifelong Health

Children's health: "The extent to which individual children or groups of children are able or enabled to (a) develop and realize their potential, (b) satisfy their needs, and (c) develop the capacities that allow them to interact successfully with their biological, physical, and social environments."[1]

Social determinants of health: "Health starts in our homes, schools, workplaces, neighborhoods, and communities. We know that taking care of ourselves by eating well and staying active, not smoking, getting the recommended immunizations and screening tests, and seeing a doctor when we are sick all influence our health. Our health is also determined in part by access to social and economic opportunities; the resources and supports available in our homes, neighborhoods, and communities; the quality of our schooling; the safety of our workplaces; the cleanliness of our water, food, and air; and the nature of our social interactions and relationships. The conditions in which we live explain in part why some Americans are healthier than others and why Americans more generally are not as healthy as they could be."[2]

Health equity: Attainment of the highest level of health for all people. Achieving health equity requires valuing everyone equally, with focused and ongoing societal efforts to address avoidable inequalities, historical and contemporary injustices, and the elimination of health and health care disparities.[3]

Health disparity: "A particular type of health difference that is closely linked with social, economic, and/or environmental disadvantage. Health disparities adversely affect groups of people who have systematically experienced greater obstacles to health based on their racial or ethnic group; religion; socioeconomic status; gender; age; mental health; cognitive, sensory, or physical disability; sexual or gender orientation; geographic location; or other characteristics historically tied to discrimination or exclusion."[4]

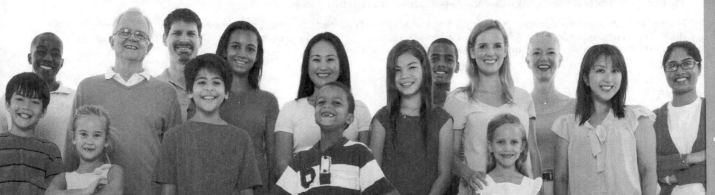

PROMOTING LIFELONG HEALTH FOR FAMILIES AND COMMUNITIES

Accumulating research in behavioral neuroscience has shown that an infant's biological heritage interacts with his life experiences to affect the developing architecture of the brain and shown how the systems rewire in response to changes in the environment (plasticity). Basic neuronal pathways lay the foundation for more complex circuits, similar to how developmental skills pave the way for more sophisticated skills. Positive early experiences establish a sturdy foundation for a lifetime of learning, healthy behaviors, and wellness.[5,6]

Although individual health trajectories vary, population patterns can be predicted according to social, psychological, environmental, and economic exposures and experiences. For example, children and adolescents living in poverty (20% of all US children ≤17 years[7]) are exposed to a cluster of determinants of health that result in high rates of infant mortality, developmental delays, asthma, ear infections, obesity, and child abuse and neglect.[8] Research results from numerous scientific disciplines suggest that "many adult diseases should be viewed as developmental disorders that begin early in life, and that persistent health disparities associated with poverty, discrimination, or maltreatment could be reduced by alleviating toxic stress (exposure to severe and chronic adversity) in childhood."[9]

Because of the powerful influence of various determinants of health early in life, the American Academy of Pediatrics (AAP) has adopted an eco-bio-developmental model of human health and disease (Figure 1).

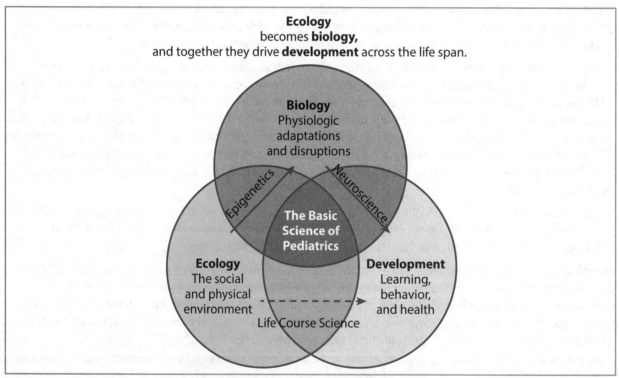

Figure 1: Eco-Bio-Developmental Model of Human Health and Disease[9]

Modified with permission from Shonkoff JP, Garner AS; American Academy of Pediatrics Committee on Psychosocial Aspects of Child and Family Health; Committee on Early Childhood, Adoption, and Dependent Care; Section on Developmental and Behavioral Pediatrics. The lifelong effects of early childhood adversity and toxic stress. *Pediatrics*. 2012;129(1):e232-e246.

The model invites health care professionals to be guardians of healthy child development and to function as community leaders to help build strong foundations for positive social interactions, educational achievement, economic productivity, responsible citizenship, and lifelong health.[9] Partnership with families is key to reaching this goal. This combined focus of efforts will result in preventive care that is more developmentally relevant and that reflects the growing evidence that programs and interventions targeting the early years have the greatest promise and provide the highest return on investment (Figure 2). However, health care professionals cannot be guardians of child health alone. Just as every surgery requires a team working in concert, pediatric health care professionals need a team focused on assessing children's and families' strengths and risks and intervening at various time points across the continuum of care. They also need strong links to community resources that can support the work done in the medical home. Health care professionals need skills and resources to build effective partnerships with families, and families need knowledge and support to become effective partners in achieving these goals.

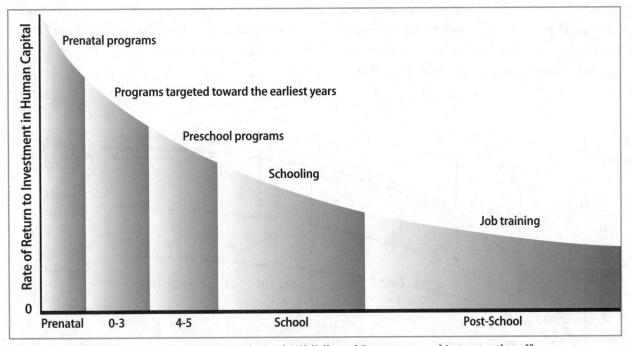

Figure 2: Rate of Return on Investments in Early Childhood Programs and Interventions[10]

Reproduced with permission from Heckman JJ. Schools, skills, and synapses. *Econ Inq.* 2008;46(3):289-324. Also, see Heckman J. The Heckman Curve: Early Childhood Development Is a Smart Investment. Heckman Equation Web site. http://heckmanequation.org. Accessed November 14, 2016.

PROMOTING LIFELONG HEALTH FOR FAMILIES AND COMMUNITIES

The Life Course Framework

Life course is a conceptual framework, consistent with the eco-bio-developmental model, that identifies and explains how the complex interplay of biological, behavioral, psychological, social, and environmental factors can shape health across an entire lifetime and for future generations. Bright Futures has adopted the life course framework to help health care professionals understand how these factors influence children's capacity to reach their full potential for health and why health disparities persist across populations. Figure 3 illustrates that higher or lower health development trajectories are influenced by the relative number and magnitude of risk and protective factors. Applying this framework in practice gives health care professionals an unprecedented opportunity to positively influence the future health and well-being of patients and their families.

Pediatric health care professionals have historically focused on development, from birth through adolescence. The life course framework incorporates and expands on this traditional perspective. Fine and Kotelchuck have summarized key life course concepts.[12]

- Health trajectories are largely shaped by events during critical periods of early development.
- The cumulative effect of experiences and exposures influences adult health.
- Biological, physical, and social environments influence the capacity to be healthy by creating risk factors and strengths and protective factors for children and families.

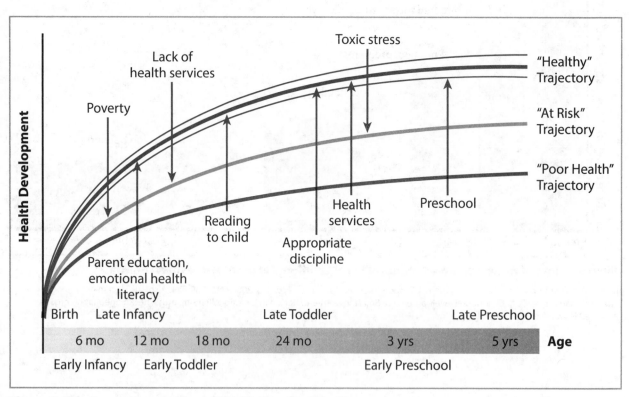

Figure 3: Life Course Perspective of Health Development[11]

Reproduced with permission from Halfon N, Larson K, Lu M, et al. *Matern Child Health J.* 2014;18(2):344-365. doi:10.1007/s10995-013-1346-2.

Critical Periods and Early Programming

An important component of the life course framework is recognizing the critical time periods when exposures can have protective or adverse effects on learning, behavior, and future health. Barker notes that "[c]ritical periods for systems and organs are usually brief, and many of them occur in utero."[13] During these periods, certain exposures can change gene expression or activity without altering the DNA sequence. This emerging field of study, called epigenetics, has shown that events during critical periods change the process by which the physical, psychological, and social environments influence the expression of DNA. This phenomenon determines body and brain architecture and function.[5,14]

Beneficial in utero environments, in which fetuses are nourished, exposed to normal levels of maternal stress hormones, and protected from toxins, provide an environment in which the fetus is able to develop optimally during times when the architecture of the brain is created and full expression of genes occurs. Evidence also shows that adverse experiences before birth have similarly important effects on development but in a negative way. These consequences include diminished physiologic responses (eg, immune system) and altered brain architecture.[1,9,13-19]

Cumulative Effects

The life course literature also stresses that the effects of early experiences are cumulative, influencing health in adulthood. Ongoing adversity in childhood can increase the risk of common chronic diseases of adulthood.[16,18,20] Environmental risks, such as chronic exposure to lead, also can be significant. Other adult health outcomes associated with adverse events of childhood include

- Cardiovascular disease[21-24]
- Obesity[25-28]
- Type 2 diabetes[29,30]
- Alcohol or drug use disorder[31]
- Depression[32]

The Adverse Childhood Experiences (ACE) Study (Box 2) has identified many associations between childhood stressors and later negative health outcomes in adulthood. The ACE Study was only the

---

Box 2

The Adverse Childhood Experiences Study[33]

The ACE Study was conducted at Kaiser Permanente from 1995–1997. More than 17,000 participants had a standardized examination and reported the number of adverse experiences they had during childhood, such as

- Childhood physical, emotional, or sexual abuse
- Emotional or physical neglect
- Being a witness to IPV
- Loss of birth parent by parental divorce, abandonment, or other reason
- Growing up with household substance use disorder, mental disorder, or an incarcerated household member

The total number of ACEs was used as a measure of cumulative childhood stress. The study identified many associations between traumatic and abusive events during childhood and adult health conditions, such as chronic lung disease, cancer, depression, and alcohol use disorder. Many of these effects were dose dependent; that is, negative exposures accumulated over time and increased future risks.[34] For example, persons who had experienced ≥2 adverse events had a 100% increased risk of developing a rheumatic disease—a result that supports mounting evidence on the effect of early life stress on adult inflammatory responses.[35] Chapman and colleagues[32] found a dose-response relationship for the probability of depressive disorders decades after the exposures. The study also found a strong relationship between the ACE score and the use of psychotropic medications, suggesting a clear association between ACEs and adult mental disorder.[36]

Abbreviations: ACE, Adverse Childhood Experiences; IPV, intimate partner violence.

beginning of our understanding of toxic stress, and it is important that health care professionals keep a broader concept of adversity in mind when addressing and caring for children and families. Many other factors can negatively affect a child's developmental trajectory. The AAP defines these factors, or toxic stresses, as "strong, frequent, or prolonged activations of the body's stress response systems in the absence of the buffering protection of a supportive adult relationship."[9]

Moderating Factors

Despite growing evidence about biological embedding and the negative effects of early adverse experiences, studies also demonstrate that caring relationships and improvements in children's environments can do much to moderate adverse effects. Because the biological systems of young children are still developing, carefully chosen positive interventions can offset negative experiences that occur during gestation or when children are very young. For example, foster children who have been hit, shaken, or threatened often do not have normal hypothalamic-pituitary-adrenal (HPA) axis activity. However, several studies have shown that the disrupted cortisol secretion caused by adversity early in life can be reversed by interventions that improve caregiving.[37-39] For example, early child maltreatment can cause dysregulation of the HPA axis, which can lead to emotional, behavioral, and physical problems. But placing children with foster parents who are taught behavioral parent training techniques can reverse this dysregulation,[40] and children who report strong social supports are less likely to experience the consequent problems of HPA dysregulation.[37-39,41]

In another example, every stage of life is affected by nutrition, including the mother's nutrition before and during pregnancy. Efforts to improve maternal nutrition and increase the availability of a variety of healthful food for children can increase the likelihood of health throughout life.[42,43] Other environmental factors that can be moderated include

- Exposure to chemicals in the home (eg, lead in paint or toys) and in the air (eg, tobacco smoke, industrial pollutants)
- Access to drinking water, whether from a municipal or private source, that meets all established health standards

All families go through difficult times, and factors such as strong and loving relationships, personal resiliency, and adequate support systems also can be important moderating factors to help families withstand these situations.[44] Two families may have similar life circumstances and incomes but may have very different outcomes after a personal tragedy or natural disaster. For example, research has shown that environmental and relational factors played major roles in accelerating or impeding recovery of children and their families affected by Hurricane Katrina. Some characteristics that positively influenced families' ability to cope were pre-disaster functioning, spirituality, social connectedness, and post-disaster consultation with a mental health professional. Factors that made recovery more difficult for children were loss of resources, school problems, and long-term family or community disruption.[45-48]

Efforts to decrease parental stress, improve parenting, provide safe and predictable routines, and bolster relationships with warm and responsive adults can buffer stressful events and situations and promote healthy development.

The Life Course Framework in Bright Futures

A central concept of the life course framework is that children and families are affected by a variety of biological (ie, "nature") and ecological (ie, "nurture") exposures that can either promote healthy development or increase risk of impairment or disease. Viewing health care through this lens allows health care professionals to identify family, neighborhood, and community determinants that affect the lifelong health of their patients. Recognizing these influences allows health care professionals to tailor their entire scope of practice (ie, screening, care coordination, formulation of treatment plans, and health promotion) to mitigate the risks that imperil a child's current and future health and promote the strengths and protective factors that secure a child's current and future health. The life course framework also encourages families, in collaboration with health care professionals, to seek support from community and other resources outside the practice to create a family-centered, culturally and linguistically competent, community-oriented, team-based medical home that promotes robust health in children within the context of their families and communities.

The goal of Bright Futures is to support a life course in which the strengths and protective factors outweigh the risk factors. To support this goal, the next 2 sections provide greater detail on the biological and ecological determinants that so profoundly influence child and family health. This discussion allows health care professionals to actively promote strengths and protective factors by assessing determinants of health within the scope of their practice.

Biological Determinants

A child's development is initially determined by the genes inherited from both parents, the expression of which can be altered in utero. A child's life course can be optimized even before birth by excellent nutrition from a healthy mother and a uterine environment that allows full expression of genes.

Conversely, the likelihood of optimal development is negatively affected by a stressed or depressed mother, intrauterine exposures to toxins, poor nutrition in utero, and birth trauma. Certain toxins affect fetal development. For example, exposure to lead, found in lead-based paints, soil, dust, and some toys, is a known danger to healthy cognitive development.[49,50] Drinking alcohol during pregnancy is one of the leading preventable causes of birth defects, intellectual disabilities, and other developmental disabilities in infants, children, and adolescents.[51] Babies born to mothers who smoke cigarettes are at higher risk of being born early, having a low birth weight, having an orofacial cleft of the lip or palate, or experiencing a sudden unexplained death during infancy.[52] Many of these determinants have been well-known for decades, and anticipatory guidance includes screening for them and counseling parents about them.

Emerging science has shown powerful and previously unknown effects of gestational influences on adult health, which go far beyond inherited genes and personal choices.[12] Figure 4 illustrates that if early childhood experiences are protective and personal, adaptive or healthy coping skills are more likely. If early experiences are insecure or impersonal, maladaptive or unhealthy coping skills are more likely. For example, recent research on the toxic effects of maternal stress and depression illustrate in utero biological determinants of health.

PROMOTING LIFELONG HEALTH FOR FAMILIES AND COMMUNITIES

- Children exposed to normal levels of maternal stress usually develop the ability to have appropriate reactions (ie, mild and brief) to stress, especially when supported by caring and responsive adults who help them learn to cope.[9] However, when a fetus is exposed to high levels of maternal stress, the developing architecture of the brain is disrupted, which results in a weakened foundation for later learning, behavior, and health.[53,54]

- High cortisol levels in the mother during pregnancy also can disrupt development of the immune, inflammatory, and vascular pathways, setting the stage for adult diseases decades after the exposures.[55]

- Expectant mothers who live in stressful environments tend to have lower-birth-weight babies, putting the child at risk for numerous conditions later in life.[55]

- Inadequate nutrition at certain time points in pregnancy results in elevated risks for adult diseases decades after birth. Low-birth-weight babies are at risk of having obesity during childhood and for hypertension, cardiovascular disease, and stroke as adults.[56]

- In addition, very low-birth-weight babies are often born with insulin resistance and other metabolic changes that put them at risk for developing diabetes later in life.[57]

- Maternal depression during the third trimester is epigenetically associated with later increased infant stress responsiveness.[58]

These and other findings from developmental neuroscience suggest that emphasizing protective factors during pregnancy and infancy can alter the trajectory of health of a mother and her baby

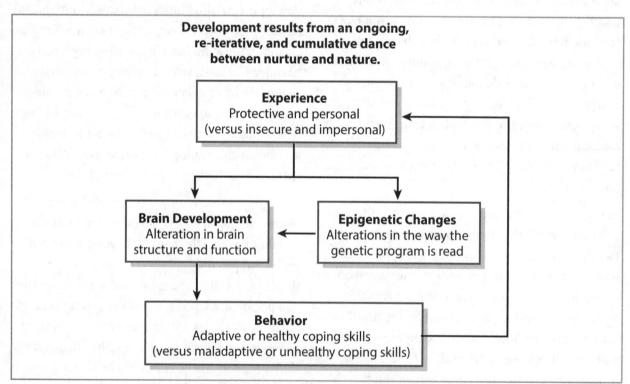

Figure 4: Interactions Between Experience, Epigenetics, Brain Development, and Behavior[59]

Modified with permission from Garner A, Forkey H, Stirling J, Nalven L, Schilling S; American Academy of Pediatrics, Dave Thomas Foundation for Adoption. *Helping Foster and Adoptive Families Cope With Trauma*. Elk Grove Village, IL: American Academy of Pediatrics; 2015. https://www.aap.org/traumaguide. Accessed November 14, 2016.

toward improved health and well-being. This emphasis can take the form of

- Supporting the nutrition and health of women before and during pregnancy
- Identifying prenatal exposures to toxic substances (eg, lead, mercury, alcohol, tobacco) and working with parents to reduce or eliminate them
- Helping identify and treat depression in women early in pregnancy
- Screening pregnant women for stress and linking them to community resources for help
- Promoting proper nutrition for underweight infants that optimizes healthy growth and minimizes potential for obesity
- Encouraging and supporting a pregnant woman's decision to breastfeed her child and providing ongoing encouragement and support postpartum and throughout the breastfeeding experience

Ecological Determinants: Social

Just as biological factors provide the foundation for a child's future health in certain key respects, social determinants—the web of interpersonal and community relationships experienced by children, parents, and families—also play a critical role. And, like biological determinants, social determinants can be characterized as strengths and protective factors or as risk factors.

Strengths and Protective Factors in Social Determinants

Children cared for with safe, predictable routines and by nurturing and responsive adults gain protection from risks to health. Children in loving families who have strong social connectedness are better able to withstand the stressors in life and strengthen adaptability. Core family members provide reassurance and confidence (a secure base) for children, allowing them to learn to trust and successfully separate from parents.[19,54,60,61]

Future health also is rooted in exposure to developmentally appropriate experiences that can be provided in the home and at child care, early childhood education, and schools. For example, a policy statement from the AAP states that regularly reading with young children stimulates optimal patterns of brain development and strengthens parent-child relationships at a critical time in child development, which, in turn, builds language, literacy, and social and emotional skills that last a lifetime.[62] High-quality early childhood education and quality-rated preschool programs, including Early Head Start and Head Start, benefit typically developing children and children with disabilities.[63] An emerging literature suggests that health-promoting family routines and practices as well as the positive effects associated with music are of value.[64]

To be able to nurture children and provide a strong foundation for healthy development, parents and other caregivers (eg, foster parents, parenting grandparents, early care and education professionals) need basic knowledge about child development and parenting skills, including the ability to

- Respond and attend appropriately to children's needs.
- Provide stimulation.
- Notice developmental delays.
- Meet children's need for self-confidence and competence.
- Display and teach resilience in the face of adversity.
- Demonstrate effective problem-solving and independent decision-making skills.
- Promote social and emotional competence.
- Help children learn to identify and manage their emotions.

In addition to the ability to nurture children, parents who have positive social connections and concrete support in times of need are better able to prepare their children for life stressors.

> In order to develop normally, a child requires progressively more complex joint activity with one or more adults who have an irrational emotional relationship with the child. Somebody's got to be crazy about that kid. That's number one. First, last, and always.
>
> —Urie Bronfenbrenner[65]

Parents are more able to create healthy norms (eg, positive family traditions, exercising as a family, always wearing seat belts) if they have these basic skills and supports.

Other adults who can support parents and provide warm, sensitive, and consistent influence on children of all ages include members of the extended family or clan, friends, neighbors, early care and education professionals, teachers, coaches, club leaders, and mentors.[66-70] Cultural continuity for foster children and children who are immigrants can positively contribute to the richness of individual identity and family or cultural traditions. In many cultures, intergenerational influence can be a powerful support for children.

Common sense dictates and research demonstrates that children do best in strong and healthy families and communities because they provide a buffer against life stresses and are fundamental to healthy brain development. The elements necessary for youth to thrive include competence, confidence, connection, character, caring, compassion, and contribution.[66-71]

Research has identified that the more strengths or developmental assets young people have in their lives, the less likely they are to engage in health risk behaviors (Box 3).[72-74] Studies of children at risk (eg, children in foster care, children of

---

Box 3

Individual Protective Factors, Strengths, and Developmental Tasks of Adolescence[70]

Focusing on protective factors for youth is a positive way to engage with families because it highlights their strengths. It also provides a mechanism by which children can reach their full potential and, as they grow into adolescence, engage in strength-based health protective behaviors, such as

1. Forming caring and supportive relationships with family members, other adults, and peers
2. Engaging in a positive way with the life of the community
3. Engaging in behaviors that optimize wellness and contribute to a healthy lifestyle
   a. Engaging in healthy nutrition and physical activity behaviors
   b. Choosing safety (eg, bike helmets, seat belts, avoidance of alcohol and drugs)
4. Demonstrating physical, cognitive, emotional, social, and moral competencies (including self-regulation)
5. Exhibiting compassion and empathy
6. Exhibiting resiliency when confronted with life stressors
7. Using independent decision-making skills (including problem-solving skills)
8. Displaying a sense of self-confidence, hopefulness, and well-being

For more information on these behaviors, see the *Promoting Healthy Development theme.*

child abuse and neglect, and homeless children) reinforce the importance of these strengths and protective factors. Relational, self-regulation, and problem-solving skills; involvement in positive activities; and relationships with positive peers and caring adults are associated with improved health and educational outcomes and fewer problem behaviors (eg, substance use disorder, delinquency, and violence). This work also identifies the critical importance of positive school and community environment and economic opportunities for these populations.[75]

Health protective behaviors grow from an awareness of self and others that begins in infancy and expands as children grow. When health care professionals are alert to any problems in this domain, opportunities for objective developmental and social and emotional screenings and referral arise, as do opportunities for early intervention. In addition to self-regulation, self-control, and self-awareness, the strength-based health protective behaviors listed in Box 3 increase a child's interpersonal connectedness with the community (ie, "social capital"). Children and adolescents develop in healthy ways and are protected from harm by their accumulated social capital and their connection to members of their extended family, faith community, neighborhood, school, and clubs.

In addition to these protective factors for healthy youth development, research has identified parental, family, and community strengths and protective factors that are associated with optimal child development, improved outcomes, and lower rates of child abuse and neglect (Box 4).

Risk Factors in Social Determinants

At the other end of the social determinants spectrum, severe or chronic adversity that occurs because of poverty, homelessness, parental dysfunction, separation or divorce, or abuse and neglect can inhibit the development of the

elements necessary for thriving and increase the risk that children and youth will engage in risky behaviors (Figure 5).

Children exposed to excessive and repeated stress in their family and social relationships are at elevated risk for disrupted development and long-term negative consequences for learning, behavioral, and physical and mental health.[15]

Chronic stresses in social relationships that children may frequently experience are intimate partner violence (IPV) and separation and divorce.

Intimate Partner Violence

Intimate partner violence is prevalent across all socioeconomic groups. According to the Centers for Disease Control and Prevention National Intimate Partner and Sexual Violence Survey released in 2010, more than 1 in 3 women (35.6%) and more than 1 in 4 men (28.5%) in the United States have experienced rape, physical violence, or stalking by an intimate partner in their lifetime.[80]

According to the National Survey of Children's Exposure to Violence, more than 8.2 million children witnessed violence between their parents in 2008.[81] Substantial evidence has accumulated regarding the toxic effects of IPV on the child. Infants and toddlers who witness violence in their homes or community show excessive irritability, immature behavior, sleep disturbances, emotional distress, fear of being alone, and regression in toileting and language. In school-aged children, overall functioning, attitudes, social competence, and school performance are often affected negatively. Moreover, the presence of violence in the home creates a significant risk of participation in youth violence activities even if the child is not abused by the family.[82] Abuse of the child is far more likely to happen in families in which violence exists between the parents.[83,84]

PROMOTING LIFELONG HEALTH FOR FAMILIES AND COMMUNITIES

Box 4

Desired Protective Factors for Families and Communities

Protective Factors Desired for Parents

In *Strengthening Families,* the Center for the Study of Social Policy identified the following protective factors for parents[76]:

- **Concrete support in times of need:** Identifying, seeking, accessing, advocating for, and receiving needed adult, child, and family services. Receiving a quality of service designed to preserve parents' dignity and promote healthy development.

- **Social connections:** Having healthy, sustained relationships with people, institutions, the community, or a force greater than oneself.

- **Knowledge of parenting and child development:** Understanding the unique aspects of child development. Implementing developmentally and contextually appropriate best parenting practices.

- **Personal resilience:** Managing both general life and parenting stress and functioning well when faced with stressors, challenges, or adversity. The outcome is positive change and growth.

- **The ability to enhance social and emotional competence of children:** Providing an environment and experiences that enable the child to form close and secure adult and peer relationships and to experience, regulate, and express emotions.

The Children's Bureau, within the Administration on Children, Youth and Families, added this sixth protective factor to their programs.

- **The ability to foster nurturing and attachment:** A child's early experience of being nurtured and developing a bond with a caring adult during early experiences affects all aspects of a child's behavior and development.[75]

Protective Factors Desired for Families[77]

The CDC National Center for Injury Prevention and Control, Division of Violence Prevention, recommends these additional family strengths that parents provide to their children.

- **Nurturing:** Nurturing adults sensitively and consistently respond to the needs of children.

- **Stability:** Stability is created when parents provide predictability and consistency in their children's physical, social, and emotional environments.

- **Safety:** Children are safe when they are free from fear and protected from physical or psychological harm.

Protective Factors Desired for Communities[78]

Awareness of the importance of community-level protective factors is growing. To have a solid foundation for health, communities must seek to provide

- Safe neighborhoods in which parents can visit with friends and children can play outdoors

- Schools in which children are physically safe and can obtain an excellent education

- Stable and safe housing that is heated in winter, free from vermin and hazards (physical and chemical), and available long-term

- Access to nutritious food

- Access to job opportunities and transportation to get to those jobs

- Access to medical care, including behavioral health and wellness care

America's Promise[79] has conceptualized the protective factors as

- Caring adults

- Safe places

- A healthy start

- Effective education

- Opportunities to help others

Abbreviation: CDC, Centers for Disease Control and Prevention.

CHILD / INDIVIDUAL STRESSORS
- Abuse, neglect, chronic fear state
- Other traumas
  - natural disasters
  - accidents and illness
  - exposure to violence
- Disabilities/chronic disease

PARENTAL / FAMILY STRESSORS
- Parental dysfunction
  - substance abuse
  - domestic violence
  - mental illness
- Divorce/single parenting
- Poverty

SOURCES OF RESILIENCE[a]
Temperament, social-emotional supports, and learned social-emotional skills

OTHER VULNERABILITIES[a]
Temperament, delays in development, and limited social-emotional supports

Physiologic STRESS in Childhood			
STRESS RESPONSE	Positive	Tolerable	Toxic
DURATION	Brief	Sustained	Sustained
SEVERITY	Mild/moderate	Moderate/severe	Severe
SOCIAL-EMOTIONAL BUFFERING	Sufficient	Sufficient	Insufficient
LONG-TERM EFFECT ON STRESS RESPONSE SYSTEM	Return to baseline	Return to baseline	Changes to baseline

[a] Sources of Resilience and Other Vulnerabilities are able to mitigate or exacerbate the physiologic stress response

TRAUMATIC ALTERATIONS
- Epigenetic modifications
- Changes in brain structure and function
- Behavioral attempts to cope
  - May be maladaptive in other contexts

Figure 5: Precipitants and Consequences of Physiologic Stress in Childhood[59]

Health care professionals must be alert to the signs of IPV and be prepared to ask questions in a sensitive manner about the safety of all family members. Routine assessment can focus on early identification of all families and persons experiencing IPV.[85] They also should discuss options that are available to parents who are being abused. Health care professionals should understand that women can be afraid to divulge they have been abused by a partner because they fear violent reprisals or losing the children.

The **National Domestic Violence Hotline** at **800-799-SAFE (7233)** provides information about local resources on IPV. Health care professionals also should be aware that state laws may mandate reporting of some incidents with certain characteristics of children exposed to IPV. If clinicians report IPV to child protective services, the child's caregiver must be informed and a plan made for the safety of the person being abused and the child.[85]

Separation and Divorce

Today, more than 1 million children per year are newly involved in parental divorce. Overall, the rate of divorce is about 50% the rate of marriage every year.[86] In 2009, 27.3% of children lived in single-parent homes and 7.5% of children lived in stepfamilies.[87] The process of separation or divorce, parental dating, and stepfamilies or blended families requires many periods of adjustment for the child or adolescent, and separation and divorce are associated with negative reactions for all members of the family. Children who joined their families by adoption or children in foster or kinship families may struggle even more with parental separation, as it may resurrect old feelings of abandonment or loss. Practical concerns, such as plans for child care, shared parenting if possible, support, custody, and emergency contacts, should be clarified. The health care professional should assess the child's reaction to the separation or divorce and refer a poorly adapting child for counseling.

If the family does not remain intact, the health care professional can seek to decrease negative effects for the parents and child by being an important resource and support for both. This can be done by[88]

- Encouraging open discussion about separation and divorce with and between parents
- Suggesting positive and supportive ways to deal with children's reactions
- Reminding parents that parental fighting leads to poor outcomes in children
- Acting as the child's advocate
- Offering support and age-appropriate advice to the child and parents regarding reactions to divorce, especially guilt, anger, sadness, and perceived loss of love
- Referring families to mental health resources with expertise in divorce, if necessary

Ecological Determinants: Physical

Physical determinants—stable housing, safe neighborhoods, nutritious and affordable foods, quality of air and water, built environment (places and spaces created or modified by people), and geographic access to resources such as health care, employment, and safe places to be physically active and socialize—can alter health trajectories in significant ways.[89] Children whose families live in safe and stable places and who have access to a variety of nutritious foods are likely to stay healthy and develop optimally. In contrast, children who grow up in areas of concentrated poverty are often subject to ecological disruptions, including psychosocial stressors, poor physical environmental factors, and harsh parenting, that increase their vulnerability to a variety of health and social problems.[19,90] The child poverty rate of African American children is 39%, almost 3 times the rate for non-Hispanic white children (14%).[91] The literature suggests that population health disparities are driven by lack of access to resources and by segregation by setting (eg, living in high-poverty neighborhoods and working in hazardous occupations).[92]

Children need safe and stable housing to thrive, and stable housing requires an adequate income. The US Department of Health and Human Services has described 5 conditions that contribute to housing instability.[93]

- High housing costs (ie, >30% of monthly income)
- Poor housing quality (eg, lack of plumbing or kitchen)
- Unstable neighborhoods (eg, poverty, crime, lack of jobs)
- Overcrowding
- Homelessness

Some researchers include multiple moves in the definition of housing insecurity.[94] Housing instability is associated with numerous problems for children, such as poor health, greater likelihood of food insecurity, and increased developmental risk.[94] Children who are homeless or whose families move frequently often do not have access to a stable, family-centered medical home, further increasing health risks.[94]

The neighborhoods in which children live can promote or impair health, so much so that the authors of *Time to Act: Investing in the Health of Our Children and Communities* stated, "when it comes to health, your ZIP code may be more important than your genetic code."[95] Nearly one-fifth of Americans live in unhealthy neighborhoods that have limited access to a high-quality education, nutritious and affordable food, safe and affordable housing, safe places for physical activity, job opportunities, and transportation to get to work or medical care.[96]

Neighborhoods with parks, sidewalks, green spaces, and safe places to play provide opportunities for physical activity and social interactions both among children and parents.[19] Living in these types of neighborhoods has been linked to lower levels of obesity, less crime, and better adult mental health.[78,97] In some neighborhoods, however, parents and children feel trapped in their houses because of crime on the streets and lack of safe places for children to play and adults to connect with their neighbors. Lifelong health can take root only in neighborhoods that are safe, are free from violence, and allow healthy choices.

Neighborhood-level access to a variety of affordable and nutritious foods is central to health and well-being, but socioeconomic conditions drastically affect food availability and diet choices.[98] In the United States, many food deserts exist—areas in which families do not have access to affordable and healthful foods, such as fruits, vegetables, whole grains, and low-fat milk, or must travel long distances to purchase them.[99] Numerous studies have found that residents of low-income, minority, and rural areas often do not have supermarkets or healthful food in their neighborhoods.[100,101] Food insecurity, which is a lack of food or a lack of variety, is linked to malnutrition and deficiency diseases,[98] and access to only poor-quality food increases the risk of obesity.[101]

Children's health also is greatly influenced by the air they breathe indoors and out, the water they drink, and the places where they live. Children in the United States usually spend most of their time indoors, and they have little control over their physical environments. The presence of pets, pests (eg, cockroaches, rodents), water leaks, or mold in homes is associated with higher allergen loads and increased rates of asthma.[102] Residential exposures are believed to contribute to 44% of diagnosed cases of asthma among children and adolescents.[103] In addition, children living in rural and farm communities are often exposed to indoor and outdoor pesticides.[104] Jacobs[105] described types of risks to children's health in built environments, including

- Physical conditions, such as heat, cold, radon exposure, noise, fine particulates in the home, and inadequate light and ventilation
- Chemical conditions, such as carbon monoxide, volatile organic chemicals, secondhand smoke, and lead
- Biological conditions, such as rodents, house dust mites, cockroaches, humidity, and mold
- Building and equipment conditions (eg, access to sewer services)

Many well-known, evidence-based interventions can decrease illness and injuries related to housing (Box 5).

The quality of outdoor air and drinking water poses health risks for many children and expectant mothers. In 2005, nearly all US children were exposed to hazardous air pollutant (HAP) concentrations that exceeded the 1-in-100,000 cancer risk benchmark. In addition, 56% of children lived in areas in which at least one HAP exceeded the benchmark for health effects other than cancer. In almost all cases, these exposures were emissions from wood-burning fires, cars, trucks, buses, planes, and construction equipment.[110] The Environmental Protection Agency estimated that 7% of children in 2009 were served by community drinking water systems that did not meet health-based standards. This estimate does not include the approximately 15% of children in the United States who obtain water from nonpublic drinking water systems, such as wells.[110] Thus, advocacy for clean air and water can improve the health of many children.

On a larger scale, changing environmental conditions—global climate change and man-made and natural disasters—increase environmental vulnerabilities for children, particularly low-income children and children of color.[111] Global climate change, a result of greenhouse gas emissions, has resulted in climate variability and weather extremes.[112] Man-made disasters such as war, oil spills, wild fires in the western United States, and large industrial chemical spills over the past decade also have affected broad geographic areas, resulting in unknown toxicant exposure risks for large populations of children.[113]

Implications for the Health Care Professional and the Medical Home

Knowledge about life course theory and the biological and ecological determinants of health can be integrated into the work of the health care professional within the context of the family-centered medical home. Identifying family and child strengths and protective factors as well as

---

Box 5

Evidence-Based Interventions to Reduce Housing-Related Illness and Injuries in Children

Local health and housing departments and other community resources are important partners in addressing housing-related illness and preventing injury,[105-109] such as

- Home environment interventions for asthma
- Integrated pest management
- Elimination of moisture
- Removal of mold
- Radon mitigation
- Smoke-free policies

- Making homes lead-safe through remediation of lead hazards
- Installation of working smoke alarms
- Fencing around pools
- Preset safe-temperature water heaters
- Testing of private wells

risks, understanding a family's cultural and personal beliefs and desired roles in shared decision-making, and linking families to community resources are all necessary components of a community system of care that promotes children's development and life-long health. In addition, health care professionals can join with other community members and organizations to advocate for strategies to address the physical determinants of health—housing stability; home health hazards; neighborhood safety; health-fulness of food, air, and water; built environment; and geographic access to resources such as health care, employment, and safe places to be physically active and socialize.

Identify Strengths and Protective Factors and Risks

The Bright Futures Health Supervision Visits provide various opportunities for health care professionals to identify and address strengths and protective factors, to identify risks, and to work with children and their families to promote the strengths and protective factors and minimize the risks.

Promote Strengths and Protective Factors

- Identify family and youth strengths and protective factors.
- Give patients and families feedback about their strengths and what they are doing well and provide other suggestions, as appropriate.

The strength-based approach with adolescents has been well described, including strategies for empowering parents and including staff of the medical home.[69,114-116] *(For additional details, see the Ecological Determinants: Social section.)*

Address Risks

- Ask about unsafe housing or neighborhood, homelessness, joblessness, transportation problems, and food insecurity.
- Consider IPV, family tobacco use, and maternal depression.

- Consider family substance use disorder and mental health issues.
- Ask about prenatal history that may pose risks, such as maternal nutrition; intrauterine exposure to toxins; maternal alcohol, drug, and tobacco use; and birth trauma.
- Consider ACEs that may affect the parent's ability to parent.

Establish Shared Decision-making

A partnership between health care professionals and family members is based on recognizing the critical role of each partner (child, parent, health care professional, and community) in promoting health and preventing illness. When a health behavior needs to change, shared decision-making strategies and motivational interviewing can be used to put a strength-based approach in action. It indicates respect for the parent or young person as an expert on her family and her situation. It also provides an opportunity to include the strengths that already have been identified as a solid foundation from which the change can be made. People, especially those in difficult situations, often do not recognize or believe they have strengths. Guiding them through a shared problem-solving session to a successful plan can be an empowering experience. It also can serve as a model for parents and youth to use when a problem arises in daily life. To achieve a true partnership, health care professionals can model and practice open, respectful, and encouraging communication while recognizing that parents are given many recommendations and they choose which to follow and which to ignore. As a result, recommendations need to be tailored to fit the life situation of the particular family. Taking steps such as the following ones fosters the growth of trust, empathy, and understanding between the health care professional and the family:

- Greet each member of the family by name.
- Allow child and parents to state concerns without interruption.
- Acknowledge concerns, fears, and feelings.

- Show interest and attention.
- Demonstrate empathy.
- Use ordinary language, not medical jargon.
- Query patient's level of understanding and allow sufficient time for response.
- Encourage questions and answer them completely.

To identify health issues, health care professionals can use Bright Futures anticipatory guidance questions. During the conversation, understanding of the issues should be expressed and feedback given. Partnerships are enhanced if verbal recognition of the strengths of both child and parents is frequently and genuinely provided. After affirming the strengths of the family, shared goals can be identified and ways to achieve those goals discussed (eg, review the linkages among the health issue, the goal, and available personal and community resources to achieve the goal).

The next step in shared decision-making is to jointly develop a simple and achievable plan of action based on the stated goals.[117] To ensure buy-in from all partners, the health care professional can

- Make sure that each partner helped develop the plan.
- Use family-friendly negotiation skills to reach an agreement.
- Set measurable goals with a specific time line.
- Plan follow-up.

Follow-up is needed to sustain the partnership. It can take place through the health care professional or a member of the medical home team, such as a care coordinator, who can help the family identify their needs and connect with helpful services and also help the family follow through on the plan. It usually occurs through phone calls or appointments, during which progress is shared, successes are celebrated, and challenges are acknowledged. During follow-up calls or appointments, the plan of action is discussed and sometimes adjusted. These communications provide an opportunity for ongoing support and referrals to community resources.

Identify and Build on Community Supports

Effective coordination of care in the family-centered medical home is rooted in establishing relationships in the community and keeping abreast of all resources and services that might help children and their parents. In addition to the traditional primary care that is essential for all children, family members can benefit from referrals to community-based services, such as family-run resource organizations, for peer support, information, and training or to evidence-based home visitation programs, parenting programs, or local preschool programs.[39] Other community resources are listed in Box 6. These services, coupled with primary care provided in a medical home, constitute a community-based system of care that is critical to promoting family well-being.

Promoting community relationships involves more than just knowing enough about local providers and agencies to make referrals, however. Health care professionals can help create safe and supportive communities by promoting local policies that ameliorate inequities and protect children (eg, smoke-free laws; violence-reduction initiatives; efforts to promote after-school activities, safe places to play, living wages, and supportive environments for lesbian, gay, bisexual, transgender, or questioning youth; efforts to eliminate food deserts). Health care professionals can serve as community educators and spokespersons. They can speak out to educate and advocate for local programs and policies (eg, the Safe Sleep campaign, foster care policies, and Reach Out and Read). Inclusion of legal aid and other family psychosocial and family support services in the medical home can support parents and help reduce their stress levels.[120-122] Additional support for parents also can come from neighborhood organizations, faith-based organizations, school and early care and education programs, and recreational services.

Box 6
Local Community Resources

Health

- Environmental health units in public health departments
- Pediatric Environmental Health Specialty Units of the Association of Occupational and Environmental Clinics (**www.pehsu.net**)[118]
- Health literacy resources
- Help Me Grow programs
- Local Child and Family Health Plus providers
- Medical assistance programs
- Medical specialty care

- Mental health resources
- Physical activity resources
- School-based health centers and school nurses
- Public health nurses
- SCHIP
- Substance use disorder treatment
- Title V Services for Children and Youth with Special Health Care Needs
- Local boards of health

Development

- Early care and education programs
- Early intervention programs
- Head Start and Early Head Start
- Playgroups

- Recreation programs
- School-based or school-linked programs
- Starting Early Starting Smart programs

Family Support

- Bereavement and related supports (for SIDS, SUID, or other causes of infant and child death)
- Child care health consultants
- Child care resource and referral agencies
- IPV resources
- Faith-based organizations
- Food banks
- Homeless shelters and housing authorities
- Language assistance programs
- Respite care services
- Home visiting services

- National Center for Medical-Legal Partnership
- Health insurance coverage resources
- Social service agencies and child protective services
- Parenting programs or support groups
  - Parents Helping Parents organizations for children with special health care needs
  - Family Voices (**www.familyvoices.org**)
- 2-generation programs that enroll parents in education or job training when children are enrolled in child care
- WIC[119] and SNAP

Adult Assistance

- Adult education and literacy resources
- Adult education for English-language instruction
- Immigration services
- Job training resources
- Substance use disorder treatment programs
- Legal aid

- Parent support programs (eg, Parents Anonymous, Circle of Parents)
- Racial- and ethnic-specific support and community development organizations
- Volunteering opportunities

Abbreviations: IPV, intimate partner violence; SCHIP, State Children's Health Insurance Program; SIDS, sudden infant death syndrome; SNAP, Supplemental Nutrition Assistance Program, formerly known as Food Stamps; SUID, sudden unexpected infant death; WIC, Special Supplemental Nutrition Program for Women, Infants, and Children.

Health care professionals can pursue a number of options to increase their understanding of the community, strengthen relationships with community organizations and service providers, and foster positive health-promoting change at the community level (Figure 6). These options include

- Learning about the community, understanding its cultures, and collaborating with community partners.

- Recognizing the special needs of certain groups (eg, people who have recently immigrated to the United States, families of children with special health care needs).

- Linking families to needed services.[123]

- Establishing relationships and partnerships with organizations and agencies that serve as local community resources, including schools and early care and education programs.

- Encouraging adoption of referral networks that have demonstrated effective partnership with the medical home and parents of young children.[123]

- Consulting and advocating in partnership with groups and organizations that serve the community, such as schools, parks and recreation agencies, businesses, and faith groups.

- Encouraging parents to find support in family, friends, and neighborhood.

- Encouraging families and all children, especially adolescents, to become active in community endeavors to improve the health of their communities. (*For more information on this topic, see the Promoting Family Support theme.*)

- Considering co-location in the medical home of mental health, care coordination, oral health, legal, social service, or parenting education professionals to address unmet needs of families.[120-122,124,125]

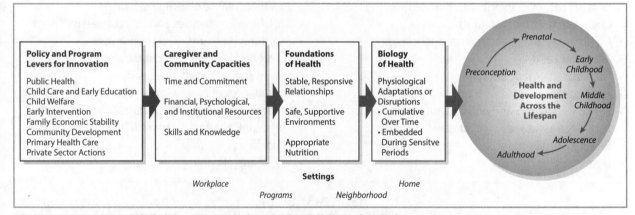

Figure 6: A Framework for Conceptualizing Early Childhood Policies and Programs to Strengthen Lifelong Health[19]

Reproduced with permission from National Scientific Council on the Developing Child, National Forum on Early Childhood Policy and Programs. The Foundations of Lifelong Health Are Built in Early Childhood. Center on the Developing Child, Harvard University, Web site. http://developingchild.harvard.edu. Published July 2010. Accessed November 14, 2016.

- Describing successful medical home partnerships with community professionals and programs that have demonstrated effectiveness with specific populations (eg, home visiting).[126]
- Working with community education and mental health professionals to ensure access to family-focused prevention programs that have been demonstrated to be effective in both reducing risks and enhancing protective factors for behavioral health. These could be integrated into medical homes or copresented in the community.

The role of families in helping the health care professional increase understanding of the community should not be underestimated. Families—especially those with children and youth with special health care needs—are often aware of community resources that the health care professional may not know. Families also can provide important information on their culture and traditions that may affect the health and well-being of the child.

Promoting Lifelong Health: Infancy (Birth Through 11 Months) and Early Childhood (1 Through 4 Years)

Incorporating the compelling data described earlier in this theme into screening and anticipatory guidance requires an organized approach. The family and environmental conditions that can infuse strength into or pose a risk for the child's healthy development are now compiled into the first anticipatory guidance priority for most visits. The Social Determinants of Health priority introduced into the fourth edition's anticipatory guidance is intended to assist health care professionals and their staff to address these important topics in a systematic way with all families and children.

Screening and anticipatory guidance are included for family, social, community, and environmental risks. To encourage family strengths, the components of the Strengthening Families Protective Factors Framework (ie, concrete help in times of need, social connections, knowledge of parenting and child development, personal resilience, and social and emotional competence) and the additional family strengths identified (ie, presence of nurturing adults, stability, and safety) have been incorporated into anticipatory guidance. *(For more information, see Box 4 of this theme.)*

Promoting Lifelong Health: Middle Childhood (5 Through 10 Years) and Adolescence (11 Through 21 Years)

School-aged children and adolescents need opportunities to do well in school and other activities and to have positive relationships with their parents, other supportive adults, and their peers. It is important to help patients and their parents appreciate that opportunities to develop caring relationships represent progress in the developmental tasks of adolescence *(see Box 3 of this theme)* and prepare them for a healthy adulthood.

Essential developmental competencies also include becoming problem-solvers, learning to cope with stress, and participating in employment, school, faith-based, and community activities. These strengths are associated with lower rates of youth risk-taking behaviors and can help young people stay on a positive life course trajectory even in the face of difficult circumstances. *(For more information on this topic, see the Promoting Healthy Development theme.)*

PROMOTING LIFELONG HEALTH FOR FAMILIES AND COMMUNITIES

References

1. Institute of Medicine, National Research Council. *Children's Health, the Nation's Wealth: Assessing and Improving Child Health*. Washington, DC: National Academies Press; 2004. http://www.ncbi.nlm.nih.gov/books/NBK92206. Accessed August 15, 2016

2. Social Determinants of Health. Healthy People 2020 Web site. http://www.healthypeople.gov/2020/topics-objectives/topic/social-determinants-health. Accessed August 15, 2016

3. Health Equity. Centers for Disease Control and Prevention Web site. http://www.cdc.gov/chronicdisease/healthequity/index.HTM. Updated February 10, 2015. Accessed August 15, 2016

4. National Partnership for Action to End Health Disparities Web site. http://minorityhealth.hhs.gov/npa/templates/browse.aspx?lvl=1&lvlid=34. Accessed August 15, 2016

5. Garner AS, Shonkoff JP; American Academy of Pediatrics Committee on Psychosocial Aspects of Child and Family Health; Committee on Early Childhood, Adoption, and Dependent Care; Section on Developmental Behavioral Pediatrics. Early childhood adversity, toxic stress, and the role of the pediatrician: translating developmental science into lifelong health. *Pediatrics*. 2012;129(1):e224-e231

6. Early Brain and Child Development. Eco-Bio-Developmental Model of Human Health and Disease. American Academy of Pediatrics Web site. https://www.aap.org/en-us/advocacy-and-policy/aap-health-initiatives/EBCD/Pages/Eco-Bio-Developmental.aspx#sthash.DALx5coB.dpuf. Accessed August 15, 2016

7. DeNavas-Walt C, Proctor BD. Income and poverty in the United States: 2013. *Current Population Reports*. 2014:1-61. https://www.census.gov/content/dam/Census/library/publications/2014/demo/p60-249.pdf. Accessed August 15, 2016

8. Agenda for Children Strategic Plan: Poverty and Child Health. American Academy of Pediatrics Web site. http://www.aap.org/en-us/about-the-aap/aap-facts/AAP-Agenda-for-Children-Strategic-Plan/Pages/AAP-Agenda-for-Children-Strategic-Plan-Poverty-Child-Health.aspx. Accessed August 15, 2016

9. Shonkoff JP, Garner AS; American Academy of Pediatrics Committee on Psychosocial Aspects of Child and Family Health; Committee on Early Childhood, Adoption, and Dependent Care; Section on Developmental and Behavioral Pediatrics. The lifelong effects of early childhood adversity and toxic stress. *Pediatrics*. 2012;129(1):e232-e246

10. Heckman JJ. Schools, skills, and synapses. *Econ Inq*. 2008;46(3):289-324. Also, see Heckman J. The Heckman Curve: Early Childhood Development Is a Smart Investment. Heckman Equation Web site. http://heckmanequation.org/content/resource/heckman-curve. Accessed September 16, 2016

11. Halfon N, Larson K, Lu M, Tullis E, Russ S. Lifecourse health development: past, present and future. *Matern Child Health J*. 2014;18(2):344-365

12. Fine A, Kotelchuck M. Rethinking MCH: the life course model as an organizing framework: concept paper. Maternal and Child Health Bureau Web site. http://www.hrsa.gov/ourstories/mchb75th/images/rethinkingmch.pdf. Published November 2010. Accessed September 14, 2016

13. Barker DJ, Thornburg KL. The obstetric origins of health for a lifetime. *Clin Obstet Gynecol*. 2013;56(3):511-519

14. National Scientific Council on the Developing Child. Early experiences can alter gene expression and affect long-term development: working paper 10. Center on the Developing Child, Harvard University, Web site. http://developingchild.harvard.edu/resources/early-experiences-can-alter-gene-expression-and-affect-long-term-development. Published May 2010. Accessed August 15, 2016

15. National Scientific Council on the Developing Child. Excessive stress disrupts the architecture of the developing brain: working paper 3. Center on the Developing Child, Harvard University, Web site. http://developingchild.harvard.edu/resources/wp3. Published January 2014. Accessed August 15, 2016

16. Barker DJ. Sir Richard Doll Lecture. Developmental origins of chronic disease. *Public Health*. 2012;126(3):185-189

17. Barker DJ, Eriksson JG, Forsen T, Osmond C. Fetal origins of adult disease: strength of effects and biological basis. *Int J Epidemiol*. 2002;31(6):1235-1239

18. Barker DJ, Forsen T, Eriksson JG, Osmond C. Growth and living conditions in childhood and hypertension in adult life: a longitudinal study. *J Hypertens*. 2002;20(10):1951-1956

19. National Scientific Council on the Developing Child, National Forum on Early Childhood Policy and Programs. The Foundations of Lifelong Health Are Built in Early Childhood. Center on the Developing Child, Harvard University, Web site. http://developingchild.harvard.edu. Published July 2010. Accessed November 14, 2016

20. Mann SL, Wadsworth ME, Colley JR. Accumulation of factors influencing respiratory illness in members of a national birth cohort and their offspring. *J Epidemiol Community Health*. 1992;43(3):286-292

21. Rosvall M, Östergren PO, Hedblad B, Isacsson SO, Janzon L, Berglund G. Life-course perspective on socioeconomic differences in carotid atherosclerosis. *Arterioscler Thromb Vasc Biol*. 2002;22(10):1704-1711

22. Lawlor DA, Batty GD, Morton SM, Clark H, Macintyre S, Leon DA. Childhood socioeconomic position, educational attainment, and adult cardiovascular risk factors: the Aberdeen children of the 1950s cohort study. *Am J Public Health*. 2005;95(7):1245-1251

23. Wamala SP, Lynch J, Kaplan GA. Women's exposure to early and later life socioeconomic disadvantage and coronary heart disease risk: the Stockholm Female Coronary Risk Study. *Int J Epidemiol*. 2001;30(2):275-284

24. Glymour MM, Avendaño M, Haas S, Berkman LF. Lifecourse social conditions and racial disparities in incidence of first stroke. *Ann Epidemiol*. 2008;18(12):904-912

25. Giskes K, van Lenthe FJ, Turrell G, Kamphuis CB, Brug J, Mackenbach JP. Socioeconomic position at different stages of the life course and its influence on body weight and weight gain in adulthood: a longitudinal study with 13-year follow-up. *Obesity (Silver Spring)*. 2008;16(6):1377-1381

26. James SA, Fowler-Brown A, Raghunathan TE, Van Hoewyk J. Life-course socioeconomic position and obesity in African American women: the Pitt County Study. *Am J Public Health*. 2006;96(3):554-560

27. Laitinen J, Power C, Jarvelin MR. Family social class, maternal body mass index, childhood body mass index, and age at menarche as predictors of adult obesity. *Am J Clin Nutr*. 2001;74(3):287-294

28. Power C, Manor O, Matthews S. Child to adult socioeconomic conditions and obesity in a national cohort. *Int J Obes Relat Metab Disord.* 2003;27(9):1081-1086

29. Lidfeldt J, Li TY, Hu FB, Manson JE, Kawachi I. A prospective study of childhood and adult socioeconomic status and incidence of type 2 diabetes in women. *Am J Epidemiol.* 2007;165(8):882-889

30. Maty SC, Lynch JW, Raghunathan TE, Kaplan GA. Childhood socioeconomic position, gender, adult body mass index, and incidence of type 2 diabetes mellitus over 34 years in the Alameda County Study. *Am J Public Health.* 2008;98(8):1486-1494

31. Melchior M, Moffitt TE, Milne BJ, Poulton R, Caspi A. Why do children from socioeconomically disadvantaged families suffer from poor health when they reach adulthood? A life-course study. *Am J Epidemiol.* 2007;166(8):966-974

32. Chapman DP, Whitfield CL, Felitti VJ, Dube SR, Edwards VJ, Anda RF. Adverse childhood experiences and the risk of depressive disorders in adulthood. *J Affect Disord.* 2004;82(2):217-225

33. About the CDC-Kaiser ACE Study. Centers for Disease Control and Prevention Web site. http://www.cdc.gov/violenceprevention/acestudy/about.html. Updated March 8, 2016. Accessed August 15, 2016

34. Edwards VJ, Holden GW, Felitti VJ, Anda RF. Relationship between multiple forms of childhood maltreatment and adult mental health in community respondents: results from the Adverse Childhood Experiences Study. *Am J Psychiatry.* 2003;160(8):1453-1460

35. Dube SR, Fairweather D, Pearson WS, Felitti VJ, Anda RF, Croft JB. Cumulative childhood stress and autoimmune diseases in adults. *Psychosom Med.* 2009;71(2):243-250

36. Anda RF, Brown DW, Felitti VJ, Bremner JD, Dube SR, Giles WH. Adverse childhood experiences and prescribed psychotropic medications in adults. *Am J Prev Med.* 2007;32(5):389-394

37. Fisher PA, Stoolmiller M, Gunnar MR, Burraston BO. Effects of a therapeutic intervention for foster preschoolers on diurnal cortisol activity. *Psychoneuroendocrinology.* 2007;32(8-10):892-905

38. Laurent HK, Gilliam KS, Bruce J, Fisher PA. HPA stability for children in foster care: mental health implications and moderation by early intervention. *Dev Psychobiol.* 2014;56(6):1406-1415

39. Woodrow Wilson School of Public and International Affairs at Princeton University and the Brookings Institution. Helping parents, helping children: two-generation mechanisms. *Future Child.* 2014;24(1, theme issue):1-170

40. Fisher PA, Van Ryzin MJ, Gunnar MR. Mitigating HPA axis dysregulation associated with placement changes in foster care. *Psychoneuroendocrinology.* 2011;36(4):531-539

41. Kaufman J, Yang BZ, Douglas-Palumberi H, et al. Brain-derived neurotrophic factor-5-HTTLPR gene interactions and environmental modifiers of depression in children. *Biol Psychiatry.* 2006;59(8):673-680

42. Fall C. Maternal nutrition: effects on health in the next generation. *Indian J Med Res.* 2009;130(5):593-599

43. Godfrey KM, Barker DJ. Fetal nutrition and adult disease. *Am J Clin Nutr.* 2000;71(5 suppl):1344s-1352s

44. National Scientific Council on the Developing Child. Supportive relationships and active skill-building strengthen the foundations of resilience: working paper 13. Center on the Developing Child, Harvard University, Web site. http://developingchild.harvard.edu/resources/supportive-relationships-and-active-skill-building-strengthen-the-foundations-of-resilience. Published 2015. Accessed August 15, 2016

45. Abramson D, Stehling-Ariza T, Garfield R, Redlener I. Prevalence and predictors of mental health distress post-Katrina: findings from the Gulf Coast Child and Family Health Study. *Disaster Med Public Health Prep.* 2008;2(2):77-86

46. Glandon DM, Muller J, Almedom AM. Resilience in post-Katrina New Orleans, Louisiana: a preliminary study. *Afr Health Sci.* 2008;8(suppl 1):s21-s27

47. Hackbarth M, Pavkov T, Wetchler J, Flannery M. Natural disasters: an assessment of family resiliency following Hurricane Katrina. *J Marital Fam Ther.* 2012;38(2):340-351

48. Kronenberg ME, Hansel TC, Brennan AM, Osofsky HJ, Osofsky JD, Lawrason B. Children of Katrina: lessons learned about postdisaster symptoms and recovery patterns. *Child Dev.* 2010;81(4):1241-1259

49. Cleveland LM, Minter ML, Cobb KA, Scott AA, German VF. Lead hazards for pregnant women and children: part 1; immigrants and the poor shoulder most of the burden of lead exposure in this country. Part 1 of a two-part article details how exposure happens, whom it affects, and the harm it can do. *Am J Nurs.* 2008;108(10):40-50

50. Weidenhamer JD. Lead contamination of inexpensive seasonal and holiday products. *Sci Total Environ.* 2009;407(7):2447-2450

51. Fetal Alcohol Spectrum Disorders Program Toolkit. American Academy of Pediatrics Web site. https://www.aap.org/en-us/advocacy-and-policy/aap-health-initiatives/fetal-alcohol-spectrum-disorders-toolkit/Pages/default.aspx. Accessed August 15, 2016

52. Best D; American Academy of Pediatrics Committee on Environmental Health, Committee on Native American Child Health, Committee on Adolescence. Secondhand and prenatal tobacco smoke exposure. *Pediatrics.* 2009;124(5):e1017-e1044

53. McEwen BS. Central effects of stress hormones in health and disease: understanding the protective and damaging effects of stress and stress mediators. *Eur J Pharmacol.* 2008;583(2-3):174-185

54. National Scientific Council on the Developing Child. Young children develop in an environment of relationships: working paper 1. Center on the Developing Child, Harvard University, Web site. http://developingchild.harvard.edu/resources/wp1. Published October 2009. Accessed August 15, 2016

55. Braveman P, Barclay C. Health disparities beginning in childhood: a life-course perspective. *Pediatrics.* 2009;124(suppl 3):S163-S175

56. Barker DJ. The developmental origins of well-being. *Philos Trans R Soc Lond B Biol Sci.* 2004;359(1449):1359-1366

57. Kanaka-Gantenbein C. Fetal origins of adult diabetes. *Ann N Y Acad Sci.* 2010;1205:99-105

58. Oberlander TF, Weinberg J, Papsdorf M, Grunau R, Misri S, Devlin AM. Prenatal exposure to maternal depression, neonatal methylation of human glucocorticoid receptor gene (*NR3C1*) and infant cortisol stress responses. *Epigenetics.* 2008;3(2):97-106

59. Garner AS, Forkey H, Stirling J, Nalven L, Schilling S; American Academy of Pediatrics, Dave Thomas Foundation for Adoption. *Helping Foster and Adoptive Families Cope With Trauma.* Elk Grove Village, IL: American Academy of Pediatrics; 2015. https://www.aap.org/traumaguide. Accessed August 15, 2016

60. Waters E, Kondo-Ikemura K, Posada G, Richters JE. Learning to love: mechanisms and milestones. In: Gunnar MR, Sroufe LA, eds. *Minnesota Symposia on Child Psychology.* Hillsdale, NJ: Lawrence Erlbaum Associates; 1991:217-255. *Self Processes and Development;* vol 23

61. Winnicott DW. The theory of the parent-infant relationship. *Int J Psychoanal.* 1960;41:585-595

62. High PC, Klass P; American Academy of Pediatrics Council on Early Childhood. Literacy promotion: an essential component of primary care pediatric practice. *Pediatrics.* 2014;134(2):404-409

63. Educational Interventions for Children Affected by Lead. Centers for Disease Control and Prevention Web site. http://www.cdc.gov/nceh/lead/publications/Educational_Interventions_Children_Affected_by_Lead.pdf. Published April 2015. Accessed August 15, 2016

64. Hudziak JJ, Ivanova MY. The Vermont Family Based Approach: family based health promotion, illness prevention, and intervention. *Child Adolesc Psychiatr Clin N Am.* 2016;25(2):167-178

65. Bronfenbrenner U. *The Ecology of Human Development: Experiments by Nature and Design.* Cambridge, MA: Harvard University Press; 1979

66. Lerner RM, Lerner JV. *The Positive Development of Youth: Report of the Findings from the First Seven Years of the 4-H Study of Positive Youth Development.* Boston, MA: Tufts University; 2011. http://ase.tufts.edu/iaryd/documents/4hpydstudywave7.pdf. Accessed August 15, 2016

67. 40 Developmental Assets for Adolescents. Search Institute Web site. http://www.search-institute.org/content/40-developmental-assets-adolescents-ages-12-18. Published 2007. Accessed August 15, 2016

68. Harper Browne C. *Youth Thrive: Advancing Healthy Adolescent Development and Well-Being.* Washington, DC: Center for the Study of Social Policy; 2014. http://www.cssp.org/reform/child-welfare/youth-thrive/2014/Youth-Thrive_Advancing-Healthy-Adolescent-Development-and-Well-Being.pdf. Accessed August 15, 2016

69. Ginsburg KR, Kinsman SB. *Reaching Teens: Strength-Based Communication Strategies to Build Resilience and Support Healthy Adolescent Development.* Elk Grove Village, IL: American Academy of Pediatrics; 2014

70. Fine A, Large R. *A Conceptual Framework for Adolescent Health: A Collaborative Project of the Association of Maternal and Child Health Programs and the National Network of State Adolescent Health Coordinators.* Washington, DC: Association of Maternal and Child Health Programs; 2005. http://www.amchp.org/programsandtopics/AdolescentHealth/Documents/conc-framework.pdf. Accessed August 15, 2016

71. Pittman K, Irby M, Tolman J, Yohalem N, Ferber T. *Preventing Problems, Promoting Development, Encouraging Engagement: Competing Priorities or Inseparable Goals?* Washington, DC: The Forum for Youth Investment; 2003. http://forumfyi.org/files/Preventing%20Problems,%20Promoting%20Development,%20Encouraging%20Engagement.pdf. Accessed August 15, 2016

72. Leffert N, Benson PL, Scales PC, et al. Developmental assets: measurement and prediction of risk behaviors among adolescents. *Appl Dev Sci.* 1998;2(4):209-230

73. Murphey DA, Lamonda KH, Carney JK, Duncan P. Relationships of a brief measure of youth assets to health-promoting and risk behaviors. *J Adolesc Health.* 2004;34(3):184-191

74. Scales PC, Benson PL, Leffert N, Blyth DA. Contribution of developmental assets to the prediction of thriving among adolescents. *Appl Dev Sci.* 2000;4(1):27-46

75. Child Welfare Information Gateway. *Protective Factors Approaches in Child Welfare.* Washington, DC: US Department of Health and Human Services, Children's Bureau; 2014. https://www.childwelfare.gov/pubs/issue-briefs/protective-factors. Accessed August 15, 2016

76. Harper Browne C. Knowledge of parenting and child development. *The Strengthening Families Approach and Protective Factors Framework: Branching Out and Reaching Deeper.* Washington, DC: Center for the Study of Social Policy; 2014:29-35. http://www.cssp.org/reform/strengtheningfamilies/branching-out-and-reaching-deeper. Accessed August 15, 2016

77. Essentials for Childhood Framework: Steps to Create Safe, Stable, and Nurturing Relationships and Environments for All Children. Centers for Disease Control and Prevention Web site. http://www.cdc.gov/violenceprevention/childmaltreatment/essentials.html. Updated April 5, 2016. Accessed August 15, 2016

78. Araya R, Dunstan F, Playle R, Thomas H, Palmer S, Lewis G. Perceptions of social capital and the built environment and mental health. *Soc Sci Med.* 2006;62(12):3072-3083

79. The Five Promises Change Lives. America's Promise Alliance Web site. http://www.americaspromise.org/promises. Accessed August 15, 2016

80. Black MC, Basile KC, Breiding MJ, et al. *National Intimate Partner and Sexual Violence Survey (NISVS): 2010 Summary Report.* Atlanta, GA: Centers for Disease Control and Prevention, National Center for Injury Prevention and Control; 2011. http://www.cdc.gov/violenceprevention/pdf/nisvs_report2010-a.pdf. Accessed August 15, 2016

81. Hamby S, Finkelhor D, Turner H, Ormrod R. Children's exposure to intimate partner violence and other family violence. *Juvenile Justice Bulletin.* 2011:1-12. http://www.ncjrs.gov/pdffiles1/ojjdp/232272.pdf. Accessed August 15, 2016

82. Holt S, Buckley H, Whelan S. The impact of exposure to domestic violence on children and young people: a review of the literature. *Child Abuse Negl.* 2008;32(8):797-810

83. Herrenkohl TI, Sousa C, Tajima EA, Herrenkohl RC, Moylan CA. Intersection of child abuse and children's exposure to domestic violence. *Trauma Violence Abuse.* 2008;9(2):84-99

84. Holden GW. Children exposed to domestic violence and child abuse: terminology and taxonomy. *Clin Child Fam Psychol Rev.* 2003;6(3):151-160

85. Thackeray JD, Hibbard R, Dowd MD; American Academy of Pediatrics Committee on Child Abuse and Neglect; Committee on Injury, Violence, and Poison Prevention. Intimate partner violence: the role of the pediatrician. *Pediatrics.* 2010;125(5):1094-1100

86. Table 133. Marriages and divorces—number and rate by state: 1990 to 2009. In: US Census Bureau. *Statistical Abstract of the United States: 2012.* Washington, DC: US Census Bureau; 2011:98. http://www2.census.gov/library/publications/2011/compendia/statab/131ed/2012-statab.pdf. Accessed August 15, 2016

87. Kreider RM, Ellis R. Living arrangements of children: 2009.

Current Population Reports. 2011:1-25. https://www.census. gov/prod/2011pubs/p70-126.pdf. Accessed August 15, 2016

88. Cohen GJ; American Academy of Pediatrics Committee on Psychosocial Aspects of Child and Family Health. Helping children and families deal with divorce and separation. *Pediatrics.* 2002;110(5):1019-1023

89. Braveman P, Gottlieb L. The social determinants of health: it's time to consider the causes of the causes. *Public Health Rep.* 2014;129(suppl 2):19-31

90. Evans GW. The environment of childhood poverty. *Am Psychol.* 2004;59(2):77-92

91. Annie E. Casey Foundation. *2013 KIDSCOUNT Data Book: State Trends in Child Well-Being.* Baltimore, MD: Annie E. Casey Foundation; 2013. http://datacenter.kidscount.org/files/ 2013KIDSCOUNTDataBook.pdf. Accessed August 15, 2016

92. Payne-Sturges D, Gee GC. National environmental health measures for minority and low-income populations: tracking social disparities in environmental health. *Environ Res.* 2006;102(2):154-171

93. Housing Instability. US Department of Health and Human Services Office of the Assistant Secretary for Planning and Evaluation Web site. https://aspe.hhs.gov/legacy-page/ancillary-services-support-welfare-work-housing-instability-153121. Accessed August 15, 2016

94. Cutts DB, Meyers AF, Black MM, et al. US housing insecurity and the health of very young children. *Am J Public Health.* 2011;101(8):1508-1514

95. Robert Wood Johnson Foundation Commission to Build a Healthier America. *Time to Act: Investing in the Health of Our Children and Communities.* Princeton, NJ: Robert Wood Johnson Foundation; 2014. http://www.rwjf.org/content/dam/farm/ reports/reports/2014/rwjf409002. Accessed August 15, 2016

96. Robert Wood Johnson Foundation Commission to Build a Healthier America. Where we live matters for our health: the links between housing and health. *Neighborhoods and Health.* 2008. http://www.commissiononhealth.org/PDF/fff21abf-e208-46dd-a110-e757c3c6cdd7/Issue%20Brief%203%20Sept%20 08%20-%20Neighborhoods%20and%20Health.pdf. Accessed August 15, 2016

97. Cohen DA, Finch BK, Bower A, Sastry N. Collective efficacy and obesity: the potential influence of social factors on health. *Soc Sci Med.* 2006;62(3):769-778

98. Wilkinson R, Marmot M. *Social Determinants of Health: The Solid Facts.* 2nd ed. Copenhagen, Denmark: World Health Organization Regional Office for Europe; 2003. http://www. euro.who.int/en/publications/abstracts/social-determinants-of-health.-the-solid-facts. Accessed August 15, 2016

99. Ver Ploeg M, Breneman V, Farrigan T, et al. *Access to Affordable and Nutritious Food: Measuring and Understanding Food Deserts and Their Consequences: Report to Congress.* Washington, DC: US Department of Agriculture; 2009. http:// www.ers.usda.gov/media/242675/ap036_1_.pdf. Accessed August 15, 2016

100. Larson NI, Story MT, Nelson MC. Neighborhood environments: disparities in access to healthy foods in the U.S. *Am J Prev Med.* 2009;36(1):74-81

101. Food Research & Action Center. Why Low-Income and Food Insecure People are Vulnerable to Obesity. FRAC Web site. http://frac.org/initiatives/hunger-and-obesity/why-are-low-income-and-food-insecure-people-vulnerable-to-obesity. Accessed September 15, 2016

102. Wilson J, Dixon SL, Breysse P, et al. Housing and allergens: a pooled analysis of nine US studies. *Environ Res.* 2010;110(2):189-198

103. Lanphear BP, Kahn RS, Berger O, Auinger P, Bortnick SM, Nahhas RW. Contribution of residential exposures to asthma in US children and adolescents. *Pediatrics.* 2001;107(6):E98

104. Quirós-Alcalá L, Bradman A, Nishioka M, et al. Pesticides in house dust from urban and farmworker households in California: an observational measurement study. *Environ Health.* 2011;10:19

105. Jacobs DE. Environmental health disparities in housing. *Am J Public Health.* 2011;101(suppl 1):S115-S122

106. Krieger J, Jacobs DE, Ashley PJ, et al. Housing interventions and control of asthma-related indoor biologic agents: a review of the evidence. *J Public Health Manag Pract.* 2010;16(5 suppl):S11-S20

107. DiGuiseppi C, Jacobs DE, Phelan KJ, Mickalide A, Ormandy D. Housing interventions and control of injury-related structural deficiencies: a review of the evidence. *J Public Health Manag Pract.* 2010;16(5 suppl):S34-S43

108. Lindberg RA, Shenassa ED, Acevedo-Garcia D, Popkin SJ, Villaveces A, Morley RL. Housing interventions at the neighborhood level and health: a review of the evidence. *J Public Health Manag Pract.* 2010;16(5 suppl):S44-S52

109. Sandel M, Baeder A, Bradman A, et al. Housing interventions and control of health-related chemical agents: a review of the evidence. *J Public Health Manag Pract.* 2010;16(5 suppl):S24-S33

110. US Environmental Protection Agency. *America's Children and the Environment.* 3rd ed. Washington, DC: US Environmental Protection Agency; 2013. http://www.epa.gov/ace. Accessed August 15, 2016

111. Committee on the Effect of Climate Change on Indoor Air Quality and Public Health, Institute of Medicine. *Climate Change, the Indoor Environment, and Health.* Washington, DC: National Academies Press; 2011

112. van Aalst MK. The impacts of climate change on the risk of natural disasters. *Disasters.* 2006;30(1):5-18

113. Turner-Henson A, Vessey JA. Environmental disasters and children. *J Pediatr Nurs.* 2010;25(5):315-316

114. Duncan P, Frankowski B, Carey P, et al. Improvement in adolescent screening and counseling rates for risk behaviors and developmental tasks. *Pediatrics.* 2012;130(5):e1345-e1351

115. Frankowski BL, Brendtro LK, Van Bockern S, Duncan PM. Strength-based interviewing: the circle of courage. In: Ginsburg KR, Kinsman SB, eds. *Reaching Teens: Strength-Based Communication Strategies to Build Resilience and Support Healthy Adolescent Development.* Elk Grove Village, IL: American Academy of Pediatrics; 2014:237-242

116. Frankowski BL, Leader IC, Duncan PM. Strength-based interviewing. *Adolesc Med State Art Rev.* 2009;20(1):22-40, vii-viii

117. Motivational Interviewing. American Academy of Pediatrics Web site. https://www.aap.org/en-us/advocacy-and-policy/ aap-health-initiatives/HALF-Implementation-Guide/ communicating-with-families/pages/Motivational-Interviewing.aspx. Accessed August 15, 2016

118. Pediatric Environmental Health Specialty Units Web site. http://www.pehsu.net. Accessed August 15, 2016

119. US Department of Agriculture, Food and Nutrition Service. Women, Infants, and Children (WIC) Web site. http://www.fns. usda.gov/wic/women-infants-and-children-wic. Published April 19, 2016. Accessed August 15, 2016

PROMOTING LIFELONG HEALTH FOR FAMILIES AND COMMUNITIES

120. Garg A, Butz AM, Dworkin PH, Lewis RA, Thompson RE, Serwint JR. Improving the management of family psychosocial problems at low-income children's well-child care visits: the WE CARE Project. *Pediatrics.* 2007;120(3):547-558

121. Sege R, Preer G, Morton SJ, et al. Medical-legal strategies to improve infant health care: a randomized trial. *Pediatrics.* 2015;136(1):97-106

122. Dubowitz H, Feigelman S, Lane W, Kim J. Pediatric primary care to help prevent child maltreatment: the Safe Environment for Every Kid (SEEK) model. *Pediatrics.* 2009;123(3):858-864

123. Help Me Grow National Center Web site. http://www.helpmegrownational.org. Accessed August 15, 2016

124. Perrin EC, Sheldrick RC, McMenamy JM, Henson BS, Carter AS. Improving parenting skills for families of young children in pediatric settings: a randomized clinical trial. *JAMA Pediatr.* 2014;168(1):16-24

125. Minkovitz CS, Hughart N, Strobino D, et al. A practice-based intervention to enhance quality of care in the first 3 years of life: the Healthy Steps for Young Children Program. *JAMA.* 2003;290(23):3081-3091

126. Home Visiting Models. US Department of Health and Human Services Maternal and Child Health Bureau Web site. http://mchb.hrsa.gov/maternal-child-health-initiatives/home-visiting. Accessed August 15, 2016

Promoting Family Support

The Family: A Description

We all come from families.

Families are big, small, extended, nuclear, multi-generational, with one parent, two parents, and grandparents.

We live under one roof or many.

A family can be as temporary as a few weeks, as permanent as forever.

We become part of a family by birth, adoption, marriage, or from a desire for mutual support.

As family members, we nurture, protect, and influence each other.

Families are dynamic and are cultures unto themselves, with different values and unique ways of realizing dreams.

Together, our families become the source of our rich cultural heritage and spiritual diversity.

Each family has strengths and qualities that flow from individual members and from the family as a unit.

Our families create neighborhoods, communities, states, and nations.

Developed and adopted by the Young Children's Continuum
of the New Mexico State Legislature

June 20, 1990

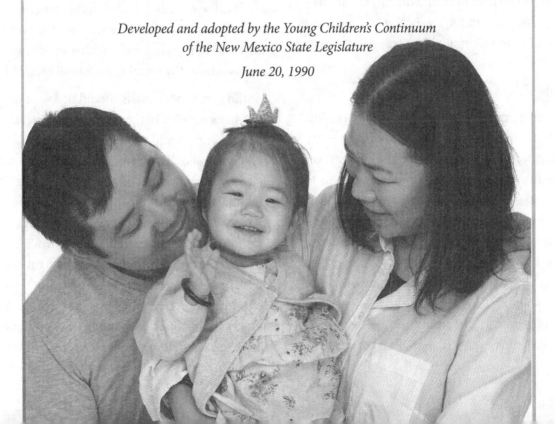

The health and well-being of infants, children, and adolescents depend on their parents, families, and other caregivers. Focusing on the family's growth and development along with the growth and development of the child is a central activity of Bright Futures for all health care professionals. It is the basis of the partnership with parents and families. Putting this approach into practice at health supervision visits involves

- Being aware of the composition of the family
- Understanding the cultural and ethnic beliefs and traditions of each family
- Assessing the well-being of parents or other caregivers
- Asking about and addressing parent-identified needs and concerns
- Assessing the family's well-being
- Identifying and building on the parents' and family's strengths and protective factors
- Assessing and addressing the family's risks
- Providing information, support, and access to community resources
- Delivering family-centered care in the medical home[1]

The essential effect of family on child health is further discussed in the *Promoting Lifelong Health for Families and Communities theme.*

The Family Constellation

Just as every child is different, so is every family. Families can include one child and one parent or guardian, or several children plus parents or guardians who range in age from adolescents to senior citizens. They might be extended families, foster families, adoptive families, or blended families with stepparents and stepchildren. Parents can be married or unmarried couples, single parents, or parents who live apart and share child-rearing responsibilities. Parents may be opposite-sex or same-sex couples.[2] The family unit can be relatively static, or it can be quite changeable if parents divorce

or remarry or if outside caregivers change. Families also can include a parent or caregiver who is of a different racial or ethnic group than the child.[3]

In some families, grandparents play a central role in the daily care of young and growing children. Intergenerational parenting occurs when grandparents and other family members assume the care for children whose birth parents are not present or not capable of caring for their children because of extended work-related absences, illness or death, drug use, neglect, abandonment, or incarceration.

Children in immigrant families now represent a quarter of the children in the United States, and they are a growing sector of the population.[4] These children experience a number of unique and powerful family-level influences as well as unique strengths.

Although it has predictable patterns, the family reshapes its daily life and support systems with the birth of each child in a way that fits with its unique mix of strengths and challenges. For families living in difficult situations, such as poverty, homelessness, divorce, separation, deployment in the military, or illness, resilience varies tremendously and is not always predictable. Two themes common to all families are that parents want the best for their children and significant change or stress that affects one family member affects all members.

Health care professionals should be aware of the characteristics of the family to which a child belongs and should be sensitive to differences among families. Establishing a relationship with a family involves open inquiry about key family members in the child's life and identification of parents, co-parents, and extended supports. The health care professional and family form a partnership in the medical home that is based on respect, trust, honest communication, and cultural competence. Becoming a culturally effective professional requires being open to multiple ways of thinking about, understanding, and interacting with the world.[5] Health care professionals can better understand their patients and facilitate communication if they integrate the family's cultural background into the general health assessment.[6] *(For more information on this topic, see the Bright Futures introduction.)*

The Role of Fathers

Providers of pediatric health care most often interact with mothers, because women are typically the primary caregivers of children. Social changes in this country have altered traditional father roles substantially, however, and increasingly, parents now share the care of their children. Moreover, a growing number of single fathers today are raising children on their own; 16% of single parents were men as of 2013.[7] Research on the effect of a father on his child's development and psychological growth has shown a range of important effects on the child's well-being, cognitive development, social competence, and later school success.[8,9]

A variety of non-nuclear family arrangements also are on the rise, in which the primary father figure is a stepfather, partner, fiancé, grandfather, or other extended family member. At the same time, more children than ever are growing up in families with only a mother and no father (24% in 2014).[10] For all these reasons, health care professionals must increase their understanding of the roles of their patients' fathers, as well as the mothers. When inviting a father to become an integral part of his newborn's health supervision visits, the health care professional is sending a clear message about his importance to the child's long-term health and development. When both parents attend health supervision visits, the health care professional can observe parent-child and parent-parent interactions and any important differences that might affect the care and support of the child. Encouraging fathers to attend health supervision visits gives the health care professional an opportunity to gain insight through direct observation and inquiry into

- The nature of the father's involvement with the child, including his views, concerns, and questions
- Some aspects of his support for the mother (and consequently support for the mother-child relationship)
- The father's general physical and mental health
- Cultural values that can contribute to the father's role and involvement with his child

Families With Adolescent Parents

Adolescent parents face a variety of specific challenges. While needing to build a nurturing relationship with their infant, they still require nurturing relationships for themselves. During a time when their children are growing and developing, adolescent parents are still growing and developing themselves, presenting unique challenges and opportunities within the parenting role. They often want to return to school and attempt to reengage with their previous friends and activities. Many lack resources, including ready transportation to health care appointments.

In most cases, the adolescent parent lives with her own parents, and the grandparent shares some aspects of child care and child-rearing. The health care professional's inquiry into the individual roles of different family caregivers, including the baby's father, will provide an opportunity to discuss individual needs and expectations. The result can be especially powerful when the adolescent and her parents meet with the health care professional to discuss their roles, differences, and mutual goals.

Many adolescents adapt well to parenting when they have a supportive and encouraging environment. Focusing on their specific parenting strengths in front of other family members during visits and providing anticipatory guidance builds confidence and competence. These young parents also may be helped by parenting classes, peer support programs, home visitation programs, and other community support services. Role models and mentors—both male and female—can be an important source of support for the adolescent parents. Schools with on-site child care and programs for adolescent parents are wonderful resources if they are available in the community.[11]

Families With Same-sex Parents

About 2 million children live in families headed by a parent identified as lesbian, gay, bisexual, or transgender (LGBT) or in families with two parents of the same sex.[2,12] The Williams Institute of the UCLA School of Law found that approximately 2% of Americans have an LGBT-identified parent.[13] Fear of discrimination, violence, or loss of custody is believed to lead to underreporting, and a considerably greater number of children are likely to currently live in families headed by LGBT-identified parents.

Children of LGBT-identified parents may be intentionally conceived when same-sex couples seek alternative reproductive technologies now available, or they may come from a previous heterosexual union, be foster children, or be adopted. Community acceptance of all these families and laws that empower partners of the same sex to marry bring legitimacy to these families and legal protections to both parents and children.[2,12,14]

It is important that health care professionals caring for the children of LGBT-identified parents value these relationships, just as they seek to understand all families. A careful review of the literature by the American Academy of Pediatrics (AAP) concluded that the children of same-sex parents were developmentally and psychologically like all other children,[2] and this has been confirmed by subsequent studies.[15] One consistent finding in children of these families is greater compassion, resilience, and tolerance than is shown by their peers, suggesting that their recognition that their family constellation is less typical makes them more accepting of social differences.[2]

Families With Adopted Children

Adoption is a broad term that can include international or domestic arrangements, adoption from foster care, placement with relatives other than parents (kinship care), open adoptions, adoption from biological families, and adoption within and across ethnic and cultural groups. Health care professionals can play a supportive role by helping families with the many issues associated with adoption. For example, families who are pursuing an international adoption may need support in dealing with unknown developmental and cognitive status or the risk of infectious diseases for the children,[16] cultural and linguistic differences, foreign travel, and numerous rules that often require exceptional parental patience and persistence.

Adoption presents special challenges and lifelong transitions for the adopted child, her biological family, and her adoptive family. All adopted children need a thorough assessment of their physical, emotional, and psychological needs at the time of adoption and as they develop because they are at increased risk for developing behavioral, emotional, and social problems. Children who are placed into families from foster care may exhibit behaviors that reflect their earlier abandonment, neglect, or biological influences, such as prenatal exposure to toxins. They might behave more like children younger than their own age because their childhood experiences have been atypical. Adopted children who are of a different race or ethnicity than their parents may encounter identity issues. In addition, an adoption affects other siblings and their acceptance of the new family members, whether these siblings are biological or they themselves are adopted.

As the child develops, parents commonly have ongoing questions and uncertainties related to the adoption. Thus, the continuity of care, developmental monitoring, and health care professional's openness to the parent's questions become all-important sources of support for adoptive parents.

Health care professionals also can offer vitally important anticipatory guidance on the development of the child's perspectives on adoption. Like everything else children learn, the understanding of adoption develops over time. The adopted infant or child will not be aware of the difference between biological and adoptive families before the age of 3 years.

Children understand simple concepts initially and gradually come to understand nuances and abstract thoughts about adoption as they grow older. Health care professionals should encourage families to talk about adoption with their children just as they talk about other complex ideas—repeatedly, over time, and with increasing detail as the child develops more advanced thought capabilities.

Parents who have adopted young children should be advised to introduce the words *adoption* and *adopted* as soon as the child begins to develop language and to elaborate, for the child, the personal story of her birth and adoption in positive, developmentally appropriate terms, thus providing the child with an opportunity to integrate the concept into her thinking from an early stage. For some school-aged children, perceptions of a sense of loss and self-esteem issues can occur during middle childhood. A struggle with concepts of identity can arise during adolescence. Health care professionals also can emphasize to families the need to provide children with truthful information regarding the adoption process, a discussion that is best initiated with parents during the child's early years.[17]

Families With Foster Care Children

Each year in the United States, more than 250,000 children are placed in foster care because of abuse or neglect, with approximately 400,000 children in the foster care system at one time.[18] These out-of-home placements for children who are unable to remain with their birth parents can be temporary or extended. Foster care ultimately may lead to family reunification; permanent severance of parental custody, thereby creating the possibility of adoption by another family; or a cycle of moving in and out of foster care until the child reaches adulthood. Children may be placed in kinship care with caregivers who are relatives, with nonrelative foster families, in a treatment or therapeutic foster care home, or in a group or congregate care home. Strong and consistent data indicate that children in foster care have special needs.

- Most children in foster care have been abused or neglected and have not experienced a stable, nurturing environment during their early life.
- Many children in foster care have experienced unrecognized fetal harm from prenatal alcohol exposure or from other teratogenic substances, from poor prenatal nutrition and perhaps from the toxic stresses experienced by the mother during her pregnancy.
- Slightly more than a half of the children return to their parent or principal caregiver. Supports to the family environment are essential to reunification success.[18]
- The length of time in foster care varies, but, on average, 46% of the children are in foster care for less than 1 year; 27%, between 1 and 2 years; 22%, from 2 to 4 years; and 5%, for more than 5 years.[18]

Thousands of children live in an informal version of foster care, in which they live with relatives other than parents. Children in kinship care outside the state foster care system are not guaranteed the special protection or monitoring that is provided to children in official foster care programs.[19] Relatives who provide informal kinship care usually receive no training or financial support for doing so.

Children who are placed in foster care during the years of active brain development are at risk of developing special health concerns, often because of the abuse and neglect that resulted in the foster care placement, in addition to the impermanence of the foster situation. For infants, an environment that is devoid of age-appropriate stimulation, nurturing, and communication or an environment of trauma affects cognitive and communication skills and alters attachment relationships. *(For more information on this topic, see the Promoting Mental Health and the Promoting Lifelong Health for Families and Communities themes.)* Young children who are placed in foster care because of parental neglect can experience profound and long-lasting consequences on all aspects of their development (eg, poor attachment formation, under-stimulation, developmental delay, poor physical development, and antisocial behavior).

Placements into foster care that occur between the ages of 6 months and about 3 years, especially if prompted by family discord and disruption, can result in subsequent emotional disturbances in the child because of the young child's limited capacity for understanding the constraints of time and place that accompany the foster care experience. The development of these disturbances depends on the nature of the attachment relationships before and after separation from the biological parents and the child's response to stress. If separation from biological parents during the first year of life (especially during the first 6 months) is followed by quality, trauma-informed care, placement in foster care may not have a deleterious effect on social or emotional functioning.[20] The traumas (or toxic stressors) children experience before and upon placement in foster care result in adaptive responses by children. These responses can employ healthy and unhealthy coping mechanisms. Health care professionals should be attentive to these responses and actively engage foster families to address these responses and behaviors.

Several developmental issues are important to consider for young children in foster care.

- The effect of traumas such as abuse, neglect, and inadequate or multiple foster care placements on brain development
- The nature of the attachment relationships before and after separation from the biological parents
- The young child's limited capacity for understanding the constraints of time and place that accompany the foster care experience
- The child's response to stress[21]

In addition to these mental health concerns that can lead to later problems, including difficulty in forming adult relationships, many children in foster care have unmet physical health care needs, including missed immunizations, poor medical history, undiagnosed infections or illnesses, and undiagnosed developmental delays.[22] Foster parents often are excluded from supports and information that are provided to birth or adoptive parents about their children's health and development. They often do not have any background information or essential medical records regarding the children in their care and may have to suddenly deal with a health crisis that they did not anticipate. Health care professionals need to create partnerships and processes to support these needs. The foster care agency caseworker is an important resource.

Health care professionals have a responsibility to comprehensively assess, treat, refer, and advocate for these vulnerable children and their caregivers.[23] By acknowledging the emotional rewards and challenges of foster parenting and addressing the multiple needs and concerns of foster families, health care professionals can greatly assist foster parents and the children in their care.

Among the approximately 402,000 children and adolescents in foster care in 2013, 160,800 were 11 years or older. Teens in foster care present a special challenge to health care professionals. Of those who "age out" of the system, 38% have emotional problems, 50% have used illicit drugs, 25% have been involved in the legal system, and only 48% have graduated from high school.[24] Thirty-six percent of children and adolescents 16 years and older in foster care live in group homes or institutional settings, compared with 1% of children aged 1 to 5.[25] Of additional concern for health care professionals is that adolescent girls in foster care are substantially more likely than other girls to have become pregnant (48% versus 20%) and nearly 3 times more likely to have had a child (32% versus 12%). Almost twice as many girls in foster care (65%) have had sexual intercourse compared to girls not in foster care (35%).[26] Ensuring continuity of reproductive health services is especially challenging for youth in foster care who move frequently from home to home.

Families With Children and Youth With Special Health Care Needs

Health care professionals who have pediatric patients with special health care needs should seek to understand the family's composition and social circumstances and the effect that the special needs have on family functioning. Family-centered care that promotes positive relationships and honest communication among all parties (families, children, and health care professionals) is critical. Because children and youth with special health care needs tend to require frequent visits with health care professionals and because most children with these special needs now live into adulthood, families find it especially important to build strong partnerships with the health care professionals who see their children, to feel comfortable asking questions and seeking advice as they face transitions and decision points along the continuum of their child's health care. Health care professionals can assist the family in helping the child reach her potential by focusing on the strengths of the child and her family.

The lives of the parents, siblings, and other caregivers are affected by the child's medical care and the need for episodic or recurrent hospitalizations, specialized procedures, and treatments. The child's interactions with multiple specialists and other service providers, including the education system, and the financial effect of the child's condition on the family also can have a profound effect on the family. Helping families identify natural support networks and community resources is essential. Peer and community networks can provide support not only for medical concerns but also for logistical and emotional issues. Community resources can include respite care; home visitor programs; early intervention programs; family resource and support centers; libraries; faith-based organizations; peer support and education programs, such as Family-to-Family Health Information Centers and Parent to Parent matching programs[27]; and recreation centers. These resources may be more easily accessed if the child or youth with special health care needs is cared for in a medical home. *(For more information on this topic, see the Promoting Health for Children and Youth With Special Health Care Needs theme.)*

Recognizing the Effect of Environment on Families

Many parents may not have control over their home environment because of living arrangements or culture or gender roles. *(For more information on the home environment, see the Promoting Safety and Injury Prevention theme.)* The health care professional can work with parents to develop strategies for ensuring a healthy living environment for the benefit of their child's health and well-being. Neighborhood and community environments directly support or challenge the well-being of families and the goals that parents have for their children. *(For more information on this topic, see the Promoting Lifelong Health for Families and Communities theme.)* Special consideration may be needed for immigrant or refugee families, especially in relation to legal status and concerns about deportation and the risk of family separation, which can affect their children's access to health care and housing. The health care professional should work with families and professional and community resources to help families create and maintain a healthy, safe environment for their children.

Forming an Effective Partnership With Families

Family-Centered Care

The health care professional plays an important role in supporting a child's health by promoting healthy family development. The health care professional also can be helpful to a child and her family in ways that go beyond the provision of expert, sensitive health care. An effective partnership includes information, support, and links to community resources. In general, most parents of young children are satisfied with their well-child care. In a national study, approximately 96% of parents of young children reported asking all their questions during their checkup, and 91% reported adequate time with the health care professional during their well-child visit.[28]

Getting to know the family requires knowing household members and the relatives who play important roles in the child's life. Although a visit naturally focuses on the child who is present, the health care professional also must understand that, in many cases, at least one additional child may be in the home, and the age and health condition of that sibling can affect both the child being examined and the family as a whole. It also is important for health care professionals to understand the cultural beliefs and values that the family holds, especially in regard to health care, diagnosis, and treatment.

By knowing the family or asking questions, the health care professional will have a better sense

of the health and well-being of the child and her family. Examples of relevant questions are as follows:

- How is your family adjusting to the new baby?
- Tell me about your child. What are her favorite activities?
- What do you enjoy doing together as a family? Do you or your children participate in neighborhood or community activities (eg, parent groups or playgroups, faith communities)?
- Who cares for your child during the day? Do you care for other people's children in your home?
- What responsibilities does your child have at home?

Information about the person who cares for the child and how the care is provided also is important for the health care professional. Child care arrangements can fluctuate during the child's early years. Whether parents and other caregivers agree or disagree on issues related to the child's care gives the health care professional insight into sources of stress and uncertainty for parents. How the siblings are adjusting and how the parents' relationship is faring under the pressure of the many needs of the young child are relevant to the well-being of the child and family. Knowledge about parental vulnerabilities, such as physical illness or mental disorder, provides additional insights for the health care professional.

An AAP Task Force on the Family 2003 policy statement remains a valid and essential summary of the literature and professional experience showing the importance of family-centered care.[6] In family-centered care, health care professionals recognize that the family is the constant in a child's life, while health care and other professionals are involved on an as-needed basis. In partnership with the family, the health care professional can promote family and child development. A central theme of family-centered care is the strong and respectful partnership between a child's family and the health care professional. This bond promotes meaningful communication and trust, which leads to mutual decision-making and a medical home in which the patient, family, and health care professional are free to discuss all issues and can expect their issues to be addressed. The elements of a successful family-professional partnership are mutual commitment, respect, trust, open and honest communication, cultural competence, and an ability to negotiate.

Complementary and Alternative Care

Collaboration with families in a clinical practice is a series of communications, agreements, and negotiations to ensure the best possible health care for the child. In the Bright Futures vision of family-centered care, families must be empowered as care participants. Their unique ability to choose what is best for their children must be recognized. Families do all they can to protect their children from sickness or harm.

The health care professional must be aware of the disciplines or philosophies that are chosen by the child's family, especially if the family chooses a therapy that is unfamiliar or a treatment belief system that the health care professional does not endorse or share. An understanding of the family's cultural beliefs and traditions can help the health care professional work with the family to create a health care plan with which both are comfortable. Families may seek second opinions or services in standard pediatric medical and surgical care fields or may choose care from alternative or complementary care providers. Families generally seek additional care from other disciplines rather than replacement care. Alternative therapies generally replace standard treatments. Complementary therapies are used in addition to standard treatments. Health care professionals should seek to determine whether complementary and alternative therapies indeed improve the standard treatments being used by a family. Families should be empowered

to say whether they choose not to carry out prescribed treatments. This empowerment is derived from the sense of trust that is built over time. They must be assured that the health care professional will not take offense at their choice but will work with the family to choose therapies that are acceptable to the family, appropriate to the problem, and safe and effective in the shared goal of the child's best health. Practitioners of standard or allopathic medicine and complementary and alternative care are driven and guided by the mandate to do no harm and to do good. Just because a chosen therapy is out of the standard scope of care does not define it as harmful or without potential benefit. Therapies can be safe and effective, safe and ineffective, or unsafe. The AAP Committee on Children With Disabilities suggests that "to best serve the interests of children, it is important to maintain a scientific perspective, to provide balanced advice about therapeutic options, to guard against bias, and to establish and maintain a trusting relationship with families."[29] Providers of standard care need not be threatened by such choices.

The use of complementary and alternative care in children is particularly common when a child has a chronic illness or condition, particularly autism spectrum disorder.[30,31] Alternative therapies are increasingly described on the Internet, with no assurance of safety or efficacy. Parents are often reluctant to tell their health care professional about such therapies, fearing disapproval. Health care professionals should ask parents directly about the use of complementary and alternative care. The health care professional's approach to this subject is equally important (ie, ask in a nonjudgmental manner to allow free discussion about the claims, hopes, and potential harm, if any, of such therapies).

The health care professional should discuss with the family its goals and reasons for the choice of alternative therapies and ask whether the family culture or religion prohibits or recommends certain health care procedures. Faith-based or religious therapeutic systems are likely to be very important to the family and its sense of health and well-being. The following issues may be considered in these discussions:

- What additional benefit is the family seeking? Are these benefits solely within the realm of complementary and alternative care, or has the standard care plan overlooked an essential family need?
- Are therapy and treatment interactions likely? This issue is especially important if herbal, nutritional, or homeopathic remedies are planned. Just as adverse drug-drug interactions must be avoided, interactions between medically prescribed drugs and complementary and alternative remedies also must be considered.
- Are the proposed interventions generally safe and effective? Are the therapies generally applied to children or is their use typically for adults? Are child-specific safety data available? Are they safe for the child's specific condition?
- Will the intervention take away from other interventions? All therapeutic interventions have a monetary and time cost. Will therapies and treatments compete with one another? If so, how will the family address conflicting or overwhelming demands?

In developing a treatment plan for the child with the family, health care professionals can

- Provide families with a range of treatment options.
- Educate the family on the importance of the proposed (standard) medical treatment and discuss the treatment in the context of the family's perception of the severity of their child's problem or illness and their beliefs about the meaning of illness. Ask the family what they think about this approach.

- Avoid dismissing complementary and alternative care in ways that suggest a lack of sensitivity or concern for the family's perspective.
- Recognize the feeling of being threatened or challenged professionally and guard against becoming defensive.
- Identify and use reliable reference sources and colleagues to ensure up-to-date information regarding the efficacy and risks of complementary and alternative care in children.
- Consult with colleagues who are knowledgeable about complementary and alternative care.

Immunization Refusal

Parental refusal of standard preventive immunizations is a frustrating and challenging occurrence in current practice. Health care professionals are trained to understand the critical importance and safety of modern immunizations and are well aware of the significant danger of not immunizing. Conversations about immunization refusal are difficult and can challenge the desired partnership with parents.

As with any therapeutic intervention, it is the health care professional's responsibility to provide clear information about the intended immunization and the disease it seeks to prevent, the efficacy of the immunization and duration of action, and the benefit to child and family. Any common adverse effects must be discussed and parental questions sought so parents are equipped to make an informed decision. For many vaccine-cautious parents, an unhurried conversation reassures their anxieties and empowers them to make the safe and appropriate decision to immunize.

Some parents cannot be reassured. They have done their own research, been swayed by media figures, or been victimized by conspiracy theorists. In these situations, consent is highly unlikely and even opening a discussion is difficult. This presents a professional dilemma for pediatric health care professionals.[32,33] It is one of the rare times when health care professionals must, with respect, not only disagree with the parents' decision but also clearly communicate that they believe the parents are in error and that they are placing their child at unnecessary risk of harm. This conversation must be repeated at each subsequent visit when immunizations are indicated. This professional disapproval may negatively affect the partnership with this family.

Parental Well-being

Some aspects of parenting are specific to the developmental stage of the child, but several general issues affect families with children at all ages.

- The physical and emotional health of the parents, siblings, and other family members
- The physical safety and emotional tone of the home environment and neighborhood
- The family's cultural and religious beliefs
- Parenting beliefs, education, and strategies
- The parents' ability to deal with life stresses
- The parents' concerns about no or inadequate health insurance caused by unaffordable high deductibles

All these issues have significant implications for the successful development of the children in the family. *(For more information on this topic, see the Promoting Lifelong Health for Families and Communities theme.)* To assess parental well-being, the health care professional can

- Observe the parents' pleasure and pride in their child.
- Note any indications of their general level of anxiety, overload, irritability, self-doubt, or depression.
- Screen for maternal depression.
- Ask about stress in the family (including intergenerational stress) or in the parents' relationship.
- Discuss the parents' work, its satisfactions for them, and the conflicts that arise between work and home.

- Ask about parents' physical and mental health, including current substance use, and emphasize the importance of preventive health care for them.
- Ask about parents' sources of support, including personal, financial, and community. Ask what they need and what they think will help them.
- Ask about other environmental stressors, including poverty, unemployment, low literacy, community violence, housing insecurity, or lack of heat and food.

In discussing these issues, it is best if the health care professional uses open-ended questions rather than closed-ended questions. Closed-ended questions require only defined answers, such as yes or no. Open-ended questions, such as, "Tell me how you manage to raise two children on your own," are designed to encourage discussion. Such questions often begin with how, what, when, where, or why.

Family Stress and Change

Major family changes and chronic family stressors are among the most prevalent and important influences on the developmental and psychological well-being of young children. In addition to parental separation and divorce, major changes can include birth of a sibling, especially if the new baby has special health care needs or a diagnosis of such needs, change to single-parent status, remarriage, illness or death of a parent or other family member, loss of job, combat deployment of a military parent, or a move to a new family home. Family issues, such as parental substance use disorder, domestic violence, and parental depression, dramatically affect the child's developmental progress. These parental issues may not come up in the course of the usual pediatric history taking, but they can seriously impair parents' ability to provide a healthy environment for a growing child. For children of all ages, the goal after such an event is to return to a life that is secure and predictable, with ensured or reestablished close ties to loved ones.

Health care professionals can support parents during these challenging times through awareness of family events and focused monitoring of the child's and the family's adaptation. The health care professional's most important intervention may be to help parents develop problem-solving skills. These skills will serve them well in managing important stressors or navigating periods of change or crisis. Suggesting strategies, posing questions, and providing tools and resources are 3 ways that health care professionals can encourage these discussions of child, parent, and family well-being and safety within the family. When parents were asked about why they attend health supervision visits, they report valuing the ongoing relationship with their health care professional and view the visit as a time for reassurance and an opportunity to discuss their priorities.[34]

Parental Depression

The mental health of all adult caregivers is important and should be addressed by the health care professional. Maternal depression has received most of the attention, but that is because of limited data on paternal depression.

Depression is common. The lifetime prevalence of major depressive disorders is 17.3%.[35] On the third or fourth day after delivery, an estimated 70% of all new mothers experience depression, and it generally does not impair functioning.

Recognition also is growing that adoptive parents may experience a similar post-adoption depression. When it becomes clear that the realities of parenting are different than the long-imagined dreams, feelings of despair and being overwhelmed can occur in both biological and adoptive parents. Some adoptive parents may again experience grieving for the biologically related child they do not have, and guilt over that feeling can add to their already complex emotions.

Parental depression or isolation is one of the greatest risk factors for child behavioral and mental health problems.[36] Identifying maternal depression is especially important during early childhood because of the vulnerability of young children. For the child, short-term behavioral reactions to maternal depression can include withdrawal, reduced activity, reduced self-control, increased aggression, poor peer relationships, greater difficulties adapting to school, and general unhappiness. Long-term effects on the child include a significantly higher chance of developing an affective disorder.

Screening for Depression

Screening for postpartum depression has been recommended by the US Preventative Services Task Force and the AAP. Universal screening for postpartum depression is now recommended at the 1 Month through 6 Month Visits.[36,37]

Health care professionals sometimes can observe signs of depression in the mother, such as a lack of energy, chronic fatigue, feelings of hopelessness, low self-esteem, poor concentration, or indecisiveness. A mother may say that she is feeling blue or experiencing somatic symptoms, such as insomnia, hypersomnia, poor appetite, or overeating. Culturally specific manifestations of depression also may occur, and the health care professional should seek to learn about those factors in relation to the populations served. Mothers may be willing to talk with their child's health care professional about their own state of well-being but only in the context of a trusting relationship with a health care professional who demonstrates care and concern for her and for her child.[38]

Certain risk factors, such as poverty, chronic maternal health conditions, domestic violence, exposure to community violence, alcohol and other substance use, and marital discord, should alert health care professionals to the higher likelihood of maternal depression and greater risk for the child's development. A history of illicit drug use or alcohol or tobacco use during pregnancy should be explored. Health care professionals should be aware that parents of children with special health care needs may go through periods of mourning, which has features similar to depression.

The health care professional can screen[37] for postpartum depression using the following 2 questions:

1. Over the past 2 weeks, have you ever felt down, depressed, or hopeless?
2. Over the past 2 weeks, have you felt little interest or pleasure in doing things?

This screening is considered positive if a woman answers yes to either of the questions.[36]

Longer questionnaires, such as the 10-question Edinburgh Postnatal Depression Scale,[39,40] also may be useful.

For parents who are experiencing depression, the health care professional can

- Provide understanding and support.
- Ask how the depressive symptoms interfere with everyday life, including caring for the child.
- Explore problems and stressors, including use of alcohol or tobacco, during pregnancy.
- Ask about a past history of depression and treatment.
- Assess the severity of the depression, *including risk for suicidal behavior.* Inquire about the presence of firearms in the home.
- Offer to speak with other family members to better understand the parent's situation and to encourage support.
- Refer to a mental health professional.
- Refer to parent's primary care professional.
- Refer to other community resources.

Parents with depressive symptoms should be asked directly about whether they have had suicidal thoughts. Parents who continue to have such thoughts should be asked whether they have a plan to harm themselves. Positive responses to these questions require an immediate referral for a

mental health evaluation. *(For more information on this topic, see the Promoting Mental Health theme.)*

Understanding and Building on the Strengths of Children and Youth

In addition to helping their children avoid unsafe and unhealthy behaviors, parents can foster healthy development in their children by promoting positive physical, ethical, and emotional behaviors and development. The following 4 positive attributes, drawn from Brendtro's Circle of Courage,[41] are particularly related to decreased risk-taking behaviors among youth. *(For more information on this topic, see the Promoting Healthy Development and Promoting Lifelong Health for Families and Communities themes.)* Strength-based parenting fosters opportunities for growth in the following attributes[42-45]:

- **Competence and mastery.** Children and youth who have a chance to gain skills and knowledge grow in competence. For instance, young children learn to sit, walk, and talk. By school age, children have acquired the ability to share, take turns, and listen. For school-aged children and youth, school success becomes an important marker for mastery. Other accomplishments in areas such as the arts, athletic activities, and community service are equally important examples of this attribute. The specific areas of accomplishment may be determined by family and community cultural values. Parents, extended family, educators, and mentors can be most helpful in assisting children and youth find and participate in activities they enjoy.
- **Empathy.** Being able to understand the feelings of others is an important developmental task for children and youth to accomplish by adulthood. Young children can demonstrate empathy as generosity when they help at home with age-appropriate tasks or play with younger siblings

and neighbors. In adolescents, this skill often manifests itself in babysitting, relationships with peers, or volunteer activities with a community or faith-based group.

- **Connectedness.** This concept refers to relationships with caring adults, relationships with other children and youth, and belonging. Research demonstrates the value of parental involvement and quality parent-adolescent communication on healthy adolescent development.[46,47] Adolescents who are involved in extracurricular and community activities and whose parents are authoritative, rather than authoritarian or passive,[44,48] appear to progress through adolescence with relatively little turmoil.

- **Autonomy and independence.** Autonomy is a goal for youth as they mature to adulthood. Children who have experience with making decisions throughout childhood and who have guidance from their parents and other caregivers in these efforts are well positioned to make this transition effectively. It is crucial to encourage appropriate self-care and self-advocacy for children with special health care needs. The rate at which children and youth are expected to make decisions and the areas over which families cede control may vary with the values and culture of the family.

Attention to these developmental tasks is equally important in children with special needs because it puts the emphasis on universal themes that are possible in almost all children as they grow. Growing in independence and having the opportunity to do things for others are two of the developmental tasks that often require focused effort for youth who have health issues.

Family Culture and Behaviors

Understanding and building on the strengths of families requires health care professionals to combine well-honed clinical interview skills with a willingness to learn from families. Families demonstrate a wide range of beliefs and priorities in how they structure daily routines and rituals for their children and how they use health care resources. These attitudes often reflect traditional family or cultural influences, which are important for health care professionals to understand if they hope to work in effective partnership with families to maximize the health and development of children. Families need ways to learn about the following factors and how they can contribute positively to their child's development:

- **Daily routines and rituals.** These include mealtimes, food choices, sleep schedules, bowel and bladder elimination habits, general cleanliness and personal hygiene, attention to dental health, tolerance for risk-taking activities, customary ways of expressing illness or distress, and parental or family use of tobacco, alcohol, or illicit drugs. For example, family meals are associated with higher dietary quality and psychological health in children and adolescents.[49] Children can thrive in families with widely varying traditions of health beliefs and practices. Emotional support, structure, and safety are the key ingredients of the environments and routines for young children at home.[50] When families hold to routines or rituals that seem to cause or exacerbate a problem, the health care professional should learn more about the history of the routine within the family and, possibly, within the family's culture.

- **Culture, beliefs, and behaviors connected with health and illness.** Families tend to use available health care resources for their young children on the basis of their knowledge, beliefs, traditions, and past experiences with health systems. Visiting a health care professional on behalf of their child reflects a family's desire to seek help or share concerns. At the same time, the family might view typical clinical guidance or use medications in unexpected ways. One family might believe that only a prescription or a shot will help, whereas another might first consult community elders and then combine medicine from the drugstore with traditional healing methods. This makes it important for health care professionals who serve children and families from backgrounds other than their own to listen and observe carefully, to learn from the family, to build trust and respect, and not to assume that a safety checklist will be followed (not out of ignorance or disrespect but rather out of adherence to tradition and past experience). Health care professionals also should understand that families and cultures tend to approach the concept of disability and chronic conditions in different ways. If possible, the presence of a staff member who is familiar with a family's community and fluent in the family's language is helpful during these discussions.

- **Nutrition and physical activity.** Families should emphasize healthy eating behaviors and physical activity beginning early in a child's life. Parents can be positive role models by eating healthfully themselves, participating in physical activity with their children, and being physically active themselves. Both regular physical activity *(for more information on this topic, see the Promoting Physical Activity theme)* and healthful dietary behaviors *(for more information on this topic, see the Promoting Healthy Nutrition theme)* are essential to prevent a sedentary lifestyle and to avoid excessive pediatric weight gain *(for more information on this topic, see the Promoting Healthy Weight theme).* Food insecurity or hunger *(for more information on this topic, see the Promoting Healthy Nutrition theme)* affects almost 1 in 5 families.[51] Health care professionals

should identify any problems the family may have in obtaining nutritious food and connect families with appropriate community resources when needed.

- **Health behaviors.** Parents are powerful role models for their children. From wearing seat belts and bicycle helmets to modeling community involvement, anger management, or responsible drinking, parents play a significant role in influencing their children's and adolescents' health protective and risk behaviors.[52]
- **Television, computer, and media viewing.** Television (TV) viewing is an established daily routine in most families. Some studies have shown positive influences of age-appropriate, curriculum-based educational TV on children's cognitive abilities and school readiness.[53,54] On the other hand, most effects of TV viewing are not positive, and TV viewing patterns have raised concern because of the effects of media violence and physical inactivity on children and adolescents. Health care professionals should support the recommendation that infants and children younger than 18 months should not watch TV or any digital media, and children 18 months through 4 years should watch no more than 1 hour of high-quality programming per day.[55] In addition, parents should be cautioned to avoid leaving the TV on in the background in the home throughout the day. For school-aged children and adolescents, parents can consider making a family media use plan.[56] The family media use plan is an online tool that parents and children can all fill out together. The tool prompts the family to enter daily health priorities, such as an hour for physical activity, 8 to 11 hours of sleep, time for homework and school activities, and unplugged time each day for independent time and time with family. The family can then consider the time left over and decide on rules around the quantity, quality, and location of media use.

- **Smoking, drinking, and substance use.** It is important to discuss with parents their attitude toward drug or alcohol use and ask how they plan to talk about drugs and alcohol with their children and adolescents.[57] Children and adolescents can be affected by substance use directly (when they use substances themselves, are exposed in utero, or are exposed through the air, such as smoke from crack cocaine) or indirectly (when they experience the consequences of substance use by family members or other adults). Parental alcohol use disorder increases the risk of adolescent alcohol use disorder because of genetic and environmental factors.[58,59]

Promoting Family Support: The Preconception and Prenatal Periods

In recent years, information on issues that are important to a woman's health before and during pregnancy has helped focus attention on the importance of these periods to the health of her children.

The Preconception Period

Health care professionals who offer pre-conceptional or inter-conceptional guidance to older adolescent girls, young adult women, and families during health supervision visits contribute to healthy pregnancies, healthy infants, and healthy outcomes for adults. Interacting with parents of young children also gives health care professionals an opportunity to discuss the desired timing and spacing of future pregnancies.

Maternal health and well-being are vital to a safe pregnancy and the birth of a healthy baby. A nutritious diet and physical activity before pregnancy benefit the mother and fetus during pregnancy and delivery. Health care professionals can educate prospective parents (those having unprotected intercourse and those who are actively planning a pregnancy) about health-promoting choices before conception that can significantly improve pregnancy outcomes for mother and infant. Choices

related to the use of alcohol, tobacco, or illicit drugs; exposure to domestic violence; and medications,[60] including over-the-counter medicines and herbal preparations that have potential teratogenic effects, are particularly important. It is essential to inform women that teratogenic injury by many agents, especially alcohol, can and does occur early in pregnancy, often even *before a woman knows of her pregnancy*.[61] Similarly, all females of childbearing age should be advised to consume adequate amounts of folic acid (400 µg per day) before conceiving to prevent neural tube defects.

The Prenatal Period

Prenatal care is effective in improving the health of mother and baby and is the major factor in preventing infant death and disease. Newborns of women who receive early prenatal care generally have better birth outcomes than those who do not.[62]

Establishing a trusting relationship between the health care professional and the family during this time, when many families need and welcome support, can be especially productive. Pregnancy is a time of initial family adaptation, which can predict later parental coping. The health care professional can gather basic information about the family and its values, beliefs, prior experiences, goals, and concerns and can provide reassurance and key information about what to expect during the newborn period. Discussing expectations and concerns with the health care professional allows parents to share their excitement and sort out their concerns. Guidance that is provided to families also should be personalized by acknowledging their beliefs, values, experiences, and needs and should be interwoven in discussions with parents. Engaging members of the family and community who provide natural support and guidance to new mothers (eg, grandmothers, aunts, and other older women) also is important because it can help foster adherence to health care. Extended family can play an important role—positively or negatively—on a mother's initiation and adherence to breastfeeding. Many home visiting programs enroll families prenatally, and some offer doula services to assist women during the prenatal period.

Optimally, during the last trimester of pregnancy, expectant parents should schedule a visit with the health care professional who will care for their baby after birth. Provided that parents have sufficient literacy and materials are written in easily understandable words in their primary language, a printed questionnaire that parents can complete in the waiting room before the appointment can suggest issues that should be emphasized during the visit.

An essential component of this initial visit is to emphasize the valuable role family has in ensuring the child's health and well-being. Whenever possible, the health care professional should encourage families to participate actively in the decision-making process. In some families, the grandparents, or a family member other than the parents, may be the decision-makers. Therefore, any discussions about decision-making for the child should include eliciting how decisions are made within the family and with whom information should be shared.

Education is particularly powerful during the prenatal period. It is an ideal time to advise prospective parents on

- Lifelong health issues, such as the importance of positive and loving relationships, a healthy diet, physical activity, immunizations (especially against pertussis and influenza), and dental health. *(For more information on this topic, see the Promoting Lifelong Health for Families and Communities, Promoting Healthy Nutrition, Promoting Physical Activity, and Promoting Oral Health themes.)*
- The importance of using seat belts and avoiding alcohol, drugs, or tobacco or any other environmental toxicants or hazards.

- The importance of the prenatal care visits with the woman's own health care professional; appropriate rate of weight gain during pregnancy; appropriate dental care; appropriate nutrient intake; healthy hygiene practices, including handwashing; preparation for childbirth; and sibling preparation and the presence of the father, partner, or other family member during delivery.
- Immediate postpartum care issues, including benefits of breastfeeding, rooming-in, and completion of newborn metabolic, hearing, and critical congenital heart disease screening. Immediate postpartum care issues include planning for the care of mother and baby after birth.
- Other newborn care topics, including safe sleep practices, newborn temperament, holding and cuddling the baby, getting siblings ready for the new baby, pets in the home, and using an appropriate car safety seat for the baby.
- Safety issues, such as intimate partner violence, the presence of guns in the home, and exposure to lead, tobacco, and mercury. *(For more information on this topic, see the Promoting Safety and Injury Prevention theme.)*

Reducing Pregnancy Complications

Pregnancy complications are often secondary to common underlying medical conditions, such as obesity, diabetes, and hypertension, and to dental conditions, such as periodontal disease. Preventable causes of developmental disability include prenatal exposure to teratogens, such as alcohol, and environmental toxins, such as tobacco smoke. Fetal alcohol spectrum disorder, which results from prenatal exposure to alcohol and is the most common known cause of intellectual disability in the United States, is entirely preventable.[63] Because no known amount of alcohol is safe for the developing fetus, women who may become pregnant because they are having unprotected intercourse or who are actively trying to become pregnant should be counseled to avoid alcohol during the preconception period and throughout pregnancy.

Smoking during pregnancy and exposure to secondhand smoke are significant contributors to infant mortality, low birth weight, and sudden infant death syndrome. Health care professionals should encourage women who smoke to stop before they become pregnant and should give them information about smoking cessation programs, including "quit lines" and smoke-free text programs,[64] and community resources. Extended or augmented smoking cessation counseling (5–15 minutes) that uses messages and self-help materials tailored to pregnant smokers, when compared with brief generic counseling interventions alone, substantially increases abstinence rates during pregnancy and leads to higher birth weights. Although stopping smoking is recommended, even reducing smoking during pregnancy will have significant health benefits for the baby and the pregnant woman.[65] Health care professionals also can mention the importance of staying tobacco-free postpartum because of the risks of exposing the baby to secondhand smoke.

Although health care professionals should caution families about avoiding or limiting environmental exposures that pose a risk to the developing fetus, they also should recognize that some environmental factors, such as poor housing, pollution, or poverty, can be beyond the family's control.[66] Health care professionals' involvement with community advocacy for better living conditions can be a way to influence the health of mothers and infants. *(For more information on this topic, see the Promoting Lifelong Health for Families and Communities theme.)*

Promoting Family Support: Infancy—Birth Through 11 Months

Ideally, parents care for their infants with the support and assistance of others. Being cognizant of the family's culture, the health care professional should ask about caregiver roles and responsibilities of the parents and other important adults in the child's life.

The family's home setting can have a major influence on parental well-being when parents and other caregivers feel alone and have limited opportunity for social interaction. Living in rural areas with distance between neighbors, in an inner city area that seems unsafe, or in a suburban neighborhood with uninterested neighbors can cause a new parent to feel unsupported. Parents who are comfortable in their new roles and who support one another physically and emotionally will have a positive effect on their infant's emotional development.

Fathers (whether biological fathers, adoptive fathers, stepfathers, or foster fathers) are important caregivers and teachers for their infants. A father's participation in newborn and infant care is enhanced if he is present at delivery, has early newborn contact, and learns about his newborn's abilities. New fathers should learn they have a unique role, distinct from that of the mother, in caring for and parenting the infant. For families who have recently arrived in this country, any changes in gender roles can be more difficult than for those who are more acculturated. The health care professional may need to discover the roles for fathers in the family's culture and build on them in discussions of other possible roles.

According to the US Department of Labor, labor force participation rate—the percentage of the population working or looking for work—for all mothers with infants, children, and adolescents younger than 18 years was 70.3% in 2014.[67] With new mothers returning to the workforce, the responsibility for providing infant care and developmental stimulation of the infant is often shared by others. High-quality child care provided by nonfamily members can be as nurturing and educational as parental care, but it requires responsive, loving, consistent caregiving by a few adults. Advising parents in their choice of child care options is an important role for health care professionals. Emotional support between the parents powerfully affects adaptation to parenting. Parents can disagree and even feel angry with each other, and they should be offered help, either by the health care professional or a mental health professional, to resolve difficulties in a positive way. Parents need to know that they should call for help immediately if they feel they may hurt each other or the baby.

Continuous attention to the quality of the parent-child relationship is an important element of health surveillance for the infant. Because an infant completely depends on his parents and because his learning and experience occur within the interpersonal context of his relationships with his caregivers, the infant is vulnerable to his parents' mood states. Postpartum depression screening is recommended.[36,37] Unanticipated events, such as illness, death, or other catastrophes, can affect the infant because the parent is upset, anxious, overwhelmed, or traumatized by the event and is unable to buffer the infant from those feelings or is unable to give the infant consistent comfort and nurturing.

Promoting Family Support: Early Childhood—1 Through 4 Years

Families approach the early childhood years of each child in the family differently. With a first child, many parents still feel tentative about their new role. They often face each stage of their child's development (eg, standing, walking, babbling, holding a cup, playing, saying first words, exploring, throwing tantrums, adjusting to new faces, sleeping alone, making friends, and going to preschool) with shifting senses of worry and wonderment.

During early childhood, fathers become increasingly engaged with their children. As their children move into toddlerhood, parents often are confronted with new pressures to balance the competing needs of their child and family with those of job and career. The child's increasing push for autonomy and the

constant vigilance that is needed to ensure safety add to the stress of this period. Established routines and family rules may help reduce continual developmental stresses common to this age. The health care professional can provide valuable encouragement and support to parents during this time by helping them understand their child's temperament and develop appropriate expectations for their child's developmental stage and level of understanding.

Promoting Family Support: Middle Childhood—5 Through 10 Years

A child is quite different in the early years of middle childhood than in the later years. A child who gets along well with caregivers and siblings at age 5 years may not do so at age 10. Caregivers and parents need to be reassured that these changes are a typical part of the child's growing independence from the family. The family should be encouraged to continue to give plenty of support, attention, and supervision as the child nears early adolescence.

In addition to evaluating parental well-being, health care professionals can encourage the parents of children in middle childhood to model healthy behaviors for their children. Encourage them not to smoke, to wear a seat belt and a bike or ski helmet, to consume alcohol responsibly, and never to drive after consuming alcohol. Also, encourage them to maintain a healthy weight through proper nutrition and regular physical activity. Family activities that include physical activity can be especially beneficial for children in this age group.

The health care professional should inquire about changes and stresses in the family, such as illness in a parent or child, job loss or other change in employment, loss of an older family member, starting school, or moving to a new school or location. Changes and stresses can have a significant effect on the child's moods, behaviors, and school performance. Children react to stress in myriad ways; some children are resilient, whereas others are slow to adapt to change. In addition, children will act out or demonstrate stress in different ways. *(For more information on this topic, see the Promoting Mental Health theme.)* Parents will need to offer extra support to their child during a particularly difficult time and may have to balance providing support to all children in the family as well as to themselves.

School is a key experience for children in middle childhood. Families can play a major supportive role by encouraging the child's educational experiences and being involved in school activities. Families who are new to this country and its educational system (especially those with low English proficiency) and families with children with special health care needs may need additional support and guidance to navigate the school system.

Promoting Family Support: Adolescence—11 Through 21 Years

The changes that occur in contemporary family life are particularly significant for adolescents. The decreased amount of time that many parents, extended family members, and neighbors are able to spend with adolescents leads to decreased communication, support, and supervision from adults at a critical period in their development, when adolescents are most likely to experiment with behaviors that can have serious health consequences.

Families are better able to support young people when they receive accurate information on the physical, cognitive, social, and emotional changes that occur during adolescence. New understanding of adolescent brain development is of interest to parents. Parents should be encouraged to maintain an interest in their adolescent's daily activities and concerns. Families who are stressed because of

economic issues or families who are new to this country and do not understand the schools and social institutions can have trouble staying involved in their adolescents' lives but should be encouraged to do so. Although adolescence is characterized by growing independence and separation from parental authority, the adolescent still needs the family's love, support, and availability. Young people are more likely to become healthy, fulfilled adults if their families remain actively involved and provide loving parenting, needed limits, and respect for the process of developing maturity. Good parent-adolescent relationships can affect the development of other social relationships, including the practice of conflict-resolution skills, pro-social behaviors, intimacy skills, self-control, social confidence, and empathy. *(For more information on this topic, see the Promoting Healthy Development and Promoting Lifelong Health for Families and Communities themes.)* The more assets young people demonstrate, the fewer at-risk behaviors they display.[68]

The health care professional also can affirm the parents as ethical and behavioral role models for their adolescent and can encourage parents to communicate their expectations clearly and respectfully. For adolescents who do not have a strong connection to family or other adults, health care professionals can play a pivotal role in providing key information on health issues, screening for emotional problems, and making referrals to community resources.

This same guidance needs to be given to parents of adolescents with special health care needs. The young person's special needs create demands that affect parents, the financial status of families, and family and social relationships, including relationships with siblings, but the developmental tasks of independence and mastery must receive equal attention for healthy outcomes. Support for healthy development for youth with special health care needs can come from other members of their interdisciplinary care team: school nurses, social workers, occupational health professionals, educators, and pediatric subspecialists. Health care professionals can help families find balance in meeting the physical and psychological needs of the adolescent with special needs and other family members while maintaining typical family routines and rituals.[69] Informal and formal support networks are key factors to supporting families with adolescents who have a chronic illness, a disability, or other risk factors. Community resources, financial support, and emotional, spiritual, and informational support help families cope and be resilient.[70] *(For more information on this topic, see the Promoting Health for Children and Youth With Special Health Care Needs theme.)*

PROMOTING FAMILY SUPPORT

References

1. American Academy of Pediatrics Medical Home Initiatives for Children With Special Needs Project Advisory Committee. The medical home. *Pediatrics.* 2002;110(1):184-186

2. Perrin EC, Siegel BS; American Academy of Pediatrics Committee on Psychosocial Aspects of Child and Family Health. Promoting the well-being of children whose parents are gay or lesbian. *Pediatrics.* 2013;131(4):e1374-e1383

3. Jones VF, Schulte EE; American Academy of Pediatrics Committee on Early Childhood; Council on Foster Care, Adoption, and Kinship Care. The pediatrician's role in supporting adoptive families. *Pediatrics.* 2012;130(4):e1040-e1049

4. Immigrant Children: Indicators on Children and Youth. Child Trends Data Bank Web site. http://childtrends. org/?indicators=immigrant-children. Updated October 2014. Accessed August 16, 2016

5. Kodjo C. Cultural competence in clinician communication. *Pediatr Rev.* 2009;30(2):57-64

6. Schor EL; American Academy of Pediatrics Task Force on the Family. Family pediatrics: report of the Task Force on the Family. *Pediatrics.* 2003;111(6 pt 2):1541-1571

7. America's Families and Living Arrangements: Table FG6. One-parent Unmarried Family Groups With Own Children Under 18, by Marital Status of the Reference Person; 2014. United States Census Bureau Web site. https://www.census.gov/hhes/families/data/cps2014FG.html. Accessed August 16, 2016

8. Cabrera NJ, Tamis-Lemonda CS. *Handbook of Father Involvement: Multidisciplinary Perspectives.* 2nd ed. London: Routledge; 2013

9. Coleman WL, Garfield C; American Academy of Pediatrics Committee on Psychosocial Aspects of Child and Family Health. Fathers and pediatricians: enhancing men's roles in the care and development of their children. *Pediatrics.* 2004;113(5):1406-1411

10. America's Families and Living Arrangements: C2. Household Relationship and Living Arrangements of Children Under 18 Years, by Age and Sex; 2014. United States Census Bureau Web site. https://www.census.gov/hhes/families/data/cps2014C.html. Accessed August 16, 2016

11. Sadler LS, Swartz MK, Ryan-Krause P, et al. Promising outcomes in teen mothers enrolled in a school-based parent support program and child care center. *J Sch Health.* 2007;77(3):121-130

12. All children matter: how legal and social inequalities hurt LGBT families; full report. Movement Advancement Project Web site. https://www.lgbtmap.org/file/all-children-matter-full-report.pdf. Published October 2011. Accessed August 16, 2016

13. Gates GJ. LGBT parenting in the United States. The Williams Institute, UCLA School of Law, Web site. http://williamsinstitute. law.ucla.edu/wp-content/uploads/LGBT-Parenting.pdf. Published February 2013. Accessed August 16, 2016

14. Obergefell v. Hodges. Slip Opinion 14-556 in Supreme Court of the United States. June 26, 2015. http://www.supremecourt.gov/opinions/14pdf/14-556_3204.pdf. Accessed August 16, 2016

15. Gartrell N, Bos H. US National Longitudinal Lesbian Family Study: psychological adjustment of 17-year-old adolescents. *Pediatrics.* 2010;126(1):28-36

16. American Academy of Pediatrics. Medical evaluation for infectious diseases for internationally adopted, refugee, and immigrant children. In: Kimberlin DW, Brady MT, Jackson MA, Long SS, eds. *Red Book: 2015 Report of the Committee on Infectious Diseases.* 30th ed. Elk Grove Village, IL: American Academy of Pediatrics; 2015:194-200

17. Jones VF; American Academy of Pediatrics Committee on Early Childhood, Adoption, and Dependent Care. Comprehensive health evaluation of the newly adopted child. *Pediatrics.* 2012;129(1):e214-e223

18. Foster care statistics 2014. Child Welfare Information Gateway Web site. https://www.childwelfare.gov/pubPDFs/foster.pdf. Published March 2016. Accessed August 16, 2016

19. Placement of children with relatives. Child Welfare Information Gateway Web site. https://www.childwelfare.gov/pubPDFs/placement.pdf. Published July 2013. Accessed August 16, 2016

20. Mekonnen R, Noonan K, Rubin D. Achieving better health care outcomes for children in foster care. *Pediatr Clin North Am.* 2009;56(2):405-415

21. Garner AS, Shonkoff JP; American Academy of Pediatrics Committee on Psychosocial Aspects of Child Family Health; Committee on Early Childhood, Adoption, and Dependent Care; Section on Developmental and Behavioral Pediatrics. Early childhood adversity, toxic stress, and the role of the pediatrician: translating developmental science into lifelong health. *Pediatrics.* 2012;129(1):e224-e231

22. Szilagyi MA, Rosen DS, Rubin D, Zlotnik S; American Academy of Pediatrics Council on Foster Care, Adoption, and Kinship Care; Committee on Adolescence; Council on Early Childhood. Health care issues for children and adolescents in foster care and kinship care. *Pediatrics.* 2015;136(4):e1142-e1166

23. American Academy of Pediatrics Task Force on Health Care for Children in Foster Care, District II, New York State. *Fostering Health: Health Care for Children and Adolescents in Foster Care.* 2nd ed. Elk Grove Village, IL: American Academy of Pediatrics; 2005

24. Foster Care: Indicators on Children and Youth. Child Trends Databank Web site. http://www.childtrends.org/wp-content/uploads/2014/07/12_Foster_Care.pdf. Updated December 2015. Accessed August 16, 2016

25. Kids Count Data Center. Data Snapshot on Foster Care Placement. Annie E. Casey Foundation Web site. http://www.aecf.org/m/resourcedoc/AECF-DataSnapshotOnFosterCarePlacement-2011.pdf. Published May 2011. Accessed August 16, 2016

26. Manlove J, Welti K, McCoy-Roth M, Berger A, Malm K. Teen Parents in Foster Care: Risk Factors and Outcomes for Teens and Their Children. Child Trends Research Brief. November 2011. http://www.childtrends.org/wp-content/uploads/2011/11/Child_Trends-2011_11_01_RB_TeenParentsFC.pdf. Accessed August 16, 2016

27. Parent to Parent USA Web site. http://www.p2pusa.org/p2pusa/SitePages/p2p-home.aspx. Accessed August 16, 2016

28. Halfon N, Stevens GD, Larson K, Olson LM. Duration of a well-child visit: association with content, family-centeredness, and satisfaction. *Pediatrics.* 2011;128(4):657-664

29. American Academy of Pediatrics Committee on Children With Disabilities. Counseling families who choose complementary and alternative medicine for their child with chronic illness or disability. *Pediatrics.* 2001;107(3):598-601

30. Valicenti-McDermott M, Burrows B, Bernstein L, et al. Use of complementary and alternative medicine in children with autism and other developmental disabilities: associations with ethnicity, child comorbid symptoms, and parental stress. *J Child Neurol.* 2014;29(3):360-367

31. National Institutes of Health National Center for Complementary and Integrative Health Web site. https://nccih.nih.gov. Accessed August 16, 2016

32. Immunization: Refusal to Vaccinate and Liability. American Academy of Pediatrics Web site. https://www.aap.org/en-us/advocacy-and-policy/aap-health-initiatives/immunization/Pages/refusal-to-vaccinate.aspx. Updated April 2016. Accessed August 16, 2016

33. American Academy of Pediatrics Section on Infectious Diseases. Documenting Parental Refusal to Have Their Children Vaccinated. American Academy of Pediatrics Web site. https//www.aap.org/en-us/Documents/immunization_refusaltovaccinate.pdf. Published 2013. Accessed August 16, 2016

34. Radecki L, Olson LM, Frintner MP, Tanner JL, Stein MT. What do families want from well-child care? Including parents in the rethinking discussion. *Pediatrics*. 2009;124(3):858-865

35. National Research Council. *Depression in Parents, Parenting, and Children: Opportunities to Improve Identificaiton, Treatment, and Prevention*. Washington, DC: National Academies Press; 2009

36. Earls MF; American Academy of Pediatrics Committee on Psychosocial Aspects of Child Family Health. Incorporating recognition and management of perinatal and postpartum depression into pediatric practice. *Pediatrics*. 2010;126(5): 1032-1039

37. Siu AL; US Preventive Services Task Force. Screening for depression in adults: US Preventive Services Task Force recommendation statement. *JAMA*. 2016;315(4):380-387

38. Heneghan AM, Mercer M, DeLeone NL. Will mothers discuss parenting stress and depressive symptoms with their child's pediatrician? *Pediatrics*. 2004;113(3 pt 1):460-467

39. Cox JL, Holden JM, Sagovsky R. Detection of postnatal depression. Development of the 10-item Edinburgh Postnatal Depression Scale. *Br J Psychiatry*. 1987;150:782-786

40. Venkatesh KK, Zlotnick C, Triche EW, Ware C, Phipps MG. Accuracy of brief screening tools for identifying postpartum depression among adolescent mothers. *Pediatrics*. 2014;133(1):e45-e53

41. Brendtro LK, Brokenleg M, Van Bockern S. *Reclaiming Youth At Risk: Our Hope for the Future*. Rev ed. Bloomington, IN: Solution Tree; 2009

42. Ginsburg KR, Jablow MM. *Building Resilience in Children and Teens: Giving Kids Roots and Wings*. 3rd ed. Elk Grove Villiage, IL: American Academy of Pediatrics; 2015

43. Steinburg LD. *The Age of Opportunity: Lessons from the New Science of Adolescence*. Boston, MA: Eamon Dolan/Houghton Mifflin Harcourt; 2014

44. DeVore ER, Ginsburg KR. The protective effects of good parenting on adolescents. *Curr Opin Pediatr*. 2005;17(4):460-465

45. Frankowski BL, Brendtro LK, Van Bockern S, Duncan PM. Strength-based interviewing: the circle of courage. In: Ginsburg KR, Kinsman SB, eds. *Reaching Teens: Strength-Based Communication Strategies to Build Resilience and Support Healthy Adolescent Development*. Elk Grove Village, IL: American Academy of Pediatrics; 2014

46. Hair EC, Moore KA, Garrett SB, Ling T, Cleveland K. The continued importance of quality parent–adolescent relationships during late adolescence. *J Res Adolesc*. 2008;18(1):187-200

47. Brooks RB. The power of parenting. In: Goldstein S, Brooks RB, eds. *Handbook of Resilience in Children*. New York, NY: Springer US; 2013:443-458

48. Milevsky A, Schlechter M, Netter S, Keehn D. Maternal and paternal parenting styles in adolescents: associations with self-esteem, depression and life-satisfaction. *J Child Fam Stud*. 2007;16(1):39-47

49. Martin-Biggers J, Spaccarotella K, Berhaupt-Glickstein A, Hongu N, Worobey J, Byrd-Bredbenner C. Come and get it! A discussion of family mealtime literature and factors affecting obesity risk. *Adv Nutr*. 2014;5(3):235-247

50. Spagnola M, Fiese BH. Family routines and rituals: a context for development in the lives of young children. *Infants Young Child*. 2007;20(4):284-299

51. Coleman-Jensen A, Rabbitt MP, Gregory C, Singh A. *Household Food Security in the United States in 2014*. Washington, DC: US Department of Agriculture, Economic Research Service; 2015. Publication ERR-194. http://www.ers.usda.gov/media/1896841/err194.pdf. Accessed August 16, 2016

52. Quraishi AY, Mickalide AD, Cody BF. *Follow the Leader: A National Study of Safety Role Modeling Among Parents and Children*. Washington, DC: National SAFE KIDS Campaign; 2005

53. Christakis DA. Interactive media use at younger than the age of 2 years: time to rethink the American Academy of Pediatrics guideline? *JAMA Pediatr*. 2014;168(5):399-400

54. Mares ML, Pan Z. Effects of *Sesame Street*: a meta-analysis of children's learning in 15 countries. *J Appl Dev Psychol*. 2013;34(3):140-151

55. American Academy of Pediatrics Council on Communications and Media. Media and young minds. *Pediatrics*. 2016;138(5):e20162591

56. How to make a family media use plan. HealthyChildren.org Web site. https://www.healthychildren.org/English/family-life/Media/Pages/How-to-Make-a-Family-Media-Use-Plan.aspx. Updated October 21, 2016. Accessed December 14, 2016

57. Jellinek M, Patel BP, Froehle MC. How to help your child or adolescent resist drugs. In: Jellinek M, Patel BP, Froehle MC, eds. *Bright Futures in Practice: Mental Health, Volume II, Toolkit*. Arlington, VA: National Center for Education in Maternal and Child Health; 2002:148

58. Duncan SC, Duncan TE, Strycker LA. Alcohol use from ages 9 to 16: a cohort-sequential latent growth model. *Drug Alcohol Depend*. 2006;81(1):71-81

59. Latendresse SJ, Rose RJ, Viken RJ, Pulkkinen L, Kaprio J, Dick DM. Parenting mechanisms in links between parents' and adolescents' alcohol use behaviors. *Alcohol Clin Exp Res*. 2008;32(2):322-330

60. Medications and Pregnancy. Centers for Disease Control and Prevention Web site. http://www.cdc.gov/pregnancy/meds/index.html. Accessed August 16, 2016

61. Cannon MJ, Guo J, Denny CH, et al. Prevalence and characteristics of women at risk for an alcohol-exposed pregnancy (AEP) in the United States: estimates from the National Survey of Family Growth. *Matern Child Health J*. 2015;19(4):776-782

62. Debiec KE, Paul KJ, Mitchell CM, Hitti JE. Inadequate prenatal care and risk of preterm delivery among adolescents: a retrospective study over 10 years. *Am J Obstet Gynecol*. 2010;203(2):122.e1-122.e6

63. Williams JF, Smith VC; American Academy of Pediatrics Committee on Substance Abuse. Fetal alcohol spectrum disorders. *Pediatrics*. 2015;136(5):e1395-e1406

64. I'm Ready to Quit. Centers for Disease Control and Prevention Web site. http://www.cdc.gov/tobacco/campaign/tips/quit-smoking. Updated August 28, 2015. Accessed August 16, 2016

PROMOTING FAMILY SUPPORT

PROMOTING FAMILY SUPPORT

65. Siu AL; US Preventive Services Task Force. Behavioral and pharmacotherapy interventions for tobacco smoking cessation in adults, including pregnant women: US Preventive Services Task Force recommendation statement. *Ann Intern Med.* 2015;163(8):622-634

66. Gorski PA, Kuo AA, Granado-Villar DC, et al; American Academy of Pediatrics Council on Community Pediatrics. Community pediatrics: navigating the intersection of medicine, public health, and social determinants of children's health. *Pediatrics.* 2013;131(3):623-628

67. US Bureau of Labor Statistics. Women in the labor force: a databook. *BLS Reports.* Report 1059. December 2015. http://www.bls.gov/opub/reports/womens-databook/archive/women-in-the-labor-force-a-databook-2015.pdf. Accessed August 16, 2016

68. Murphey DA, Lamonda KH, Carney JK, Duncan P. Relationships of a brief measure of youth assets to health-promoting and risk behaviors. *J Adolesc Health.* 2004;34(3):184-191

69. Seligman M, Darling RB. *Ordinary Families, Special Children: A Systems Approach to Childhood Disability.* 3rd ed. New York, NY: Guilford Press; 2009

70. Case-Smith J. Parenting a child with a chronic medical condition. In: Marini I, Stebnicki MA, eds. *The Psychological and Social Impact of Illness and Disability.* 6th ed. New York, NY: Springer Publishing Company; 2012:219-231

Promoting Health for Children and Youth With Special Health Care Needs

Children and youth with special health care needs share many health supervision needs in common with typically developing children. They also have unique needs related to their specific health condition. Birth defects, inherited syndromes, developmental disabilities, and disorders acquired later in life, such as asthma, are relatively common; children with special health care needs represent nearly 20% of the childhood population, or 14.6 million children.[1] In addition, an increasing number of children are receiving diagnoses of developmental disabilities and conduct disorders, which may indicate special health care needs.

The US Department of Health and Human Services Maternal and Child Health Bureau defines children and youth with special health care needs as children "…who have or are at increased risk for chronic physical, developmental, behavioral, or emotional conditions, and who require health and related services of a type or amount beyond that

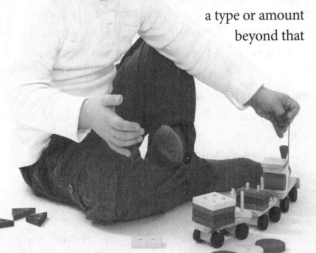

required generally."[2] Children with special health care needs and their families represent an increasing respon- sibility for primary care practices. The growing numbers of children with special health needs and the increasing complexity of their care demand new practice models for care and support for families. For example, infants diagnosed prenatally or at birth may have complex morbidities and conditions that were not previously cared for in the primary care setting. Although children with special health

care needs may present unique challenges for care provision, their survival and integration into home and community settings reflect enormous advances made in the basic sciences and technology and the expansion of pediatric home care in the recent past.

Approximately 0.1% of children and youth with special health care needs may need assistance from various forms of technology for some or all of the day and may need the help of multiple health and community providers. Among children with chronic health conditions who require hospitalization, more than 40% depend on technology, including medications, devices (eg, feeding tubes, central venous catheters, and tracheostomies), or both.[3] This includes 12% to 20% of hospitalized children with special needs who require devices, one-third of children who require medications, and 10% of children who require devices and medications. Hospitalization rates for children with more than one complex condition are significantly higher than for children with only one complex condition.[4]

In the previous century, many children with severe disorders did not survive, much less achieve adulthood or function as active members of a family. Now they and their families receive services in the community and schools that were previously unavailable and often rely on their medical home as a primary support. However, the necessary resources are all too often not introduced or discussed, not accessible, or not coordinated, and many families are not connected to adequate support systems in their communities. When referred for supportive services, many families experience difficulties following through because of misunderstandings, misgivings, financial concerns, perceived inadequate support through the process of referral and engagement, and other challenges.

Each age or developmental stage presents children and families with different developmental tasks. Developmental progress and medical management can be complicated for children with special health care needs. The medical home considers the unique trajectories of the child and his family along with the regular preventive and primary care needs of the child and family according to the guidelines for all children.

Implementing a Shared Plan of Care and Care Coordination

The individual health care professional or practice cannot meet the needs of the child with special needs and her family alone. High-quality pediatric care occurs when children, families, and professionals forge trusting, caring partnerships that fully use the knowledge and expertise of all. Frequently, a multidisciplinary team designed to meet multiple interdisciplinary needs must be involved in the child's care, thereby creating the structure of an integrated medical home that collaborates with community partners. This kind of integrated medical home can develop a team-based,

integrated, continuously updated plan of care for the child or youth with special needs. Such a plan can be an effective tool that links activities from visit to visit and coordinates the child's care across the health care continuum.[5,6] A shared plan of care (SPoC) typically is developed in partnership with the family and multiple care providers and describes the child and family's priorities and plans to support optimal health (Box 1).[7] It takes into consideration the child's medical information, development plan, Individual Family Service Plan for young children, and educational plan (ie, the Individualized Education Program).

An SPoC enables all partners to operate from the same family-centered perspective and to be accountable for desired outcomes. Parent partnerships with professionals can be achieved through the mutual sharing of goals, timely communication, and planned monitoring of care plans with targeted follow-up. Family-centered team care in the SPoC model enables the primary care team and the family to capitalize on blended family and provider goals and draw on supportive community resources and supports. This process is known as care coordination.

Care coordination provided within the medical home supports continuity and longitudinal care needs as critical primary care functions.[5,8-10] A care coordination framework builds on characteristics and functions consistent with the primary care medical home.[10] Pre-visit assessments or pre-visit contacts with the family can help team members prepare for a visit that effectively addresses the child's health care needs. Such pre-visit contact can assist the family to prepare for a visit, describe what to expect in preventive care, and identify topics about which they may wish to ask questions.[11] All children need routine health supervision as well as sick or condition-related care. Pre-visit planning allows time to review progress in achieving identified goals and follow-up from referrals. Families

Box 1

Principles for Successful Use of a Shared Plan of Care

1. Children, youth, and families are actively engaged in their care.

2. Communication with and among their medical home team is clear, frequent, and timely.

3. Providers or team members base their patient and family assessments on a full understanding of child, youth, and family needs, strengths, history, and preferences.

4. Youth, families, health care professionals, and their community partners have strong relationships characterized by mutual trust and respect.

5. Family-centered care teams can access the information they need to make shared, informed decisions.

6. Family-centered care teams use a selected plan of care characterized by shared goals and negotiated actions; all partners understand the care planning process, their individual responsibilities, and related accountabilities.

7. The team monitors progress against goals, provides feedback, and adjusts the plan of care on an ongoing basis to ensure that it is effectively implemented.

8. Team members anticipate, prepare, and plan for all transitions (eg, early intervention to school, hospital to home, pediatric to adult care).

9. The plan of care is systematized as a common, shared document; it is used consistently by every health care professional within an organization and by acknowledged health care professionals across organizations.

10. Care is subsequently well coordinated across all involved organizations and systems.

Reproduced with permission from McAllister JW. *Achieving a Shared Plan of Care with Children and Youth with Special Health Care Needs: An Implementation Guide.* Palo Alto, CA: Lucile Packard Foundation for Children's Health; 2014.

can be asked about their family needs and expectations in culturally sensitive ways and about roles they wish to play in shared decision-making. Visits can therefore focus on obtaining a medical history, administering questionnaires or screening tools, reviewing the existing SPoC, performing a physical examination, entering into discussions, providing anticipatory guidance, and planning next steps. Responsibilities should be clarified and accountability determined for the various condition-specific health care and follow-up and resource needs.

Table 1 depicts the work flow of a family-centered team in partnership with the family; pre-visit, visit, and post-visit activities are detailed.

Highly effective care coordination extends the medical home and makes use of community partnerships and resources, building a relationship among families, specialty health care professionals, schools, and community resources. An eco-map provides a concise visual representation of the many entities involved in caring for the child and family.

Table 1

Work Flow of a Family-Centered Team Approach to Care			
Roles of Care Partnership	**Pre-Visit Activities: Anticipation and Preparation**	**Visit Activities: Building Partnership Relationships**	**Post-Visit Activities: Following Through With Accountability**
Care Coordinator, or Providers of Care Coordination	• Reach out to patient/family • Complete a pre-visit assessment • Review priorities • Review and/or initiate a **plan of care;** summarizing progress/gaps • Huddle with team • Communicate/share ideas, concerns	• Assess and discuss needs, strengths, goals, and priorities • Educate and share information • Inform the **plan of care** in real time • Facilitate communications • Set time for next visit or contact	• Update/share the **plan of care** and implement accountable tasks • Ensure quality access and communication loops with resource contacts • Create opportunities for the ongoing engagement of patients/families • *Repeat these steps accordingly*
Youth and Family	• Prepare for visit or contact, review recent events, insights, expectations, goals, and hopes • Review existing **plan of care** for progress, gaps, successes, failures, and frame questions • Prioritize topics to address at visit	• Share priorities with team • Discuss care options together • Contribute to current **plan of care** development and/or revision • Ask for/acquire needed caregiving/self-care skills • Offer feedback and ideas • Set time for next visit/contact	• Review care information and instructions • Access and communicate with team as desired or needed • Use, share, and implement the **plan of care** with health partners • Complete tasks responsible for • *Repeat these steps accordingly*
Pediatric Clinician	• Huddle with team • Review pre-visit assessment data • Review **plan of care** and other data • Identify the need for a **plan of care** if none exists • Attend to team readiness/gaps for holding a prepared/planned visit	• Meet with family, engage them as part of the medical home core team • Complete screenings and/or assessments • Evaluate, listen, learn, and plan • Frame family and clinical goals: bio-psychosocial, functional, environmental • Co-create, update **plan of care** • Link with referrals/resources • Set time for next visit or contact	• Update/implement the **plan of care** completing accountable tasks • Monitor communications • Huddle with team frequently • Help guide team conferences • Supervise continuous care coordination and ensure plan of care oversight • *Repeat these steps accordingly*

Reproduced with permission from McAllister JW. *Achieving a Shared Plan of Care with Children and Youth with Special Health Care Needs: An Implementation Guide.* Palo Alto, CA: Lucile Packard Foundation for Children's Health; 2014.

It enables practices and families to delineate the existing plan of care coordination, assess the current supports surrounding a family, and identify gaps in services. Creating the eco-map brings together the team of resource and service providers that can potentially care for the child and family, including caregivers (day, night, weekdays, and weekends); physicians; legal and financial consultants and institutions; psychological and counseling support; diet and nutrition support; hearing, vision, speech therapy; physical therapy; occupational therapy; toileting; and school, religious, educational, and community supports. Figure 1 shows an example of a completed eco-map.

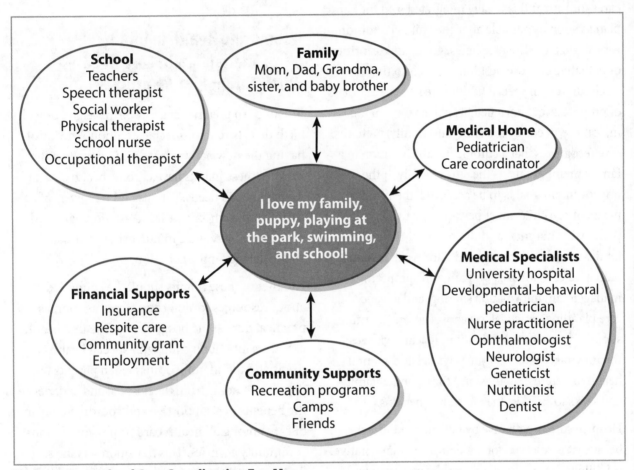

Figure 1: Example of Care Coordination Eco-Map

Palliative and Hospice Care

Infants, children, and adolescents with chronic, life-threatening, or life-limiting conditions may benefit from palliative care, and consultation with experienced palliative care providers can be considered.[12] The goal of palliative care is to improve the life of the affected child and of the family that cares for him and is ideally integrated into the care plan as soon as possible after the child's condition is recognized.[13] The principles, goals, and priorities of palliative care are best integrated into the care of all children with special health care needs, regardless of prognosis for shortened life expectancy. In focusing on the needs of the child and family, palliative care recognizes that a chronic health condition in a family member affects the entire family. If the life improvement goal is to be achieved, the physical needs of the child must be cared for in a comprehensive manner, and the needs of the child's family must be identified and addressed. Pediatric palliative care focuses on pain and symptom management, information sharing, and advanced care planning; practical, psychosocial, and spiritual support; and care coordination. It acknowledges the inevitable effect on the physical and mental health of parents, siblings, and the extended family and seeks to support these essential persons.

Hospice care is palliative by nature, but it differs because it is reserved for patients for whom curative treatments are no longer available or chosen and for whom death in the foreseeable future would not come as a surprise to caregivers and health care professionals. The primary treatment goal shifts from cure to comfort, while continuing the management of the special health care need. Emphasis is focused on assisting the family and, when possible, the child to identify goals for care and living that account for their needs for comfort and support and prioritizes their wishes and desires. Special attention is given to pain management; alleviation of nausea, shortness of breath, and other uncomfortable symptoms; management of disturbed sleep; and alleviation of anxiety in the patient. The family is helped with their own uncertainty, anxiety, and grief, and supports are identified. The needs of siblings are addressed and end-of-life planning is discussed. Both palliative care and hospice care can significantly enhance the care provided in the medical home.[12-14]

Promoting Health in Infants With Special Health Care Needs— Birth Through 11 Months

Infants born preterm, at a low birth weight, or with birth defects require special attention. The joy of having the new baby is tempered by the fact that many of these infants have chronic health care and developmental needs. Parents and caregivers of an infant with a chronic health condition will need support and guidance in nurturing the infant and fostering family cohesion.

Families of these infants should be counseled about resources for long-term care as soon as practical during the hospital stay. The first health care transition for a child with special health care needs and their family occurs when parents take their infant home from the hospital and experience the benefits of a supportive and coordinated plan of care among all health care professionals and community agencies. This transition sets the stage for the parent-professional partnership and builds trust that the health care system will provide support when parents have questions and concerns.

Anticipatory guidance should be structured around the parents' concerns, goals, and expectations. Specific guidance can include information on growth and development, feeding concerns, specialized health care needs for the infant, expectations and plans for achieving developmental milestones, and any specific vulnerability that the family will need to address. Health care professionals also can discuss the infant's integration into the family structure and family dynamic and ways other children in the family can be introduced to the possibility that their sibling can have different challenges because of her disability and circumstances.

The health care professional should explore with the family their understanding of their infant's health condition, its effect on the family, their expectations on issues such as family supports and care coordination, and their cultural beliefs and their hopes for the child. The health care professional plays an important role in helping the family develop expectations and plans for their child's future. Many families may need assistance with referrals to community services, financial assistance, and other types of supports. This assistance is vital because many high-risk infants with chronic disorders have significant unmet health care and resource needs.[15] The health care professional plays an important role in identifying conditions that place the infant at risk of disability and warrant immediate referral to early intervention services or other community resources (Box 2). It is important for the medical home team to follow up to be sure that connections to community services have been successful. Health care professionals should note children who require enhanced developmental surveillance and

periodic standardized developmental screening to permit the earliest identification of their need for intervention services.

The health care professional also plays an important and continuing role in providing informed clinical opinion in determining the scope of services that are needed by the child and family and in helping the family meet state, federal, or insurance company eligibility criteria for appropriate services. Hospital-based integrated primary care and specialty care teams for infants with medical complexity are available in some communities.[16] Care coordination of services, follow-up, and collaboration with other community agencies in the context of the medical home are important.

Professionals should be aware that some families may not recognize the early developmental delays or concerns of the pediatrician or may not view early intervention as positive. They may see efforts to screen and evaluate as efforts to stigmatize their child, or they may belong to a culture or religion in which differences are tolerated and accepted and are not addressed. Each family experiences readiness for developmental intervention services differently. However, they may be open to other support services and resources, such as culturally competent parent supports.

Box 2

Program for Infants and Toddlers with Disabilities (Part C of Individuals with Disabilities Education Act)

Children from birth–age 3 years who exhibit, or are at risk of, delays in development are eligible under federal law for early intervention services that will foster age-appropriate development. The Program for Infants and Toddlers with Disabilities (Part C of IDEA) assists states in operating a comprehensive, statewide program of early intervention services for infants and toddlers with disabilities, from birth–age 3, and their families. A diagnosis is not necessary for enrollment in early intervention programs. Children can be on waiting lists for an evaluation while receiving services. Children from the age of 3–school age and beyond also are eligible for early intervention services through the educational system (Part B of IDEA, also called Section 619) or through developmental services. Eligibility criteria for infants, children, and adolescents can be found at **http://ectacenter.org.**

Abbreviation: IDEA, Individuals with Disabilities Education Act.

Developmental surveillance, screening, and observations are important in all aspects of any child's growth and development. Formal developmental evaluation is indicated if a developmental screen is failed and if any signs of developmental delay exist, if the parents express concern or questions about their child's development, or if the child is at risk of developmental challenges because of factors such as prematurity or prenatal exposure to alcohol, drugs, or other toxins. *(For more information on this topic, see the Promoting Healthy Development theme.)*

Many parents are aware of developmental delays or irregularities before they are told about them by a health care professional. Their concerns must be promptly addressed and appropriate evaluation must be initiated. This evaluation might begin in the primary care office and might include an immediate referral to an early intervention program, a developmental specialist, or, for most cases, both. Follow-up of referrals with the parents is especially important in case delays in accessing intervention services occur or if the infant's condition is determined ineligible. In this situation, the health care professional can help parents obtain other sources of support and intervention.

The parent-child relationship is the most important factor in supporting every child's development, particularly for infants or children with chronic health conditions or special health care needs. Yet parents may be under significant stress related to the provision of their infant's care needs. The health care professional plays an important role in assessing the family's strengths and their predicament, including concerns about the parent-child relationship or parental lack of knowledge about parenting or infant care, which may place the infant at further risk of developmental, behavioral, or physical disabilities and that warrant referral to early intervention services or other community supports.

Long-term outcomes for all infants are improved when the strengths of the infant and families are recognized and opportunities are provided for parents to have early physical contact through rooming-in, breastfeeding, holding skin-to-skin, cuddling the infant, and understanding infant cues and sleep and awake states. Infants with special health care needs frequently provide parents with cues or signals that are more difficult to interpret, poor sleep, crying and fussiness, and feeding challenges. These concerns need to be addressed, and they may indicate the need for early intervention.[17,18]

Promoting Health in Children With Special Health Care Needs: Early Childhood—1 Through 4 Years

Health care professionals who take care of children between the ages of 1 and 4 years have a responsibility to follow through with addressing known disorders and to diagnose and manage new special health care needs as they arise over time. Because children in this age group grow and progress rapidly, parents anticipate and analyze how their child is reaching developmental milestones such as walking, talking, and socializing. Developing pleasurable activities for the child and family and keeping a sense of the joy of childhood accentuates the child's strengths and achievements.

When parents express concerns about how their child is developing, the health care professional should listen and observe carefully. A wait-and-see attitude will not suffice, particularly if the child falls into an at-risk group. A proactive approach is essential. Some disorders have well-organized societies, such as the National Down Syndrome Society[19] to offer specific guidance on Down syndrome, while other problems or less common congenital anomalies may require individualized expertise.

Parental concerns are highly accurate markers for developmental disability. The health care professional must be sensitive to these concerns. Several tools are available to assess parent concerns about learning, development, and behavior. If developmental screening suggests problems or if developmental delay or disability is suspected, a referral should be made to an appropriate early intervention program or developmental specialist for evaluation. If significant developmental delay or disability is confirmed or if a delay in diagnostic confirmation is likely, the child also should be referred for early intervention services matched to the child's and family's needs. With the appropriate services in place, the primary health care professional provides a medical home for the child and, in partnership with the family, assists with ongoing care planning, monitoring, and management across agencies and professionals. The primary care practice team carries out these activities by providing care coordination services while at the same time helping with the normally encountered developmental hurdles and health supervision, including timely immunization.

Participation in enjoyable activities like playgroups, singing, reading, and games to the extent of the child's abilities should be emphasized. Barriers to easy access to these services, such as inadequate health care coverage plans, family finances, access to resources, parental health and well-being, and sibling issues, also must be addressed.

Young children with special health care needs often have working parents and require child care and preschool just like typically developing children of the same age. As in all settings where these children spend their time, accommodations will be needed. Coordination with all caregivers and family members, including siblings, and a clear plan for how to manage acute problems, such as hypoglycemia or a seizure, lessen the fear that such events always entail. Families whose young children have special health care needs usually find that referrals to parent-to-parent support programs and family organizations are helpful. The transition between services described in Part C of the Individuals with Disabilities Education Act and

Part B (see Box 2) can be an especially difficult time for parents as they learn to negotiate the system requirements, which now include education, or find that their child's condition is no longer eligible for services.[20] The pediatric provider must understand the importance of this transition and provide parent support or alternative community supports for the family.

The health care professional caring for a child with a special health care need, while perhaps having received little training in this domain during residency, will come to an understanding of the crucial roles that additional professionals play in the lives of these children. These include occupational, physical, speech, behavioral, and respiratory therapists; education and child life specialists; personal care aides and assistants; and home care licensed practical or registered nurses. The medical home may be the ideal setting for responses to requests for guidance, clarification, or attention to concerns raised by all these home care personnel. The extent of responses will be influenced by the capacity of the health care professional or practice to provide care coordination if sources of support for the time and work required are limited or absent.

Promoting Health in Children With Special Health Care Needs: Middle Childhood—5 Through 10 Years

Middle childhood is a critical time for children with special health care needs to be actively involved in their own care so they can adapt successfully to their conditions. Two major transitions occur during this period—entrance into kindergarten at the beginning of middle childhood and entrance into middle school at the end. These are significant milestones for parents and the child as they adapt to increasing educational and social demands and the child begins to assume self-care responsibilities. During this period, children with special needs continue to define their sense of self and improve their ability to care for their own health, supported by their interactions with their care providers. Children adapt best to chronic illness when health care professionals, families, schools, and communities work together to foster their emerging independence. Inclusion in school and community life allows children with special health care needs to feel valued and to integrate their specific care needs with other aspects of their lives. Many children and youth with special health care needs require extra support from their schools, including resource room services, special classes and aides, and adaptations in the school environment, including accommodations for physical activity and sports. They and their families may experience prejudice and misunderstanding, both in the social and academic worlds. Their families frequently experience increased levels of emotional and financial stress and isolation.

It is important to discuss family perspectives because families may have various beliefs and values regarding the independence of children with special health care needs based on culture and history. Further, families should have appropriate supports if they need to cope with certain difficult tasks, such as hospitalizations or painful tests, illness, or possibly death.

When families have children with special health care needs, the health care professional may need to work with the family to provide information to the school and teachers on how best to meet the child's needs. Information effectively shared about what issues are and are not expected because of the underlying condition may help improve a child's school performance and schoolmate acceptance. Parents and child care providers should be sensitive to these issues and responsive to the needs of medically fragile children and their healthy siblings. At the same time, children with special health care needs should not be given special privileges simply because of their condition. Instead, outlining rules and responsibilities is extremely important for the child's development and the family's functioning.

Child care providers and teachers can play an important supportive role and be a source of information for parents and their children.

Promoting Health in Adolescents With Special Health Care Needs— 11 Through 21 Years

As children with special health care needs enter adolescence and experience puberty and rapid physical and emotional development, new levels of functionality in the face of their special need can bring important and remarkable gains in independence and autonomy. Alternatively, limitations related to their illness can further underscore their physical dependence and threaten autonomy, which can limit the development of emotional independence. Pubertal development may be affected, influencing healthy sexual development and perceived sexual autonomy.

Careful assessment of medical conditions, strengths, and risk-taking behaviors, followed by sensitive discussions of the youth's perceived needs and goals, can assist the adolescent with a special health care need to maximize physical and emotional development and support the attainment of full emotional development and maturity. Assessing physical abilities and carefully analyzing risks can foster participation in adaptive or interscholastic sports activities. The health care professional's expectations and opportunities for the adolescent to take active roles in their care decisions are important.

Entrance into high school is a significant transition for youth and their parents as they experience adapting to increasing educational and social demands, assumption of self-care responsibilities, and greater independence with the long-term goal of a happy, rewarding adolescence. The pediatric health care professional must understand the importance of this transition and provide parent support or alternative community supports for the family. Just as in the care of adolescents whose overall health status and development are more typical, adolescents with special health care needs require time alone with the health care professional to discuss, as able, topics germane to reproductive health, sexuality, relationships, mood, and the use of nicotine, alcohol, marijuana, and other drugs. Particularly important issues include discussion of academic performance, substance use, and sexuality.

Transitioning to Adult Care

Optimal health care for youth includes a formal plan for the transition to an adult health care provider. Transition is a flexible process, allowing youth to move to increasing levels of adult specialty care as they are ready, with the anticipation of completing the process by 25 years of age. Successful transition involves the early engagement and participation of the youth and family with the pediatric and adult health care teams in developing a formal plan. Health care professionals who care for adolescents with special health care needs and providers of pediatric specialty care for issues such as human immunodeficiency virus (known as HIV), chronic illness, and other special health care needs should have a policy for the transfer of the adolescent to adult care. The plan can be introduced to the youth in early adolescence and modified as the youth approaches transition.

Before initiating the transfer to adult care, it is important to assess developmental milestones to define the youth's readiness to assume responsibility for her own care. A successful transition from pediatric- to adult-oriented health care depends on the youth acquiring disease self-management skills, except for youth who lack the decisional capacity to guide their own health care and are under legal guardianship. The process should be as seamless as possible. Communication between the adolescent and adult care professionals is essential and may include personal contact and a written medical summary.[21]

It may be difficult to identify health care professionals with the expertise that the family and youth have experienced in the pediatric arena. Youth may find that the adult care services may not be as nurturing in providing support as they are accustomed to in the pediatric and adolescent medicine settings. Although the literature describes several transitioning care models, no research exists comparing these models or the patient satisfaction attributed to each.[22]

References

1. National Survey of Children's Health 2011/12 data. Data Resource Center for Child and Adolescent Health Web site. http://www.childhealthdata.org/learn/NSCH. Accessed September 19, 2016

2. McPherson M, Arango P, Fox H, et al. A new definition of children with special health care needs. *Pediatrics.* 1998;102(1):137-140

3. Feudtner C, Villareale NL, Morray B, Sharp V, Hays RM, Neff JM. Technology-dependency among patients discharged from a children's hospital: a retrospective cohort study. *BMC Pediatr.* 2005;5(1):8

4. Burns KH, Casey PH, Lyle RE, Bird TM, Fussell JJ, Robbins JM. Increasing prevalence of medically complex children in US hospitals. *Pediatrics.* 2010;126(4):638-646

5. Palfrey JS, Sofis LA, Davidson EJ, Liu J, Freeman L, Ganz ML. The Pediatric Alliance for Coordinated Care: evaluation of a medical home model. *Pediatrics.* 2004;113(5 suppl 4):1507-1516

6. Turchi RM, Berhane Z, Bethell C, Pomponio A, Antonelli R, Minkovitz CS. Care coordination for CSHCN: associations with family-provider relations and family/child outcomes. *Pediatrics.* 2009;124(6 suppl 4):S428-S434

7. McAllister JW. *Achieving a Shared Plan of Care with Children and Youth with Special Health Care Needs: An Implementation Guide.* Palo Alto, CA: Lucile Packard Foundation for Children's Health; 2014. http://www.lpfch.org/sites/default/files/field/publications/achieving_a_shared_plan_of_care_implementation.pdf. Accessed September 19, 2016

8. Starfield B, Shi L. The medical home, access to care, and insurance: a review of evidence. *Pediatrics.* 2004;113(5 suppl 4):1493-1498

9. Homer CJ, Klatka K, Romm D, et al. A review of the evidence for the medical home for children with special health care needs. *Pediatrics.* 2008;122(4):e922-e937

10. Antonelli RC, McAllister JW, Popp J. *Making Care Coordination a Critical Component of the Pediatric Health System: A Multidisciplinary Framework.* New York, NY: The Commonwealth Fund; 2009. http://www.lpfch.org/sites/default/files/care_coordination_a_multidisciplinary_framework.pdf. Accessed September 19, 2016

11. McAllister JW, Presler E, Turchi RM, Antonelli RC. Achieving effective care coordination in the medical home. *Pediatr Ann.* 2009;38(9):491-497

12. American Academy of Pediatrics Committee on Bioethics, Committee on Hospital Care. Palliative care for children. *Pediatrics.* 2000;106(2 pt 1):351-357

13. What is palliative care. American Academy of Pediatrics Section on Hospice and Palliative Medicine Web site. http://www2.aap.org/sections/palliative/WhatIsPalliativeCare.html. Accessed September 19, 2016

14. American Academy of Pediatrics Section on Hospice and Palliative Medicine, Committee on Hospital Care. Pediatric palliative care and hospice care commitments, guidelines, and recommendations. *Pediatrics.* 2013;132(5):966-972

15. Hintz SR, Kendrick DE, Vohr BR, et al. Community supports after surviving extremely low-birth-weight, extremely preterm birth: special outpatient services in early childhood. *Arch Pediatr Adolesc Med.* 2008;162(8):748-755

16. Cohen E, Kuo DZ, Agrawal R, et al. Children with medical complexity: an emerging population for clinical and research initiatives. *Pediatrics.* 2011;127(3):529-538

17. Hemmi MH, Wolke D, Schneider S. Associations between problems with crying, sleeping and/or feeding in infancy and long-term behavioural outcomes in childhood: a meta-analysis. *Arch Dis Child.* 2011;96(7):622-629

18. Tauman R, Levine A, Avni H, Nehama H, Greenfeld M, Sivan Y. Coexistence of sleep and feeding disturbances in young children. *Pediatrics.* 2011;127(3):e615-e621

19. National Down Syndrome Society Web site. http://www.ndss.org. Accessed November 8, 2016

20. Adams RC, Tapia C; American Academy of Pediatrics Council on Children With Disabilities. Early intervention, IDEA Part C services, and the medical home: collaboration for best practice and best outcomes. *Pediatrics.* 2013;132(4):e1073-e1088

21. American Academy of Pediatrics, American Academy of Family Physicians, American College of Physicians, Transitions Clinical Report Authoring Group. Supporting the health care transition from adolescence to adulthood in the medical home. *Pediatrics.* 2011;128(1):182-200

22. Crowley R, Wolfe I, Lock K, McKee M. Improving the transition between paediatric and adult healthcare: a systematic review. *Arch Dis Child.* 2011;96(6):548-553

Promoting Healthy Development

Some of the most influential medical research over the past decades illuminates the nature of the developmental origins and progression of the pervasive causes of morbidity and mortality in adults. In actuality, chronic diseases often get seeded and begin their pathological trajectories during gestation or childhood, sometimes decades before clinical manifestations create functional limitations. In other instances, conditions formerly seen only in older adult populations are now affecting people at younger ages. Scientific insights into epigenetics, psychoneuroimmunology, and biological stress reactivity further inform our understanding of causal links among the social determinants of health, emotion, biological risk, and health over the lifespan. *(For more information on this topic, see the Promoting Lifelong Health for Families and Communities theme.)*

Every health supervision encounter with children involves promoting healthy child development. Understanding child development and the application of its principles sets the care of children apart from that of adults. Infants grow to be children, then adolescents, and then adults. Health promotion to ensure physical, cognitive, and social and emotional health, as well as to protect the child from infectious diseases and injuries (intentional and unintentional) and harmful environmental exposures, supports the healthy development of the child. Successful health promotion efforts should take into account the developmental reality of the child now, as well as her developmental expectations for the next months and her developmental potential for growth over time.

Encouraging the development of the growing child references early brain growth and development. Physical health and growth is essential to support brain development. Even more important are the influences of stimulation and positive social ties with family, culture, and community.

The development of the infant, child, or youth with special health care needs is addressed in separate sections within this theme. Even a child whose brain growth and function have been impaired by injury or early neglect has a developmental potential that must be discerned and supported to achieve the best possible outcome for that child.

Monitoring Healthy Child and Adolescent Development

Developmental surveillance and screening of children and adolescents are integral components of health care supervision within the context of the family-centered medical home. Surveillance of children and adolescents is a continuous and cumulative process that is used to ensure optimal health outcomes; it is essential in identifying and treating children with developmental and behavioral problems. During all encounters, the pediatric health care team must listen carefully to parental concerns and observations about a child's development.[1]

Early identification of children with developmental delay is critical for diagnosing problems and providing early therapeutic interventions.[1] The parents' report of current skills can accurately identify developmental delay, even though they may not recognize it as such. Standardized developmental parent-completed questionnaires make it easier for health care professionals to systematically elicit information that is reliable and valid.[2]

Comprehensive child development surveillance may include

- Eliciting and attending to the parents' concerns
- Maintaining a developmental history
- Making accurate and informed observations of the child
- Identifying the presence of risk and protective factors
- Periodically using screening tests
- Documenting the process and findings

Developmental Surveillance and Screening in Infancy and Early Childhood

In monitoring development during infancy and early childhood, ongoing surveillance is supplemented and strengthened by standardized developmental screening tests that may be used at certain visits (9 Month, 18 Month, and 2½ Year) and at other times at which concerns are identified.[2] Commonly used developmental screening tools include the *Ages and Stages Questionnaires (ASQ)*,[3] the *Parents' Evaluation of Developmental Status (PEDStest)*,[4] and the *Survey of Well-being of Young Children (SWYC)*.[5] Autism spectrum disorder screening occurs at the 18 Month and 2 Year Visits, and the most common tool is the *Modified Checklist for Autism in Toddlers Revised, with Follow-Up* (known as *M-CHAT-R/F*).[6] The *SWYC*, which also includes autism screening; *PEDStest*; and *ASQ* all include psychosocial screening that can be used to identify cognitive, emotional, and behavioral concerns from birth through age 5 years.

Developmental Surveillance in Middle Childhood and Adolescence

Currently, no comprehensive developmental screening tests exist for use during the Middle Childhood or Adolescence Visits. However, several tools have been developed that are useful in screening for particular problems. For example, the Pediatric Symptom Checklist includes a psychosocial screening that can be used to identify cognitive, emotional, and behavioral problems.[7] The CRAFFT (car, relax, alone, forget, friends, and trouble) is a validated, 6-item screening tool that can distinguish between "low" and "high" risk substance use among adolescents who have already begun to use substances.[8,9]

In addition to assessing youth for risk behaviors, health care professionals monitor school-aged children's and adolescents' progress on the developmental tasks of adolescence. This developmental surveillance addresses youth attributes and choices associated with healthy emotional and physical outcomes as well as decreased health risk behavior during adolescence.[10-14] These are the things youth need to say yes to as they move toward adulthood. The child or adolescent should

1. Demonstrate social and emotional competence (including self-regulation).
2. Exhibit resiliency when confronted with life stressors.
3. Use independent decision-making skills (including problem-solving skills).
4. Display a sense of self-confidence and hopefulness.
5. Form caring and supportive relationships with family members, other adults, and peers.
6. Engage in a positive way with the life of the community.
7. Exhibit compassion and empathy.
8. Engage in healthy nutrition and physical activity behaviors.
9. Choose safety (eg, bike helmets, seat belts, avoidance of alcohol and drugs).[15]

During the health supervision visit, most practitioners identify these strengths as they conduct their general and developmental history. Commenting on the child's or adolescent's progress on these developmental tasks helps the youth and family understand their areas of strength and can help the health care professional tailor anticipatory guidance. It is important for parents to know that children who have these strengths or protective factors in their lives are more likely to do well in school and less likely to be involved in health risk behaviors.[16] Discussion about successes allows youth to realize what strategies have worked, so they can use them again.

Health care professionals can use the context of "opportunities" to frame discussions of areas in which things are not going well. If deficits in developmental progress are identified during Middle Childhood Visits, a strength-based conversation with the parents can focus on providing *opportunities* for the child to grow in these areas. When concerns are identified during an Adolescence Visit, clinicians can seek to determine whether the youth has had an opportunity to grow in each one of the desired outcomes listed previously. If that opportunity has not yet occurred, the use of shared decision-making, a problem-solving approach, motivational interviewing, or another brief intervention may help identify at least one new thing to try.

Parents can benefit from the knowledge that these are the areas they can prioritize for their children—giving them opportunities to grow in these positive aspects. As with all developmental surveillance, if a young person is lacking progress on one or more developmental tasks, it can be helpful to assure him that he is a "work in progress."

Promoting Healthy Development: Infancy—Birth Through 11 Months

The first year of life continues the prenatal period of neural plasticity and rapid adjustment to stimuli that allows the infant's brain to develop to its maximum potential, or not, depending on his experiences.[17] Beginning with the Prenatal Visit, developmentally focused anticipatory guidance should include information on attachment and the importance of healthy relationships. Long-term outcomes for all infants are improved when health care professionals emphasize the abilities of the infant and facilitate opportunities for the parents to have early physical contact through breastfeeding, rooming-in, holding skin-to-skin, and cuddling the infant.[18,19]

Preventive topics include safety related to the child's developmental abilities and physical capabilities, sudden unexpected infant death (known as SUID), coping with the stressors that make infants vulnerable to abuse (eg, infant crying, maternal postpartum depression, paternal depression, substance use by a parent, economic pressures, and social isolation), and parenting an infant with special or developmental health care needs. Cultural considerations influence parental perspectives about infant temperament and the parental or caregiver role in supporting the infant's self-regulation. The health care professional must try to understand the complex interrelationship of the family's beliefs, values, abilities, behaviors, culture, and traditions, which affect how a family protects, teaches, and socializes an infant. Parents' perspectives about the needs of their children and whether they view the infant's behaviors as normal or typical for the child's age are equally important considerations. Because families vary in their responses and behaviors, the health care professional must learn about these customs and seek to understand parents' responses and behaviors, even if they differ from those expected in the community context.

Infants With Special Health Care Needs

Most infants are born healthy, but some are born early, at a low birth weight, or with congenital conditions or develop special health care needs. Parents and other caregivers of an infant with special health care needs will need support and guidance in nurturing the infant and fostering family cohesion. Anticipatory guidance should be structured around the parents' goals and expectations. Specific guidance can include information on growth and development, feeding concerns, specialized health and developmental care needs for the infant, expectations for achieving developmental milestones, and any specific vulnerability that the family will need to know. The health care professional should document developmental and prenatal history to facilitate appropriate diagnoses as well as explore with families their understanding of their infant's health condition, its effect on the family, their expectations on issues such as family supports and care coordination, and their hopes for the child. Additionally, many families may need assistance with referrals, financial assistance, and other types of supports. *(For more information about this topic, see the Promoting Health for Children and Youth With Special Health Care Needs theme.)*

The health care professional plays an important role in identifying conditions that place the infant at risk of disability and warrant immediate referral to early intervention services (Box 1). Health care professionals should note children who require close developmental surveillance and periodic standardized developmental screening to permit the earliest identification of their need for intervention services. The health care professional also plays an important and continuing role in providing informed clinical opinion in determining the child's eligibility and the scope of services that are needed by the child and family. Care coordination of screening services and follow-up in the context of the medical home are important. Professionals should, however, be aware that some families may not view early intervention as positive (eg, they may see efforts to screen and evaluate as efforts to stigmatize their child, or they may belong to a culture or religion in which differences are tolerated and accepted and are not "fixed").

Developmental surveillance, screening, and observations are important in all aspects of the child's growth and development. Formal developmental evaluation is indicated if any signs of developmental delay exist, if the parents express concern or questions about their child's development, or if the child is at risk of developmental challenges because of factors such as prematurity or prenatal exposure to alcohol, drugs, or other toxins. It is a federal requirement that, as a primary referral source, a physician make a referral to Part C Early Intervention within 7 days of an identified developmental concern.[20] Many parents are aware of

Box 1

Program for Infants and Toddlers with Disabilities (Part C of Individuals with Disabilities Education Act)

Children from birth–age 3 years who exhibit, or are at risk of, delays in development are eligible under federal law for early intervention services that will foster age-appropriate development. The Program for Infants and Toddlers with Disabilities (Part C of IDEA) assists states in operating a comprehensive, statewide program of early intervention services for infants and toddlers with disabilities, from birth–age 3, and their families. A diagnosis is not necessary for enrollment in early intervention programs. Children can be on waiting lists for an evaluation while receiving services. Children from the age of 3–school age and beyond also are eligible for early intervention services through the educational system (Part B of IDEA, also called Section 619) or through developmental services. Eligibility criteria for infants, children, and adolescents can be found at **http://ectacenter.org.**

Abbreviation: IDEA, Individual with Disabilities Education Act.

developmental delays or irregularities before they are told about them by a health care professional. Their concerns must be promptly addressed, and appropriate evaluation must be initiated. This evaluation might begin in the primary care office or might result in an immediate referral to an early intervention program for immediate care and a developmental specialist for evaluation.

Domains of Development

During a child's life, the most dramatic growth—physical, motor, cognitive, communicative, and social and emotional—occurs during infancy. By 1 year of age, the infant has nearly tripled his birth weight, added almost 50% to his length, and doubled his brain weight. By the age of 2, the brain has twice as many synapses as it will have in adulthood. During the remainder of childhood and adolescence, the brain is actively engaged in pruning,[21] developing, and refining the efficiency of its neural networks, especially in the prefrontal cortex, the critical brain region responsible for decision-making, judgment, and impulse control. This dynamic process of neuronal maturation continues into early adulthood.[22] Outcomes for infants who are prenatally exposed to toxins (eg, alcohol, lead, and illicit drugs) are determined by the specific toxin; degree, pattern, or timing of exposure; and the quality of the nurturing environment.[17,23]

Studies on early brain development confirm the importance of positive early experiences in the formation of brain cell connections. These early experiences, especially parent-child interactions, have a significant effect on a child's emotional development and learning abilities.

Gross Motor Skills

From birth to the end of the first year of life, major changes occur in the infant's gross motor skills. As tone, strength, and coordination improve sequentially from head to heel, the infant attains head control, rolls, sits, crawls, pulls to a stand, cruises, and may even walk by 1 year of age. Delays in gross motor milestones, asymmetry of movement, or muscle hypertonia or hypotonia should be identified and evaluated for early intervention referrals.[24] Within the framework of safe sleep guidelines,[25] it is important to promote age-appropriate and safe opportunities for tummy-time play to allow young infants to master their early motor skills.

Fine Motor Skills

Hand-eye coordination and fine motor skills also change dramatically during infancy. These abilities progress from reflexive grasping to voluntary grasp and release, midline play, transferring an object from one hand to the other, shaping the hand to an object, inferior and then superior pincer grasp, using the fingers to point, self-feeding, and even marking with a crayon by 1 year of age. Babies should be given opportunities to play with toys and food to advance their fine motor skills.

Cognitive, Linguistic, and Communication Skills

Environmental factors influence the infant's developing brain significantly during the first year of life. When parents provide consistent and predictable daily routines, the infant learns to anticipate and trust his environment. An infant's brain development is affected by daily experiences with parents and other caregivers during feeding, play, consoling, and sleep routines.[26]

At birth, newborns already hear as well as adults do, but their responses can be difficult for parents to understand. For most infants, hearing provides the foundation for language development, but 1 to 3 babies per thousand are born with a hearing loss and 9 to 10 per thousand will have identifiable permanent hearing loss in one or both ears by school age.[27,28] Newborns will have a screening test for hearing before discharge from the hospital or should be screened before 1 month of age if not born in a hospital. Thereafter, hearing should be screened regularly and whenever parents express concern about hearing or language development.[29] Newborns can recognize their parents' voices at birth. By 3 days of age, they can distinguish their mother's voice from others.

Newborns also have color vision, can see in 3 dimensions, and can track visually. Close up, they show a preference for the pattern of human faces. Visual acuity progresses rapidly from newborn hyperopia to adult levels of 20/20 vision when the child is 5 to 6 years of age. Delays in development of fine motor skills or cognitive, linguistic, or communication skills may be caused by a deficit in the child's vision. A comprehensive eye examination should be performed as soon as possible to determine whether a vision problem is the root cause of any developmental delay.[30]

Newborns copy facial expressions from birth, use the emotional expressions of others to interpret events, and understand and use gestures by 8 months of age. By 8 weeks, infants coo; by 6 to 8 months, they begin to babble with vowel-consonant combinations; and by 1 year, they usually speak a few single words. The normal range for the acquisition of these pre-linguistic skills is broad. Families in which each parent has a separate native language should have each parent speak to the children in that parent's own language to promote bilingualism.

Beyond babbling, language acquisition progress depends on reciprocal stimulation a child receives.[31] Children who are frequently talked, signed, or read to have larger and richer vocabularies than children who have not received this stimulation. Reading is important for all children, including infants. Health care professionals should educate parents about how to read to infants and the importance of language stimulation, including singing songs to infants and children, reading to them, storytelling, and talking to them. Parents and pediatricians also need to appreciate the transition from the parent talking about pictures in a book to engaging the child in

reciprocally talking and pointing to pictures in a book. This technique, known as "dialogic reading," has been shown to encourage emergent literacy skills.[32] Health care professionals also should identify feeding issues related to oromotor function and coordination because these are integral to early pre-linguistic and later communication skills. Special discussions could be used with parents who are unable to communicate verbally or who have a child with special communication needs (eg, a child with hearing loss) to help the parents support normal language development in their children. Exposure to language from a live person has been shown to have a positive effect on early child development, whereas television screen exposure increasingly shows adverse effects.[33,34]

Children who live in print-rich environments and who are read to during the first years of life are more likely to learn to read on schedule than children who are not exposed in this way.[35] Giving an age- and culturally appropriate book to the child, along with anticipatory guidance to the parent about reading aloud, at each health supervision visit from birth to 5 years, has been shown to improve the home environment and the child's language development, especially in children at socioeconomic risk.[35-40] Parents should make reading with their children part of the daily routine. Reading together in the evening can become an important part of the bedtime ritual, beginning in infancy and continuing for years. Books and reading encourage development in multiple domains and are especially important for cognitive and linguistic development. Book-handling skills in young children also reflect fine motor skills, and parent-child reading promotes social and emotional development as well. Reading to a young child is often a source of great warmth and good memories for parents and children alike. Parents can use books in various ways, and health care professionals can emphasize to parents with low or no literacy skills that having conversations with their young children about the pictures in books (ie, interactive reading) also is an important way to encourage language development (Box 2).

Social and Emotional Skills

As parents learn to recognize their infant's behavior cues for engagement, disengagement, or distress and consistently respond appropriately to their infant's needs (eg, being fed when hungry or comforted when crying), babies learn to trust and love their parents.

Children with special health care needs may not exhibit the same responses as other children. This difficulty can cause parents to feel inadequate because they cannot discern their child's needs. Helping a family recognize even the small gains their child is making provides support to the family and acknowledges the progress and growth in their child with special needs.

By 3 months of age, infants may interact differently with different people. At about 8 months, an infant shows social referencing, looking to his parents in ambiguous or unfamiliar situations to figure out how to respond. At about the same age, his capacity to discriminate between familiar and unfamiliar people shows itself as stranger anxiety. By 14 months, he develops enough assurance and communication ability to contain his stranger anxiety and deal successfully with a new person. During the first year, the infant's social awareness advances from a tendency to cry when he hears crying to attempts to offer food, initiate games, and even take turns by 1 year. As autonomy emerges, babies may begin to bite, pinch, and grab what they want. Health care professionals should tell parents to anticipate these infant behaviors and advise on consistent, appropriate (firm but gentle) responses to redirect the infant's behavior.

Box 2

Promoting Literacy

To help parents promote healthy language and cognitive development in young children, *Bright Futures: Guidelines for Health Supervision of Infants, Children, and Adolescents* recommends anticipatory guidance on reading aloud at every health supervision visit from birth to 5 years[41] and strongly encourages giving a book that is developmentally and linguistically appropriate, as well as culturally responsive to the family, at these visits, whenever possible, to children at socioeconomic risk. The provision of the book directly into the hands of the child should be accompanied by intentional, skilled observation of the child and family's response to and handling of the book, all as a route for developmental surveillance and assessment of relational health in the family.

The AAP recommends health care professionals promote early literacy in the following ways:

1. Advising all parents that reading aloud with their young children can enrich parent-child interactions and relationships, which enhances their children's social and emotional development while building brain circuits to prepare children to learn language and acquire early literacy skills.

2. Counseling all parents about developmentally appropriate reading activities that are enjoyable for the child and the parents and offer language-rich exposure to books and pictures and the written word.

3. Providing developmentally, culturally, and linguistically appropriate books at health supervision visits for all high-risk, low-income children and identifying mechanisms to obtain these books so this does not become a financial burden for pediatric practices.

4. Additional community and advocacy recommendations are available.[41] For example, Reach Out and Read (**www.reachoutandread.org**)[42] is a national nonprofit organization that, for more than 25 years, has promoted early literacy by making books a routine part of pediatric primary care so children grow up with books and a love of reading.[35,36] The evidence-based model, delivered in the context of patient and family-centered care, offers training for providers and technical assistance for practices or clinics that are interested in implementing a Reach Out and Read program. In addition, many organizations provide support to make books available at low or no cost.

Abbreviation: AAP, American Academy of Pediatrics.

Different cultures may have various expectations about the age at which children will achieve socially mediated milestones. It is therefore important to ask not only what the child can do but also what the family expects and allows.

Separation Anxiety

Parents need to know that infants as young as 4 to 5 months of age may be anxious, when they are separated from their parents, when meeting strangers or even familiar relatives. Even grandparents need to allow the infant to warm up to them before taking the infant from the mother. This anxiety peaks at about 8 months. This is not a rejection but a normal developmental phase.

Providing time for the infant to get to know a new caregiver in the presence of the mother, before separation, is critically important. There must be consistency in this relationship. Transitions will be easier if a child is encouraged to have a special stuffed animal, blanket, or similar favorite object, which she holds on to as an important companion. Young children use this transitional object to comfort them.

Transition is often as difficult for the parent as it is for the child. If the parent is going back to work or school and using child care on a consistent basis, the parent often feels a combination of intense longing for the child, intense guilt, and jealousy. Parents need to be reassured that they will remain the most important people to their infant's happiness, well-being, and health. The infant may have intense emotions, including crying and irritability, that are saved for times when she is within the safe embrace of her mother. These expressions reflect the intensity of attachment to the mother. Guidance for both the child and parent may be needed to ease transitions and promote healthy adaptations.

Early Care and Education

Early care and education describes programs available for children before school entry. Child care is one option in an array of settings that includes family child care homes, center-based child care, and in-home relative care, as well as home visiting programs. Regardless of the location or person providing care, young children benefit when they receive high-quality care. Care that fosters children's healthy development should be offered by caregivers who relate consistently to the children; who are available, physically and emotionally, to respond to each child's needs and interests; and who provide care in a clean, safe, nurturing, and stimulating environment. The fewer children cared for by each provider, the better the situation is for the child. For large child care centers, parents should ask whether the center adheres to national standards and is accredited by organizations such as the National Association for the Education of Young Children (**www.naeyc.org**).[43] In addition, resources are available to parents for assessing the quality and services available in child care settings.[44-46]

Developmental Highlights of Infancy

The Influence of Culture on Development

Health care professionals should understand that what are often considered milestones are less "stones" than "markers," and these markers shift according to upbringing. The timing for acquisition of any developmental task is determined by surveying many infants to determine the range of accomplishment dates. The populations surveyed are typically the population of convenience. So milestones must be understood as normed to a population (Table 1). Cultural expectations shape development such that children from different cultures may have different (but still healthy) development timelines.[47] However, it is important to note that children are still held to the same standards once they reach kindergarten. Therefore, once a child reaches preschool age, developmental differences should be viewed in light of overall population means.

Table 1

Developmental Milestones for Developmental Surveillance at Preventive Care Visits[a]				
Age	Social Language and Self-help	Verbal Language (Expressive and Receptive)	Gross Motor	Fine Motor
Newborn–1 week	Makes brief eye contact with adult when held	Cries with discomfort Calms to adult voice	Reflexively moves arms and legs Turns head to side when on stomach	Holds fingers closed Grasps reflexively
1 month	Calms when picked up or spoken to Looks briefly at objects	Alerts to unexpected sound Makes brief short vowel sounds	Holds chin up in prone	Holds fingers more open at rest
2 months	Smiles responsively (ie, social smile)	Vocalizes with simple cooing	Lifts head and chest in prone	Opens and shuts hands
4 months	Laughs aloud	Turns to voice Vocalizes with extended cooing	Rolls over prone to supine Supports on elbows and wrists in prone	Keeps hands unfisted Plays with fingers in midline Grasps object
6 months	Pats or smiles at reflection Begins to turn when name called	Babbles	Rolls over supine to prone Sits briefly without support	Reaches for objects and transfers Rakes small object with 4 fingers Bangs small object on surface
9 months[b]	Uses basic gestures (holds arms out to be picked up, waves "bye-bye") Looks for dropped objects Picks up food with fingers and eats it Turns when name called	Says "Dada" or "Mama" nonspecifically	Sits well without support Pulls to stand Transitions well between sitting and lying Balances on hands and knees Crawls	Picks up small object with 3 fingers and thumb Releases objects intentionally Bangs objects together
12 months	Looks for hidden objects Imitates new gestures	Says "Dada" or "Mama" specifically Uses 1 word other than *Mama, Dada,* or personal names Follows a verbal command that includes a gesture	Takes first independent steps Stands without support	Drops object in a cup Picks up small object with 2-finger pincer grasp

continued

PROMOTING HEALTHY DEVELOPMENT

Table 1 *(continued)*

Age	Social Language and Self-help	Verbal Language (Expressive and Receptive)	Gross Motor	Fine Motor
15 months	Imitates scribbling Drinks from cup with little spilling Points to ask for something or to get help	Uses 3 words other than names Speaks in jargon Follows a verbal command without a gesture	Squats to pick up objects Climbs onto furniture Begins to run	Makes mark with crayon Drops object in and takes object out of a container
18 months[b,c]	Engages with others for play Helps dress and undress self Points to pictures in book Points to object of interest to draw attention to it Turns and looks at adult if something new happens Begins to scoop with spoon	Uses 6–10 words other than names Identifies at least 2 body parts	Walks up with 2 feet per step with hand held Sits in small chair Carries toy while walking	Scribbles spontaneously Throws small ball a few feet while standing
2 years[c]	Plays alongside other children (parallel) Takes off some clothing Scoops well with spoon	Uses 50 words Combines 2 words into short phrase or sentence Follows 2-step command Uses words that are 50% intelligible to strangers	Kicks ball Jumps off ground with 2 feet Runs with coordination	Stacks objects Turns book pages Uses hands to turn objects (eg, knobs, toys, and lids)
2½ years[b]	Urinates in a potty or toilet Engages in pretend or imitative play Spears food with fork	Uses pronouns correctly	Begins to walk up steps alternating feet Runs well without falling	Grasps crayon with thumb and fingers instead of fist Catches large balls
3 years	Enters bathroom and urinates by self Plays in cooperation and shares Puts on coat, jacket, or shirt by self Engages in beginning imaginative play Eats independently	Uses 3-word sentences Uses words that are 75% intelligible to strangers Understands simple prepositions (eg, *on, under*)	Pedals tricycle Climbs on and off couch or chair Jumps forward	Draws a single circle Draws a person with head and 1 other body part Cuts with child scissors

continued

Table 1 *(continued)*

Age	Social Language and Self-help	Verbal Language (Expressive and Receptive)	Gross Motor	Fine Motor
4 years	Enters bathroom and has bowel movement by self Brushes teeth Dresses and undresses without much help Engages in well-developed imaginative play	Uses 4-word sentences Uses words that are 100% intelligible to strangers	Climbs stairs alternating feet without support Skips on 1 foot	Draws a person with at least 3 body parts Draws simple cross Unbuttons and buttons medium-sized buttons Grasps pencil with thumb and fingers instead of fist

[a] Developmental milestones are intended for discussion with parents for the purposes of surveillance of a child's developmental progress and for developmental promotion for the child. They are not intended or validated for use as a developmental screening test in the pediatric medical home or in early childhood day care or educational settings. Milestones are also commonly used for instructional purposes on early child development for pediatric and child development professional trainees.

These milestones generally represent the mean or average age of performance of these skills when available. When not available, the milestones offered are based on review and consensus from multiple measures as noted.

[b] It is recommended that a standardized developmental test be performed at these visits.

[c] It is recommended that a standardized autism screening test be performed at these visits.

Sources: Capute AJ, Shapiro BK, Palmer FB, Ross A, Wachtel RC. Normal gross motor development: the influences of race, sex and socio-economic status. *Dev Med Child Neurol.* 1985;27(5):635-643; Accardo PJ, Capute AJ. *The Capute Scales: Cognitive Adaptive Test/Clinical Linguistic and Auditory Milestone Scale (CAT/CLAMS).* Baltimore, MD: Paul H. Brooks Publishing Co; 2005; Beery KE, Buktenica NA, Beery NA. *The Beery-Buktenica Developmental Test of Visual-Motor Integration, Sixth Edition (BEERY VMI).* San Antonio, TX: Pearson Education Inc; 2010; Schum TR, Kolb TM, McAuliffe TL, Simms MD, Underhill RL, Lewis M. Sequential acquisition of toilet-training skills: a descriptive study of gender and age differences in normal children. *Pediatrics.* 2002;109(3):E48; Oller JW Jr, Oller SD, Oller SN. *Milestones: Normal Speech and Language Development Across the Lifespan.* 2nd ed. San Diego, CA: Plural Publishing Inc; 2012; Robins DL, Casagrande K, Barton M, Chen CM, Dumont-Mathieu T, Fein D. *Validation of the Modified Checklist for Autism in Toddlers, Revised with Follow-Up (M-CHAT-R/F). Pediatrics.* 2014;133(1):37-45; Aylward GP. *Bayley Infant Neurodevelopmental Screener.* San Antonio, TX: The Psychological Corporation; 1995; Squires J, Bricker D. *Ages & Stages Questionnaires, Third Edition (ASQ-3): A Parent-Completed Child Monitoring System.* Baltimore, MD: Paul H. Brookes Publishing Co; 2009; and Bly L. Motor Skills Acquisition Checklist. Psychological Corporation; 2000.

Suggested citation: Lipkin P, Macias M. Developmental milestones for developmental surveillance at preventive care visits. In: Hagan JF, Shaw JS, Duncan PM, eds. *Bright Futures: Guidelines for Health Supervision of Infants, Children, and Adolescents.* 4th ed. Elk Grove Village, IL: American Academy of Pediatrics; 2017.

Self-regulation

Infants generally are born with unstable physiologic functions. With maturation and sensitive caregiving, physiologic stability; temperature regulation; sustained suck; coordinated suck, swallow, breath sequences; and consistent sleep-wake cycles will improve. During the first year, the infant's ability to self-regulate (eg, transition from awake to sleep) and modulate her behavior in response to stress are influenced by the environment, particularly by the consistency and predictability of the caregivers. The consistency and predictability of responses to the infant feeding cues and encouragement for regular sleep helps establish an infant's diurnal pattern of waking and sleeping. The infant also develops ways to calm herself and expands her ability to selectively focus on a particular activity. Large individual differences exist in self-regulatory abilities. Infants who are born with special health care needs, such as those who are of low birth weight or small for gestational age, or those born to mothers with diabetes or mothers who misused drugs or alcohol during pregnancy are at particular risk of problems with self-regulation.

A major component of infant health supervision consists of counseling parents about their infant's temperament, colic, tantrums, and sleep disturbances. The "goodness of fit" between parents and infant can influence their interaction. Helping parents understand their infant's temperament and their own can help them respond effectively to their infant.

Crying is stressful for families and frustrating for parents. Health care professionals will want to help parents discover calming techniques and understand that a certain amount of crying is inevitable. A crying baby should be checked because she may need attention. But when an infant cries, she is never angry. The crying is not a parent's fault. Helping a parent recognize this is important in preventing abusive head trauma or other physical abuse. Parents should consider whom they can ask for help if they are having trouble coping or if they fear they might harm their baby.

Sleep

Parents need guidance on differentiating between active and quiet sleep because they may assume their infant is getting adequate sleep when taken to the mall, taken to a party, or left in a carrier or swing all day. During these times, infants are more apt to be in active sleep. Active sleep alone is not adequate for appropriate rest and often results in a fussy baby. Health care professionals should help parents understand their infant's need for a consistent, predictable, quiet sleep location, including for naptime. Table 2 presents the key characteristics of various infant states. Table 3 lists typical infant sleep patterns. *(For more information on sleep-related topics, including room sharing, bed sharing, and sleep position, see the Promoting Safety and Injury Prevention theme.)*

Table 2

Key Characteristics of Various Infant States[48]	
Infant States	**Characteristics**
Quiet sleep	Very difficult to awaken; regular respirations; little movements; may startle
Active sleep	May awaken and go back to sleep; body movements, eyelid movements; irregular respirations
Drowsy	Increasing body movements, eyelid opening; more easily awakened for a feeding but may return to sleep with comforting
Alert	Alert expression, open eyes, and surveys surroundings, especially faces; optimum state for feedings
Active alert	Beginning to fuss and show need for a diaper change. If needs are not met, fussing escalates to crying.
Crying	Crying that lasts for >20 seconds. Usually, infant can be comforted with holding, feeding, or diaper change; exploring the duration, intensity, and frequency of crying is needed to determine strategies for interventions.

Table 3

Typical Infant Sleep Patterns and Sleep Location[a]						
Activities	**Birth–3 Months**	**3–6 Months**	**6–9 Months**	**9–12 Months**	**12–18 Months**	**18–48 Months**
Average sleep, hours	14	13	13	13	12–13	12–13 in 24 hours
Range of sleep, hours	12–16	12–15	10–14	10–14	12–14	12–14 in 24 hours
Night awakenings	Depends on feeding routine	2–3	1–3	1–2	0–1	0
Number of naps per day	Depends on feeding	2–4 (am and pm)	2 (am and pm)	1–2 (am and pm)	1–2	1
Length of naps, hours	1–3	2–3 each	1–3 each	1–3 each	1–3 each	1–2 each
Sleep location	Bassinette or crib in parents' room	Crib, ideally in parents room[a]			Crib	In own bed at 2–3 years

[a] AAP recommends that "infants sleep in the parents' room, close to the parents' bed but on a separate surface designed for infants, ideally for the first year of life, but, at least for the first 6 months."[25]

Derived from American Academy of Pediatrics Task Force on Sudden Infant Death Syndrome. SIDS and other sleep-related infant deaths: updated 2016 recommendations for a safe sleeping environment. *Pediatrics*. 2016;138(5):e20162938; Barnard KE, Thomas KA. *Beginning Rhythms: The Emerging Process of Sleep Wake Behavior and Self-Regulation*. 2nd ed. Seattle, WA: NCAST Programs, University of Washington; 2014; and Bright Futures Infancy and Early Childhood Expert Panels.

Discipline, Behavioral Guidance, and Teaching

The interaction between parents and their infant is central to the infant's physical, cognitive, social, and emotional development, as well as her self-regulation abilities. The infant brings her temperament style, physical attentiveness, health, and vigor to this interaction.

Parents need to understand the differences among discipline, teaching, and punishment so they can introduce appropriate measures for correcting and guiding their infant's behavior. All behavior has meaning, and for an infant, the motive for behavior is often based on a need, such as hunger or comfort. Correcting an infant's behavior is about teaching and guiding, not punishment and discipline. It is important to discuss distraction as a developmentally appropriate discipline for infants. It also may be beneficial to discuss strategies to prevent the need for disciplinary measures by avoiding overtiredness through consistent daily routines for feeding and

sleep and by providing a developmentally appropriate safe home environment.

Parents' ability to respond appropriately to their child's behavior is determined by their own life stresses, their past experiences with other children, their knowledge, their temperament, their own experiences of being nurtured in childhood, and other responsibilities, such as other children in the household, work, and daily household tasks. Their perceptions of the infant also can influence the interaction. These perceptions come from their own expectations, needs, and desires, as well as from the reaction of other people to the child.

Parents' emotional health also significantly influences their ability to provide appropriate discipline, behavioral guidance, and teaching. Depression is common in many mothers of infants and can seriously impair the baby's emotional and even physical well-being. Babies of depressed mothers show delays in growth and development, diminished responsiveness to facial expressions, reduced play and exploratory behaviors, and decreased motor skills.[49,50] Parental substance use disorder can have similar negative effects. Health supervision for the child must include monitoring the emotional health of the parents or primary caregivers. The health care professional should recognize and provide assistance if parents demonstrate or acknowledge their difficulty in responding to their infant's needs. *(For more information on this topic, see the Promoting Lifelong Health for Families and Communities theme.)*

Promoting Healthy Development: Early Childhood—1 Through 4 Years

At the beginning of this developmental period, a child's understanding of the world, people, and objects is bound by what he can see, hear, feel, and manipulate physically. By the end of early childhood, the process of thinking moves beyond the here and now to incorporate the use of mental symbols and the development of fantasy. For the infant, mobility is a goal to be mastered. For the active young child, it is a mechanism for exploration and increasing independence. The 1-year-old is beginning to use the art of imitation in his repetition of familiar sounds and physical gestures. The 4-year-old has mastered most of the complex rules of the languages that are spoken in the home and can communicate thoughts and ideas effectively (see Table 1).

The young child is beginning to develop a sense of himself as separate from his parents or primary caregivers. By the end of early childhood, the well-adjusted child, having internalized the security of early bonds, pursues new relationships outside the family as an individual in his own right. Understanding and respecting this evolving independence is a common parental challenge.

Because children in this age group grow and progress rapidly, parents anticipate and analyze how their child is reaching developmental milestones such as walking, talking, and socializing. When parents express concerns about how their child is developing, the health care professional should listen and observe carefully. A wait-and-see attitude will not suffice, particularly if the child falls into an at-risk group. A proactive approach is essential.

Young Children With Special Health Care Needs

Health care professionals who take care of children between the ages of 1 and 4 years have a responsibility to diagnose special health care needs. Parental concerns are highly accurate markers for developmental disability, and it is essential for the health care professional to be sensitive to these concerns. Several tools are available for identifying a child with special health care needs. If developmental delay or disability is suspected, a referral should be made to an appropriate early intervention program or developmental specialist for evaluation. The child should simultaneously be referred to an early intervention program that is matched to the child's and family's concerns. If significant developmental delay or disability is confirmed, appropriate services are in place and can be modified as indicated.

The health care professional provides a medical home for the child and, in partnership with the family, assists with ongoing care planning, monitoring, and management across agencies and professionals. The primary care practice team carries out these activities by providing care coordination services. *(For more information on this topic, see the Promoting Health for Children and Youth With Special Health Care Needs theme.)* Complicating factors, such as family finances, access to resources, language and culture, parental health and well-being, and sibling issues, also should be considered. Families whose young children have special health care needs usually find that referrals to parent-to-parent support programs are helpful.

Domains of Development

Gross and Fine Motor Skills

The physical abilities of children in the 1- through 4-year age range vary considerably. Some are endowed with natural grace and agility; others demonstrate less fine-tuning in their physical prowess, yet they "get the job done." As a fearless and tireless explorer and experimenter, the toddler is vulnerable to injury, but appropriate adult supervision and a physically safe environment provide the child with the freedom to take controlled risks.

Many children do not live in safe environments. Parents may try to provide a safe environment within the confines of their own dwelling, but the immediate community may be characterized by substandard housing conditions, overcrowding, residence in a shelter, or violence. Health care professionals who are aware of these circumstances can access or serve as a bridge to community resources to better support parents' efforts to find developmentally appropriate surroundings and experiences that allow their children to safely develop their motor skills.

Cognitive, Linguistic, and Communication Skills

Young children learn through play. If the toddler experienced nurturing and attachment during infancy, he now has a strong base from which to explore the world. The self-centered focus of the young child is related less to a sense of selfishness than to a cognitive inability to see things from the perspective of others. The child's growth in understanding the world around him is evidenced by his linguistic development (ie, by his capacity for naming and remembering the objects that surround him and his ability to communicate his wishes and feelings to important others).

Young children live largely in a world of magic; they often have difficulty differentiating what is real from what is make-believe. Such fantasies, unless scary to

the child, are to be expected and encouraged at this stage of development. Some children have imaginary friends. Many children engage in elaborate fantasy play. Learning to identify the boundaries between fantasy and reality and developing an elementary ability to think logically are 2 of the most important developmental tasks of this age.

Parents and other caregivers need to provide a safe environment for these young learners to explore. Children need access to a variety of tools (books and toys) and experiences. They need opportunities to learn through trial and error, as well as through planned effort. Their seemingly endless string of repetitive questions can test the limits of the most patient parents. These queries, however, must be acknowledged and responded to in a manner that not only provides answers but also validates and reinforces the child's curiosity.

The development of language and communication during the early childhood years is of central importance to the child's later growth in social, cognitive, and academic domains. Communication is built on interaction and relationships. The greater the nurturing and the stronger the connection between parents and child, the greater the child's motivation to communicate will be, first with gestures and then with spoken or signed language. Unstructured, creative, face-to-face, and hands-on play and reading are wonderful forums for language enhancement.

Language

Language development usually is described in 3 separate categories: (1) speech, or the ability to produce sound, a concept that encompasses rhythm, fluency, and articulation; (2) expressive language, or the ability to convey information, feelings, thoughts, and ideas through verbal and other means, including facial expressions, hand gestures, and writing; and (3) receptive language, or the ability to understand what one hears and sees. Children can have problems in one area but not in another. Exposure to books and reading aloud during the time that precedes the formal teaching and learning of reading are central to language development. Watching for vocalizations or naming of colors and objects when the child is given a book in the examination room can be helpful in assessing language development. Typical expressive and receptive language acquisitions in the early years include

- Between the ages of 12 and 18 months, children make the leap from sound imitation and babbling to the acquisition of a few meaningful words (eg, *Dada, Mama, mine, shoe*). Through repeated use, these first words teach them how words are used in communication. At the same time that the child gains expressive language, he also shows increased comprehension of simple commands (eg, "say bye-bye") and the names of familiar people and objects. Toddlers expand their communicative repertoire through a variety of gestures (eg, pointing, waving, and playing pat-a-cake) with and without vocalizations. The child's demonstration of "communicative intent" or proto-declarative pointing (ie, pointing to a desired object and watching to see whether the parent sees it) is an indication of normal social and language development. The absence of pointing and establishing joint attention is a red flag and merits screening for autism spectrum disorder. At about 18 months of age, most toddlers have begun a word-learning explosion, acquiring an understanding, on average, of 9 new words every day. This pattern continues throughout the preschool years.
- Between the ages of 18 months and 2 years, children recognize many nouns and understand simple questions. By the age of 2 years, the expressive language of most children includes 2-word phrases, especially noun-verb combinations that indicate actions desired or observed (eg, "drink juice," "Mommy give").

- Between the ages of 2 and 3 years, children usually are speaking in sentences of at least 4 to 5 words. They are able to tell stories and use what and where questions. They have absorbed the rules for regular plural word forms and for the use of past tense. Their speech can still be difficult for a nonfamily member to understand, but it becomes increasingly clear after 3 years of age. A good rule of thumb for normal development is that 75% to 80% of a 3-year-old's speech should be intelligible to a stranger.
- Between the ages of 3 and 4 years, children are learning fundamental grammar rules. They have a vocabulary that exceeds 1,000 words, and their pronunciation should be generally understandable. They frequently ask why and how questions. Their exuberant use of language in play and social interaction often suggests a process of "thinking out loud."

Parents may ask health care professionals about the effects of being raised in a bilingual home. They can be reassured that this situation permits the child to learn both languages simultaneously as though each language were the mother tongue. In the less common scenario when the child experiences language delays, however, language that is spoken by all caregivers or that is consistent to specific settings (ie, in the home, in child care settings) may be preferred.

Many aspects of language development seem to be robust because they develop normally despite environmental conditions. Certain aspects, notably vocabulary and language usage, however, depend heavily on the family and early school experiences if the child is to become proficient.[17] Thus, the young child who is exposed to an everyday environment that is rich in language through stories, word games, rhymes and songs, questions and conversation in the family and during play, and books will be well prepared for the language-laden world of school. *(For more information on this topic, see the Literacy section later in this theme.)*

Objective screening at birth and during early childhood, followed by timely assessment, makes it possible for hearing loss to be identified and intervention begun before language delays arise. Whenever language delays are present, an audiological evaluation is recommended even if hearing screening results were negative. A referral should also be made to early intervention services to optimize language development.

Social and Emotional Skills

Temperament and Individual Differences

The temperamental differences that were manifested in the feeding, sleeping, and self-regulatory behaviors of the infant are transformed into the varied styles of coping and adaptation demonstrated by the young child. The range of normal behavior is broad. Some young children appear to think before they act, whereas others are impetuous. Some children are slow to warm up to other people; others are friendly and outgoing. Some children accept limits and rules more easily than others. Some children are highly reactive to changes in their environment and to sensory experiences of all kinds, whereas others are less reactive. Some children tend to express themselves loudly and intensely; others are quieter.

Understanding the unique temperament profile of the child will better prepare the health care professional to assist parents and other caregivers in understanding the child's behavior, especially when the child's behavioral reactions are confusing or problematic. Discussing with parents how the child's behavior is interpreted within the family and counseling them when concerns or conflicts emerge between the child's temperament and their personal styles may prevent significant problems later on. Reading books or telling stories that some children can identify with may assist them in expressing feelings they are as yet unable to articulate.

Culture

The culture of the family and community provide a framework within which the socialization process unfolds. Children are heavily influenced by the culture, opinions, and attitudes of their families as they are taught to act, believe, and feel in ways that are consistent with the values of their communities.[51] Culture influences the roles of parents and extended family members in child-rearing practices and the ways in which parents and other adults interact with children. Cultural groups approach parenting in different ways. In some cultures, the mother is expected to be primarily responsible for all aspects of an infant's or a toddler's care. In other cultures, the care and nurturing of children is shared among mother, father, and extended family, including aunts, uncles, grandparents, and cousins. This wide circle of caregivers also may have responsibility for disciplining and making other decisions about a child's upbringing.

The increasingly self-aware young child grapples with complex issues, such as gender roles, peer or sibling competition, cooperation, and the difference between right and wrong, within this cultural milieu. Aggression, acting out, excessive risk-taking, and antisocial behaviors can appear at this time. Caregivers need to respond with a variety of interventions that set constructive limits and help children achieve self-discipline. Fun-filled family activities, such as playing games, reading, vacations, or holiday gatherings, serve as reminders of the joy and laughter the child brings to all. Ultimately, healthy social and emotional development depends on how children view themselves and the extent to which they feel valued by others. The quality of the parent-child relationship is the foundation for emotional well-being and the emerging sense of mastery and self-esteem. The pediatrician can learn from each family the culture and traditions that are important to them and that affect how the child is raised and nurtured.

Developmental Highlights of Early Childhood

Self-regulation and Daily Living Tasks

During the early childhood years, the relative dominance of biological rhythms is reduced through the development of self-control. Satisfactory self-control allows children to respond appropriately to events in their lives through delaying gratification until important facets of the situation are considered, modulating their responses, remaining calm, focusing on the task, recognizing that their responses have consequences, and behaving in the expected manner to adhere to rules and expectations established by their significant caregivers.[52] Usually, these behaviors begin to manifest by 2 to 3 years of age.

Children with inadequate self-control can be impulsive or hyperactive, heightening concerns for safety. At the opposite extreme, children with excessive self-control tend to be anxious or have fixed behaviors. Of course, behavior varies so that a child may exhibit a great variety of behaviors at any given time in response to the same external cues.

Mastering activities in daily life shows that the child is moving toward achieving self-control. Chief among these are learning how to calm himself (which is needed to establish a regular sleep pattern), feed himself, toilet train, and take the major step of attending school. Health care professionals should actively prepare parents and their toddlers for achieving these milestones through discussing these topics and, when concerns persist after counseling, should make referrals for appropriate consultation.

Sleep

By the end of the first year of life, most children should be able to sustain or return to sleep throughout the night, and most parents should allow children to regulate their own nighttime sleep patterns. A bedtime routine that promotes relaxation (eg, bath, book, or song) and the use of a transitional object are extremely helpful. Toddlers and preschoolers generally sleep 8 to 12 hours each night. Exact duration of nighttime sleep varies with the child's temperament, activity levels, health, and growth. The duration and timing of naps will affect nighttime sleeping. Most children awaken from sleep at times during the night but can return to sleep quickly and peacefully without parental intervention. Sleep problems sometimes reflect separation fears on the part of parents and children. Parents who feel especially anxious, depressed, or frightened can be reluctant to permit their young child to exercise self-control over sleep patterns at night. Children from 1 to 4 years of age should be allowed to sleep through the night without a nighttime feeding. Dreams and nightmares can accompany active stages of sleep beginning at these ages. At such times, children may require reassurance that they are protected from the dangers that stir their imagination and intrude on their calm sleep. Changes, such as acute illness, birth of siblings, and visits from friends and relatives, also can interfere temporarily with established sleep routines. Disorders, such as obstructive sleep apnea, and parasomnias, such as sleepwalking, can begin during these early years, and health care professionals should consider such a possibility in any child who has persistent sleep difficulties.

If health care professionals ask about sleep patterns at each of the visits during early childhood, they will gain rich insights into the child's and family's development. When parents have concerns about their child's sleep, the health care professional should explore, in more depth, the child's daytime behavior, temperament, and mood, as well as events, experiences, conditions, and feelings of family members. Although most issues lend themselves to open dialogue and counseling within the primary care relationship, some conflicts may require further exploration and intervention by a developmental-behavioral or mental health professional.

Toilet Training

For a child to successfully toilet train, he must have the cognitive capacity to respond to social cues and the neurologic ability to respond to bowel and bladder signals. Parents often want advice about when and how to toilet train a child. The first discussion about toilet training is best introduced at around the 18 Month Visit. Such early counseling can prevent harmful battles between the parents who might be focused on early toilet training and the child who is not yet physically or cognitively ready. In-depth discussion usually begins at the 2 Year Visit. The health care professional should explore the parents' thoughts about this task and provide guidance to fill in the gaps.

Control of urination and bowel movements is a major step forward in developmental integrity. Successful completion of this task is a source of pride and respect for the child and the parents.

Daytime control usually is achieved before night-time dryness. Bed-wetting (nocturnal enuresis) is a common disorder with many possible therapies.[53] It is more common in boys and deep sleepers. Bed-wetting should be discussed with the child and family and investigation considered if the child continues to wet the bed after age 7 years, if bed-wetting results in problems within the family, or if infection or anatomic abnormalities are suspected. Fortunately, with time, most children with bed-wetting develop nighttime urination control. Bowel control is usually completely achieved by age 3 years.

Socialization

When provided the opportunity, toddlers and preschoolers acquire socialization skills and the ability to appropriately interact with other children and adults. Social interaction in early childhood promotes comfort and competence with relationships later in life. The social competencies are developmental assets[12] and therefore should be encouraged in children of these ages. Social

competencies include planning and decision-making with others, positive and appropriate interpersonal interactions, exposure to other cultures and ethnicities, behavioral resistance to inappropriate or dangerous behavior, and peaceful conflict resolution. Young toddlers will observe these behaviors in others, and preschoolers will begin to practice them. Toddlers also are inclined to internalize positive or negative attitudes toward themselves and others. Children note differences between groups of people (eg, they express understanding of racial identity as early as 3 years of age[54]), but they do not ascribe a value; they learn that from the adults in their environments. Opportunities for social interaction can be encouraged in the home with visitors, in playgroups, in faith-based organizations, and in public places, such as the park or early care and education programs.

Discipline, Behavioral Guidance, and Teaching

Discipline is one tool parents can use to help modify and structure a child's behavior. It encompasses positive reinforcement of admired behavior (eg, praise for picking up toys) and negative reinforcement of undesirable behavior (eg, a time-out for fighting with a sibling). The eventual incorporation of a functional sense of discipline that reinforces social norms is critical to the child's development. Although often thought of in negative terms, positive discipline helps a child fit into the daily family schedule and makes childhood and child-rearing pleasant and fun. In fact, the Latin root for *discipline* means "to teach."

Family structure, values, beliefs, and cultural background influence approaches to behavioral guidance and teaching. Health care professionals should discuss with the parents how they were disciplined, how that discipline made them feel, and the most and least effective methods of discipline. In all families and cultures, discipline is a process whereby caregivers and other family members teach the young child, by instruction and example, how to behave and what is expected of him. What the child learns at this stage and how the parent-child interactions surrounding discipline take form can have long-term effects on the child's and family's development.

Exploring the roles that siblings play in development also should be addressed. The methods parents use to guide siblings in helping raise the other family members should be reviewed. The special requirements of children and youth with special health care needs and foster care or adopted children are best discussed openly with all the family members, so everyone is aware of parental expectations.

Although parents often look to the health care professional as a resource for developing strategies related to behavioral guidance and teaching, many cultures also look to family, particularly elders. In most cases, discussions with parents regarding behavioral guidance should explore the parents' goals for the child, as well as the meaning behind the behaviors they wish to modify. Consideration of the child's developmental capacities and temperament profile should be a key component of this discussion. For instance, parents of a 2-year-old frequently overestimate the child's capacity to integrate rules into everyday behavior, because of their observations of the child's growing understanding of language. With respect to temperament, parents can misinterpret a child's intense and reactive responses as intentionally oppositional rather than as part of his inborn behavioral style. Through explaining these developmental attributes, the health care professional plays a crucially important role in helping parents understand the meaning of their child's behavior and in assessing the developmental readiness of the child to absorb new lessons about behavioral expectations.

Discussion of discipline is a high priority for the Bright Futures 15 and 18 Month Visits because it is important, for later child development, to establish a positive and successful foundation of

parent-child interactions regarding behavior. Established negative behaviors can be extremely difficult to change, and, without help, many parents are not able to see the long-term effects of their child's behavior and their own choices in guiding them.

At times, the behavior of the child pushes all parents to their emotional limits. Many adverse behaviors, such as aggressive acts in the school-aged child, have their roots in behavior established in early childhood. Maintaining a sense of humor and taking time away can help parents deal with stressful events. Discussing dilemmas and sharing frustrations with other involved adults are important in maintaining a sense of perspective and humor during difficult periods with the young child. Referring parents to home visiting programs, early care and education programs, or parent support groups can also help them learn to cope with challenging situations, learn strategies and skills to assist their child, and learn about child development.

General features of effective behavioral guidance include several essential components, all of which are necessary for successful discipline.[55]

- A positive, supportive, loving relationship between the parents and child (Children want to please their parents.)
- Clear expectations communicated to the child in a developmentally appropriate manner
- Positive reinforcement strategies to increase desired behaviors (eg, having fun with the child and other family members, which sets the stage to reward and reinforce good behaviors with time together in enjoyable activities)
- Removal of reinforcements or use of logical consequences to reduce or eliminate undesired behaviors

Parents can increase the likelihood of achieving their behavioral goals for their child by establishing predictable daily routines and providing consistent responses to their child's behavior. Especially during early childhood, consequences should be administered within close temporal proximity to the target behavior and, if possible, related to the behavior (eg, bring the child in from playtime if she is throwing sand when asked not to).[55] Some families (eg, first-time parents or adolescent parents) experience pressure from elders to use harsh or physical means of punishment. Culturally, it may be inappropriate to ignore what an elder has proposed. Parents may feel conflicted when they attempt to use new or different methods of discipline that are not supported within their families or communities.

The most potent tool for effective discipline is attention. By paying attention to desired behaviors and ignoring undesired ones, parents can use the following techniques to help foster good behavior in their child:

- Praise the child frequently for good behavior. Specific acknowledgment (rather than global praise) helps teach the child appropriate behaviors (eg, "Wow, you did a good job putting that toy away!" rather than "Great!"). Time spent together in an enjoyable activity is a valuable reward for desired behavior.

- Communicate expectations in positive terms. By noting when the child is doing something good, parents will help the child understand what they like and expect. Statements such as, "I like it when you play quietly with your brother," or, "I like that you climb into your car seat when I ask you to," are nonjudgmental and communicate to the child that these are behaviors the parents like.

- Model and role-play the desired behaviors.

- Prepare the child for change in the daily routine by discussing upcoming activities and expected behaviors.

- State behavioral expectations and limits for the child clearly and in a developmentally appropriate manner. These expectations should be few, realistic, and consistently enforced.

- Allow the child time for fun activities, especially as a reward for positive behaviors.

- Remove or avoid the places and objects that contribute to unwanted behavior.

- Use time-out or logical consequences to deal with undesirable behavior. Time-out is a structured method of avoiding paying attention to undesired behaviors.

- Promote consistent discipline practices across caregivers, but recognize that complete agreement is not always possible, and most children can learn more than one set of rules that are reasonable and logical.

- Ensure that the child understands the discipline is about his behavior and not about his worth as a person.

- Avoid responding to the child's anger with anger. This reaction teaches the wrong lesson and may escalate the child's response.

- Take time to reflect on their own physical and emotional response to the child's behavior so they can choose the most appropriate discipline technique.

Conventional disciplinary methods do not work well with children with certain physical or developmental conditions. The following examples illustrate the point that "one size does not fit all" with respect to behavioral guidance:

- Children with poor communication skills and language delay often use behavior as a means of communication. Caregivers should make every effort to help them develop more effective communication skills.

- Children who have hyperacute responses to their sensory environment require proactive interventions.

Because corporal punishment is no more effective than other approaches for managing undesired behavior in children, the American Academy of Pediatrics recommends that parents be encouraged and assisted in developing methods other than spanking in response to undesired behavior (Box 3).[55,56] Other forms of corporal punishment, such as shaking or striking a child with an object,

---

Box 3

Discipline: Key Messages for Parents

- Discipline means teaching, not punishing.
- All children need guidance, and most children need occasional discipline.
- Discipline is about a child's behavior, not about his worth as a person.
- Discipline is effective when it is consistent; it is ineffective when it is not consistent.
- Parents' discipline should be geared to the child's developmental level.
- Discipline is most effective when the parent can understand the child's point of view.
- Discipline should help a child learn from his mistakes. The child should understand why he is being disciplined.
- Disciplinary methods should not cause a child to feel afraid of his parents.
- A parent should not physically discipline a child if the parent feels out of control.

---

should never be used. In many jurisdictions, corporal punishment that leaves a mark or a bruise mandates a report to child protective services. Referral to high-quality parenting programs and counseling should be considered for children with difficult behavioral problems or any parent struggling with parenting strategies.

Literacy

Learning to read and write is a complex process that takes time and represents the coming together of a variety of skills and pathways in the brain. It requires that children have good, consistent relationships with caring adults who provide one-on-one interactions and who support the development of oral language. Literacy skills begin to develop in infancy, when parents and other caregivers talk or sign to their baby, and continue to develop in early childhood, when toddlers learn to communicate through language, explore their world through imaginary play, and listen to stories, whether read from books or spoken in an oral tradition. Because young children are active learners, they find joy in exploring and learning the meaning of language and communicating in increasingly sophisticated ways as they move toward literacy.

Parents' and health care professionals' expectations for a young child's literacy accomplishments should be based on developmentally appropriate activities, such as the encouragement of talking, singing, and imaginative play; simple art projects; easy access to books; and frequent reading times. Reading and writing are so linked to development, relationships, and environment that children will vary greatly in when and how they learn to read and write. This is true for other complex skills as well.

It is important to identify the literacy level of parents—not only when providing written educational materials but when encouraging parents to read to their child. Books do not have to be read to encourage literacy in children. Parents can use the books to tell stories, point out pictures, and let children make up their own story. Parents who use books in this way encourage their child in learning to read.

Health care professionals can support literacy by encouraging parents to tell stories, create or visit environments filled with books, find a place at home for imaginary play and art projects, ask their child questions and invite him to talk about his ideas, give time for reading daily, and set aside quiet times each day for reading with their child (eg, just before bed). By encouraging parents at every health supervision visit to find age-appropriate ways of incorporating books and reading aloud into children's daily routines, the health care professional can give parents a way to help their children grow up associating books with positive parental attention. These discussions also can help parents understand the role that child care and preschool programs play in helping children get ready to read and write.[57]

The health care professional's office should reflect reading as a priority, with a specific area set aside to encourage imaginative play, a place with a collection of quality books and magazines in which children can look at books or be read to and a place with information about community libraries and adult and family literacy opportunities. *(For more information on this topic, see Box 2 of this theme.)* The presence of screen media in a waiting room can give a contradictory message. The evidence-based Reach Out and Read Program has increased the likelihood that parents will read to their children even among families at risk because of low-literacy among parents.[39,40] By giving a book at every health supervision visit from birth through age 5 years, especially to children at socioeconomic risk, the health care professional can intentionally build the skills of parents to actively participate in their children's cognitive and language development by increasing the frequency of parental reading aloud, improving the home environment, and helping parents increase children's language development.[35,39,40]

Play

A hallmark of the passage through early childhood is the emergence and steady elaboration of play activities. For the young toddler, play centers on direct explorations into the surrounding world, including the manipulation of objects to create interesting outcomes (eg, the sounds that banging a pot may produce or the interesting results of pouring water into a sandbox). With the development of language, from around age 18 months, play becomes progressively more reflective of the child's remembered experiences and imagined possibilities, as enacted through symbolic play.

Thus, a doll comes to represent a living, imaginary person who can be fed, bathed, or scolded—just as the young child has personally experienced in real life.

In representational or symbolic play, which usually is evident by 2 years of age, the child has a new way of "replaying" the events in his life. Unlike real life, play allows him to control the events and their outcomes. Challenging experiences can be better understood through their re-creation as play. Play can enable the child to better cope with stressful experiences by taking charge and developing a preferred story. Confusing or difficult experiences can be mastered through the practice in experimentation and planning that play permits.

Many children at this age become attached to transitional objects and use them to help them fall asleep, comfort them when they are hurt or upset, and join them in their world of make-believe. The transitional object is a prime example of how the child's active imagination plays a central role in development toward independence and self-regulation.

From 3 to 5 years of age, the child's developmental gains in language and speech, cognitive ability, and fine and gross motor skills allow for increasingly complex forms of play. Play becomes an important modality for practicing and enhancing a broad range of skills, such as the motor skills and spatial understanding that comes with building with blocks or working with puzzles.

Play is a critical part of development, and toys are a critical part of play. Health care professionals often are asked to recommend appropriate toys for their patients. Toys should be educational and should promote creativity. Parents and health care professionals should avoid toys that make loud or shrill noises; toys with small parts, loose strings, cords, rope, or sharp edges; and toys that contain potentially toxic materials. Toys that promote violence, social distinctions, gender stereotypes, or racial bias also should be avoided. Video games are not recommended for young children, but if used they should be screened for inappropriate content. Health care professionals can advise parents on distinguishing between safe and unsafe toys, choosing age-appropriate toys that help promote learning, and using books and magazines to read together.[58]

Play provides a window into many aspects of the child's developmental progress and into how she is attempting to understand the events, transitions, and stresses of everyday life. Parents and other caregivers should recognize the importance of play for the development of their young children. Play requires that children feel secure and that the play environment be sufficiently protected from intrusion and disruption. Parent-child play, in which the child takes the lead and the parent is attentive and responsive, elaborating but not controlling the events of play, is an excellent technique for enhancing the parent-child relationship and language development. When typical play is missing or delayed, the health care professional should consider the possibility of a developmental disability or emotional disorder, possible significant stresses in the child's environment, or both. The child's relationship to the family pets, if any, should be discussed and should include queries about attachment, responsibilities for pet care, and pet safety.

Play is no less important for children with physical or cognitive disabilities, but adaptations may be needed to allow such children to use the toy. These may include switches to allow the toy to activate or modifications to keep the toy in reach for children with limited mobility or dexterity. Therapists can be helpful in identifying and adapting toys for individual children.

Separation and Individuation

By the child's first birthday, he has likely secured a reasonably firm sense of trust that his primary caregivers are reliable, protective, and encouraging. In turn, the young toddler should begin to feel as though he can trust others enough to feel

comfortable in communicating his feelings, needs, and interests. From this base of emotional security, the young child can dedicate his second year to begin growing increasingly independent from his caregivers—in actions, words, and thoughts. Periodically checking in with his parents for guidance and reassurance about safe and socially acceptable limits, the toddler waffles between testing bold new behaviors and exploring new environments and demanding to be consoled and protected. During this stage of development, parents can help their child by providing safe opportunities for freedom and encouragement with support. As the young child develops increasing comfort in exploring time, space, and relationships with adults and peers, he begins to discover more about his own identity, effectiveness, and free will. The more positive experiences a preschool-aged child enjoys with other children and adults, the better prepared he becomes for his subsequent adventures at school.

Early Care and Education

According to the *Child Health USA 2014* report, 64.8% of mothers with preschool-aged children were in the labor force (either employed or looking for employment) in 2013.[59] Census Bureau data show that children are cared for in a variety of settings. For example, nearly a half of preschool-aged children are cared for by family members. Other settings include day care centers, nursery schools, preschools, federal Head Start, kindergarten and grade schools, family day care, and nonrelatives (eg, babysitters, nannies, and housekeepers). All of these settings come under the comprehensive rubric of *early care and education,* and they vary across states, ages, health status, and family income levels. Children from lower-income families are less likely to be cared for in centers than are children from higher-income families and are more likely to be in the care of relatives.[60] Families with young children, especially those living at or near the poverty level and those with several children in child care, often find that child care costs strain their budget, requiring them to balance competing family needs. Although federal subsidies for child care exist, most communities have waiting lists for openings. The health care professional and support staff who are familiar with community resources and sensitive to families' financial struggles can guide families as they make child care decisions.

Because child care for children with special health care needs is the most difficult to find and is in the shortest supply in most communities, a family's search for suitable child care can be frustrating and can sometimes cause a parent to stop working. This problem is compounded for families with low incomes, children who have more severe special health care needs, or both. In these situations, the health care professional and staff can help families by understanding their unique needs and the available community resources. Parents may benefit from being connected to local public health resources as well as contacts through the local Early Intervention Program agency, often referred to as IDEA Part C. These contacts can help with developmental concerns and also provide links to other community resources. The health care professional and staff also can work with the child care provider to ensure that the setting is appropriate and the staff has the training necessary to give the child a safe and healthy environment.

Preschools should never have more than 10 children per teacher. Providers for children with special health care needs may require specialized training and support. Parents should inquire whether their preschools adhere to national standards and are accredited by organizations such as the National Association for the Education of Young Children (**www.naeyc.org**).[43]

Quality child care gives young children valuable opportunities to learn to relate effectively with peers and adults, to explore the diverse physical and social world, and to develop confidence in their abilities to learn new skills, form trusting bonds of friendship, and process information from a variety of sources. High-quality early care and education and home visiting programs also are linked to positive health outcomes, supporting the foundations of health, which include stable and responsive relationships, secure and safe environments, nutrition, health-promoting behaviors, and healthy child development.[61] Health care professionals should learn about the health, developmental, and behavioral issues of their patients as they are manifested in child care. Health care professionals can integrate this information in their assessment, counseling, and advocacy for children and families in their practice and their community. The more sources of insight into the child's life the health care professional has, the better prepared the professional will be to support the child's health and development as he takes his first steps beyond the family. Many health care professionals provide formal consultative services to child care centers in their communities.

School Readiness

At the end of the early childhood developmental stage, the young child and his parents will begin the transition into kindergarten. The child will be challenged to demonstrate developmental capacities, including

- Language and speech or signing that is sufficient for communication and learning
- Cognitive abilities that are necessary for learning sound-letter associations, spatial relations, and number concepts
- Ability to separate from family and caregivers (especially for the child who has not already participated in preschool activities)
- Self-regulation with respect to behavior, emotions, attention, and motor movement
- Ability to make friends and get along with peers
- Ability to participate in group activities
- Ability to follow rules and directions
- Skills that others appreciate, such as singing or drawing

However, too many children today enter kindergarten significantly behind their peers in one or more of these abilities. Problems in self-regulation of emotions and behavior and problems in maintaining attention and focus are common at kindergarten entry and predict future educational and social problems.[62,63]

In an extensive survey, kindergarten teachers reported that roughly a half of kindergartners have difficulty following directions, and a third lack academic skills and have problems with working in a group.[64] Socioeconomic, racial, and ethnic cognitive gaps have been shown to exist at kindergarten entry and, if unaddressed, have the potential to persist and grow over time.[65]

Social and emotional development during early childhood (which was neglected in past research on school readiness) has been shown to be strongly connected to later academic success. Qualities that are crucial to learning and depend on early emotional and social development include self-confidence, curiosity, self-control of strong emotions, motivation to learn, and the ability to make friends and become engaged in a social group.[17,63]

The goal of having every child ready for school is a task that encompasses all of early childhood and depends on the efforts of everyone involved in the care of the young child during his first 5 years (Box 4). Throughout these years, the health care professional plays a vital role in promoting this goal through assessing and monitoring the

- General health of the child, including vision and hearing
- Child's developmental trajectory
- Emotional health of the child and family, especially when based on the health care professional's long-term knowledge of child-family relationships
- Child's social development (both skills and difficulties)
- Specific child-based, family-based, school-based, and community-based risk factors

Health care professionals have a unique opportunity to recognize problems and, when possible, to intervene early with effective referral for specific services as well as general evaluation so as to enhance the child's readiness for learning by the start of school. Intervention services for eligible children can begin at birth and continue through age 21 years. For details on eligibility and services, refer to the US Department of Education Office of Special Education and Rehabilitative Services (**www2.ed.gov/about/offices/list/osers/osep**).[66]

Box 4
Promoting School Readiness

In assessing school readiness, the AAP recommends that health care professionals encourage the 5 Rs.[67]

1. Reading together as a daily fun family activity
2. Rhyming, playing, talking, singing, and cuddling together throughout the day
3. Routines and regular times for meals, play, and sleeping, which help children know what they can expect and what is expected from them
4. Rewards for everyday successes, particularly for effort toward worthwhile goals such as helping, realizing that praise from those closest to a child is a potent reward
5. Relationships that are reciprocal, nurturing, purposeful, and enduring, which are the foundation of a healthy early brain and child development

---

Abbreviation: AAP, American Academy of Pediatrics.

Promoting Healthy Development: Middle Childhood—5 Through 10 Years

The middle childhood years are an important transitional period during which children build on the skills developed in the various domains of early childhood in preparation for adolescence. Middle childhood is an important time for families to strengthen their ties and to help children consolidate and build on their cognitive and emotional attributes, such as communication skills, sensitivity to others, ability to form positive peer relationships, self-esteem, and independence. These attributes will help them cope with the stresses and potential risks of adolescence. Parents should be encouraged to appreciate the individual maturity level of their child. As a result, they can celebrate the child's evolving autonomy by granting new privileges. Parents who match each new entitlement with a new responsibility signal their respect for the child's growing capability to contribute to the family and the community.

Middle childhood is also a period when children become increasingly exposed to the world outside of their family through school and extended social interactions. Parents must begin to allow their child a degree of independence she had not experienced before.

Children and Youth With Special Health Care Needs

Children with special health care needs continue to define their sense of self in middle childhood and improve their ability to care for their own health. They will have emotional maturity that is appropriately reflective of their needs, developmental level, and physical challenges (Table 4). It is important to discuss family perspectives because families may have cultural beliefs and values regarding the independence of their special children. Inclusion in school and community life allows children with special health care needs to feel valued, develop friendships, and integrate their specific care needs with other aspects of their lives. Children adapt best to chronic illness when health care professionals, families, schools, and communities work together to foster their emerging independence. Child care providers and teachers can play an important supportive role and be a source of information for the parents and the children. *(For more information on this topic, see the Promoting Health for Children and Youth With Special Health Care Needs theme.)*

Domains of Development

Gross and Fine Motor Skills

Monitoring the child's growth patterns and conducting periodic physical examinations to assess growth and development are important components of health supervision. Major increases in strength and improvements in motor coordination occur during middle childhood. These changes contribute to the child's growing sense of competence in relation to her physical abilities and enhance her potential for participating in sports, dance, gymnastics, and other physical pursuits. A child's participation in sports or other physical activities can reinforce positive interaction skills and the establishment of a positive self-image that will serve the child throughout her life. Efforts to maintain good physical health and exercise patterns are important to achieving and maintaining a healthy weight. *(For more information on this topic, see the Promoting Healthy Weight theme.)*

Children develop at slightly different rates depending on their unique physical characteristics and experiences. Parental concerns are highly accurate markers for developmental problems. Parental observation of the child in relation to peers and concerns over loss of function or skills established earlier should be addressed immediately.

To support children's healthy physical development, health care professionals can work with communities to ensure that children have access to safe, well-supervised play areas; recreation centers; team sports and organized activities; parks; and schools. For children to flourish, communities must provide carefully maintained facilities to help their bodies and minds develop in a healthy way. Health care professionals can support their guidance by advocating for community facilities available to all children. *(For more information on this topic, see the Promoting Physical Activity theme.)*

Cognitive, Linguistic, and Communication Skills

Children's readiness to learn in school depends on cognitive maturation as well as their individual experiences. During middle childhood, the child moves from magical thinking to more logical thought processes. The synthesis of basic language, perception, and abstraction allows the child to read, write, and communicate thoughts of increasing complexity and creativity. Progress can appear subtle from month to month, but it is dramatic from one school year to the next. As the child's cognitive skills grow, she matures in her ability to understand the world and people around her and to function independently. Occasionally, children are impaired in their development because of learning problems, behavioral and emotional problems, or both. The health care professional can offer support by ensuring screening and evaluation for any suspected delays or problems.

The major developmental achievement of this age is self-efficacy, or the knowledge of what to do and the confidence and ability to do it. Success at school is most likely to occur when this achievement is encouraged by parents and valued by families. Families who reward children with enthusiasm and warmth for putting forth their best effort ensure their steady educational progress and prepare them to use their intelligence and knowledge productively. Through awareness of individual learning styles, including the need for necessary accommodations, parents and teachers can adapt materials and experiences to each child. School success is an important factor in the development of a child's self-esteem. In families in which parents have had unsuccessful educational experiences or have had limited education, support from health care professionals and others in the community is critical in supporting their children through the educational process.

Social and Emotional Skills

As children become increasingly independent and demonstrate initiative, they develop their own sense of personhood (Table 4). They begin to discern where they fit among their peers and in their family, school class, neighborhood, and community. When the fit is good and comfortable, children see themselves as effective and competent members of their family, group, team, school, and community. When the fit is tenuous or poor, the dissonance can be a source of distress and can predispose children to emotional illnesses with long-term consequences. *(For more information on this topic, see the Promoting Mental Health theme.)* Ongoing support for the child provides the best opportunity for acceptance and forms the basis for a strong self-worth. Support is especially important for children with special health care needs.

Children need both the freedom of personal expression and the structure of expectations and guidelines that they can understand and accept. Families should provide opportunities for the child to interact with other children in play environments without excessive adult interference. However, not all cultures accept this perspective. The health care professional and the family should discuss these issues. Most experts believe that children benefit from the experience of independent play with peers. Unfortunately, some neighborhoods or living arrangements restrict these opportunities. In addition, some children with special health care needs may need adaptive equipment or facilities to allow for inclusive play experiences. Children also need to have positive interactions with adults, reinforcing their sense of self-esteem, self-worth, and belief in their capability of personal success.

The child's sense of self evolves in a social context. Health care professionals can help families understand this dynamic and encourage specific roles for the children within the family. Parents who consciously assess their child's emotional maturity and role in the family at each birthday will appreciate the changes that have occurred subtly over time.

Table 4

Social and Emotional Development in Middle Childhood	
Topics	**Key Areas** (*Key areas in italics are especially important for children with special health care needs.*)
Self	**Self-esteem** • Experiences of success • Reasonable risk-taking behavior • Resilience and ability to handle failure • Supportive family and peer relationships
	Self-image • Body image, celebrating different body images • Prepubertal changes; initiating discussion about sexuality and reproduction; *prepubertal changes related to physical care issues*
Family	**What matters at home** • Expectation and limit setting • Family times together • Communication • Family responsibilities • Family transitions • Sibling relationships • *Caregiver relationships*
Friends	**Friendships** • Making friends, friendships with peers with and without special health care needs • Family support of friendships, *family support to have typical friendship activities, as appropriate*
School	**School** • Expectation for school performance; school performance developed and defined in IEP or Section 504 Plan • Homework • Child-teacher conflicts, building relationships with teachers • Parent-teacher communication • Ability of schools to address the needs of children from diverse backgrounds • Awareness of aggression, bullying, and being bullied • Absenteeism
Community	**Community strengths** • Community organizations • Religious groups • Cultural groups
	High-risk behaviors and environments • Substance use • Unsafe friendships • Unsafe community environments • *Particular awareness of risk-taking behaviors and unsafe environments because children may be easily abused or bullied*

Abbreviation: IEP, Individualized Education Program.

Developmental Highlights of Middle Childhood

Moral and Spiritual Development

The child's development as an individual involves an understanding of the life cycle—birth, growth and maturation, aging, and death. She becomes increasingly aware that an individual's life fits into a larger scheme of relationships among individuals, groups of people, other living creatures, and the earth itself. School-aged children become keenly interested in these topics, especially if they experience life events such as the birth of a sibling or the death of a grandparent. Children also become aware of violent death, on the highways or on street corners. When a death occurs, parents should be encouraged to discuss the loss with their children and provide assistance to children who are having difficulty with the grieving process.

As children experience these events and learn to view their personal encounters as part of a larger whole, families and communities provide an important structure. These experiences provide children with a basic foundation of value systems and encourage them to examine their personal actions in the context of those around them.

The relationship among values, competence, self-esteem, and personal responsibility needs to be modeled and affirmed by the child's parents, teachers, and communities. Parents need to help their child maintain a balance of responsibilities at school and home, time spent with family and friends, extracurricular and community activities, and personal leisure. Achieving this balance is essential for healthy development. Failures must be acknowledged, and supports might need to be offered. Transgressions may require discipline for accountability and trust to be learned. Genuine competence and self-esteem are strengthened when goals and standards are clear and the child is recognized for working hard in school, successfully completing chores and special projects, and participating in school and community activities.

Promoting Healthy Development: Adolescence—11 Through 21 Years

Adolescence is a dynamic experience, not a homogenous period of life. Adolescents differ widely in their physical, social, and emotional maturity because they enter puberty at different ages, progress at different paces, and experience different challenges in their developmental trajectories. To complicate the adolescent experience, parents also can experience changes in health, employment, geographic relocation, marital relationships, or the health of their parents and other family members. These experiences can be very formative in the lives of adolescents as they begin to understand more about effects of these changes on their family. However, although they may understand the changes intellectually, they may still lack the coping skills to deal with them.

Viewing adolescence in stages—early adolescence (11–14 years of age), middle adolescence (15–17 years of age), and late adolescence (18–21 years of age)—yields a better understanding of physical and psychological development and potential problems. Three key transitional domains (physiological, psychological, and social) can be used to chart adolescent changes and challenges (Table 5). The nature, length, and course of typical adolescent development can be viewed differently by families because cultural expectations for independence and self-sufficiency can differ. The health care professional should discern from families how they view this stage of life and note potential conflicts between the family's values and culture as opposed to those of the developing adolescent.

Youth With Special Health Care Needs

Like all youth, those with a special health care establish autonomy during adolescence, the final stage of development leading to adulthood. Limitations related to illness may further underscore physical dependence, which can limit the development of emotional independence. These adolescents may fear that their special need precludes autonomy.

Careful assessment of medical conditions, strengths, and risk-taking behaviors can allow sensitive discussions of the youth's perceived needs and goals. As with their typically developing peers, sexuality is an essential topic of concern for discussion. A goal of health supervision for adolescents with special needs is to maximize their physical development and support attainment of full emotional development and maturity. *(For more information on this topic, see the Promoting Health for Children and Youth With Special Health Care Needs theme.)*

Table 5

Domains of Adolescent Development			
	Early Adolescence (11–14 Years)	**Middle Adolescence (15–17 Years)**	**Late Adolescence (18–21 Years)**
Physiological	Onset of puberty, growth spurt, menarche (girls)	Ovulation (girls), growth spurt (boys)	Growth completed
Psychological	Concrete thought, preoccupation with rapid body changes, sexual identity, questioning independence, parental controls that remain strong	Competence in abstract and future thought, idealism, sense of invincibility or narcissism, sexual identity, beginning of cognitive capacity to provide legal consent	Future orientation; emotional independence; capacity for empathy, intimacy, and reciprocity in interpersonal relationships; self-identity; recognized as legally capable of providing consent[68]; attainment of legal age for some issues (eg, voting) but not all issues (eg, drinking alcohol)
Social	Search for same-sex peer affiliation, good parental relationships, and other adults as role models; transition to middle school, involvement in extracurricular activities; sensitivity to differences between home culture and culture of others	Beginning emotional emancipation, increased power of peer group, conflicts over parental control, interest in sexual relationships, initiation of driving, risk-taking behavior, transition to high school, involvement in extracurricular activities, possible cultural conflict as adolescent navigates between family's values and values of broader culture and peer culture	Individual over peer relationships; transition in parent-adolescent relationship, transition out of home; may begin preparation for further education, career, marriage, and parenting
Potential problems	Delayed puberty; acne; orthopedic problems; school problems; psychosomatic concerns; depression; unintended pregnancy; initiation of tobacco, alcohol, or other substance use	Experimentation with health risk behaviors (eg, sex; tobacco, alcohol, or other substance use), motor vehicle crashes, menstrual disorders, unintended pregnancy, acne, short stature (boys), conflicts with parents, overweight, physical inactivity, poor eating behaviors, eating disorders (eg, purging, binge-eating, and anorexia nervosa)	Eating disorders, depression, suicide, motor vehicle crashes, unintended pregnancy, acne; tobacco, alcohol, or other substance use disorder

Domains of Development

Gross and Fine Motor Skills

Pubertal growth brings completion of physical development. Adult height and muscle mass are attained. Increasing size and strength are accompanied by enhanced coordination of both gross and fine motor skills. The boy or girl who can barely make the high school junior varsity basketball team as a ninth grader has the agility and strength necessary for varsity performance by 10th or 11th grade. Motor development continues into the final stage of development.

Cognitive, Linguistic, and Communication Skills

Success in school contributes substantially to the adolescent's self-esteem and progress toward becoming a socially competent adult. The National Longitudinal Study for Adolescent Health[69,70] found that school performance and choice of free-time activities were the most important determinants for every risky behavior studied, regardless of socioeconomic status, race, or if living in a 1- or 2-parent household. Students who have a high academic self-concept tend to have higher academic achievement and less test anxiety, take more advanced classes, and are less likely to drop out of school. Parental involvement and expectations and participation in extracurricular activities enhance adolescent academic achievement and educational attainment. Health care professionals should encourage conversations between parents and their adolescents on these issues.

Adolescents who feel connected to their school and who have a high academic self-concept are motivated to achieve. Peer relationships also influence adolescents' attitudes. Adolescents whose peers have or are perceived to have higher educational aspirations tend to be more engaged in school and to have higher hopes for continuing their education. Adolescents who work more than 20 hours

a week tend to have a lower level of engagement in school.[71] The health care professional should encourage youth to participate in extracurricular activities. Factors such as disability and limited English proficiency can interfere with school success and need attention.

Some adolescents make the academic and social transition from middle school to high school easily. Others find this transition overwhelming, with an effect on motivation, self-esteem, and academic performance.

The Centers for Disease Control and Prevention National Center for Health Statistics estimates that among adolescents aged 12 to 17 years, nearly 10% have a learning disability.[72] Adolescents with a fair or poor health status were 6.5 times as likely to have a learning disability than adolescents with an excellent or a very good health status.[72] Students with learning disabilities can have difficulty with academics as well as social relationships. These students are more prone to depression and a lack of confidence.[73] Health care professionals should screen youth for declining grades and attendance issues, signs of learning disorders, and social adjustment concerns. With attention to adherence to specific school district policies, heath care professionals can interact with the school nurse, psychologist, counselor, or administrator to identify and address academic, social, and emotional difficulties that can interfere with school success.

Social and Emotional Skills

A consistent, supportive environment for the adolescent, with graded steps toward autonomy, is necessary to foster emotional and social well-being. This supportive environment requires the participation of the family, school, health care professional, and community and the adolescent himself.[10] Parents will struggle for a balance for their adolescent between restrictions that are designed to protect him and freedom that is intended to enhance growth. The adolescent will struggle for this balance too. Parental difficulty with this balance may be recognized by excess anxiety regarding appropriate adolescent progress in separation and individuation or by apparent over-involvement in their adolescent's planning and decision-making. Discussion with parents may be indicated.

The emotional well-being of adolescents is tied to their sense of self-esteem. High self-esteem is generally associated with feelings of life satisfaction and a sense of control over one's life, whereas low self-esteem is correlated with lower reports of happiness and higher reports of feeling as if one is not in control of one's life. Adolescents who demonstrate good social and problem-solving skills also usually have enhanced self-esteem because these skills increase their sense of control over their world. This asset is essential in deriving the ability to handle stress and cope with challenging situations.

Another important developmental milestone that is critical to emotional well-being is the adolescent's growing sense of self. Long hours spent talking, grooming, being alone, and rushing to be part of a group—any group—are all part of the adolescent's search for a conception of self. Intelligence, in the narrow sense of the term, also is significant to the cognitive self. During adolescence, the individual has to learn the accumulated wisdom of society. As the adolescent becomes facile in using concepts and abstractions, he begins to combine new ideas in new ways to arrive at creative solutions.

Normal fluctuations of mood now are the adolescent's responsibility. With increasing autonomy, he may become unwilling to share feelings and, to a point, unconsciously seek to avoid dependence on family for mood modulation. Like other skills he acquires, managing feelings of sadness and anxiety requires guidance, practice, and experience.

During the course of adolescence, the increasingly autonomous and socially competent youth finds his place in family and community. Social competence can be defined as "the ability to achieve personal goals in social interaction while at the same time maintaining positive relationships with others over time and across situations."[74] The specific behaviors that characterize social competence will vary with the situation in which the adolescent is functioning. Socially competent youth are able to decode and interpret social cues and consider alternative responses along with their consequences.

To function in an adult world, a youth must become aware of his relations to others and learn the personal effect of relationships on his daily activities. Accordingly, he must appreciate the effects of his actions toward others if relationships are to be mature and reciprocal. Understanding how others might interpret a situation, recognizing another's predicament, and comfortably appreciating another's feelings are new and important experiences. Empathy must be achieved for healthy adult relationships to flourish.

The adolescent's social and emotional skills also are influenced by the young adult's growing interactions with the wider community through travel, higher education, volunteer activities, or structured job experiences. These activities can help adolescents realize that they have meaningful roles and can contribute productively to society. Through these activities, youth learn the importance of general adherence to rules and authority. External mandates are internalized in an appreciation of right or wrong and consequences.

PROMOTING HEALTHY DEVELOPMENT

109

Developmental Highlights of Adolescence

Assets

Health advocates have begun to look at the family and community factors that promote healthy development. This asset model, or strength-based approach, provides a broader perspective on adolescent development than the more traditional deficit model, which looks at the problems experienced by adolescents and develops preventive interventions (Table 6). The asset model reinforces health-promoting interactions or social involvement (eg, good parent-adolescent communication and participation in extracurricular activities[75]) and assists adolescents and their parents in setting goals to achieve healthy development.

Research demonstrates the value of parental involvement and quality parent-adolescent communication on healthy adolescent development.[76-78] Adolescents whose parents are authoritative, rather than authoritarian or passive, and who are involved in extracurricular and community activities appear to progress through adolescence with relatively little turmoil.[79]

Models of Care

On-site integrated health services in the schools—with referrals to health care professionals and community agencies and mental health centers for supplementary services—are an increasingly prevalent model for delivery of adolescent health care. In some situations, the school-based health center is the medical home for the youth enrolled in the center. School-based health centers can be especially effective in ensuring immunizations, promoting sports safety, and providing access for students with special health care needs. All services and programs should work to improve communication between school and home so parents stay involved in their adolescents' lives away from home and learn effective strategies to deal with some of the challenges that their adolescents face.

Health care professionals might ask young people how they learn about healthy living. Health promotion programs in schools help adolescents establish good health habits and avoid those that can lead to morbidity and mortality. Health promotion curricula can include family life education and social skills training, as well as information on pregnancy prevention, abstinence, conflict resolution, healthy nutrition and physical activity practices, and avoidance of unhealthy habits such as the use of tobacco products, alcohol, or other drugs. Referrals to appropriate, culturally respectful, and accessible community resources also help adolescents learn about and address mental health concerns, nutrition and physical health, and sexual health issues. When young people decide to seek assistance beyond their family, those resources should provide appropriate confidential counseling and support to them in making healthy choices while encouraging good communication with parents and family.

Table 6

Comparison of Asset and Deficit Models	
Asset Model	**Deficit Model**
• Positive family environment	• Abuse or neglect
• Relationships with caring adults	• Witness to domestic violence
• Religious and spiritual anchors	• Family discord and divorce
• Involvement in school, faith-based organization, or community	• Parents with poor health habits
• Accessible recreational opportunities	• Unsafe schools
	• Unsafe neighborhood

References

1. Glascoe FP, Marks KP. Detecting children with developmental-behavioral problems: the value of collaborating with parents. *Psychol Test Assess Model.* 2011;53(2):258-279

2. American Academy of Pediatrics Council on Children With Disabilities, Section on Developmental Behavioral Pediatrics, Bright Futures Steering Committee, Medical Home Initiatives for Children With Special Needs Project Advisory Committee. Identifying infants and young children with developmental disorders in the medical home: an algorithm for developmental surveillance and screening. *Pediatrics.* 2006;118(1):405-420

3. Paul H. Brookes Publishing Company. *Ages and Stages Questionaires.* http://agesandstages.com. Accessed November 8, 2016

4. Glascoe FP. PEDStest.com Web site. http://www.pedstest.com/default.aspx. Accessed November 8, 2016

5. Floating Hospital for Children at Tufts Medical Center. *The Survey of Well-being of Young Children.* https://sites.google.com/site/swyc2016. Accessed November 8, 2016

6. Robins D, Fein D, Barton M. M-CHAT.org Web site. https://m-chat.org. Accessed November 8, 2016

7. Jellinek M, Patel BP, Froehle MC, eds. *Bright Futures in Practice: Mental Health, Volume II, Toolkit.* Arlington, VA: National Center for Education in Maternal and Child Health; 2002

8. The CRAFFT Screening Tool. Center for Adolescent Substance Abuse Research Web site. http://www.childrenshospital.org/ceasar/crafft. Accessed September 16, 2016

9. Knight JR, Sherritt L, Shrier LA, Harris SK, Chang G. Validity of the CRAFFT substance abuse screening test among adolescent clinic patients. *Arch Pediatr Adolesc Med.* 2002;156(6):607-614

10. Harper Browne C. *Youth Thrive: Advancing Healthy Adolescent Development and Well-Being.* Washington, DC: Center for the Study of Social Policy; 2014. http://www.cssp.org/reform/child-welfare/youth-thrive/2014/Youth-Thrive_Advancing-Healthy-Adolescent-Development-and-Well-Being.pdf. Accessed November 8, 2016

11. Benson PL, Scales PC, Syvertsen AK. The contribution of the developmental assets framework to positive youth development theory and practice. *Adv Child Dev Behav.* 2011;41:197-230

12. Scales PC, Benson PL, Roehlkepartain EC, Sesma A Jr, van Dulmen M. The role of developmental assets in predicting academic achievement: a longitudinal study. *J Adolesc.* 2006;29(5):691-708

13. Murphey DA, Lamonda KH, Carney JK, Duncan P. Relationships of a brief measure of youth assets to health-promoting and risk behaviors. *J Adolesc Health.* 2004;34(3):184-191

14. Lerner RM, Lerner JV. *The Positive Development of Youth: Report of the Findings from the First Seven Years of the 4-H Study of Positive Youth Development.* Boston, MA: Tufts University; 2011. http://ase.tufts.edu/iaryd/documents/4hpydstudywave7.pdf. Accessed November 8, 2016

15. Fine A, Large R. *A Conceptual Framework for Adolescent Health: A Collaborative Project of the Association of Maternal and Child Health Programs and the National Network of State Adolescent Health Coordinators.* Washington, DC: Association of Maternal and Child Health Programs; 2005. http://www.amchp.org/programsandtopics/AdolescentHealth/Documents/conc-framework.pdf. Accessed November 8, 2016

16. Duncan PM, Garcia AC, Frankowski BL, et al. Inspiring healthy adolescent choices: a rationale for and guide to strength promotion in primary care. *J Adolesc Health.* 2007;41(6):525-535

17. Shonkoff JP, Phillips DA, eds. *From Neurons to Neighborhoods: The Science of Early Childhood Development.* Washington, DC: National Academy Press; 2000

18. American Academy of Pediatrics Section on Breastfeeding. Breastfeeding and the use of human milk. *Pediatrics.* 2012;129(3):e827-e841

19. Moore ER, Anderson GC, Bergman N, Dowswell T. Early skin-to-skin contact for mothers and their healthy newborn infants. *Cochrane Database Syst Rev.* 2012;(5):CD003519

20. US Department of Education Office of Special Education and Rehabilitative Services. Early intervention program for infants and toddlers with disabilities. Final regulations. *Fed Regist.* 2011;76(188):60140-60309

21. Davies D. *Child Development: A Practitioner's Guide.* 3rd ed. New York, NY: The Guilford Press; 2011

22. Weinberger DR, Elvevag B, Giedd JN. *The Adolescent Brain: A Work in Progress.* Washington, DC: The National Campaign to Prevent Teen Pregnancy; 2005. http://web.calstatela.edu/faculty/dherz/Teenagebrain.workinprogress.pdf. Accessed November 8, 2016

23. US Environmental Protection Agency. *America's Children and the Environment.* 3rd ed. Washington, DC: US Environmental Protection Agency; 2013. http://www.epa.gov/ace. Accessed November 8, 2016

24. Noritz GH, Murphy NA; American Academy of Pediatrics Neuromotor Screening Expert Panel. Motor delays: early identification and evaluation. *Pediatrics.* 2013;131(6):e2016-e2017

25. American Academy of Pediatrics Task Force on Sudden Infant Death Syndrome. SIDS and other sleep-related infant deaths: updated 2016 recommendations for a safe infant sleeping environment. *Pediatrics.* 2016;138(5):e20162938

26. Gorski PA. Contemporary pediatric practice: in support of infant mental health (imaging and imagining). *Infant Ment Health J.* 2001;22(1-2):188-200

27. Bhatia P, Mintz S, Hecht BF, Deavenport A, Kuo AA. Early identification of young children with hearing loss in federally qualified health centers. *J Dev Behav Pediatr.* 2013;34(1):15-21

28. American Academy of Audiology Subcommittee on Childhood Hearing Screening. Childhood Hearing Screening Guidelines. Centers for Disease Control and Prevention Web site. http://www.cdc.gov/ncbddd/hearingloss/documents/AAA_Childhood%20Hearing%20Guidelines_2011.pdf. Published September 2011. Accessed November 8, 2016

29. Foust T, Eiserman W, Shisler L, Geroso A. Using otoacoustic emissions to screen young children for hearing loss in primary care settings. *Pediatrics.* 2013;132(1):118-123

30. Miller JM, Lessin HR; American Academy of Pediatrics Section on Ophthalmology, Committee on Practice and Ambulatory Medicine; American Academy of Ophthalmology; American Association for Pediatric Ophthalmology and Strabismus; American Association of Certified Orthoptists. Instrument-based pediatric vision screening policy statement. *Pediatrics.* 2012;130(5):983-986

31. Tamis-LeMonda CS, Kuchirko Y, Song L. Why is infant language learning facilitated by parental responsiveness? *Curr Dir Psychol Sci.* 2014;23(2):121-126

32. Lever R, Sénéchal M. Discussing stories: on how a dialogic reading intervention improves kindergartners' oral narrative construction. *J Exp Child Psychol.* 2011;108(1):1-24

PROMOTING HEALTHY DEVELOPMENT

33. Jordan AB, Robinson TN. Children, television viewing, and weight status: summary and recommendations from an expert panel meeting. *Ann Am Acad Pol Soc Sci.* 2008;615(1):119-132

34. Mistry KB, Minkovitz CS, Strobino DM, Borzekowski DL. Children's television exposure and behavioral and social outcomes at 5.5 years: does timing of exposure matter? *Pediatrics.* 2007;120(4):762-769

35. Zuckerman B. Promoting early literacy in pediatric practice: twenty years of Reach Out and Read. *Pediatrics.* 2009;124(6):1660-1665

36. Zuckerman B, Khandekar A. Reach Out and Read: evidence based approach to promoting early child development. *Curr Opin Pediatr.* 2010;22(4):539-544

37. Sharif I, Rieber S, Ozuah PO. Exposure to Reach Out and Read and vocabulary outcomes in inner city preschoolers [published correction appears in *J Natl Med Assoc.* 2002;94(9):following table of contents]. *J Natl Med Assoc.* 2002;94(3):171-177

38. Weitzman CC, Roy L, Walls T, Tomlin R. More evidence for Reach Out and Read: a home-based study. *Pediatrics.* 2004;113(5):1248-1253

39. Needlman R, Toker KH, Dreyer BP, Klass P, Mendelsohn AL. Effectiveness of a primary care intervention to support reading aloud: a multicenter evaluation. *Ambul Pediatr.* 2005;5(4):209-215

40. Needlman R, Silverstein M. Pediatric interventions to support reading aloud: how good is the evidence? *J Dev Behav Pediatr.* 2004;25(5):352-363

41. High PC, Klass P; American Academy of Pediatrics Council on Early Childhood. Literacy promotion: an essential component of primary care pediatric practice. *Pediatrics.* 2014;134(2):404-409

42. Reach Out and Read Web site. http://www.reachoutandread.org. Accessed November 9, 2016

43. National Association for the Education of Young Children Web site. http://www.naeyc.org. Accessed November 9, 2016

44. American Academy of Pediatrics. Healthy Child Care America Web site. http://www.healthychildcare.org. Accessed November 9, 2016

45. Parents and Families. Child Care Aware America Web site. http://www.childcareaware.org/parents-and-guardians. Accessed November 9, 2016

46. Choosing Child Care. Child Care Aware America Web site. http://childcareaware.org/parents-and-guardians/child-care-101/choosing-child-care. Accessed November 9, 2016

47. Adolph KE, Berger SE. Motor development. In: Damon W, Lerner RM, Kuhn D, Siegler R, eds. *Handbook of Child Psychology.* 6th ed. Hoboken, NJ: John Wiley & Sons; 2006:161-213. *Cognition, Perception, and Language;* vol 2

48. Perinatal Nursing Education: Understanding the Behavior of Term Infants. States of the Term Newborn. March of Dimes Web site. http://www.marchofdimes.org/nursing/modnemedia/othermedia/states.pdf. Accessed November 9, 2016

49. Goodman SH, Rouse MH, Connell AM, Broth MR, Hall CM, Heyward D. Maternal depression and child psychopathology: a meta-analytic review. *Clin Child Fam Psychol Rev.* 2011;14(1):1-27

50. Raposa E, Hammen C, Brennan P, Najman J. The long-term effects of maternal depression: early childhood physical health as a pathway to offspring depression. *J Adolesc Health.* 2014;54(1):88-93

51. Tomasello M. The ontogeny of cultural learning. *Curr Opin Psychol.* 2016;8:1-4

52. McClelland MM, Cameron CE. Self-regulation in early childhood: improving conceptual clarity and developing ecologically valid measures. *Child Dev Perspect.* 2012;6(2):136-142

53. Ramakrishnan K. Evaluation and treatment of enuresis. *Am Fam Physician.* 2008;78(4):489-496

54. Alejandro-Wright MN. The child's conception of racial classification: a socio-cognitive developmental model. In: Spencer MB, Brookins GK, Allen WR, eds. *Beginnings: The Social and Affective Development of Black Children.* Hillsdale, NJ: Lawrence Erlbaum Associates; 1985:185-200

55. American Academy of Pediatrics Committee on Psychosocial Aspects of Child and Family Health. Guidance for effective discipline [published correction appears in *Pediatrics.* 1998;102(2 pt 1):433]. *Pediatrics.* 1998;101(4 pt 1):723-728

56. American Academy of Pediatrics. HealthyChildren.org Web site. https://healthychildren.org. Accessed November 9, 2016

57. Podhajski B, Nathan J. A pathway to reading success: building blocks for literacy. *N Engl Read Assoc J.* 2005;41(2):24

58. Glassy D, Romano J; American Academy of Pediatrics Committee on Early Childhood, Adoption, and Dependent Care. Selecting appropriate toys for young children: the pediatrician's role. *Pediatrics.* 2003;111(4 pt 1):911-913

59. US Department of Health and Human Services, Health Resources and Services Administration, Maternal and Child Health Bureau. *Child Health USA 2014.* Rockville, MD: US Department of Health and Human Services; 2015. http://www.mchb.hrsa.gov/chusa14/dl/chusa14.pdf. Accessed November 9, 2016

60. Laughlin L. Who's Minding the Kids? Child Care Arrangements: Spring 2011. Washington, DC: US Census Bureau; 2013. Publication P70-135. https://www.census.gov/content/dam/Census/library/publications/2013/demo/p70-135.pdf. Accessed November 9, 2016

61. Fisher B, Hanson A, Raden T. *Start Early to Build A Healthy Future: The Research Linking Early Learning and Health.* Chicago, IL: Ounce of Prevention Fund; 2014. http://www.theounce.org/pubs/Ounce-Health-Paper-2016.pdf. Accessed November 9, 2016

62. Sabol TJ, Pianta RC. Patterns of school readiness forecast achievement and socioemotional development at the end of elementary school. *Child Dev.* 2012;83(1):282-299

63. Blair C, Raver CC. School readiness and self-regulation: a developmental psychobiological approach. *Annu Rev Psychol.* 2015;66:711-731

64. Rimm-Kaufman SE, Pianta RC, Cox MJ. Teachers' judgments of problems in the transition to kindergarten. *Early Child Res Q.* 2000;15(2):147-166

65. Garcia E. *Inequalities at the Starting Gate: Cognitive and Noncognitive Skills Gaps between 2010–2011 Kindergarten Classmates.* Washington, DC: Economic Policy Institute; 2015. http://www.epi.org/files/pdf/85032c.pdf. Accessed November 9, 2016

66. US Department of Education Office of Special Education and Rehabilitative Services Web site. http://www2.ed.gov/about/offices/list/osers/osep/index.html. Accessed November 9, 2016

67. High PC; American Academy of Pediatrics Committee on Early Childhood, Adoption, and Dependent Care; Council on School Health. School readiness. *Pediatrics.* 2008;121(4):e1008-e1015

68. English A, Bass L, Boyle AD, Eshragh F. *State Minor Consent Laws: A Summary.* 3rd ed. Chapel Hill, NC: Center for Adolescent Health & the Law; 2010

69. Resnick MD, Bearman PS, Blum RW, et al. Protecting adolescents from harm. Findings from the National Longitudinal Study on Adolescent Health. *JAMA.* 1997;278(10):823-832

70. Add Health. National Longitudinal Study of Adolescent to Adult Health Web site. http://www.cpc.unc.edu/projects/addhealth. Accessed November 9, 2016

71. Staff J, Schulenberg JE, Bachman JG. Adolescent work intensity, school performance, and academic engagement. *Sociol Educ.* 2010;83(3):183-200

72. Bloom B, Jones LI, Freeman G. Summary health statistics for U.S. children: National Health Interview Survey, 2012. *Vital Health Stat 10.* 2013;(258):1-81

73. Alesi M, Rappo G, Pepi A. Depression, anxiety at school and self-esteem in children with learning disabilities. *J Psychol Abnorm Child.* 2014;3:3

74. Rubin KH, Rose-Krasnor L. Interpersonal problem solving and social competence in children. In: Van Hasselt VB, Hersen M, eds. *Handbook of Social Development: A Lifespan Perspective.* New York, NY: Springer; 1992:283-323

75. Fredricks JA, Eccles JS. Extracurricular involvement and adolescent adjustment: impact of duration, number of activities, and breadth of participation. *Appl Dev Sci.* 2006;10(3):132-146

76. Viner RM, Ozer EM, Denny S, et al. Adolescence and the social determinants of health. *Lancet.* 2012;379(9826):1641-1652

77. Eisenberg ME, Sieving RE, Bearinger LH, Swain C, Resnick MD. Parents' communication with adolescents about sexual behavior: a missed opportunity for prevention? *J Youth Adolesc.* 2006;35(6):893-902

78. DeVore ER, Ginsburg KR. The protective effects of good parenting on adolescents. *Curr Opin Pediatr.* 2005;17(4):460-465

79. Huver RM, Otten R, de Vries H, Engels RC. Personality and parenting style in parents of adolescents. *J Adolesc.* 2010;33(3):395-402

Promoting Mental Health

Establishing mental health and emotional well-being is arguably a core task for developing children and adolescents and those who care for them. Mental health is not merely the absence of mental disorder but is composed of social, emotional, and behavioral health and wellness and should be considered in the same context as physical health. Because cultures may differ in their conceptions of mental health, it is important for the health care professional to learn about family members' perceptions of a mentally healthy individual and their goals for raising children. In their shared work to raise a child, parents, family, community, and professionals commit to fostering the development of that child's sense of connectedness, self-worth and joyfulness, intellectual growth, and mental health. Shonkoff and Phillips[1] describe that marvelous process of the child's development of mental health in their book *From Neurons to Neighborhoods.* Each Bright Futures Health Supervision Visit addresses the physical and mental health of the child or adolescent. This theme highlights opportunities for promoting mental health in every child, including specific suggestions for each age and stage of development.

Mental health can be compromised at many critical times in development, beginning prenatally with the mental health of the mother, through infancy with the importance of attachments, through early childhood, and beyond. The health care professional, therefore, is challenged to promote mental health through activities that are aimed at prevention, risk assessment, and diagnosis and to offer an array of appropriate interventions. Common risk factors for child behavioral and mental health problems include[2-4]

- Prenatal risk factors
  - Developmental trauma
  - Alcohol exposure
  - Drug exposure
  - Lead exposure
  - Environmental toxins
- Genetic risk factors (eg, congenital developmental disability)
- Chronic medical illness or developmental disability
- Social and environmental risk factors
  - Poverty or homelessness
  - Exposure to intimate partner violence (IPV) or child maltreatment
  - Foster care placement
  - Disasters or other life trauma
- Family risk factors
  - Parental depression and social isolation
  - Bereavement
  - Separation or divorce
  - Chronic physical illness or mental disorder or death involving family members
  - Substance misuse by a family member
  - Incarceration of a family member
  - Military service of a family member
- Skills deficiencies
  - Lack of parenting knowledge or performance deficits
  - Child social skills deficits
  - School failure and learning problem or disability

PROMOTING MENTAL HEALTH

Common challenges to child, adolescent, and family mental health are further described in this theme by age of highest prevalence. *(For additional discussions on these issues, see the Promoting Lifelong Health for Families and Communities theme.)*

In 2004, the American Academy of Pediatrics (AAP) convened a Task Force on Mental Health to help health care professionals enhance the mental health care they provide.[5] The goals of this task force were to build health care professional skills and enhance services through systems change in clinical practice and in the family's community of care. The task force developed a report for health care professionals, which includes 2 algorithms for care, and a companion toolkit.[6] The algorithms are (1) "Promoting Social-Emotional Health, Identifying Mental Health and Substance Use Concerns, Engaging the Family, and Providing Early Intervention in Primary Care" and (2) "Assessment and Care of Children With Identified Social-Emotional, Mental Health, or Substance Abuse Concerns, Ages 0 to 21 Years." The AAP has compiled a collection of mental health competencies and encourages health care professionals to integrate mental health into primary care and specialty care practice.[7]

Prevalence and Trends in Mental Health Problems Among Children and Adolescents

One-half of all the lifetime cases of mental disorder begin by age 14 years, and three-quarters are apparent by age 24.[8] Therefore, most mental health problems are chronic, with roots of origin during youth. For example, the median age of onset for anxiety and impulse control disorders is about age 11.[8] One in 5 teens experiences significant symptoms of emotional distress, and nearly 1 in 10 is emotionally impaired, with the most common disorders including depression, anxiety disorders, attention-deficit/hyperactivity disorder (ADHD),

and substance use disorders.[9] Among vulnerable populations of youth, such as those involved in the juvenile justice system, high rates of psychiatric disorders (66% of boys and 74% of girls) exist.[10] Unfortunately, under-detection of mental health problems in pediatric practice has been well-documented and recognized,[11,12] and even among youth who have been identified, many do not seek, find, or receive treatment services.[13,14]

Screening and Referral

Primary care professionals meet with children and families at regular intervals, and this frequent access to a primary care medical home is more available than access to specific mental health services. Primary care professionals are therefore ideally situated to begin the process of identifying children with problem behaviors that might indicate mental disorders, as well as identifying parents and caregivers struggling with mental health concerns that may affect the child. Consistent with the US Preventive Services Task Force (USPSTF) recommendation, screening for depression among adolescents in primary care is now included in the *Bright Futures: Guidelines for Health Supervision of Infants, Children, and Adolescents* Adolescence Visits.[15] Building a solid collaboration among the health care professional and other service providers (eg, psychiatrists, psychologists, social workers, and other therapists) and agencies (eg, schools, mental health agencies, state departments of health, mentoring groups, agencies serving children and youth with special health care needs, and child protective services) improves the effectiveness of support for children and, ultimately, the possibilities of positive outcomes for the children. *(For more information on this topic, see the Promoting Lifelong Health for Families and Communities theme.)* This need is illustrated by a study showing that although psychosocial problems identified in pediatric offices increased from 6.8% to 18.7% in the 17-year period of 1979–1996,[16] the National Institute for Health

Care Management estimates that 75% of children diagnosed as having mental disorders are treated by primary care professionals.[17] These professionals often have limited access to mental health professionals with appropriate training and skills to assist them with behavior screening, treatment, and referral issues.[18] Collaborative or integrated mental health care in pediatric practice offers improved access to mental health care and improved outcomes.[19]

Pediatric behavioral, developmental, and mental health issues are more common than childhood cancers, cardiac problems, and renal problems combined. However, research has repeatedly shown that primary care professionals recognize less than 30% of children with substantial dysfunction.[20] This lack of recognition is caused by the necessary brevity of pediatric appointments and stigma associated with mental health concerns, which result in hesitancy to bring up subject areas for which no quick fix exists. However, in some cases, the primary care professional can assess the child's problem and provide appropriate and successful intervention. The health care professional should try to determine whether the nature of the problem falls within her areas of interest and expertise before offering interventions. In other instances, when a problem is identified outside the realm of her expertise, the health care professional must be able to refer the family to experts who can provide a complete evaluation and treatment plan.

Existing screening tools can help the health care professional recognize possible mental health concerns. Screening for postpartum depression has been recommended by the USPSTF and the AAP. Universal screening for postpartum depression is now recommended at the 1 Month through 6 Month Visits. [21,22]

One of the most efficient ways for health care professionals to improve the recognition and treatment of psychosocial problems in children

and adolescents is by using a mental health screening test, such as the 35-item *Pediatric Symptom Checklist* (*PSC*)[23] or the more brief *PSC-17*,[24] which can be completed in the waiting room by a parent. A positive score on the *PSC* suggests the need for further evaluation. *The Survey of Well-being of Young Children* (known as *SWYC*) screens child development from birth to age 5 by assessing 3 domains of psychosocial health: the developmental domain, the social and emotional domain, and the family context.[25] *The Patient Health Questionnaire-2* (*PHQ-2*) has been successfully used to screen for adolescent depression in clinical settings with adequate sensitivity and specificity.[26] All of these tools are available in the public domain. All tools should be administered in the family's primary language.

Screening does not provide a diagnosis for a mental disorder, however. Screening indicates the severity of symptoms, assesses the severity within a given time period, and provides a way to begin a conversation about mental health issues. Health care professionals must be adept at identifying mental health concerns and determining whether they are leading to impaired functioning at home, at school, with peers, or in the community. Providing education to the patient and parent about mental disorders, symptoms, causes, and treatments is an important first step in helping the family take charge of its management if a disorder exists. It also helps the family avoid placing blame and allows for reasonable expectations to be set.

Pediatric health care professionals can provide high-quality care for mental disorders[27] by providing in-office treatment, comanaging care with a mental health professional, or referring the patient. Training and past experience will guide the decision to treat or refer, but time constraints to provide ongoing management also are a consideration.[28] The presence of a trusting relationship between the child, adolescent, or parent and the health care professional often predicts a successful

PROMOTING MENTAL HEALTH

treatment or referral process. Pediatric health care professionals in primary care should assess their ability to manage mild, moderate, and severe emotional problems with or without consultation. The level of health care professional competence, clinical need, and availability of mental health referral should help dictate the conditions for referral. Referral may be appropriate in the following situations:

- Emotional dysfunction is evident in more than one of the following critical areas of the child's or adolescent's life: home, school, peers, activities, and mood.
- The patient is acutely suicidal or has signs of psychosis.
- Diagnostic uncertainty exists.
- The patient has not responded to treatment.
- The parent requests referral.
- An adolescent's behavior creates discomfort for the health care professional, potentially precluding an objective evaluation (eg, adolescents with acting-out or seductive behaviors).
- The patient, or his family, has a social relationship with the treating health care professional; in some instances, the nature of the mental or behavioral health problem indicates or demands referral.

When the possibility of referral is brought up early in the process, acceptance of mental health treatment may be better. The health care professional should discuss with the family members their views on referral to a mental health professional and acknowledge that stigma often is associated with such referral. Understanding how the family's culture can affect the view of treatment for mental health issues and knowing resources that will support those views can greatly enhance the success of the referral process. The health care professional should learn how the family's culture views mental wellness and emotional and behavioral problems and should connect the family with culturally appropriate services. Even after a patient

is referred to a mental health professional, ongoing involvement by and surveillance of symptoms by the primary health care professional are of value.

Children and Youth With Special Health Care Needs

Children and adolescents with chronic health conditions require special consideration concerning their mental health needs. Many syndromes that are primarily neurologic, genetic, or developmental in nature include mental health symptoms or conditions. Other chronic health conditions share comorbidity with mental health diagnoses. Attention to these components of the child's or adolescent's special health care need is a basic and essential part of care.

In addition, any chronic health condition brings stressors to both the child and family. These stressors, while secondary to the medical problem, are essential components of the child's health. Health care professionals who care for children and youth with special health care needs must be alert to complications of anxiety, depression, or problems of adjustment. The medical home model of care brings attention to and offers treatments for these comorbidities.[29] *(For more information on this topic, see the Promoting Health for Children and Youth With Special Health Care Needs theme.)*

Promoting Mental Health and Emotional Well-being: Infancy—Birth Through 11 Months

Infant mental health is the flourishing of a baby's capacity for warm connection with his parents and caregivers. The interaction between parent and infant is central to the infant's physical, cognitive, social, and emotional development, as well as to his self-regulation abilities. The infant brings his strengths of temperamental style, the ability to engage, health, and vigor to this interaction.

The ability of the parents to respond well is determined by their own temperament, expectations, and "goodness of fit" with their child's temperament. Life stresses, past experiences with children, and their own experiences of being nurtured in childhood also influence parenting skills. Their perceptions of the infant also can color the interaction. These perceptions derive from their own expectations, needs, and desires, as well as from the projection of other people's characteristics onto the child.

The infant's emotions may be affected by the emotional and physical health of the caregiver.[21] Depression and anxiety are common in many mothers and fathers of infants and can seriously impair the baby's emotional and even physical well-being because of neglect of the infant's needs and lack of responsiveness to the infant's engagement cues. Parental substance use can have similar effects. Health supervision for the child must therefore include monitoring the emotional health of the parents or primary caregivers.

Patterns of Attachment

Attachment describes the process of interrelation between a child and his parent and is central to healthy mental and emotional development. Attachment is influenced by parental, child-related, and environmental factors. Health care professionals can teach parents the importance of the quality of their interaction with their infant and the effect of attachment on the development of the child's sense of self-worth, comfort, and trust.

Health care professionals should observe the attachment style and pattern during clinical encounters with infants and parents, although providers may not be able to observe the different attachment styles in short clinical encounters, as some children will be fearful. They should give anticipatory guidance to assist families in enhancing secure development.

Three patterns of attachment have been described by Bowlby[30] and many others in infants and young children—secure attachment, insecure and avoidant attachment, and insecure attachment characterized by ambivalence and resistance (Box 1). Increasing

Box 1
Attachment Patterns[31]

Secure Attachment
Parent: Is sensitive, responsive, and available.
Child: Feels valued and worthwhile; has a secure base; feels effective; feels able to explore and master, knowing that parent is available; and becomes autonomous. During visit, engages with health care professional and seeks and receives reassurance and comfort from parent.

Insecure and Avoidant Attachment
Parent: Is insensitive to child's cues, avoids contact, and rejects.
Child: Feels no one is there for him, cannot rely on adults to get needs met, feels he will be rejected if needs for attachment and closeness are shown and therefore asks for little to maintain some connection, and learns not to recognize his own need for closeness and connectedness. During visit, may act fearful but also angry with the parent, may seek contact but then arch away and struggle, and also may act extremely helpless or sad but not seek comfort and protection.

Insecure Attachment Characterized by Ambivalence and Resistance
Parent: Shows inconsistent patterns of care, is unpredictable, may be excessively close or intrusive but then push away. This pattern is seen frequently with depressed caregiver.
Child: Feels he should keep adult engaged because he never knows when he will get attention back and is anxious, dependent, and clingy.

evidence points to the permanent positive effect of secure attachment and the persisting negative effects of insecure patterns of attachment on development.

Challenges to the Development of Mental Health

Infant Well-being

Infant well-being and early brain development are discussed in the *Promoting Lifelong Health for Families and Communities theme.* Signs of possible problems in emotional well-being in infants include

- Poor eye contact
- Lack of brightening on seeing parent
- Lack of smiling with parent or other engaging adult
- Lack of vocalizations
- Not quieting with parent's voice
- Not turning to sound of parent's voice
- Extremely low activity level or tone
- Lack of mouthing to explore objects
- Excessive irritability with difficulty in calming
- Sad or somber facial expression (evident by 3 months of age)
- Wariness (evident by 4 months of age; precursor to fear, which is evident by 9 months of age)
- Dysregulation in sleep
- Physical dysregulation (eg, vomiting or diarrhea)
- Poor weight gain

If the infant appears to have problems with emotional development, the health care professional should determine the degree to which the parents may be experiencing depression, grief, anxiety, post-traumatic stress disorder (PTSD), other significant stress, substance use, or IPV. A mental health professional or a pediatric health care professional who is skilled in developmental behavior should then evaluate the parent-child interaction.

Child Maltreatment and Neglect

Child maltreatment or abuse can occur in any family. Without identification and intervention, unchecked acute and chronic stressors in a household can lead to child neglect or abuse.

Many factors are associated with child maltreatment, including

- A child who is perceived by parents to be demanding or difficult to satisfy
- An infant who is diagnosed as having a chronic illness or disability
- A family who is socially isolated, without community support
- Mental health needs in one or both parents that have not been diagnosed and treated
- Parental alcohol and substance misuse
- A parent with career difficulties, who may see the newborn as an impediment or burden
- Family economic hardship or poverty in combination with other factors

Infants and toddlers are at higher risk for abuse and neglect than are older children. Infants and children who are younger than 3 years account for more than a quarter of all maltreated children. Nearly three-quarters of child abuse fatalities occur before age 3, and maltreated infants younger than 1 year are 3 times more likely to die than those who pass their first birthday.[32] A disproportionate number of these children are in families that live in poverty and experience familial disruption. Their families live in high-risk environments and frequently confront substance use, mental or physical illness, family violence, or inadequate living conditions. More than three-quarters of reports to child protective services are for child neglect, yet this often can go undetected because the physical and emotional findings can be subtle.[32]

Health care professionals should learn to recognize infants who are being abused or are at risk for abuse by a parent or other member of the household. If abuse is suspected, the health care professional should ask direct questions in a respectful way to attempt to determine whether any kind of abuse might be occurring. Any unexplained bruises or other signs of abuse should be thoroughly investigated. *Suspected* cases of child abuse or neglect *must* be reported to the appropriate child welfare agency by law in all states and US territories. Health care professionals are mandated reporters and should err on the side of bringing concerns to authorities who will investigate the issues. It is best practice to share concerns with the family and to explain to the family the legal obligation to report. In general, reporting without the family's knowledge is counterproductive because it can lead the family to further distrust the health care system. However, concerns of imminent harm to the child, the potential for flight, or genuine fears for personal safety may require involving law enforcement and social service without informing the family and other caregivers.

Abuse and neglect have long-term effects on brain development and increase the likelihood of behavioral disorders in the child. The earlier in life the child is subjected to neglect or physical or emotional abuse and the longer the abuse continues, the greater the risk to his emotional and behavioral development. Recognizing the risk of maltreatment to the child's healthy physical and mental development is as vital as recognizing a nutritional deficiency or toxin exposure. Physical and mental abuse during the first few years of a child's life can cause the development of hypervigilance and fear. An infant who is under chronic stress can respond with apathy, poor feeding, withdrawal, and failure to thrive. When the infant is under acute threat, the typical "fight" response to stress can change from crying to tantrums, aggressive behaviors, or inattention and withdrawal. The child can become psychologically disengaged, leading to detachment and apathy. This response, in turn, has an effect on the child's ability to form healthy trusting relationships with adults and peers. Studies show that, as children get older, those who have been abused or neglected are more likely to perform poorly in school, commit crimes, and experience emotional problems, sexual problems, alcohol or substance use, and impaired physical health.[33-35]

Health care professionals can play an important role in preventing child maltreatment. They can help strengthen families and promote safe, stable, nurturing relationships. Health care professionals also can advocate for positive behavioral interventions and supports in schools.[36] Referring parents to home visiting programs, early care and education programs, or parent support groups can serve as an important prevention strategy because these programs are designed to help parents learn to cope with challenging situations and also learn strategies and skills to assist their child and learn about child development. Many of these programs have requirements for serving children with special needs, screen for developmental and mental health concerns, and provide additional and wraparound services, such as mental health consultants and behavioral specialists.[37,38]

Abusive Head Trauma

Abusive head trauma (AHT), previously referred to as shaken baby syndrome or shaken impact syndrome, is the nonaccidental traumatic injury that results from violent shaking of an infant or child. Head injury from AHT is the leading cause of death and long-term disability in children who are physically abused.[39,40] Patients typically are infants younger than 1 year, most often younger than 6 months. Infants who cry excessively, have difficult temperaments or colic, or who are perceived by their caregivers to require excessive attention are at increased risk. Male infants, infants with very low birth weight, premature babies, and children with disabilities are at highest risk for AHT or physical violence.

Abusive head trauma often has its roots in unrealistic expectations and parents' lack of understanding of infant development, which contribute to frustration, stress, limited tolerance, and resentment toward the infant. Normal behaviors for an infant, such as crying, can be frustrating, especially for parents who are sleep-deprived, depressed, or experiencing other stresses. Hospitalized or chronically ill children are at increased risk, as their parents experience increased levels of stress, anxiety, exhaustion, depression, perceived loss of control, anger, grief, chronic sorrow, and poor adjustment. At times, most parents feel frustrated and confused if their infant exhibits any of the following behaviors:

- Cries and can be consoled only with constant holding or rocking
- Cries and is not consoled with holding, rocking, or other parent efforts
- Will not go to sleep easily or awakens at the slightest sound and will not return to sleep
- Stays awake for extended periods or is perceived to need constant attention
- Has feeding difficulties, such as
  - Spitting up after almost every feeding or vomiting frequently
  - Poor oromotor skills, poor sucking, or feed refusal, or takes more than 30 to 40 minutes for a feeding
- Is hungry all the time or eats a large amount and spits up
- Takes only short naps during the day and is fussy in the early evening

The stressed parent or caregiver may be unaware of the infant's vulnerability. Injury can occur when the parent is frustrated by the child's normal but "irritating" behavior. Health care professionals should listen to how the family is coping with their newborn, lack of sleep, their infant's crying, and other concerns. Asking how the parent reacts to these situations can reveal that the baby has been shaken or slapped or is at risk of being shaken. In this case, health care professionals should firmly

educate the parents on the dangers of AHT and give them alternative strategies for helping the infant to stop crying, go to sleep, or feed as expected. Community resources, such as home visiting programs,[36] early intervention services, and educational programs, should be offered to support the parents.

Caring for the Family Facing Infant Illness

Caring for the parents and family of a sick infant or child with disabilities challenges the support and crisis intervention skills of the health care professional. Advances in medical science mean that an increased number of families are experiencing preterm birth or prenatal diagnosis of a significant health condition in the infant. *(For more information on this topic, see the Promoting Health for Children and Youth With Special Health Care Needs theme.)*

Premature birth or an infant's illness at delivery may mean separating the infant from the mother and family, thereby impeding the attachment process. The health care professional should recognize and validate the range of responses and the strengths and needs of parents as individuals. The extended family of grandparents and relatives, as well as individual and community beliefs, values, and expectations, affect a parent's ability to adapt to having a low-birth-weight or sick infant.

Hope, empowerment, and parent-professional partnerships are important factors in the adaptation and healing after a high-risk birth or the birth of a child with a disability. Parents benefit from guidance and practical tools for their day-to-day living. Referrals to support groups and culturally appropriate community networks of support, combined with practical information, provide important support for families.

When parents have an infant with a disability or serious health problem, health care professionals must recognize that the parents will go through a process of grieving and mourning for the anticipated and idealized child. Parents need support to understand that this is a normal and necessary process if they are to be able to form a close attachment to their infant. If their infant is critically ill, parents must learn to deal with life-and-death decisions and uncertainty and understand the realities of medical decision-making. Parents' responses can involve chronic or recurrent sorrow and sadness, regardless of the infant's clinical condition or level of health care need. The health care professional should be aware of specific red flags, such as symptoms of acute depression, agitation, or inability to carry out normal daily responsibilities, which should prompt referral for immediate medical or mental health care. The health care professional also should assess the parent-infant relationship for signs of inappropriate attachment, excessive-perceived child vulnerability, parental guilt, and infant abuse or neglect involving the infant or other children. The health care professional also should seek to understand parents' personal strengths and the strengths they may access that are related to their cultural and religious beliefs.

Some parents tend to be permissive toward a child with a medical illness and are reluctant to set disciplinary boundaries.[41] This reaction can happen because a parent feels sad for the child, but it also can lead to behavioral difficulties. These children sometimes are in the greatest need of a predictable structure regarding rules because other aspects of their life are not predictable.

Promoting Mental Health and Emotional Well-being: Early Childhood—1 Through 4 Years

Mental health in early childhood is tightly bound to healthy development in the child, healthy relationships within the family, and strong support for both child and family in the community. Between the ages of 1 and 4 years, the child makes remarkable

advances in her abilities to rely on herself, direct her energies, and interact with others. Building from a secure base of trust in her family, her growing autonomy leads to new explorations and a beginning identity as a distinct and capable person. Within the context of a positive and supportive parent-child relationship, this new growth toward autonomy and self-determined initiative forms the basis for self-esteem, curiosity about the world, and self-confidence. Steady gains are made, as well, in the capacity for self-control and more effective regulation of strong emotions, including anger, sadness, and frustration.

Maturation in emotional development, along with new communicative skills, sets the stage for dramatic growth in social understanding and behavior. Early care and education programs become the arenas for practice in social interaction and in learning to share with others and to express needs and feelings. From home and child care experiences, the child develops important early realizations regarding morality and fair play.

The increasingly self-aware young child grapples with complex issues, such as gender roles, peer or sibling competition, cooperation, and the difference between right and wrong. The temperamental differences that were manifested in the feeding, sleeping, and self-regulatory behaviors of the infant are transformed into the varied styles of coping and adaptation demonstrated by the young child. Some young children appear to think before they act; others are impetuous. Some children are slow to warm up, whereas others are friendly and outgoing. Some accept limits and rules more easily than others. The range of normal behavior is broad and highly depends on the match between the child's and the caregiver's styles. Aggression, acting out, excessive risk-taking, and antisocial behaviors can appear at this time. Caregivers need to respond with a variety of interventions that set constructive limits and help children achieve self-discipline.

Ultimately, healthy social and emotional development depends on how children view themselves and the extent to which they feel valued by others.

Mental health and behavioral concerns can coalesce around a particular behavioral symptom in the child. The health care professional will want to consider underlying child-based factors, which are described in more detail in later sections. In addition, physical, psychological, and social issues of a parent can affect the child's emerging sense of self in relation to others and must be considered in attempting to understand the origin of a child's behavior. Important parental issues include the parents' state of physical and mental health, their temperament, their past and present stressors, and their experiences as a child with their own parents.

Patterns of Attachment

Patterns of attachment between child and parent can be observed in early childhood and are useful in predicting healthy development as well as predicting behavioral problems and disorders in the child.[42] As independence and autonomy take center stage for the child, issues of caring, connectedness, and trust become increasingly important for a family. Health care professionals should seek to understand the family's perceptions of these issues from their personal and cultural perspectives to effectively assess strengths and concerns for the child's development.

As the child's world expands during this developmental stage, she will begin to interact regularly with other adults beyond her parents, including aunts and uncles, grandparents, early care and education providers, and preschool teachers. She will develop patterns of attachment with these adults as well. Secure and loving attachment in these relationships can help ensure her healthy development. The child's emotions are affected by the emotional health of the parents and caregivers. Understanding both the child's and caregiver's temperament and the goodness of fit is important.

Challenges to the Development of Mental Health
Behavioral Patterns

When a child's behavioral patterns and responses seem chronically "off track" from those expected for her age, the health care professional should assess

- Developmental capacities of the child, especially those connected with the challenges that provoke the concerning behavior
- Physical health conditions that might influence the child emotionally and behaviorally
- Temperament and sensory-processing abilities of the child
- The relationship between the child and the conditions and demands of the child's caregiving environment
- The quality of the parent-child relationship and security of the attachment
- Family understanding of the child's behavior, specifically regarding the child's underlying feelings and motivations, and the family's responses to the behavior
- Broader contextual circumstances, including family stress, family change, cultural expectations and influences, and early care and education experiences
- Depression in the child or a history of trauma

The health care professional can gain a detailed understanding of the child's behavior in any particular situation by using an ABC (antecedents, behavior, and consequences) approach,[43,44] which consists of asking the parents or other caregiver who saw what happened to explain in detail

- The antecedents, or the conditions and circumstances in which the behavior occurs (eg, biting, which mainly occurs at preschool when the child is asked to stop playing)
- The behavior itself
- The consequences of the behavior for the child, as well as for others affected, both immediate and long-term

The parents' explanations for why the child is behaving in a certain way are key to understanding their reactions to the child's difficulties. Personal and cultural norms, views on how development proceeds, and theories of motivation will affect how the parent evaluates the child's behavior. This ABC approach avoids misleading generalizations about a particular behavior and focuses on the unique elements of the child; her relationships with family, peers, or caregivers who are important to her; and the contexts for the behavior.

When concerns about behavior are noted, the health care professional might ask the parent, "Who cares for your child during the day?" Young children may act out, exhibit aggressive behaviors, or hurt other children because they are not supervised directly or are not disciplined in an appropriate and positive manner. They may exhibit negative behaviors because they spend time with someone else who acts poorly. This can occur even when the child is in a quality child care environment if the program or caregiver isn't a good fit for the child's temperament or personality. Asking about the child's environment and the program's accreditation[45] or asking for the parent's permission to speak to the caregiver directly can lead to enlightening discussions that may enable the health care professional to offer effective guidance.

Early care and education encompasses an array of programming available for children before school entry. Child care is one option in that array of settings that includes family child care homes, center-based child care, and in-home relative care, as well as home visiting programs. Regardless of the child care arrangement, it should always be of high quality. Many states have quality rating improvement systems, which offer parents the opportunity to seek quality early care and education programs based on criteria established by such systems. Additionally, each state has licensing rules for early childhood programs, monitored by state or local agencies. Knowledge of such rules also can help parents decide where they choose to enroll their child. Parents should ask whether their child care centers adhere to national standards and are accredited by organizations such as the National Association for the Education of Young Children,[46] the American Montessori Society,[47] the Council on Accreditation,[48] or the National Accreditation Commission of the Association for Early Learning Leaders.[49]

Table 1 shows ways that certain domains of influence can contribute, individually or in combination, to the development of behavioral problems and disorders in early childhood. By exploring these 4 domains of influence with the parent, the health care professional can better understand the behavioral problem, recognize the strengths that are inherent in the child, and assist the parent and other caregivers in making adjustments when needed. Parents have expressed eagerness for their child's health care professionals to spend more time with them on behavioral concerns.[50] This approach to identifying strengths, anticipating developmental challenges, and solving behavioral problems will be extremely helpful in supporting and counseling families. This evaluation is best done at the primary care level. Health care professionals can then assess the efforts that parents make in response to guidance and the effect of those efforts on the child to determine the need for further mental health referral. The time and attention the primary care professional gives to these concerns facilitate the parents' acceptance of a mental health referral when indicated.

Families from different cultures have differing developmental and behavioral expectations for their children. Discussions of these issues can begin with a dialogue about what parents expect and why. Understanding these expectations will help the health care professional provide effective and appropriate support to the parents.

Table 1

Domains of Influence				
Examples of Behavioral Concerns	Developmental/ Health Status	Temperament and Sensory Processing[51]	Family-Child Interactions	Other Environmental Influences
Bedtime struggles • Trouble getting the child to sleep • Difficulties with night waking	Does the child's capacity to calm herself and transition into a sleep state seem unusually delayed for that child's age? Are specific health conditions involved? Was there a recent illness?	What is the influence of the child's temperament, especially • Biological regularity? • Adaptability? • Reactivity to sensory input?	Has the family provided a predictable and developmentally appropriate ritual for helping the child settle into sleep? Does the family allow her to fall asleep on her own? Is the child feeling insecure because of lack of adequate time with the parent? What are the family's expectations regarding where the child sleeps? Does the child have a transitional object?	Is there a quiet room for sleeping that is free of TV and sibling activities? (For families living in small spaces, this may be unattainable.) Are any changes or tensions in the family likely to be felt by the child, such as the mother returning to work, a change in child care, or a new sibling?
Resistance to toilet training	Is the child developmentally ready, including showing interest? Is there any interest? Is there any suspicion of painful defecation or constipation?	What is the influence of the child's temperament, especially • Biological regularity? • Reactivity to sensory input? • Distractibility?	Is the parent's approach in sync with the child's developmental status and temperament? Are culturally based expectations forming the parents' expectations? Is there undue pressure or are there negative reactions from parents and others? Are there any signs of fearfulness by the child?	Is toilet training being attempted during a period of major change or high stress? What are the toileting routines at child care or preschool? Are they compatible with home routines?

continued

Table 1 *(continued)*

Examples of Behavioral Concerns	Developmental/ Health Status	Temperament and Sensory Processing[51]	Family-Child Interactions	Other Environmental Influences
Excessive tantrums	What other means does the child have for expressing frustration and anger? Can she do so through speech? Do developmental delays in self-care or other skills routinely cause frustration? Are there physical causes of chronic discomfort or pain, such as eczema or chronic rhinitis? Is the child getting sufficient sleep?	What is the influence of the child's temperament, especially • High intensity? • Negative mood? • Reactivity to sensory input? • High persistence?	What is the child trying to communicate through the tantrum? Do specific events or interactions in the family trigger the tantrums? How do the parents respond? Do their responses help calm the child or escalate the tantrum? Are the parents able to give support without giving in to unacceptable demands?	Are the tantrums linked to family change or stress? Are other family members also experiencing high levels of frustration? How is anger generally expressed in the family? Are the tantrums linked to a change in the child care setting or child care provider?
Chronic aggression	Do developmental delays contribute to chronic frustration, including deficits in expressive language and fine motor abilities?	What is the influence of the child's temperament, especially • Negative mood? • Highly impulsive? • Difficulty in adapting to changes in routine? • High intensity? • Unusually sensitive to sensory input? • Has she learned to attack before she is threatened?	Is the child needy or angry because emotional needs are unmet? What is the quality of the parent-child attachment? Is the child seeking attention? Is there overt or covert encouragement of aggression in the family, such as an indication that parents are proud of child being feisty or showing acceptance of aggression by ignoring it? Is there a parental perception that being aggressive is a survival tactic in the neighborhood or community?	Has the child witnessed violence and aggression, especially within her family? Has the child witnessed or been exposed to violence or aggression in the community or neighborhood? Has she experienced physical abuse herself, at home or in child care? Have there been significant disruptions in the life of the family that affect daily routines? Has there been unsupervised viewing of violent or mature TV or video games?

continued

PROMOTING MENTAL HEALTH

Table 1 (continued)

Examples of Behavioral Concerns	Developmental/ Health Status	Temperament and Sensory Processing[51]	Family-Child Interactions	Other Environmental Influences
Difficulty in forming friendships	Are there developmental delays, especially in expressive language and fine motor skills? (Social-skill deficits are a central feature of pervasive developmental disorders and ASD.)	What is the influence of the child's temperament, especially • Shy, inhibited, or slow to warm up? • Sensory processing abnormalities with hypersensitivities or hyposensitivities?	How does the child's social behavior differ within the family compared with that of peers? Does the child have a secure emotional base with the parent?	Does the child have opportunities to meet and play with other children? Are the conditions for those interactions optimal for the child? For example, many children who are shy do better with short play dates with one other child than with extended time with large groups.
Excessive anxiety, which can be expressed by excessive fearfulness, clingy behaviors, frequent crying, tantrums or frequent nightmares, and other sleep problems (Separation anxiety is developmentally normal during the first 3 years of life; thereafter, it should steadily lessen.)	Do developmental delays or disabilities reduce the child's capacity for expression and control? Do chronic health conditions affect sense of comfort and security? Are there perceived risks to health by the family ("the vulnerable child syndrome")?[41] Are there any acute health problems requiring separation from a parent?	What is the influence of the child's temperament, especially • Shy, inhibited, or slow to warm up? • Avoidance of new situations? • Difficulty in adapting to changes in routine? • Sensory processing abnormalities with hypersensitivities?	Is there a pattern of overprotectiveness or under-protectiveness from the parent? Does the parent accurately read the child's cues and show appropriate empathy? Or, is the parent's sensitivity to cues heightened, awkward, and tense? Does the parent demonstrate the capacity to soothe the child? Is there a family history of an anxiety disorder?	Exposure to significant traumatic events (eg, witnessing IPV) may result in chronic anxiety, such as PTSD. Major changes in the family or ongoing family stress situations may contribute to an anxious condition.

continued

Table 1 *(continued)*

Examples of Behavioral Concerns	Developmental/ Health Status	Temperament and Sensory Processing[51]	Family-Child Interactions	Other Environmental Influences
Excessive activity and impulsivity	Are there problems with sensory input or expressive and motor output? (Regulatory disorder of motor output and sensory input can lead to impulsive motor behaviors and craving of sensory stimulation. Behavior is disorganized, unfocused, and diffused. It can be accompanied by weaknesses in auditory or visual-spatial processing.)	What is the influence of the child's temperament, especially • High activity? • High distractibility? • Low persistence and attention span?	Is the parent clearly and comfortably in charge? Does the child receive positive feedback as well as clear expectations and appropriate limits from the parent? What is the quality of the parent-child attachment? Is there affection between the parent and child, or do irritation and frustration seem to predominate?	Anxiety or depression may manifest as hyperactive, impulsive behavior in the young child. Family stress and change, past traumatic experiences, and family health and mental health conditions should be explored.

Abbreviations: ASD, autism spectrum disorder; IPV, intimate partner violence; PTSD, post-traumatic stress disorder; TV, television.

Child Sexual Abuse

Health care professionals can play an important role in preventing and identifying child sexual abuse, and it is important that they are able to talk with parents about concerns and ensure that parents are aware of problem signs. Discussions with parents can include ways they can help reduce their child's vulnerability to sexual abuse. Statistics indicate that most children are sexually abused by people they know well. It is safest for parents to know where and with whom their child is spending time, including in care and education settings. Parents' use of proper names for body parts and functions can also help reduce children's vulnerability to sexual abuse. Children who are comfortable talking about their bodies are more likely to be able to disclose when something worrisome or uncomfortable is happening to them.[52]

Parents should give their child permission to tell them about any uncomfortable or threatening experiences, reassuring the child that he will be believed and will not be in trouble for telling. Health care professionals are reminded that child abuse reporting laws require them to report concerns for child sexual abuse.

Early Identification of Autism Spectrum Disorder

Autism spectrum disorder (ASD) is a neurobiologic disorder characterized by fundamental deficits in social interaction and communication skills. A range of other developmental delays and differences exist; approximately 55% of children with ASD also have intellectual disabilities.[53] Common behavioral features of ASD include hand flapping, rocking, or twirling; hypersensitivity to a wide range of sensory experiences such as sound and touch; and extreme difficulties in adjusting to transitions and change.

PROMOTING MENTAL HEALTH

With an incidence as high as 1 in 68 children,[54] ASD has become a major concern for all health care professionals, and new diagnostic categories have been adopted.[55] According to the Centers for Disease Control and Prevention (CDC), the estimated prevalence of ASD in 2010 has increased roughly 23% since 2008 and 78% since 2002.[54,56] The prognosis can be greatly improved with early and intensive treatment. Therefore, early identification is critical.

Health care professionals should consider the possibility of ASD as early as the child's first year of life. Infants with ASD can show little interest in being held and may not be comforted by physical closeness with their parents. They have significant limitations in social smiling, eye contact, vocalization, and social play.

During the first half of the child's second year, more specific deficits are often seen. Red flags include

- The child fails to orient to her name.
- The child shows impairment in joint attention skills (ie, the child's capacity to follow a caregiver's gaze or follow the caregiver's pointing or the child's own lack of showing and pointing).
- The child does not seem to notice when parents and siblings enter or leave the room.
- The child makes little or no eye contact and seems to be in her own world.
- Parents report that the child has a "hearing problem" (ie, she does not respond to speech directed at her).
- The child's speech does not develop as expected.

Because these signs of ASD are often difficult to elicit in the context of the pediatric health supervision visit, health care professionals must listen carefully to the observations of parents and they must have a high index of suspicion regarding ASD. It is important to consider ASD for children aged 12 or 15 months when communication concerns are identified in routine developmental surveillance.

Screening tests for ASD are available for use in primary care.[57] In addition, universal screening for ASD is recommended at the 18 Month and 2 Year Visits.[58]

Promoting Mental Health and Emotional Well-being: Middle Childhood—5 Through 10 Years

Middle childhood is a time of major cognitive development and mastery of cognitive, physical, and social skills. Children in this age group continue to progress from dependence on their parents and other caregivers to increasing independence and a growing interest in the development of friendships and the world around them. Children frequently compare themselves with others. During this time, children may begin to notice the cultural differences between their family and others as they begin to develop a cultural, racial, ethnic, or religious identity. Although they are initially egocentric, they become increasingly aware of other people's feelings. Concrete thinking predominates; they are concerned primarily with the present and have limited ability for abstract or future-oriented thinking. This process evolves during the middle childhood years. As children approach adolescence, their capacity for abstract thought grows, they have the ability to think and act beyond their own immediate needs, and they are better able to see the perspectives of other people.

Middle childhood also is an important time for continued development of self-esteem and in the ongoing process of attachment. All children want to feel competent and enjoy recognition for their achievements. Children of depressed parents or parents with an authoritarian parenting style are at risk of not receiving this important developmental support.

Praise is important, but realistic praise is essential. Competencies are to be celebrated but in the context of their importance. Attempted mastery should be noted and valued, as children do not learn without trying. Failures are to be acknowledged and transgressions must be noted if both are to be learning experiences.

It may be necessary to discuss developing self-esteem with certain parents to help them become comfortable with not just praise but also constructive criticism and, when appropriate, discipline. Parents can be reassured that their child's distress about the difficulty of a task often can be a motivator, and it is important to be tolerant of certain levels of their child's distress. It is an important parenting task to prepare children for adversity. For a child to achieve genuine self-esteem, he must learn the importance of trying and realize that some skills are hard and that the degree of difficulty of the skill affects his sense of accomplishment. Parents cannot change the environment; rather, they must help their children learn to adapt to it. Parents can be important supports, but children must do the work to gain from the accomplishment, both at this stage of development and later, as their increasing competencies bring increased independence.

Success at school and home is influenced by previous experience, by the child's ability to get along with others, and by expectations that fit his capabilities. Success also is influenced by the quality of the schools in the community and by the expectations of educators for children of their racial, ethnic, or socioeconomic background; for children who are not native English speakers; or for children with special health care needs. In addition, some children experience bullying and violence at school or at home. These experiences can limit the child's continued development of self-esteem. The health care professional should be aware of these developments and can support children and their families as they face the emerging challenges of greater independence and the awareness of others' needs, feelings, thoughts, and desires. *(For more information on this topic, see the Promoting Lifelong Health for Families and Communities theme.)*

Some children at this age may take on responsibilities far beyond those typical for their age. For example, children in immigrant families, particularly those who live in linguistically isolated households (defined by the US Census Bureau as a household in which no one >14 years speaks English very well[59]), may serve as interpreters for their parents in situations such as interacting with social service agencies or keeping the electric company from turning off the power. Children with a parent who has a serious physical or mental health condition, such as children of wounded veterans returned from Iraq or Afghanistan, may be helping their parent carry out even simple tasks such as taking medicines. Health care professionals should assess children in these circumstances to determine whether they may be experiencing excessive stress and social isolation. If so, the health care professional can work with families to identify community resources that can provide support and assistance.

Children with special health care needs are no different in their need to belong, anxiety about self-esteem, risk-taking behavior, and coming to terms with their entrance into the expanding world outside of their family. However, their special health care needs can present limitations or challenges to a full participation in activities with their peers. Health care professionals should be aware of these issues and the risk for mental health problems and should be prepared to respond when signs of distress emerge.

Patterns of Attachment and Connection

The concept of attachment in infancy and early childhood is more appropriately described as connectedness as the child moves through middle childhood and adolescence. Defined as a strong positive connection to parents or other caregivers, connectedness is key to emotional well-being. The Search Institute has identified family support ("high levels of love and support") and positive family communication as important components of their 40 developmental assets.[60] *(For more information on this topic, see the Promoting Family Support theme.)*

Challenges to the Development of Mental Health

Middle childhood is often the time when mental health problems first present, and it is an essential time for parents to be doing all they can to promote positive social skills and reinforce desired behavior. The rate of identification of psychosocial problems and mental disorders within a primary care setting is relatively low.

In some situations, the health care professional will not only screen for mental health concerns but also perform a thorough assessment to determine whether the child really has a problem and to refer for a more in-depth diagnostic evaluation if the screening and assessment indicate a problem. *(For more information on this topic, see the AAP Task Force on Mental Health report and toolkit.[6])* However, the reality is that few families identified as needing mental health assistance will actually receive treatment. The techniques that a health care professional uses when making a referral can help break down the stigma of a mental health referral. A minimal delay between the onset of illness and treatment likely leads to the best outcome.

Attending to these issues may be especially important for those living in poverty, but most studies have not addressed the influence of culture, race, and systemic issues on outcomes. Few evidence-based treatments have taken into account the child's social context.

Protective Factors

Research studies have revealed consistently strong relationships between the number of protective factors, or assets, present in children's lives and the extent to which their mental and emotional development will be positive and successful. Children who report more assets are less likely to

engage in risky health behaviors.[61] The fewer the number of assets present, the greater the possibility that children will engage in risky behaviors. Key adults in the child's life should promote a strengths-based model that focuses on building these assets. Although health care professionals need to recognize risks, they also should be helping the family develop the strengths that can contribute to a positive environment for the child.[62] *(For more information on this topic, see the Promoting Lifelong Health for Families and Communities theme.)*

Protective factors include[63]

- A warm and supportive relationship between parents and children
- Positive self-esteem
- Good coping skills
- Positive peer relationships
- Interest in and success at school
- Healthy engagement with adults outside the home
- An ability to articulate feelings
- Parents who are employed and are functioning well at home, at work, and in social relationships

Increasing a child's assets will help him develop resiliency in the face of adversity. Resilient children understand that they are not responsible for their parents' difficulties and are able to move forward in the face of life's challenges. The resilient child is one who is socially competent, with problem-solving skills and a sense of autonomy, purpose, and future.

In a child's early years of elementary school, adults need to do what they can to bolster his self-confidence because this is protective against depressive symptoms. Self-esteem is instrumental in helping children avoid behaviors that risk health and safety. In many cases, the development of self-esteem depends on the development of social skills. Health care professionals can help parents teach their children that failure and mistakes are an inevitable but, ultimately, a useful part of life. Problems with anxiety and depression commonly develop in middle childhood or earlier, but their prevalence increases remarkably in early adolescence.[64] Early warning signs sometimes can be identified in the elementary school years so that later mental disorders are prevented.

Learning Disabilities and Attention-Deficit/Hyperactivity Disorder

The early years of elementary school are frequently the time when learning problems and learning disabilities or ADHD first present. A learning disability is defined as a discrepancy between the actual academic achievement of a student and that student's intellectual potential. An official diagnosis of a learning disability usually cannot be made before the age of 7 years. Often, initial behavioral signs can mask the underlying neurodevelopmental disturbance. The health care professional should evaluate for any signs or symptoms of inattention, impulsivity, lack of focus, or poor academic performance that are not consistent with the child's expected cognitive abilities and should be prepared to counsel and to make referrals for evaluations. Early identification and intervention can have long-term positive effects for children with learning disabilities.

When a child demonstrates overactivity, impulsivity, and inattention that interfere with his ability to learn, have fun, or have relationships, he should be evaluated for ADHD or other conditions that impair attention. Neurobehavioral disorder associated with prenatal alcohol exposure (ND-PAE) may include ADHD symptoms. The CDC estimates that approximately 11% of children and adolescents aged 4 to 17 (6.4 million) have been diagnosed as having ADHD as of 2011, an increase of 7.8% since 2003.[65] Family and school skills should emphasize learning impulse control, building self-esteem, acquiring coping skills, and building social skills.

Mood Disorders

A mood disorder, such as dysthymic disorder or depression, can lead to dysfunction in multiple areas of a child's emotional, social, and cognitive development. Depressive disorders are characterized by disturbances in mood, symptoms of irritability and emptiness, and loss of interest in usual activities. They can be accompanied by reckless and destructive behavior; somatic concerns, including eating and sleep disturbances; and poor social and academic functioning.[66] Among prepubertal children and adolescents with mood disorders, a second mental health diagnosis, such as ADHD, anxiety, or conduct disorders, is common. A small proportion of prepubertal children with mood disorders have child-onset bipolar disorder, although it is more common in adolescence or young adulthood. Associated signs include aggressive and uncontrollable outbursts and agitated behavior that can resemble ADHD. Mood lability may be evident on the same day or over the course of days or weeks. Reckless behaviors, dangerous play, and inappropriate sexual behaviors may be present.

Disruptive mood dysregulation disorder (DMDD) occurs in children, adolescents, and adults aged 5 to 18 and is marked by frequent (>3 times per week), significant temper and rage outbursts, inconsistent with developmental level, and irritable, angry mood between outbursts, most of the day and most of the time.[67] In the *Diagnostic and Statistical Manual of Mental Disorders,* Fifth Edition (DSM-5), DMDD is a new diagnosis and describes a distinct pattern of behaviors in children who had often been considered to have bipolar disorder. Unlike children with bipolar disorder, who are likely to develop adult bipolar disorder, children with DMDD are at risk of developing depression.

Frequently, health care professionals in primary care are the main source of care for children with mild and moderate depression. All children and families need to be asked about feelings of sadness, sleep problems, and loss of interest in activities.

Depression can go undetected. A simple question, such as, "When is the last time you had a really good time?" is nonthreatening but gives much information to the interviewer. Empathetic responses from the person who is conducting the interview are important. Depression screening tools and standardized instruments for behavioral problems are available. Depression screening, using a standardized instrument, is recommended at each visit beginning at the 12 Year Visit.

Further discussion of mood disorders can be found in the AAP mental health toolkit and in the *Adolescence section of this theme.*[6,68]

Anxiety Disorders

Anxiety in childhood can be a normal feeling, but it also can lead to the appearance of symptoms that are similar to ADHD and depression. If usual coping strategies do not work or if an anxiety disorder is causing impairment in school or in relationships, differential diagnosis is to be considered.

Anxiety disorders include a heterogeneous group of internalizing disorders characterized by excessive fear or worry. Anxiety disorders frequently occur alongside depression and can have significant effect on school, social, and family activities. Child anxiety may be a precursor to depression.[69,70]

In 2009, the incidence of anxiety disorders in youth was estimated to be 8%.[71] Separation anxiety, selective mutism, and social phobia are equally common in boys and girls, with specific phobia more common among girls.[66] Children who have experienced a trauma may meet criteria for PTSD.

Conduct Disturbances

Conduct disturbances are characterized by negative or antisocial behaviors that range in severity from normal developmental variations to significant mental disorders.[72] Symptomatic behaviors of oppositional defiant disorder can include persistent tantrums, arguing with adults, refusing to adhere to reasonable adult requests, and annoying others.

Conduct disorders usually involve serious patterns of aggression toward others, destruction of property, deceitfulness or theft, and serious violations of rules.[66] Behaviors suggestive of conduct disorder require assessment, home and school interventions, and referral for mental health services.

Bullying

It is difficult to estimate the prevalence of bullying because of differences in measurement and definitions of bullying.[73] Rates as low as 13% and as high as 75% have been reported, indicating that many children are bullied some time during their school years.

Children who bully are likely to have emotional, developmental, or behavioral problems. Children usually become bullies because they are unhappy or do not know how to get along with other children. Perpetrators may have been bullied themselves or have their own mental health or self-esteem issues. Bullying is associated with poor school adjustment and academic achievement. In addition, perpetrators have increased alcohol use and smoking and enhanced risk of adult criminality.[74]

If parents, teachers, or health care professionals have a reason to believe a child is a bully, he may need assessment and support. Assessing parental mental health and promoting positive parenting behaviors are important to the care of the bullying perpetrator. *(For more information on bullying, see the Promoting Safety and Injury Prevention theme.)*

Types of bullying include

- **Verbal:** Name-calling (the most common form of bullying).
- **Physical:** Punching or pushing.
- **Relational:** Purposely leaving someone out of a game or group.
- **Extortion:** Stealing someone's money or toys.
- **Cyberbullying:** Using the Internet, social media, or text messages or other digital technology to bully others. *(For more information on this topic, see the Promoting the Healthy and Safe Use of Social Media theme.)*

Bullying hurts everyone. People who are bullied can be physically or emotionally hurt. Witnesses also can become sad or scared by what they have seen. A child who becomes withdrawn or depressed because of bullying should receive professional help. Children who are bullied experience real suffering that can interfere with their social and emotional development, as well as their school performance. Some children have even attempted suicide rather than continue to endure such harassment and punishment.

Most of the time, bullying does not occur in private; other children are watching.[75,76] A health care professional who suspects that a child is being bullied or witnessing bullying should ask the child to talk about what is happening. Responding in a positive and accepting manner and providing opportunities to talk can foster open and honest discussion about the reasons why the bullying is occurring and about possible solutions. **StopBullying.gov** is a useful resource for bullying and cyberbullying.[77,78]

The following suggestions are for parents and health care professionals in situations of bullying[77]:

- Learn what a child's school and community use to help combat bullying, such as peer mediation, conflict resolution, anger management training, and increased adult supervision.
- Identify the school's bullying policy; it is often published on the school's Web site.
- Seek help from the child's teacher or the school guidance counselor. Most bullying occurs on playgrounds, in lunchrooms, in bathrooms, on school buses, or in unsupervised halls.
- Ask what the child thinks should be done. What has already been tried? What worked and what did not? Health care professionals can help the child assertively practice what to say to the bully so he will be prepared the next time. The simple act of insisting that the bully leaves him alone may have a surprising effect. Explain to the child that the bully's true goal is to get a response.

- Encourage a popular peer to help enforce a school's no-bullying policy.

Adults can teach the child to take the following actions[79]:

- Always tell an adult. It is an adult's job to help keep children safe. Teachers or parents rarely see a bully being mean to someone else, but they want to know about it so they can help stop the bullying.
- Stay in a group when traveling back and forth from school, during shopping trips, on the school playground, or on other outings. Children who bully often pick on children who are by themselves because it is easier and they are more likely to get away with their bad behavior.
- If it feels safe, try to stand up to the bully. This does not mean the child should fight back or bully back. Often, children who bully like to see that they can make their target upset. Instead, he can calmly tell the bully that he does not like it and the bully should stop. Otherwise, the child should try walking away to avoid the bully and seek help from a teacher, coach, or other adult.
- A child who is being bullied online should not immediately reply. Instead, he should tell a family member or another trusted adult as soon as possible. The decision about whether to respond to cyberbullying is a complex one. On one hand, an appropriate response is standing up to the bully. On the other hand, responding could make the bullying worse by establishing a cyber-dialogue before an undetermined and potentially large audience.

Early Substance Use

Almost all children eventually will find themselves in a situation in which they must decide whether they will experiment with smoking, drugs, or alcohol. In their 2011 policy statement, the AAP Committee on Substance Abuse (now Committee on Substance Use and Prevention) warned: "Although it is common for adolescents and young adults to try mood-altering chemicals, including nicotine, it is important that this experimentation not be condoned, facilitated, or trivialized by adults, including parents, teachers, and health care providers."[80] Health care professionals should discuss these issues with children, and their parents, before they reach adolescence. Although most children who experiment with substances do not develop a substance use disorder, even occasional use can have serious consequences, such as an increased risk of health concerns and mistakes made because of impaired judgment. Education about the implications of substance use must begin in middle childhood. Delaying initiation of substance use may help future substance-related problems.

Parents who smoke place their children at higher risk of smoking. Parents should think about which behaviors they would like to model for their children. Positive role modeling can be established by parents by not smoking cigarettes or electronic cigarettes, banning smoking at home, limiting alcohol, avoiding drug use, and actively monitoring the attitudes and behaviors of their children. Positive and honest communication between a parent and child is one of the best ways to prevent substance use. Promotion of self-esteem and avoidance of overly critical feedback can help the child learn to resist the pressure for experimentation. If talking within the family becomes a problem, a health care professional may be able to encourage the communication.

Child Sexual Abuse

As discussed in the *Early Childhood section,* parents can help reduce their child's vulnerability to sexual abuse. Most often, children are abused by people they know well. Parents should give their child permission to tell them about any uncomfortable or threatening experiences they may have, reassuring the child that he will be believed and will not be in trouble for telling. Health care professionals are reminded that child abuse reporting laws require them to report concerns for child sexual abuse.

Promoting Mental Health and Emotional Well-being: Adolescence—11 Through 21 Years

The adolescent's progression toward optimal functional capacity and involvement in meaningful interpersonal relationships and personal activities varies depending on individual personality. Thus, health care professionals must identify normal ranges of development rather than a specified outcome or end point.

The development of emotional well-being centers on the adolescent's ability to effectively cope with multiple stressors. This trait also is called psychological resilience. The development of resilience is a primary goal of successful adolescent development. Resilient coping includes using problem-solving strategies for emotional management, being able to match strategies to specific situations, and drawing on others as resources for social support. *(For more information on this topic, see the Promoting Lifelong Health for Families and Communities theme.)* Cross-sectional data from Vermont show a striking negative correlation between the presence of protective factors and a variety of risk behaviors.[62] National longitudinal data from the National Longitudinal Study of Adolescent to Adult Health (Add Health) study demonstrate a similar, powerful effect of protective factors on subsequent violence.[81] School-based programs focused on teaching adolescents positive social development have been shown to be effective tools for risk reduction.[82] Young people should be encouraged to engage in pro-social paid or volunteer community activities to develop mastery of a particular skill or activity, thus becoming more independent in responsible ways. The adolescent should experience these activities as autonomous and self-initiated. Meaningful activities enhance satisfaction and self-esteem even in the context of poor support from parents and families. Support from after-school activity group leaders can be protective against poor relationships with primary caregivers.[83]

Mental health and developmental disabilities are often chronic conditions requiring continuing care in a medical home. Affected youth may be cared for similarly to children and youth with other special health care needs, for which collaboration with the family, school, and mental health professionals typically will be required.

Adolescents are recommended to have at least one visit per year with their health care professional, and mental health problems can be first discussed in that setting. Health care professionals should know the symptoms of common mental disorders in this population, as well as risk factors for suicide, and should ask about these symptoms during an office visit whenever appropriate.[84,85] Inquiry about school, peers, and mental health may be appropriate at illness encounters as well as health supervision visits.

Compas[86] suggests a framework to assess the mental health of adolescents (Table 2). When using this framework, the health care professional should elicit the perspectives of the adolescent herself, as well as her parents, teachers, and, if needed, mental health professionals. Sociocultural differences are a significant factor in evaluating an adolescent's emotional well-being. Appropriate social norms within a majority culture may not be shared by youth outside that culture. Youth from culturally diverse families also may experience conflicts between values and expectations at home and those that arise from the mainstream culture and peers from other backgrounds.

Table 2

Framework for Evaluating Adolescent Emotional Well-being[86]	
Domain	**Factors to Assess**
Coping with stress and adversity	• Skills and motivation to manage acute, major life stressors and recurring daily stressors • Skills to solve problems and control emotions • Flexibility and the ability to meet the demands of varying types of stressors
Involvement in meaningful activities	• Skills and motivation to engage in meaningful activities • Behaviors and activities that are experienced as autonomous • Self-directed involvement
Perspective of interested parties	• Perspectives of the adolescent, parents, teachers, and, if needed, the mental health professional • Adolescent's subjective sense of well-being • Adolescent's behavioral stability, predictability, and adherence to social rules
Developmental factors	• Prior developmental milestones and issues • Variations in adolescent's cognitive, affective, social, and biological development • Cohort differences in events and social context that affect positive mental health
Sociocultural factors	• Differences in values affecting optimal development and functioning • Differences in perceived threats to positive mental health and the risk of maladjustment • Cultural protective factors, such as religion and values

Adapted with permission from Compas BE. Promoting positive mental health during adolescence. In: Millstein SG, Petersen AC, Nightingale EO, eds. *Promoting the Health of Adolescents: New Directions for the Twenty-First Century.* New York, NY: Oxford University Press; 1993:159-179.

Patterns of Attachment and Connection

Connectedness with parents, family, and caregivers remains a critical component of the healthy development of adolescents. Most school-aged children and youth continue to spend time with their parents and maintain strong bonds with their parents. The risk of psychological problems and delinquency are higher in youth who are disconnected from their parents.[87] Studies document reduced risk-taking behavior among youth who report a close relationship with their parents.[62] The physical presence of a parent at critical times, as well as time availability, is associated with reduced risk behaviors. Even more important are feelings of warmth, love, and caring from parents. Data from Add Health have shown that parent-family connectedness and perceived school connectedness are protective factors against health risk behaviors.[81,88]

Adolescents and their parents have to prioritize conversations and communication that balance this sense of belonging with opportunities for the youth to grow in decision-making skills and sense of autonomy. Peers and siblings also can contribute positively to the youth's sense of belonging. The literature describes a positive bond with school (described as students who feel that teachers treat students fairly, are close to people at school, and feel part of their school) as a protective factor.[89]

Challenges to the Development of Mental Health

Adolescents who have major difficulties in one area of functioning often demonstrate symptoms and difficulties in other areas of daily functioning. For example, if they are having school difficulties secondary to ADHD, symptoms such as motoric activity or impulsivity will be evident at home and may interfere with other activities. Even less overt disorders, such as learning disabilities or difficulties in peer relationships, often will manifest as a depressed mood at home, tension with siblings, or low self-esteem. Health care professionals should know the symptoms of common mental disorders in this population, especially depression, as well as risk factors for suicide, and should ask about these symptoms during any office visit, whenever appropriate, in addition to the depression screening recommended for each adolescent health supervision visit.[15,85]

Some prevention programs in mental health care can strengthen protective factors, such as social skills, problem-solving skills, and social support, and reduce the consequence of risk factors, psychiatric symptoms, and substance use. Unfortunately, few studies have examined the effect of prevention programs on the incidence of new mental health cases, in part because of the large number of study participants that would be needed to ensure scientifically reliable findings.[90]

Mental Health Concerns

The most common mental health problems of adolescents are anxiety disorders; behavior disorders, including ADHD, oppositional defiant disorder, and conduct disorder; mood disorders; and learning problems. The prevalence of all mood disorders increases uniformly with age.[91] Substance use and misuse and suicidal behavior also are significant problems during this developmental stage.

Depression and Anxiety

Mood disorders are characterized by repeated, intense internal or emotional distress over a period of months or years. Unreasonable fear and anxiety, lasting sadness, low self-esteem, and worthlessness are associated with these conditions. The wide mood changes in adolescents challenge health care professionals to distinguish between a mental disorder and troubling but essentially normal behavior.

Depression and anxiety, with potentially different manifestations across cultural groups, are common and significant problems during this developmental period.[91] Depression is present in about 5% of adolescents at any given time. Having a parent with a history of depression doubles to quadruples an adolescent's risk of a depressive episode.[92] Depression also is more common among adolescents with chronic illness and after stressful life events, such as the loss of a friend, parent, or sibling. It is more common as well after exposure to community disasters or other significant traumas. Depression in adolescents is not always characterized by sadness but can be seen as irritability, anger, boredom, an inability to experience pleasure, withdrawal from social interactions or problems with peers or friends, or difficulty with family relationships, school, and work. Academic failure and risk behaviors such as substance use and dependency,[93] high-risk sexual behaviors, and violence all have been linked to depression in adolescents.

When treating an adolescent with depression, the health care professional should determine past suicidal behavior or thoughts and family history of suicide. *Parents should be advised to remove firearms and ammunition*[85] and any potentially lethal medications from the home, including such common over-the-counter drugs as acetaminophen and aspirin. Access to the Internet should be monitored for suicide content in communications and Web sites. *(For more information on this topic, see the Suicide section of this theme.)*

Like other mental health problems, symptoms of anxiety range in intensity. For some adolescents, symptoms such as excessive worry, fear, stress, or physical symptoms can cause significant distress but not impair functioning enough to warrant the diagnosis of an anxiety disorder. Mental health problems are classified as disorders when symptoms significantly affect an adolescent's functioning. The lifetime prevalence of any anxiety disorder among adolescents in the United States is about 32%, with rates for specific disorders ranging from 2.2% for generalized anxiety disorder to 19.3% for a specific phobia.[91] Studies have demonstrated a relationship between anxiety disorders and alcohol misuse in adolescents and young adults.[94] Thus, to make

appropriate diagnoses, treatment plans, and referrals, the health care professional must review the individual's risk and protective factors to better understand the adolescent's symptoms and the context within which they occur.

One strategy for improving the detection of mental health problems is to screen for anxiety and depressive disorders during routine health evaluations. The USPSTF[15] now recommends screening adolescents for depression in clinical practices that have systems in place to ensure accurate diagnosis, effective treatment, and follow-up.

A variety of measures to screen for mood disorders can be used in the primary care setting for children and adolescents.[95] The *PHQ-2* contains 2 items and is a commonly used measure in the adult population. Recent data in an adolescent population found that scores of 3 or more had a sensitivity of 74% and specificity of 75% for detecting youth who met *Diagnostic and Statistical Manual of Mental Disorders, Fourth Edition (DSM-IV)*, criteria for major depressive disorder.[26] However, the health care professional may choose to use other screening measures for adolescents that can concurrently screen for anxiety, eating disorders, and depression.

Deficits in Attention, Cognition, and Learning

Adolescents with deficits in attention, cognition, and learning are likely to present with an array of concerns that involve academic, psychosocial, and behavioral functioning.

Many children who have been diagnosed as having ADHD continue to have difficulties throughout their adolescence and adulthood.[96] Adolescents with ADHD often have comorbid oppositional defiant disorder and conduct disorder. Symptoms of ADHD also may indicate ND-PAE. In addition to having developmental and social problems, affected adolescents may have significant problems with organizational skills, work completion, and self-esteem.

Conduct Disturbances

Conduct disturbances and disorders are manifested through the same behaviors in adolescence as they are in middle childhood. These behaviors include persistent fits of temper, arguing with adults, refusing to adhere to reasonable adult requests, annoying others, aggression toward others, destruction of property, deceitfulness or theft, and serious violations of rules. Substance use, interpersonal aggression, and other problem behaviors also tend to occur in adolescents with these disorders.

Sexual Abuse

Health care professionals should counsel adolescents about healthy relationships and at the same time screen for, as well as counsel against, coercive and abusive relationships with intimate partners. Sexual abuse remains a risk for adolescents. Children and youth with disabilities are 2.2 times more likely to be sexually abused than are typically developing children, as they often depend on others for intimate care and have increased exposure to a large number of caregivers and settings. They also may have inappropriate social skills, poor judgment, and an inability to seek help or report abuse, and they often lack strategies to defend themselves against abuse.

Child sex trafficking, including commercial and sexual exploitation of children and youth, is associated with a plethora of serious physical and emotional health problems. Children and youth who are trafficked seldom self-identify, but health care professionals can remain alert to "indicators associated with the patient's presentation at the visit, history of living situation and physical findings."[97,98]

Suicide

Suicide is the third leading cause of death for adolescents. In 2013, 4,878 suicides occurred among those aged 15 to 24, including 2,210 deaths by firearm.[99] Data collected in 2013 by the CDC Youth Risk Behavior Surveillance System (YRBSS) show that 17.0% of high school students reported they had seriously considered attempting suicide, 13.6% had made a plan, and 8.0% had made a suicide attempt.[100] Although the proportion of students who reported that they have seriously considered suicide has decreased from 29% in 1991, the number of adolescents who reported attempting suicide has remained relatively stable across the last decade.[101] Completed suicides by adolescent and adult males aged 15 to 19 are 6 times greater than those by their female counterparts. However, suicide attempts are almost twice as high among girls when compared to boys.[85] In 2014, the USPSTF found insufficient evidence to recommend for or against suicide risk screening in adolescence or other age groups, even though depression screening is recommended.[102]

Health care professionals who treat suicidal adolescents should not rely solely on an adolescent's promise to not harm herself and should involve parents and other caregivers in monitoring suicidal thoughts and gestures. *Parents should be advised to remove firearms and ammunition from the home.*[85,103] Attention also should be directed to other sources of risk, such as knives and medications, including common over-the-counter drugs, such as acetaminophen and aspirin. Of importance, suicide risk seems highest at the beginning of a depressive episode, so expeditious treatment or referral is crucial. Although no evidence-based data indicate that psychiatric hospitalization prevents immediate or eventual suicide, the clinical consensus is that immediate hospitalization is a critical component in preventing adult and adolescent patients who are suicidal from dying by suicide.

Substance Use and Misuse

Use or misuse of alcohol, tobacco, and other drugs is a significant health concern during adolescence. For adolescents, smoking, drinking, and illicit drug use are leading causes of injury and death. Although the USPSTF emphasized the importance of this problem and called for continued study,[104] it was unable to find sufficient evidence for or against the universal screening of adolescents for substance use.[105] The USPSTF did find sufficient evidence to recommend screening for alcohol misuse in adults aged 18 and older.[106] The primary care setting is an opportunity for primary care professionals to assume greater responsibility for managing substance abuse treatment for their patients.[107,108] Therefore, prevention, screening, and early intervention are vitally important.

Significant changes in drug awareness take place in early adolescence, and substance use most often begins between grades 7 and 10.[109] By late adolescence 78.2% have consumed alcohol, with 15.1% meeting alcohol misuse criteria, and 42.5% use drugs with a 16.4% rate of misuse.[110]

Misuse of prescription drugs is highest among adults aged 18 to 25, with 2.2% of youth aged 12 to 17 reporting nonmedical use of prescription drugs.[111,112] Prescription and over-the-counter drugs are most commonly misused by adolescents, after alcohol and marijuana. As with alcohol, most youth who misuse medications obtain the medication from family and friends.

Addictive behavior begins in adolescence and has both biological and environmental causes. Adolescents of parents who misuse substances are particularly vulnerable to health or social problems.[113] Prevention efforts can start in the home.[111] Families should be advised to lock medications in their home and in relatives' homes.

As adolescents become older, increased access to substances and independence from parents contribute to the risk for substance use or dependence.

Substance use can interfere with judgment and decision-making, which, in turn, can increase risk-taking and contribute to motor vehicle crashes, homicides, and suicides. In addition, adolescents are at increased risk for unprotected sexual activity and interpersonal violence while under the influence of alcohol or other drugs.

The YRBSS provides valuable data on the substance-using behaviors of adolescents (Box 2). Perceived risk versus benefit, perceived social approval versus disapproval, and drug availability in the community are all influencing factors in adolescent substance use. Health care professionals may not be fully aware of all the illicit drugs available and thus should talk with adolescents about the drugs of choice in their region.

Screening and Intervention

Major transitions, such as puberty, moving, parental divorce, and school changes (eg, entering high school), are associated with increased risk of adolescent substance use.[114] Adolescents should be asked whether they or their friends have ever tried or are using tobacco, alcohol, or other drugs. The health care professional should give anticipatory guidance as part of routine health maintenance.[115]

Pediatric health care professionals also should be active in their efforts to prevent smoking cigarettes, electronic cigarettes, and chewing tobacco among their adolescent patients. Smoking prevention actions are an evidence-based intervention recommended by the USPSTF.[116] In addition, an AAP policy statement states, "Because 80% to 90% of adult smokers began during adolescence, and two thirds became regular, daily smokers before they reached 19 years of age, tobacco use may be viewed as a pediatric disease. Every year in the United States, approximately 1.4 million children and adolescents younger than 18 years start smoking, and many of them will die prematurely from a smoking-related disease. Moreover, recent evidence indicates that adolescents report symptoms of

Box 2

Youth Risk Behavior Surveillance System

Since 1991, the CDC has conducted a biannual national survey of ninth- to 12th-grade high school students. Adolescents who are in school complete the YRBSS. The actual prevalence of substance use among the general adolescent population, which includes high school dropouts, is probably higher than that reflected in the YRBSS. Findings from the 2013 YRBSS are listed below.[100]

Alcohol

- 18.6% of students first drank alcohol (other than a few sips) before the age of 13 years.

- 66.2% of students had ever drank alcohol, and 34.9% had at least one drink of alcohol on at least one day in the past 30 days.

- 20.8% reported episodic heavy drinking (ie, ≥5 drinks of alcohol on ≥1 occasions) during the previous 30 days.

- 21.9% of these high school students had ridden with a driver who had been drinking.

Tobacco Use

- 41.1% of high school students had ever tried cigarette smoking, and 8.8% had ever smoked at least one cigarette every day for 30 days (ie, ever smoked cigarettes daily).

- 9.3% of students had first smoked a whole cigarette before the age of 13 years.

- 15.7% of students reported current cigarette use (ie, used cigarettes on ≥1 of the preceding 30 days).

- During the 30 days preceding the survey, 8.8% of students had used smokeless tobacco and 12.6% had smoked cigars.

Marijuana

- 40.7% of the high school students reported having used marijuana, with 8.6% having tried the drug before the age of 13 years.

Cocaine

- 5.5% of students had ever used cocaine (eg, powder, crack, or freebase).

Inhalants, Heroin, Methamphetamines, Hallucinogens, and Nonprescription Steroids or Other Drugs

- 8.9% of students had ever used inhalants (eg, sniffing glue, breathing the contents of aerosol cans, or inhaling paints or sprays to get high, referred to as huffing).

- 6.6% of students had ever used Ecstasy (also called MDMA).

- 2.2% of students had ever used heroin (also called smack, "junk," or China white).

- 3.2% of students had ever used methamphetamines (also called speed, crystal, crank, or ice).

- 7.1% of students had ever used hallucinogenic drugs (eg, LSD, acid, PCP, angel dust, mescaline, or mushrooms).

- 3.2% of students had ever taken steroids without a physician's prescription.

- 17.8% of students had ever taken prescription drugs, other than steroids, without a physician's prescription.

Abbreviations: CDC, Centers for Disease Control and Prevention; LSD, lysergic acid diethylamide; PCP, phencyclidine hydrochloride; YRBSS, Youth Risk Behavior Surveillance System.

tobacco dependence early in the smoking process, even before becoming daily smokers."[117]

Smoking among college students is a major concern. Because smoking initiation peaks between ages 18 and 25, progression from occasional to daily smoking almost always occurs by age 26, and curbing tobacco influence on campuses could prevent a new cohort of lifetime smokers. In fact, as many of 25% of full-time college students are current smokers.[118] Health care professionals should advise their college-aged patients about the hazards of smoking, offering to aid in cessation if they are smoking, and suggest that they consider requesting a smoke-free residence hall if they have asthma or other health problems that are exacerbated by tobacco smoke.[118]

The CDC Community Guide found that Smoke-Free policies reduced the initiation of smoking among young people.[119] In 2013, the USPSTF recommended that all adolescents and young adults be screened for tobacco use and that antitobacco messages be included in health promotion counseling for children, adolescents, and young adults on the basis of the proven reduction in risk resulting from avoiding tobacco use.[120] In 2015, the USPSTF recommended behavioral counseling for adults 18 and older, including pregnant women, and Food and Drug Administration approved pharmacotherapy for adults who are not pregnant.[121]

The USPSTF continues to find that evidence is insufficient to assess the balance of benefits and harms of screening adolescents, adults, and pregnant females for illicit drug use.[122] As noted in the Substance Abuse and Mental Health Services Administration white paper,[123] although substantial research has been conducted on the effectiveness of Screening, Brief Intervention, and Referral to Treatment (SBIRT) in reducing risky alcohol consumption, evidence for the effectiveness of SBIRT in reducing risky drug use is still accumulating. In 2011, the AAP Committee on Substance Abuse recommended that pediatric health care professionals

become knowledgeable about SBIRT and the spectrum of substance use in their practice area and "to screen all adolescent patients for tobacco, alcohol, and other drug use with a formal, validated screening tool, such as the CRAFFT screen, at every health supervision visit and appropriate acute care visits, and respond to screening results with the appropriate brief intervention."[80] A comprehensive follow-up recommendation from this group was released in 2016 and includes recommendations for screening tools.[107] The Screening to Brief Intervention (known as S2BI) tool, the CRAFFT (car, relax, alone, forget, friends, and trouble) brief screening tool,[124] and others that are appropriate for use in the adolescent primary care setting are reviewed.[107] Screening for substance use is included in the Adolesent Visits of this edition.

Screening is essential for all adolescents, including those with special health care needs. Although health care professionals may tend to skip screening for adolescents with special health care needs because of the adolescent's chronic illness or developmental difference, doing so is inconsistent with the approach of the medical home and would be a missed opportunity for prevention or early intervention.

The health care professional's screening, in combination with community prevention efforts,[125] is important despite barriers that include limited time, lack of training, perceived low self-efficacy, and lack of treatment resources and reimbursement.[123,126,127] Brief primary care and school-based prevention interventions have demonstrated efficacy. Success in treating a substance use problem is more likely if treatment is begun early.[128-130] Early substance use has been correlated with an increased risk of use disorder in adulthood.[131,132] The onset of early drinking has been associated with increased risk of alcohol-related health and social problems in adults, including dependence later in life, frequent heavy drinking, unintentional

PROMOTING MENTAL HEALTH

injuries while under the influence, and motor vehicle crashes.[133]

Unlike the DSM-IV, the DSM-5 no longer categorizes substance abuse and substance dependence separately but instead considers substance use disorder as a measured continuum, from mild to severe.[66] The DSM-5 diagnoses describe each specific substance as specific entities (eg, alcohol use disorder, stimulant use disorder), with the same overarching criteria from mild to severe. Although *alcohol* or *drug dependence* has in the past been considered a less stigmatizing term for adolescents, it is no longer an accurate diagnostic category.

Prevention and Protective Factors

Substance use prevention programs have been designed for diverse target audiences in different settings. The content of prevention programs varies from didactic information about alcohol, tobacco, and other drugs to skills development for drug resistance or refusal. The prevention message needs to be consistent and from multiple sources (ie, in the home, at school, in child care, in the community, and from the medical home).[114] School-based smoking prevention programs with multiple components that teach resistance skills and engage youth in substance-free activities have been successful.[134] Involving families and communities and reinforcing school lessons with a clear, consistent social message that adolescent alcohol, tobacco, and other drug use is harmful, unacceptable, and illegal strengthens prevention efforts.[114,135]

Preventing tobacco use among adolescents and young adults remains an important activity for the pediatric health care professional. As of January 2013, more than 1,100 college or university campuses in the United States had adopted 100% smoke-free campus policies that eliminate smoking in indoor and outdoor areas across the entire campus, including residence halls. This figure was about double from a year earlier and almost triple from 2 years earlier.[118] The CDC Community Guide has found strong evidence that (1) increasing the price of tobacco products is effective in reducing tobacco use among adolescents and adults, reducing population consumption of tobacco products, and increasing tobacco use cessation and (2) mass media campaigns are effective in reducing tobacco use among adolescents when implemented in combination with tobacco price increases, school-based education, and other community education programs.[121] These recommendations provide direction for health care professionals who choose to advocate for tobacco prevention within their community or state or their health organizations.

The National Institute on Drug Abuse (NIDA) has highlighted evidence-based examples of effective prevention that targeted risk and protective factors of drug use for the individual, family, and community. On the basis of its review of the research literature, NIDA identified the following family protective factors[114]:

- A strong bond between children and their families
- Parental involvement in a child's life
- Supportive parenting
- Clear limits and consistent enforcement of discipline

Outside the family setting, the most salient protective factors were

- Age-appropriate parental monitoring (eg, curfews, adult supervision, knowing the child's friends, and enforcing household rules)
- Success in academics and involvement in extracurricular activities
- Strong bonds with pro-social institutions, such as school and religious institutions, and acceptance of conventional norms against drug use

In 1997, Simantov et al[136] conducted a cross-sectional, school-based survey of students in grades 5 through 12. Adolescents who reported connectedness to their parents were least likely to engage in high-risk behaviors. Another protective factor was participation in extracurricular activities, such as exercise or after-school sports clubs. However, although extracurricular activities decreased smoking with statistical significance, the decreased alcohol consumption was less.

Effective health supervision addresses all components of health, including physical growth and development as well as emotional development and mental health. As considered in the *Promoting Lifelong Health for Families and Communities theme,* physical brain growth and emotional development are influenced by multiple factors from the prenatal period through young adulthood. Preventable risks to healthy brain development and enhanceable protective factors to foster mental health exist. Successful health promotion demands attention to the emotional development and the mental health through each of the ages and stages of growth and development.

PROMOTING MENTAL HEALTH

References

1. Shonkoff JP, Phillips DA, eds. *From Neurons to Neighborhoods: The Science of Early Childhood Development.* Washington, DC: National Academy Press; 2000

2. Turner HA, Finkelhor D, Ormrod R. The effect of lifetime victimization on the mental health of children and adolescents. *Soc Sci Med.* 2006;62(1):13-27

3. Shim R, Koplan C, Langheim FJ, Manseau MW, Powers RA, Compton MT. The social determinants of mental health: an overview and call to action. *Psychiatr Ann.* 2014;44(1):22-26

4. Kieling C, Baker-Henningham H, Belfer M, et al. Child and adolescent mental health worldwide: evidence for action. *Lancet.* 2011;378(9801):1515-1525

5. Foy JM; American Academy of Pediatrics Task Force on Mental Health. Enhancing pediatric mental health care: algorithms for primary care. *Pediatrics.* 2010;125(suppl 3):S109-S125

6. American Academy of Pediatrics Task Force on Mental Health. *Addressing Mental Health Concerns in Primary Care: A Clinicians Toolkit.* Elk Grove Village, IL: American Academy of Pediatrics; 2010

7. American Academy of Pediatrics Committee on Psychosocial Aspects of Child and Family Health, Task Force on Mental Health. The future of pediatrics: mental health competencies for pediatric primary care. *Pediatrics.* 2009;124(1):410-421

8. Kessler RC, Berglund P, Demler O, Jin R, Merikangas KR, Walters EE. Lifetime prevalence and age-of-onset distributions of DSM-IV disorders in the National Comorbidity Survey Replication. *Arch Gen Psychiatry.* 2005;62(6):593-602

9. Knopf D, Park MJ, Mulye TP. The mental health of adolescents: a national profile, 2008. National Adolescent Health Information Center Web site. http://nahic.ucsf.edu/downloads/MentalHealthBrief.pdf. Published 2008. Accessed November 9, 2016

10. Teplin LA, Abram KM, McClelland GM, Dulcan MK, Mericle AA. Psychiatric disorders in youth in juvenile detention. *Arch Gen Psychiatry.* 2002;59(12):1133-1143

11. Zuckerbrot RA, Maxon L, Pagar D, Davies M, Fisher PW, Shaffer D. Adolescent depression screening in primary care: feasibility and acceptability. *Pediatrics.* 2007;119(1):101-108

12. Borowsky IW, Mozayeny S, Ireland M. Brief psychosocial screening at health supervision and acute care visits. *Pediatrics.* 2003;112(1):129-133

13. Murphey D, Barry M, Vaughn B. Mental health disorders. Child Trends Web site. http://www.childtrends.org/wp-content/uploads/2013/03/Child_Trends-2013_01_01_AHH_MentalDisordersl.pdf. Published January 2013. Accessed November 9, 2016

14. Improving Mental Health Services in Primary Care: A Call to Action for the Payer Community - June 2014. American Academy of Pediatrics Web site. https://www.aap.org/en-us/Documents/payeradvocacy_business_case.pdf. Accessed November 9, 2016

15. US Preventive Services Task Force. Screening and treatment for major depressive disorder in children and adolescents: US Preventive Services Task Force recommendation statement [published correction appears in *Pediatrics.* 2009;123(6):1611]. *Pediatrics.* 2009;123(4):1223-1228

16. Kelleher KJ, McInerny TK, Gardner WP, Childs GE, Wasserman RC. Increasing identification of psychosocial problems: 1979-1996. *Pediatrics.* 2000;105(6):1313-1321

17. Strategies to Support the Integration of Mental Health into Pediatric Primary Care. National Institute for Health Care Management Foundation Web site. http://www.nihcm.org/pdf/PediatricMH-FINAL.pdf. Published August 2009. Accessed November 9, 2016

18. Horwitz SM, Kelleher KJ, Stein RE, et al. Barriers to the identification and management of psychosocial issues in children and maternal depression. *Pediatrics.* 2007;119(1):e208-e218

19. Kolko DJ, Campo J, Kilbourne AM, Hart J, Sakolsky D, Wisniewski S. Collaborative care outcomes for pediatric behavioral health problems: a cluster randomized trial. *Pediatrics.* 2014;133(4):e981-e992

20. Glascoe FP. Increasing identification of psychosocial problems. *Pediatrics.* 2001;107(6):1496

21. Earls MF; American Academy of Pediatrics Committee on Psychosocial Aspects of Child and Family Health. Incorporating recognition and management of perinatal and postpartum depression into pediatric practice. *Pediatrics.* 2010;126(5):1032-1039

22. Siu AL; US Preventive Services Task Force. Screening for depression in adults: US Preventive Services Task Force recommendation statement. *JAMA.* 2016;315(4):380-387

23. Pediatric Symptom Checklist. Bright Futures Web site. http://www.brightfutures.org/mentalhealth/pdf/professionals/ped_sympton_chklst.pdf. Accessed November 9, 2016

24. Gardner W, Murphy M, Childs G, et al. The PSC-17: a brief pediatric symptom checklist with psychosocial problem subscales. A report from PROS and ASPN. *Ambul Child Health.* 1999(5):225-236

25. Floating Hospital for Children at Tufts Medical Center. *The Survey of Well-being of Young Children.* https://sites.google.com/site/swyc2016. Accessed November 9, 2016

26. Richardson LP, Rockhill C, Russo JE, et al. Evaluation of the PHQ-2 as a brief screen for detecting major depression among adolescents. *Pediatrics.* 2010;125(5):e1097-e1103

27. Asarnow JR, Jaycox LH, Anderson M. Depression among youth in primary care models for delivering mental health services. *Child Adolesc Psychiatr Clin N Am.* 2002;11(3):477-497, viii

28. Hagan JF Jr. The new morbidity: where the rubber hits the road or the practitioner's guide to the new morbidity. *Pediatrics.* 2001;108(5):1206-1210

29. American Academy of Pediatrics Medical Home Initiatives for Children With Special Needs Project Advisory Committee. The medical home. *Pediatrics.* 2002;110(1):184-186

30. Bowlby J. Separation anxiety. *Int J Psychoanal.* 1960;41:89-113

31. Cassidy J, Shaver PR. *Handbook of Attachment: Theory, Research, and Clinical Applications.* New York, NY: Guilford Press; 2008

32. US Department of Health and Human Services; Administration for Children and Families; Administration on Children, Youth and Families; Children's Bureau. Child Maltreatment 2013. Administration for Children and Families Web site. http://www.acf.hhs.gov/sites/default/files/cb/cm2013.pdf. Accessed November 9, 2016

33. Anda RF, Felitti VJ, Bremner JD, et al. The enduring effects of abuse and related adverse experiences in childhood. A convergence of evidence from neurobiology and epidemiology. *Eur Arch Psychiatry Clin Neurosci.* 2005;256(3):174-186

34. Edwards VJ, Anda RF, Dube SR, Dong M, Chapman DP, Felitti VJ. The wide-ranging health consequences of adverse childhood experiences. In: Kendall-Tackett KA, Giacomoni SM, eds. *Child Victimization: Maltreatment, Bullying and Dating Violence, Prevention and Intervention*. Kingston, NJ: Civic Research Institute; 2005:8-16

35. Long-term consequences of child abuse and neglect. Child Welfare Information Gateway Web site. https://www.childwelfare.gov/pubpdfs/long_term_consequences.pdf. Published July 2013. Accessed November 9, 2016

36. Flaherty EG, Stirling J Jr; American Academy of Pediatrics Committee on Child Abuse and Neglect. The pediatrician's role in child maltreatment prevention. *Pediatrics*. 2010;126(4):833-841

37. Grayson J, Childress A, Baker W, Hatchett K. Evidence-based treatments for childhood trauma. *VA Child Prot Newsl*. 2012;95:1-20

38. Spielberger J, Gitlow E, Winje C, Harden A, Banman A. *Building a System of Support for Evidence-Based Home Visitation Programs in Illinois: Findings from Year 3 of the Strong Foundations Evaluation*. Chicago, IL: Chapin Hall at the University of Chicago; 2013

39. Christian CW, Block R; American Academy of Pediatrics Committee on Child Abuse and Neglect. Abusive head trauma in infants and children. *Pediatrics*. 2009;123(5):1409-1411

40. Graham DI. Paediatric head injury. *Brain*. 2001;124(pt 7): 1261-1262

41. Green M, Solnit AJ. Reactions to the threatened loss of a child: a vulnerable child syndrome. Pediatric management of the dying child, part III. *Pediatrics*. 1964;34:58-66

42. Kochanska G, Kim S. Early attachment organization with both parents and future behavior problems: from infancy to middle childhood. *Child Dev*. 2013;84(1):283-296

43. Albrecht SJ, Dore DJ, Naugle AE. Common behavioral dilemmas of the school-aged child. *Pediatr Clin North Am*. 2003;50(4):841-857

44. Kazdin AE. *Behavior Modification in Applied Settings*. 7th ed. Long Grove, IL: Waveland Press; 2013

45. Accreditation. ExceleRate Web site. http://www.excelerateillinoisproviders.com/resources/accreditation. Accessed November 9, 2016

46. National Association for the Education of Young Children Web site. http://www.naeyc.org. Accessed November 9, 2016

47. American Montessori Society Education that Transforms Web site. http://amshq.org. Accessed November 9, 2016

48. Council on Accreditation Web site. http://coanet.org/home. Accessed November 9, 2016

49. Association for Early Learning Leaders National Accreditation Commission For Early Care and Education Programs Web site. http://www.earlylearningleaders.org. Accessed May 10, 2016

50. Bethell C, Peck C, Abrams M, Halfon N, Sareen H, Collins KS. Partnering with Parents to Promote the Healthy Development of Young Children Enrolled in Medicaid. Commonwealth Fund Web site. http://www.commonwealthfund.org/~/media/files/publications/fund-report/2002/sep/partnering-with-parents-to-promote-the-healthy-development-of-young-children-enrolled-in-medicaid/bethell_partnering_570-pdf. Published September 2002. Accessed November 9, 2016

51. Liss M, Timmel L, Baxley K, Killingsworth P. Sensory processing sensitivity and its relation to parental bonding, anxiety, and depression. *Pers Individ Dif*. 2005;39(8):1429-1439

52. Stop Abuse Campaign: Working Together to Stop Abuse Web site. http://stopabusecampaign.com. Accessed November 9, 2016

53. Charman T, Pickles A, Simonoff E, Chandler S, Loucas T, Baird G. IQ in children with autism spectrum disorders: data from the Special Needs and Autism Project (SNAP). *Psychol Med*. 2011;41(3):619-627

54. Centers for Disease Control and Prevention. Prevalence of autism spectrum disorder among children aged 8 years—autism and developmental disabilities monitoring network, 11 sites, United States, 2010. *MMWR Surveill Summ*. 2014;63(2):1-21

55. DSM-5 Autism Spectrum Disorder Fact Sheet. American Psychiatric Association Web site. http://www.dsm5.org/Documents/Autism%20Spectrum%20Disorder%20Fact%20Sheet.pdf. Published 2013. Accessed November 9, 2016

56. Autism and Developmental Disabilities Monitoring (ADDM) Network. Centers for Disease Control and Prevention Web site. http://www.cdc.gov/ncbddd/autism/addm.html. Updated March 31, 2016. Accessed November 9, 2016

57. Johnson CP, Myers SM; American Academy of Pediatrics Council on Children With Disabilities. Identification and evaluation of children with autism spectrum disorders. *Pediatrics*. 2007;120(5):1183-1215

58. American Academy of Pediatrics Council on Children With Disabilities, Section on Developmental Behavioral Pediatrics, Bright Futures Steering Committee, Medical Home Initiatives for Children With Special Needs Project Advisory Committee. Identifying infants and young children with developmental disorders in the medical home: an algorithm for developmental surveillance and screening. *Pediatrics*. 2006;118(1):405-420

59. Shin HB, Bruno R. Language Use and English-Speaking Ability: 2000. US Census Bureau Web site. https://www.census.gov/prod/2003pubs/c2kbr-29.pdf. Published 2003. Accessed November 9, 2016

60. Search Institute. 40 Developmental Assets for Children Grades K–3 (ages 5-9). National Dropout Prevention Center/Network at Clemson University Web site. http://dropoutprevention.org/wp-content/uploads/2015/05/40AssetsK-3.pdf. Published 2009. Accessed November 9, 2016

61. Ostaszewski K, Zimmerman MA. The effects of cumulative risks and promotive factors on urban adolescent alcohol and other drug use: a longitudinal study of resiliency. *Am J Community Psychol*. 2006;38(3-4):237-249

62. Murphey DA, Lamonda KH, Carney JK, Duncan P. Relationships of a brief measure of youth assets to health-promoting and risk behaviors. *J Adolesc Health*. 2004;34(3):184-191

63. Shea P, Shern D. *Primary Prevention in Behavioral Health: Investing in Our Nation's Future*. Alexandria, VA: National Association of State Mental Health Program Directors (NASMHPD); 2011. http://www.mentalhealthamerica.net/sites/default/files/Primary_Prevention_in_Behavioral_Health_Final_20112.pdf. Accessed November 9, 2016

64. Beesdo-Baum K, Knappe S. Developmental epidemiology of anxiety disorders. *Child Adolesc Psychiatr Clin N Am*. 2012;21(3):457-478

65. New Data: Medication and Psychological Services Among Children Ages 2-5 Years (Healthcare Claims Data). Centers for Disease Control and Prevention Web site. http://www.cdc.gov/ncbddd/adhd/data.html. Updated May 4, 2016. Accessed November 9, 2016

66. American Psychiatric Association. *Diagnostic and Statistical Manual of Mental Disorders: DSM-5*. 5th ed. Washington, DC: American Psychiatric Association; 2013

67. Leibenluft E. Severe mood dysregulation, irritability, and the diagnostic boundaries of bipolar disorder in youths. *Am J Psychiatry*. 2011;168(2):129-142

PROMOTING MENTAL HEALTH

68. Zuckerbot R, Cheung A, Jensen PS, et al. Guidelines for Adolescent Depression in Primary Care (GLAD-PC): I. Identification, assessment, and initial management. *Pediatrics.* 2007;120(5):e1299-e1312

69. Keeton CP, Kolos AC, Walkup JT. Pediatric generalized anxiety disorder: epidemiology, diagnosis, and management. *Paediatr Drugs.* 2009;11(3):171-183

70. Flannery-Schroeder EC. Reducing anxiety to prevent depression. *Am J Prev Med.* 2006;31(6 suppl 1):S136-S142

71. Merikangas KR, Nakamura EF, Kessler RC. Epidemiology of mental disorders in children and adolescents. *Dialogues Clin Neurosci.* 2009;11(1):7-20

72. Baker K. Conduct disorders in children and adolescents. *Paediatr Child Health (Oxford).* 2013;23(1):24-29

73. Gladden RM, Vivolo-Kantor AM, Hamburger ME, Lumpkin CD. Bullying surveillance among youths: uniform definitions for public health and recommended data elements. Centers for Disease Control and Prevention Web site. http://www.cdc.gov/violenceprevention/pdf/bullying-definitions-final-a.pdf. Published 2014. Accessed November 9, 2016

74. Shetgiri R, Lin H, Flores G. Trends in risk and protective factors for child bullying perpetration in the United States. *Child Psychiatry Hum Dev.* 2013;44(1):89-104

75. Jones LM, Mitchell KJ, Turner HA. Victim reports of bystander reactions to in-person and online peer harassment: a national survey of adolescents. *J Youth Adolesc.* 2015;44(12):2308-2320

76. Rivers I, Poteat VP, Noret N, Ashurst N. Observing bullying at school: the mental health implications of witness status. *Sch Psychol Q.* 2009;24(4):211-223

77. Support the Kids Involved. StopBullying.gov Web site. http://www.stopbullying.gov/respond/support-kids-involved/index.html. Accessed November 9, 2016

78. StopBullying.gov Web site. http://www.stopbullying.gov/index.html. Accessed November 9, 2016

79. What You Can Do. StopBullying.gov Web site. http://www.stopbullying.gov/kids/what-you-can-do/index.html. Accessed November 9, 2016

80. Levy SJ, Kokotailo PK; American Academy of Pediatrics Committee on Substance Abuse. Substance use screening, brief intervention, and referral to treatment for pediatricians. *Pediatrics.* 2011;128(5):e1330-e1340

81. Add Health: The National Longitudinal Study of Adolescent to Adult Health Web site. http://www.cpc.unc.edu/projects/addhealth. Accessed November 9, 2016

82. Waters L. A review of school-based positive psychology interventions. *Aust Educ Dev Psychol.* 2011;28(2):75-90

83. Mahoney JL, Schweder AE, Stattin H. Structured after-school activities as a moderator of depressed mood for adolescents with detached relations to their parents. *J Community Psychol.* 2002;30(1):69-86

84. Zametkin AJ, Alter MR, Yemini T. Suicide in teenagers: assessment, management, and prevention. *JAMA.* 2001;286(24):3120-3125

85. Shain BN; American Academy of Pediatrics Committee on Adolescence. Suicide and suicide attempts in adolescents. *Pediatrics.* 2007;120(3):669-676

86. Compas BE. Promoting positive mental health during adolescence. In: Millstein SG, Petersen AC, Nightingale EO, eds. *Promoting the Health of Adolescents: New Directions for the Twenty-First Century.* New York, NY: Oxford University Press; 1993:159-179

87. Hoeve M, Stams GJ, van Der Put CE, Dubas JS, van der Laan PH, Gerris JR. A meta-analysis of attachment to parents and delinquency. *J Abnorm Child Psychol.* 2012;40(5):771-785

88. Bartlett TR. Patterns of problem behaviors in adolescents and the effect of risk and protective factors on these patterns of behavior. Paper presented at: Southern Nursing Research Society Annual Meeting 2003; Orlando, FL

89. Oelsner J, Lippold MA, Greenberg MT. Factors influencing the development of school bonding among middle school students. *J Early Adolesc.* 2011;31(3):463-487

90. Cuijpers P. Examining the effects of prevention programs on the incidence of new cases of mental disorders: the lack of statistical power. *Am J Psychiatry.* 2003;160(8):1385-1391

91. Merikangas KR, He JP, Burstein M, et al. Lifetime prevalence of mental disorders in U.S. adolescents: results from the National Comorbidity Survey Replication—Adolescent Supplement (NCS-A). *J Am Acad Child Adolesc Psychiatry.* 2010;49(10):980-989

92. Brent DA, Birmaher B. Clinical practice. Adolescent depression. *N Engl J Med.* 2002;347(9):667-671

93. Quello SB, Brady KT, Sonne SC. Mood disorders and substance use disorder: a complex comorbidity. *Sci Pract Perspect.* 2005;3(1):13-21

94. Zimmerman P, Wittchen HU, Hofler M, Pfister H, Kessler RC, Lieb R. Primary anxiety disorders and the development of subsequent alcohol use disorders: a 4-year community study of adolescents and young adults. *Psychol Med.* 2003;33(7):1211-1222

95. Sharp LK, Lipsky MS. Screening for depression across the lifespan: a review of measures for use in primary care settings. *Am Fam Physician.* 2002;66(6):1001-1008

96. Barkley RA. Major life activity and health outcomes associated with attention-deficit/hyperactivity disorder. *J Clin Psychiatry.* 2002;63(suppl 12):10-15

97. Dovydaitis T. Human trafficking: the role of the health care provider. *J Midwifery Womens Health.* 2010;55(5):462-467

98. Greenbaum J, Crawford-Jakubiak JE; American Academy of Pediatrics Committee on Child Abuse and Neglect. Child sex trafficking and commercial sexual exploitation: health care needs of victims. *Pediatrics.* 2015;135(3):566-574

99. Xu J, Murphy SL, Kochanek KD, Bastian BA. Deaths: final data for 2013. *Natl Vital Stat Rep.* 2016;64(2):1-119

100. Kann L, Kinchen S, Shanklin SL, et al. Youth risk behavior surveillance—United States, 2013 [published correction appears in *MMWR Surveill Summ.* 2014;63(26):576]. *MMWR Surveill Summ.* 2014;63(4):1-168

101. National Center for HIV/AIDS Viral Hepatitis STD and TB Prevention, Division of Adolescent and School Health. Trends in the Prevalence of Suicide-Related Behavior National YRBS: 1991-2013. Centers for Disease Control and Prevention Web site. http://www.cdc.gov/healthyyouth/data/yrbs/pdf/trends/us_suicide_trend_yrbs.pdf. Accessed November 9, 2016

102. Lefevre ML; US Preventive Services Task Force. Screening for suicide risk in adolescents, adults, and older adults in primary care: U.S. Preventitive Services Task Force recommendation statement. *Ann Intern Med.* 2014;160(10):719-726

103. American Academy of Pediatrics Committee on Injury and Poison Prevention. Firearm-related injuries affecting the pediatric population. *Pediatrics.* 2000;105(4 pt 1):888-895

104. Patnode CD, O'Connor E, Rowland M, Burda BU, Perdue LA, Whitlock EP. Primary care behavioral interventions to prevent or reduce illicit drug use and nonmedical pharmaceutical use in children and adolescents: a systematic evidence review for the U.S. Preventive Services Task Force. *Ann Intern Med.* 2014;160(9):612-620

105. Final Recommendation Statement: Drug Use, Illicit: Primary Care Interventions for Children and Adolescents, March 2014. US Preventive Services Task Force Web site. http://www.uspreventiveservicestaskforce.org/Page/Document/UpdateSummaryFinal/drug-use-illicit-primary-care-interventions-for-children-and-adolescents?ds=1&s=drug use. Accessed September 18, 2016

106. Moyer VA; US Preventive Services Task Force. Screening and behavioral counseling interventions in primary care to reduce alcohol misuse: U.S. Preventive Services Task Force recommendation statement. *Ann Intern Med.* 2013;159(3):210-218. Also, see http://www.uspreventiveservicestaskforce.org/Page/Document/UpdateSummaryFinal/alcohol-misuse-screening-and-behavioral-counseling-interventions-in-primary-care?ds=1&s=alcohol. Accessed September 18, 2016

107. American Academy of Pediatrics Committee on Substance Use and Prevention. Substance use screening, brief intervention, and referral to treatment. *Pediatrics.* 2016;138(1):e20161210

108. Levy SJ, Williams JF; American Academy of Pediatrics Committee on Substance Use and Prevention. Substance use screening, brief intervention, and referral to treatment. *Pediatrics.* 2016;138(1):e20161211

109. 2007 Fact Sheet on Substance Use: Adolescents & Young Adults. National Adolescent Health Information Center Web site. http://nahic.ucsf.edu/downloads/SubstanceUse2007.pdf. Accessed November 9, 2016

110. Swendsen J, Burstein M, Case B, et al. Use and abuse of alcohol and illicit drugs in US adolescents: results of the National Comorbidity Survey—Adolescent Supplement. *Arch Gen Psychiatry.* 2012;69(4):390-398

111. Drugs, Brains, and Behavior. The Science of Addiction. National Institute on Drug Abuse Web site. https://www.drugabuse.gov/publications/drugs-brains-behavior-science-addiction/preface. Updated 2014. Accessed November 9, 2016

112. Substance Abuse and Mental Health Services Administration. *Results from the 2013 National Survey on Drug Use and Health: Summary of National Findings.* Rockville, MD: Substance Abuse and Mental Health Services Administration; 2014. HHS publication (SMA) 14-4863. http://www.samhsa.gov/data/sites/default/files/NSDUHmhfr2013/NSDUHmhfr2013.pdf. Accessed November 9, 2016

113. Gance-Cleveland B, Mays MZ, Steffen A. Association of adolescent physical and emotional health with perceived severity of parental substance abuse. *J Spec Pediatr Nurs.* 2008;13(1):15-25

114. Robertson EB, David SL, Rao SA. *Preventing Drug Use among Children and Adolescents: A Research-Based Guide for Parents, Educators, and Community Leaders.* 2nd ed. Bethesda, MD: National Institute on Drug Abuse; 2003. https://www.drugabuse.gov/sites/default/files/preventingdruguse_2.pdf. Accessed November 9, 2016

115. Park MJ, Macdonald TM, Ozer EM, et al. *Investing in Clinical Preventive Health Services for Adolescents.* San Francisco, CA: University of California, San Francisco, Policy Information and Analysis Center for Middle Childhood and Adolescence, & National Adolescent Health Information Center; 2001. http://nahic.ucsf.edu/downloads/CPHS.pdf. Accessed November 9, 2016

116. Moyer VA; US Preventive Services Task Force. Primary care interventions to prevent tobacco use in children and adolescents: US Preventive Services Task Force recommendation statement. *Ann Intern Med.* 2013;159(8):552-557

117. Sims TH; American Academy of Pediatrics Committee on Substance Abuse. Tobacco as a substance of abuse. *Pediatrics.* 2009;124(5):e1045-e1053

118. Going Smoke Free: Colleges and Universities. Americans for Nonsmokers' Rights Web site. http://no-smoke.org/goingsmokefree.php?id=447. Accessed November 9, 2016

119. The Guide to Community Prevention Services. Reducing Tobacco Use and Secondhand Smoke Exposure. The Community Guide Web site. http://www.thecommunityguide.org/tobacco/index.html. Updated November 10, 2014. Accessed November 9, 2016

120. Moyer VA; on behalf of the US Preventive Services Task Force. Primary care interventions to prevent tobacco use in children and adolescents: US Preventive Services Task Force recommendation statement. *Ann Intern Med.* 2013;159(8):552-557

121. Siu A; US Preventive Services Task Force. Behavioral and pharmacotherapy interventions for tobacco smoking cessation in adults, including pregnant women: US Preventive Services Task Force recommendation statement. *Ann Intern Med.* 2015;163(8):622-634. http://www.uspreventiveservicestaskforce.org/Page/Document/UpdateSummaryFinal/tobacco-use-in-children-and-adolescents-primary-care-interventions?ds=1&s=smoking cessation. Accessed September 21, 2016

122. Moyer VA; US Preventive Services Task Force. Primary care behavioral interventions to reduce illicit drug and nonmedical pharmaceutical use in children and adolescents: US Preventive Services Task Force recommendation statement. *Ann Intern Med.* 2014;160(9):634-639

123. Screening, brief intervention, and referral to treatment: new populations, new effectiveness data. *SAMHSA News.* 2009;17(6):1-20

124. Knight JR, Sherritt L, Shrier LA, Harris SK, Chang G. Validity of the CRAFFT substance abuse screening test among adolescent clinic patients. *Arch Pediatr Adolesc Med.* 2002;156(6):607-614

125. Elder RW, Nichols JL, Shults RA, Sleet DA, Barrios LC, Compton R. Effectiveness of school-based programs for reducing drinking and driving and riding with drinking drivers: a systematic review. *Am J Prev Med.* 2005;28(5 suppl):288-304

126. Van Hook S, Harris SK, Brooks T, et al. The "Six T's": barriers to screening teens for substance abuse in primary care. *J Adolesc Health.* 2007;40(5):456-461

127. Yarnall KS, Pollak KI, Ostbye T, Krause KM, Michener JL. Primary care: is there enough time for prevention? *Am J Public Health.* 2003;93(4):635-641

128. Winters KC, Fahnhorst T, Botzet A, Lee S, Lalone B. Brief intervention for drug-abusing adolescents in a school setting: outcomes and mediating factors. *J Subst Abuse Treat.* 2012;42(3):279-288

129. Stange KC, Woolf SH, Gjeltema K. One minute for prevention: the power of leveraging to fulfill the promise of health behavior counseling. *Am J Prev Med.* 2002;22(4):320-323

130. Stevens MM, Olson AL, Gaffney CA, Tosteson TD, Mott LA, Starr P. A pediatric, practice-based, randomized trial of drinking and smoking prevention and bicycle helmet, gun, and seatbelt safety promotion. *Pediatrics.* 2002;109(3):490-497

131. Hingson RW, Heeren T, Winter MR. Age at drinking onset and alcohol dependence: age at onset, duration, and severity. *Arch Pediatr Adolesc Med.* 2006;160(7):739-746

PROMOTING MENTAL HEALTH

149

132. Behrendt S, Wittchen HU, Höfler M, Lieb R, Beesdo K. Transitions from first substance use to substance use disorders in adolescence: is early onset associated with a rapid escalation? *Drug Alcohol Depend.* 2009;99(1-3):68-78

133. Hingson R, Heeren T, Zakocs R. Age of drinking onset and involvement in physical fights after drinking. *Pediatrics.* 2001;108(4):872-877

134. Bandy T, Moore KA. Child Trends Fact Sheet: What Works for Preventing and Stopping Substance Use in Adolescents: Lessons Learned from Experimental Evaluations of Programs and Interventions. Child Trends Web site. http://www.childtrends.org/wp-content/uploads/2013/03/Child_Trends-2008_05_20_FS_WhatWorksSub.pdf. Published May 2008. Accessed November 9, 2016

135. Drug Abuse Prevention Starts with Parents. HealthyChildren.org Web site. http://www.healthychildren.org/English/ages-stages/teen/substance-abuse/Pages/Drug-Abuse-Prevention-Starts-with-Parents.aspx. Updated November 21, 2015. Accessed November 9, 2016

136. Simantov E, Schoen C, Klein JD. Health-compromising behaviors: why do adolescents smoke or drink?: identifying underlying risk and protective factors. *Arch Pediatr Adolesc Med.* 2000;154(10):1025-1033

Promoting Healthy Weight

Maintaining a healthy weight during childhood and adolescence is critically important for children's and adolescents' overall health and well-being, as well as for good health in adulthood. A child's or adolescent's weight status is the result of multiple factors working together—heredity, metabolism, height, behavior, and environment.[1] Two of the most important behavioral determinants are nutrition and physical activity. How much and what a child or adolescent eats and the types and intensity of physical activity she participates in can affect weight and therefore overall health. A balanced, nutritious diet and regular physical activity are keys to preventing overweight and obesity.

Underweight is an issue for some children and adolescents, including some children and youth with special health care needs and some adolescents with eating disorders, but the overriding concern with weight status in the United States today is overweight and obesity. Therefore, this theme focuses on preventing, assessing, and treat- ing overweight and obesity in children and adolescents. It can be used in concert with the *Promoting Healthy Nutrition and Promoting Physical Activity themes.*

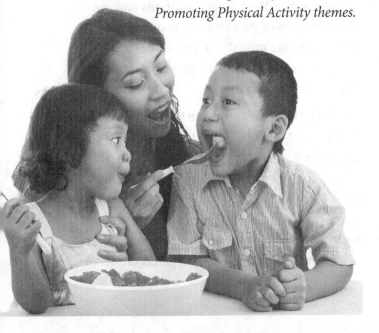

Definitions and Terminology

Body mass index (BMI) is defined as weight (kilograms) divided by the square of height (meters): weight (kg)/[height (m)]^2. Although BMI does not directly measure body fat, it is a useful screening tool because it correlates with body fat and health risks.[2] Additionally, measuring BMI is clinically feasible. In children and adolescents, BMI distribution, like weight and height distributions, changes with age. As a result, while BMI is appropriate to categorize body weight in adults, BMI percentiles specific for age and sex from reference populations define underweight, healthy weight, overweight, and obesity in children and adolescents.

Body mass index is recommended as one of several screening tools for assessing weight status. For individual children and adolescents, health care professionals need to review growth patterns, family histories, and medical conditions to assess risk and determine how to approach the child or adolescent, and family. Children and adolescents with BMI between the 85th and 94th percentiles are defined as having overweight (Table 1) and often have excess body fat and health risks, although for some, this BMI category reflects high lean body mass rather than high levels of body fat. Almost all children and adolescents with BMIs at or above the 95th percentile have obesity and have excess body fat with associated health risks. The use of 2 cut points, 85th percentile and 95th percentile BMI, captures varying risk levels and minimizes overdiagnosis and underdiagnosis.

Table 1

Body Mass Index Percentile Categories for Children and Adolescents	
Body Mass Index Percentile	**Definition**
<5th percentile	Underweight
≥5th–84th percentile	Healthy weight
≥85th–94th percentile	Overweight
≥95th percentile	Obese

Source: Centers for Disease Control and Prevention. Division of Nutrition, Physical Activity, and Obesity, National Center for Chronic Disease Prevention and Health Promotion. About Children & Teen BMI. http://www.cdc.gov/healthyweight/assessing/bmi/childrens_bmi/about_childrens_bmi.html. Updated May 15, 2015. Accessed September 18, 2016.

Prevalence of Overweight and Obesity

According to measured heights and weights from nationally representative samples of children and adolescents assessed as part of the National Health and Nutrition Examination Survey (NHANES) (1976–1980 and 2011–2012), obesity prevalence rose from 5.0% to 8.4% in children aged 2 to 5 years, from 6.5% to 17.7% in children and adolescents aged 6 to 11 years, and from 5.0% to 20.5% in adolescents aged 12 to 19 years.[3] During 2008 to 2011, a downward trend in obesity prevalence was seen among children aged 2 to 4 years participating in federal nutrition programs in 19 states and territories, whereas other states showed no change or showed increases in prevalence.[4] The obesity epidemic disproportionately affects some racial-ethnic and economic groups.[3,5] In 2011 to 2012, the obesity prevalence was particularly high among African American females aged 2 to 19 (20.5%) and among Hispanic males aged 2 to 19 (24.1%).[3] Poverty has been associated with higher obesity prevalence among adolescents. However, the prevalence among specific population subgroups has differed.[5] Health care professionals are faced with addressing this problem in an increasing number of children and adolescents.

A child or adolescent who has obesity often continues to have obesity into adulthood, with higher degrees of excess weight associated with increasing risk of persistence.[6] Obesity is associated with many chronic health conditions, including type 2 diabetes, hypertension, dyslipidemia, nonalcoholic fatty liver disease, obstructive sleep apnea, and cardiovascular disease.[7,8] These chronic conditions, previously identified only in adults, are now present in growing numbers of adolescents and even in children. These conditions lead to increased health care costs. In addition, children and adolescents who have obesity experience stigmatization and lower quality of life.

Defining Overweight and Obesity in Special Populations

Infants and Children Younger Than 24 Months

For infants and children younger than 24 months, the Centers for Disease Control and Prevention (CDC) and the American Academy of Pediatrics (AAP) recommend the use of the World Health Organization (WHO) Growth Charts (Appendix A), which more accurately reflect the recommended standard of breastfeeding than do the CDC Growth Charts (Appendix B). The WHO charts describe healthy growth in optimal conditions and are therefore growth standards. In contrast, the CDC charts are growth references, describing how populations of children grow in a particular place and time.

The WHO charts also provide BMI values for 0 to 2 years; BMI cannot be calculated with CDC charts until after 2 years. Normative values for healthy weight, underweight, overweight, and obesity differ between the CDC and WHO systems. According to the WHO, weight-for-length and BMI less than the 2nd percentile defines underweight and greater than the 98th percentile defines overweight, with no specific cut point for obesity in this age group. Reflecting a clearer understanding of normative growth in breastfed infants, the CDC highlights that "clinicians should be aware that fewer US children will be identified as having underweight using the WHO charts, slower growth among breastfed infants during ages 3 to 18 months is normal, and gaining weight more rapidly than is indicated on the WHO charts might signal early signs of overweight."[9,10]

Late Adolescents

The adult cut point for overweight (BMI = 25 kg/m²) can be used to define overweight in late adolescence even when the 85th percentile is defined by a higher absolute BMI. For example, a female adolescent aged 17 years, 4 months, with a BMI of 25.2 is at the 84th percentile. Even though her BMI is slightly below the 85th percentile, the BMI is in the overweight category because it is above the adult cut point for overweight of 25 kg/m². Similarly, the adult definition of obesity (BMI ≥30 kg/m²) can be used in late adolescence when this value is lower than the 95th percentile.

Those With Severe Obesity

The overall obesity rate is increasing, as is the prevalence of severe obesity among children and adolescents. Those who have severe obesity are at high risk of multiple cardiovascular disease risk factors and poor health.[11,12] There is no consensus on a definition of severe obesity. The AAP Expert Committee on Treatment of Child and Adolescent Obesity[13] suggested use of the 99th percentile based on cut points defined by Freedman and colleagues[12] from NHANES data. However, the sample of children and adolescents with BMI at this level was small, and more valid cut points may soon supersede this information. However, for children and adolescents with BMI at or above this level, intervention is more urgent than for children and adolescents who have lesser degrees of obesity. Health care professionals should ensure that best efforts are made to provide treatment to children and adolescents whose BMI for age and sex is above the 97th percentile, which is the highest curve available on the growth charts. (For information about treating obesity, see the Treating Overweight and Obesity section of this theme.)

Children and Youth With Special Health Care Needs

Children and youth with special health care needs may find it difficult to make healthy food choices, control their weight, and be physically active. This can be caused by difficulty with chewing or swallowing foods, medications that contribute to weight gain and changes in appetite, physical limitations that reduce the child's ability to be active, and a lack of accessible environments that enable exercise. As a result, children with mobility limitations and intellectual or learning disabilities are at increased risk of obesity.[14-16] Children and adolescents aged 10 through 17 years who have special health care needs have higher rates of obesity (20%) than do children of the same ages without these needs (15%).[17]

Preventing Overweight and Obesity

Preventing overweight and obesity should begin early. This includes encouraging women to enter pregnancy at a healthy weight and to gain weight according to current guidelines.[18] Pregnant women also are encouraged to quit smoking during pregnancy, because exposure to tobacco in utero has been independently associated with an increased risk of obesity in multiple population-based epidemiological studies.[19] Following delivery, women should be supported to exclusively breastfeed for the first 6 months of life followed by continued breastfeeding with added complementary foods for at least one year. This method of feeding prevents short-term and long-terms risks of obesity.[20]

PROMOTING HEALTHY WEIGHT

Lifestyle behaviors to prevent obesity, rather than intervention to improve weight status, should be the aim of anticipatory guidance for children and adolescents with healthy BMI for age and sex (≥5th–84th percentile) and for some children and adolescents with BMI for age and sex in the overweight category (≥85th–94th percentile), depending on their growth pattern and risk factors. Health care professionals should be aware of the increased risk of obesity in children and adolescents with parents who have obesity and in those whose mothers had diabetes during the child's gestation.

Obesity prevention is complex. It is less about the health care professional targeting a specific health behavior and more about the process of influencing families to change behaviors when habits, culture, and environment promote less physical activity and more energy intake. Health care professionals can work effectively with families and can create systems that support ongoing commitment to achieving and maintaining a healthy weight. Although limited research is available for use in clinical practice, the approaches described below may be useful guides for providing anticipatory guidance and counseling for children and adolescents and their families.

- **Communicating effectively.** Health care professionals need to convey support and empathy. They should choose words carefully, recognizing that terms such as *fat* and *obese* may be perceived as derogatory. Instead, they should consider using neutral terms, such as *weight, having excess weight,* and *high BMI.* They should learn about values or circumstances that may be common in the population they serve, especially if that culture differs from the health care professional's own culture. A health care professional's knowledge of a family's values and circumstances may be helpful in tailoring anticipatory guidance. Some parents may need help in seeking and obtaining resources such as food assistance, case management, support groups, and home visiting services.

- **Sensitivity to cultural traditions.** Culture influences perceptions of an attractive body image, ideas of a healthy weight, and the importance of physical activity, selection of foods, and parenting strategies. For example, parents may view excess weight as healthy and may be offended at suggestions their child or adolescent has excess weight, overweight, or obesity. Ensuring that a child or adolescent is not underweight may be very important to people from cultures in which poverty or insufficient food is common.[21]

- **Encouraging effective parenting.** Parents are critical to helping children and adolescents develop healthy habits, and health care professionals can encourage parents to provide age-appropriate guidance and be good role models. Health care professionals can suggest that parents establish and promote routines and structures (eg, related to family meals, physical activity, screen time, and sleep) for their child or adolescent in a nurturing and healthy environment. Inadequate sleep has been associated with increased BMI.[22]

- **Accommodating stages of change (readiness to change).** Before a person is ready to change a behavior, she needs to be aware of the problem, have a plan to address it, and then begin the new behavior.[23] Health care professionals can help children and adolescents and their families move along these stages rather than prescribing a new behavior to those who are not ready to change. For example, unsafe neighborhoods or lack of recreation areas may cause a parent to fear outside play and may be a barrier to increasing physical activity. Working with parents to devise a plan for finding alternative opportunities for safe play may help parents be more comfortable in encouraging their children to be physically active.

- **Using motivational interviewing.** Motivational interviewing (MI) uses nonjudgmental questions and reflective listening to uncover a child's, adolescent's, or parent's beliefs and values. Health care professionals can use MI to motivate rather than direct or tell families what to do. Motivational interviewing can help the child, the adolescent, or families formulate a plan that is consistent with their values and readiness to change. This approach may prevent defensiveness that can arise in response to a more directive style. Recent studies have demonstrated a reduction in BMI percentiles when MI was used by a physician, with and without the assistance of a registered dietitian.[24,25]

- **Using cognitive behavioral techniques.** Health care professionals can encourage goal setting, monitoring behaviors targeted for change, and use of positive reinforcement. Initial goals should be easily achievable, such as engaging in 15 minutes of moderate physical activity each day or cutting back on sugar-sweetened beverages by one per day over a period of time. Parents should reinforce behavior goals rather than weight change goals, and reinforcement should be verbal praise or an extra privilege, not food. Health care professionals and parents should expect imperfect adherence and should focus on successes, not failures.[26]

Although defining the contribution of specific behaviors to overweight and obesity prevention is difficult, evidence shows that certain eating and physical activity behaviors improve the balance between energy expenditure and food intake. Box 1 lists actions that health care professionals, families, communities, and school personnel, as well as legislators, policy makers, and insurance providers, can take to prevent overweight and obesity in children and adolescents.

The Role of the Health Care Professional Office or Clinic Staff

Health care professional office or clinic staff and office systems can support efforts to address obesity prevention consistently. The following practices can help ensure that all staff adopt methods to address obesity prevention[2,30]:

- Routinely document BMI for age and sex. This practice will improve early recognition of overweight and obesity, which may be more amenable to intervention than more severe obesity.[2]

- Establish procedures to deliver obesity prevention messages to children and adolescents (eg, 5-2-1-0).[42] When the child's or adolescent's individual risk of obesity is low, these messages can promote appropriate general health or wellness rather than weight management. Simple, memorable guidelines, presented early and repeated regularly with supporting educational materials, can be delivered efficiently in the office or clinic and are likely to be effective teaching tools.

- Establish procedures for intervening with children and adolescents who have overweight (≥85th–94th percentile BMI) or obesity (≥95th percentile BMI).[43] For instance, when a child or adolescent has overweight, a health care professional can review family history, the child's or adolescent's blood pressure and cholesterol, and BMI percentile over time and then assess health risk according to that information. Staff should flag charts of children and adolescents with overweight or obesity so all staff at all visits are aware of the problem and can monitor growth, risk factors, and social and emotional issues.

- Involve and train interdisciplinary teams (eg, physicians, nurses, physician assistants, dietitians, mental health professionals, and administrative staff) in their respective responsibilities in addressing obesity prevention.

Building on the prevention approach of promoting healthy weight, issues salient to each developmental period are addressed next. The emphasis during each period is on eating healthy foods, participating in physical activity, and supporting a nurturing environment in age-appropriate ways.

PROMOTING HEALTHY WEIGHT

155

Box 1

Actions to Prevent Overweight and Obesity in Children and Adolescents[27]

For Health Care Professionals

- Encourage breastfeeding.[9,28]
- Discourage smoking during pregnancy, and provide resources for females capable of becoming pregnant to quit smoking.[19]
- Plot and assess BMI percentiles routinely for early recognition of overweight and obesity.[2]
- Address increasing BMI percentiles before they reach ≥95th percentile.[2]
- Identify children and adolescents at risk of overweight and obesity,[6,13] who are those
  - Whose parents have overweight or obesity
  - With a sibling who has overweight or obesity
  - From families of lower socioeconomic status
  - With limited cognitive stimulation
  - Born to mothers who had gestational diabetes during pregnancy
  - With special health care needs
- Assess eating and physical activity behavior, amount of non-homework (recreational) screen time (eg, TV, computer, handheld device), and whether the child or adolescent has a TV or other devices with screens in the bedroom.[29]
- Assess barriers to healthy eating and physical activity.[30]
- Provide anticipatory guidance for nutrition and physical activity.[30]

For Families

- Choose healthy behaviors.
  - Ensure that "special times" do not frequently involve food or sedentary activities.
  - Use things other than food or screen time as rewards.
  - Promote physically active family time (eg, hikes, bike rides, playing outside, dancing, active indoor games).
  - Eat together as a family (≥3 times per week).[30,31]
  - Limit eating out.[30,32]
  - Eat breakfast daily.[30]
- Emphasize healthy food and drink choices.
  - Focus on nutrient-dense choices—vegetables, fruits, whole grains, fat-free or low-fat milk and dairy products, seafood, lean meats and poultry, eggs, beans and peas, and nuts and seeds.
  - Limit foods and drinks high in calories and with few nutrients—those high in added sugars, saturated fats, and refined grains (eg, sugar-sweetened beverages, baked goods, dairy desserts, pizza).
  - Limit before-bed snacks.
  - Limit between-meal snacking.
- Be physically active.
  - Encourage adults to engage in the equivalent of at least 150 minutes a week of moderate-intensity[a] aerobic physical activity and also do muscle-strengthening activities ≥2 days a week.
  - Encourage children and adolescents, aged 6–17 years, to engage in ≥60 minutes of physical activity each day. Most of the 60 minutes should be spent engaging in moderate- or vigorous[b]-intensity aerobic physical activity that generates sweating.[33]

---

[a] Moderate-intensity activity is activity that makes children's and adolescents' hearts beat faster than normal and that makes them breathe harder than normal. They should be able to talk but not sing.

[b] Vigorous-intensity activity is activity that makes children's and adolescents' hearts beat much faster than normal and that makes them breathe much harder than normal. Children and adolescents should be able to speak only in short sentences.

continued

Box 1 *(continued)*

Actions to Prevent Overweight and Obesity in Children and Adolescents[27]

- Encourage young children to engage in at least 60 minutes and up to several hours of unstructured physical activity each day.[34] Young children should not to be sedentary for >60 minutes at a time except when sleeping. For infants, physical activity should take the form of daily supervised "tummy time" when the child is awake.
- Avoid screen time in infants and children <18 months. Children 18 months through 4 years should limit screen time to no more than 1 hour per day.[35]
- Turn off the TV during mealtimes.
- Establish a family media use plan (a set of rules about media use and screen time that are written down and agreed on by all family members).[36,37] The family media use plan is an online tool that parents and children can fill out together. The tool prompts the family to enter daily health priorities, such as an hour for physical activity, 8 to 11 hours of sleep, time for homework and school activities, and unplugged time each day for independent time and time with family. The family can then consider the time left over and decide on rules around the quantity, quality, and location of media use.
- Ensure that children and adolescents get adequate sleep based on age.[22]

For Schools
- Integrate nutrition and physical activity education into school curriculum.[38]
- Promote physical activity throughout the day.[38]
- Provide recess in addition to physical education.[39]
- Encourage children and adolescents to walk or bike to school where it is safe to do so.
- Provide nutritious meals that meet National School Lunch and School Breakfast Programs standards, as mandated by the Healthy, Hunger-Free Kids Act.
- Enact policies that limit the availability of sugar-sweetened beverages in schools and competitive foods served on school campuses.[40]

For Communities
- Ensure that healthy food and beverage options are the routine, easy choice.[41]
- Provide safe playgrounds and safe neighborhoods for biking, walking, and other physical activities.[30]
- Promote physical activity outside the school day, such as after-school programs that encourage physical activity.
- Identify and deliver culturally relevant messages about healthy eating, physical activity, and weight.

For Legislators, Policy Makers, and Insurance Providers
- Support schools and communities in their activities to promote healthy weight and prevent overweight and obesity.
- Reimburse health care professionals (eg, physicians, nurse practitioners, physician assistants, dietitians) for providing anticipatory guidance about nutrition and physical activity.

Abbreviations: BMI, body mass index; TV, television.

PROMOTING HEALTHY WEIGHT

Screening for and Assessing Overweight and Obesity

Universal Assessment of Obesity Risk

Screening for obesity risk, an ongoing process,[11,13] starts with BMI evaluation (or weight-for-length if the child is <2 years) and incorporates evaluation of medical conditions and risks, current behaviors, family attitudes, socioeconomic concerns, and psychosocial situation. According to this information, health care professionals can promote obesity prevention through anticipatory guidance and by reinforcing behaviors that will promote sustained healthy weight (eg, increasing intake of vegetables and fruits; increase physical activity; decreasing intake of food high in calories, fats, and added sugars; decreasing screen time and other sedentary behaviors) or treat overweight or obesity.

In general, children and adolescents with normal BMI for their age and sex (ie, between the 5th and 85th percentile) benefit from preventive anticipatory guidance, which guides them toward healthy behaviors or reinforces current healthy behaviors. This guidance should be framed as growing healthy bodies rather than achieving specific weights. Children and adolescents whose BMI is in the overweight category (ie, 85th–94th percentile) require additional attention. Some may have a healthy body weight, but others may have excess body fat and will benefit from weight control intervention. A wait-and-see approach may result in a missed opportunity to prevent progression of overweight. Children and adolescents whose BMI is in the obese category (ie, >95th percentile) benefit from weight control intervention.

The Expert Committee for the Prevention, Assessment, and Treatment of Child and Adolescent Overweight and Obesity (convened by the Health Resources and Services Administration, CDC, and American Medical Association) recommends the following actions for screening and assessing all children for prevention and providing counseling for early intervention[11,13]:

- **Calculate BMI and plot on the appropriate growth curve at least once a year.** Identify current category of underweight (<5th percentile), healthy weight (5th–84th percentile), overweight (85th–94th percentile), or obese (≥95th percentile). Calculators, wheels, tables, and nomograms are some of the tools used to calculate BMI, which is plotted on the CDC or WHO Growth Charts.
- **Assess medical factors.** Includes family history in first- and second-degree relatives (ie, siblings, parents, aunts, uncles, and grandparents) of type 2 diabetes and cardiovascular disease risk factors, such as hypertension and dyslipidemia. In addition, the health care professional should perform a medical history and physical examination to identify any obesity-related conditions that may exist. In the case of severe obesity, the health care professional can evaluate for rare cases of underlying syndromes. Depending on BMI category, age, and family history, laboratory evaluation may be needed for several obesity-related conditions that often have no signs or symptoms, including dyslipidemia, diabetes, and nonalcoholic fatty liver disease.
- **Assess dietary, physical activity, and sedentary behaviors.** A brief assessment of foods and beverages typically consumed and the pattern of consumption can uncover modifiable behaviors associated with excess caloric intake. A dietitian can do a thorough evaluation when detail is needed or when initial obvious excesses have been addressed. An assessment of participation in age-appropriate moderate- and vigorous-intensity physical activity, both structured and unstructured, can determine approximate

amount of time spent being physically active, again with the goal of identifying opportunities for increased activity. Screen time (eg, watching television [TV] and using computers and digital devices) is associated with increased risk of obesity, and reduction of non-homework screen time is an effective strategy for weight control. Therefore, asking about hours of media or screen time will uncover a very important opportunity to modify behavior for improved energy balance.

- **Assess attitude and emotional state, including any socioeconomic stressors.** Families may not recognize excess weight or be aware of risks that obesity poses. Or, they may be unable to make behavior changes to improve eating and physical activity behaviors. This may often be caused by changes in economic, employment, or other psychosocial situations. Before providing anticipatory guidance about new behaviors, it is recommended that health care professionals assess attitude and capacity for change.

Treating Overweight and Obesity

The primary goal of obesity treatment is to improve long-term physical and psychosocial health through establishing permanent healthy lifestyle behaviors and changes to the environment where the child or adolescent lives.[11] For some children and adolescents who have overweight or obesity, implementing these habits alone will lead to improved weight (weight loss or weight maintenance during linear growth), but other children and adolescents may need additional focused efforts to achieve negative energy balance. Others may need additional help with behavior modification strategies to develop and sustain healthy habits. Emotional health (good self-esteem and an appropriate attitude toward food and the body) also is an important outcome. To achieve these goals, it has been recommended that health care professionals present a staged approach with 4

treatment stages of increasing intensity.[8] Children and adolescents can begin at the least intense stage and advance from there, depending on response to treatment, age, degree of obesity, health risks, and motivation.

Table 2 presents the 4 stages of treatment and includes the intervention strategies (the behavior changes to recommend) and the process for providing the intervention (how to offer an intervention to a family, including information about location, staffing, and support).

- **Stage 1. Prevention Plus.** As a first step, children and adolescents who have overweight or obesity and their families can focus on basic healthy eating and physical activity habits that are the foundation of obesity prevention strategies. However, unlike children and adolescents who are already at a healthy weight, the outcome is improved BMI status rather than maintained healthy BMI, and the health care professional offers more frequent monitoring to motivate the child or adolescent, and family. *Stage 1* interventions could be included in the health supervision visit.

- **Stage 2. Structured Weight Management.** This stage of treatment is accomplished in follow-up to the health supervision visit and is distinguished from Prevention Plus less by differences in targeted behaviors and more by the support and structure provided to the child or adolescent, and family, to achieve those behaviors.

- **Stage 3. Comprehensive Multidisciplinary Intervention.** This stage of treatment involves more intensive targeting behavior changes, more frequent visits, and the involvement of specialists to maximize support for behavior changes. Generally, this type of intervention is beyond what a health care professional office can offer within the typical visit structure. However, an office or several offices could organize specialists to provide this type of approach.

Table 2

Staged Approach for Treatment of Childhood and Adolescent Obesity[2,32]			
Stage	What: Recommended Behaviors for Child or Adolescent, and Family	How: Settings and Staff for Intervention	When
Stage 1. Prevention Plus	• 5+ fruits and vegetables. • <1 hour per day screen time. • ≥1 hour per day moderate or vigorous physical activity. • Reduce or eliminate sugar-sweetened beverages. • Maintain healthy eating behaviors (eg, 3 meals a day, family meals, limited eating out). • Family-based change.	• Office-based • Trained office support (eg, physician, nurse practitioner, nurse, physician assistant) • Scheduled follow-up visits	• Frequency of visits based on readiness to change or behavioral counseling. • Reevaluate in 3–6 months. • Advance to next level depending on response and interest.
Stage 2. Structured Weight Management	• Develop plan for child or adolescent, and family, to include more structure (timing and content) of daily meals and snacks. • Balanced macronutrient diet. • Reduced screen time to <1 hour per day for non-academic activities. • Increased time spent in moderate and vigorous physical activity. • Monitoring taught to improve success (eg, logs of screen time, physical activity, dietary intake, dietary patterns).	• Office-based (registered dietitian, physician, nurse) trained in assessment techniques • Motivational interviewing or behavioral counseling • Teaching parenting skills and managing family conflict • Food planning • Physical activity counseling • Support from referrals	• Monthly visits tailored to child or adolescent, and family. • Advance if needed or if no improvement after 3–6 months (improvement = weight maintenance or BMI deflection downward).

continued

Table 2 *(continued)*

Stage	What: Recommended Behaviors for Child or Adolescent, and Family	How: Settings and Staff for Intervention	When

Stage 3. Comprehensive Multidisciplinary Intervention	• Structured behavioral program (eg, food monitoring, goal-setting contingency management)
	• Improved home food environment
	• Structured dietary and physical activity interventions designed to result in negative energy balance
	• Strong parental or family involvement, especially for infants and children <12 years
		• Multidisciplinary team that includes registered dietitian, counselor or mental health care professional, and physical activity specialist
		• Dedicated pediatric weight-management program that includes nutrition, physical activity, and behavior change
			• Weekly for 8–12 weeks and then monthly
			• If no improvement after 6 months (improvement = weight loss or BMI deflection downward),
			  – For children aged 2–5 years, remain in stage 3 with continued support.
			  – For children and adolescents aged 6–11 years if >99th percentile and a comorbidity, consider stage 4.
			  – For children, adolescents, and young adults aged 12–18 years if >99th percentile with a comorbidity or with >6 months of no weight loss in stage 3, consider stage 4.

Stage 4. Tertiary Care Intervention	• Continued diet and physical activity behavioral counseling. Also, consider more aggressive approaches, such as medication, surgery, or meal replacement.	• Pediatric weight-management center operating under established protocols • Multidisciplinary team	• According to protocol

Abbreviation: BMI, body mass index.

Derived from Barton M; US Preventive Services Task Force. Screening for obesity in children and adolescents: US Preventive Services Task Force recommendation statement. *Pediatrics.* 2010;125(2):361-367; and adapted with permission from Spear BA, Barlow SE, Ervin C, et al. Recommendations for treatment of child and adolescent overweight and obesity. *Pediatrics.* 2007;120(suppl 4):S254-S288.

■ **Stage 4. Tertiary Care Intervention.** This stage of treatment, which is well beyond the purview of a health supervision visit, may include intensive interventions. These interventions, which include medications, surgery, and meal replacements, may be considered for some children and adolescents with severe obesity.

The metric for improved weight is BMI percentile, generally to below the 85th percentile, although some children and adolescents will be healthy in the overweight category (85th–94th percentile). Although improvement in BMI percentile is the goal, serial weights can reflect energy balance in the short-term. Weight maintenance leads to reduction in absolute BMI because of ongoing

linear growth, and even slow weight gain can result in lower BMI percentile because BMI for a given percentile curve rises with age. In general, younger children and those with milder obesity should change weight more gradually than older children or adolescents or those with severe obesity.

Table 3 summarizes recommendations for weight change targets for children and adolescents in obesity treatment. For children 2 years and younger, caloric restrictions designed to reduce weight are not recommended. However, health care professionals should discuss the long-term risks of obesity with parents and encourage them to establish obesity prevention strategies for this younger age.

PROMOTING HEALTHY WEIGHT

Table 3

Weight Change Targets for Children and Adolescents Based on Body Mass Index[2,32,44]				
Age, years	Body Mass Index 5th–84th Percentile	Body Mass Index 85th–94th Percentile[a]	Body Mass Index 95th–98th Percentile	Severe Obesity[b]
2–5	Maintain growth velocity.	Weight maintenance or BMI trending downward[a]	Weight maintenance or BMI trending downward	If BMI >21 gradual weight loss of not >1 lb per month until BMI <97th percentile
6–11	Maintain growth velocity.	Weight maintenance or BMI trending downward[a]	Gradual weight loss not more than 1 lb per month[c]	Weight loss maximum of an average of 2 lb per week[c]
12–18	Maintain growth velocity until linear growth complete.	Weight maintenance or BMI trending downward[a]	Weight loss of a maximum of an average of 2 lb per week[c]	Weight loss maximum of an average of 2 lb per week[c]

Abbreviations: BMI, body mass index; NHANES, National Health and Nutrition Examination Survey.

[a] These targets apply to children and adolescents who need to improve weight. Some children and adolescents who are in (or just above) the 85th–94th percentile category are unlikely to have excess body fat and should receive usual prevention counseling without a goal of lowering BMI percentile.

[b] There is no consensus on a definition of severe obesity. The expert committee suggested use of the 99th percentile based on cut points defined by Freedman et al[12] using NHANES data. However, these cut points may be imprecise. Children and adolescents with BMI at or above this level have increased health risks; therefore, intervention is more urgent.

[c] Excessive weight loss should be evaluated for high-risk behaviors.

Derived from Barton M; US Preventive Services Task Force. Screening for obesity in children and adolescents: US Preventive Services Task Force recommendation statement. *Pediatrics.* 2010;125(2):361-367; adapted with permission from Spear BA, Barlow SE, Ervin C, et al. Recommendations for treatment of child and adolescent overweight and obesity. *Pediatrics.* 2007;120(suppl 4):S254-S288; and Holt K, Wooldridge N, Story N, Sofka D. *Bright Futures: Nutrition.* 3rd ed. Elk Grove Village, IL: American Academy of Pediatrics; 2011.

Promoting a Healthy Weight: Infancy—Birth Through 11 Months

Breastfeeding[9,28] and not overfeeding (if bottle-feeding) are recommended to ensure adequate growth that is not excessive. The introduction of solid foods, as complementary additions to energy and nutrient intakes, should be delayed until around age 6 months.[9] Introducing foods with a variety of tastes and textures lays the groundwork for children's acceptance of a variety of healthy foods, including vegetables.[45,46]

The feeding relationship between the parent or other caregiver and the infant reflects a dynamic process that is initiated during infancy and extends into adolescence. Many parents and other caregivers are aware of cues from the infant suggesting hunger but need education about when to stop feeding the infant. Signs of fullness include turning away from a spoon, clamping the mouth shut, or playing with food. The interplay of signs of hunger and fullness lead to the infant's ability to self-regulate food intake in response to energy needs. Self-regulation is learned in a responsive, healthy feeding relationship that involves

- Responding early and appropriately to hunger and satiety cues
- Recognizing the infant's developmental abilities and feeding skills
- Balancing the infant's need for assistance with encouragement of self-feeding
- Allowing the infant to initiate and guide feeding interactions
- Providing the infant with multiple opportunities for back and "tummy time" and other age-appropriate physical activity
- Allowing the infant to explore his environment

Promoting a Healthy Weight: Early Childhood—1 Through 4 Years

Promoting healthy weight using a responsive parenting approach during early childhood continues building on the self-feeding and self-regulation skills initiated during infancy.[46] Healthy food choices divided into 3 meals and 2 to 3 snacks daily should provide adequate macronutrients and micronutrients for growth. *(See the For Families section of Box 1 in this theme for information on healthy eating behaviors and healthy food choices.)* Toddlers and young children typically display erratic eating behaviors that reflect growth spurts and pauses and their need to demonstrate independence. Parents and other caregivers should be guided to respond to these behaviors in ways that reflect understanding, provide structure, and support exploration. Rather than imposing how a food is served (eg, whole foods or pieces), parents can ask the child which way he would like it. They can offer two vegetables and allow the child to choose one. If a child stops eating his favorite food, parents can accept the refusal calmly, recognizing that appetite is variable and he may simply not be hungry. Alternative suggestions might be offered but not forced. If the child doesn't want to try a new food, the parent can let the child know they will be serving the food again, and maybe next time he will like it.

Parents may need guidance about age-appropriate time limits as they begin to introduce their young child to TV and other types of media. Interactive play between adults and young children prevents long periods of sedentary behaviors.

Early childhood programs have been identified as promising environments for intervention and prevention of obesity with research specifically supporting child care as an ideal context.[47] Other programs that serve young children and their families include early intervention and home visiting programs. Because of the significant number of hours a child can spend in child care and early childhood programs, the settings present ideal opportunities to prevent obesity by raising awareness about the issue, providing guidance to families and caregivers, and creating environments that support health for our youngest children.

Promoting a Healthy Weight: Middle Childhood—5 Through 10 Years

In middle childhood, children begin to broaden their experiences, and they are expected to make some of their own food choices. Out-of-home influences become more important as school routine and peers' behavior may challenge or enrich the child's and family's habits. It is recommended that health care professionals provide parents and children with information about healthy foods for lunches and snacks. In some schools, children as young as age 5 years serve themselves during school breakfast and lunch, and they should be encouraged to make healthy food choices. Parents and children may not be aware of the large number of calories consumed from juice, soft drinks, and coffee and energy drinks.

Media messages strongly influence food choices. During middle childhood, children are exposed to more media messages than at younger ages. During this period, many children increase their use of computers and handheld devices, which can increase their exposure to media messages about food and in turn influence their food choices.

When children start school, they are less active during the day. Encouraging physical activity outside the school day is critical. This activity should be free play and something the child considers fun. Although many children may begin organized sports during or before middle childhood, free play also should be encouraged.[34]

During middle childhood, children become more aware of their appearance and may express concern with their body image or weight. They may eat less to try to lose weight. Addressing the individual child's concerns may help prevent unhealthy eating behaviors.

Promoting a Healthy Weight: Adolescence—11 Through 21 Years

Adolescents spend a good deal of time away from home, and many consume fast foods and other foods that are often high in calories, saturated fats, added sugars, refined grains, and sodium. It is common for adolescents to skip meals and to snack frequently. As adolescents take increasing responsibility for what they eat, parents can support their choices by providing healthy foods at home and opportunities for the adolescent to learn about selecting, purchasing, and preparing foods. This can help the adolescent choose healthy foods. Parents, health care professionals, and others in the community can advocate for healthy food options in school cafeterias, vending machines, snack bars, school stores, and other venues at which adolescents buy food and beverages.

Health care professionals need to be sensitive to adolescents' concerns about body image and weight. Evaluating the level of body satisfaction and practices the adolescent uses to maintain or reduce body weight (eg, dieting, binge eating, physical activity patterns) will help health care professionals recognize early symptoms of eating disorders that can develop with unhealthy weight control behaviors.[48]

References

1. Pérez-Escamilla R, Obbagy JE, Altman JM, et al. Dietary energy density and body weight in adults and children: a systematic review. *J Acad Nutr Diet.* 2012;112(5):671-684

2. Barton M; US Preventive Services Task Force. Screening for obesity in children and adolescents: US Preventive Services Task Force recommendation statement. *Pediatrics.* 2010;125(2):361-367

3. Fryar CD, Carroll MD, Ogden CL; Division of Health and Nutrition Examination Surveys. Prevalence of overweight and obesity among children and adolescents: United States, 1963-1965 through 2011-2012. Centers for Disease Control and Prevention Web site. http://www.cdc.gov/nchs/data/hestat/obesity_child_11_12/obesity_child_11_12.htm. Accessed August 16, 2016

4. Ogden CL, Carroll MD, Kit BK, Flegal KM. Prevalence of childhood and adult obesity in the United States, 2011-2012. *JAMA.* 2014;311(8):806-814

5. Wang Y, Beydoun MA. The obesity epidemic in the United States—gender, age, socioeconomic, racial/ethnic, and geographic characteristics: a systematic review and meta-regression analysis. *Epidemiol Rev.* 2007;29(1):6-28

6. Singh AS, Mulder C, Twisk JW, van Mechelen W, Chinapaw MJ. Tracking of childhood overweight into adulthood: a systematic review of the literature. *Obes Rev.* 2008;9(5):474-488

7. Dietz WH, Robinson TN. Clinical practice. Overweight children and adolescents. *N Engl J Med.* 2005;352(20):2100-2109

8. Hoelscher DM, Kirk S, Ritchie L, Cunningham-Sabo L; Academy Positions Committee. Position of the Academy of Nutrition and Dietetics: interventions for the prevention and treatment of pediatric overweight and obesity. *J Acad Nutr Diet.* 2013;113(10):1375-1394

9. American Academy of Pediatrics Section on Breastfeeding. Breastfeeding and the use of human milk. *Pediatrics.* 2012;129(3):e827-e841

10. Grummer-Strawn LM, Reinold C, Krebs NF; Centers for Disease Control and Prevention. Use of World Health Organization and CDC growth charts for children aged 0-59 months in the United States. *MMWR Recomm Rep.* 2010;59(RR-9):1-15

11. Krebs NF, Himes JH, Jacobson D, Nicklas TA, Guilday P, Styne D. Assessment of child and adolescent overweight and obesity. *Pediatrics.* 2007;120(suppl 4):S193-S228

12. Freedman DS, Mei Z, Srinivasan SR, Berenson GS, Dietz WH. Cardiovascular risk factors and excess adiposity among overweight children and adolescents: the Bogalusa Heart Study. *J Pediatr.* 2007;150(1):12-17.e2

13. Barlow SE; Expert Committee. Expert committee recommendations regarding the prevention, assessment, and treatment of child and adolescent overweight and obesity: summary report. *Pediatrics.* 2007;120(suppl 4):S164-S192

14. Bandini LG, Curtin C, Hamad C, Tybor DJ, Must A. Prevalence of overweight in children with developmental disorders in the continuous National Health and Nutrition Examination Survey (NHANES) 1999-2002. *J Pediatr.* 2005;146(6):738-743

15. Chen AY, Kim SE, Houtrow AJ, Newacheck PW. Prevalence of obesity among children with chronic conditions. *Obesity (Silver Spring).* 2010;18(1):210-213

16. Ells LJ, Lang R, Shield JP, et al. Obesity and disability—a short review. *Obes Rev.* 2006;7(4):341-345

17. National Center on Birth Defects and Developmental Disabilities. Disability and obesity. Center for Disease Control and Prevention Web site. http://www.cdc.gov/ncbddd/disabilityandhealth/obesity.html. Accessed August 16, 2016

18. Rasmussen KM, Yaktine AL; Institute of Medicine. *Weight Gain During Pregnancy: Reexamining the Guidelines.* National Academies Press; 2009

19. Ino T, Shibuya T, Saito K, Inaba Y. Relationship between body mass index of offspring and maternal smoking during pregnancy. *Int J Obes (Lond).* 2012;36(4):554-558

20. Ip S, Chung M, Raman G, et al. Breastfeeding and maternal and infant health outcomes in developed countries. *Evid Rep Technol Assess (Full Rep).* 2007;(153):1-186

21. Caprio S, Daniels SR, Drewnowski A, et al. Influence of race, ethnicity, and culture on childhood obesity: implications for prevention and treatment: a consensus statement of Shaping America's Health and the Obesity Society. *Diabetes Care.* 2008;31(11):2211-2221

22. Lumeng JC, Somashekar D, Appugliese D, Kaciroti N, Corwyn RF, Bradley RH. Shorter sleep duration is associated with increased risk for being overweight at ages 9 to 12 years. *Pediatrics.* 2007;120(5):1020-1029

23. Norcross JC, Krebs PM, Prochaska JO. Stages of change. *J Clin Psychol.* 2011;67(2):143-154

24. Schwartz RP, Hamre R, Dietz WH, et al. Office-based motivational interviewing to prevent childhood obesity: a feasibility study. *Arch Pediatr Adolesc Med.* 2007;161(5):495-501

25. Davoli AM, Broccoli S, Bonvicini L, et al. Pediatrician-led motivational interviewing to treat overweight children: an RCT. *Pediatrics.* 2013;132(5):e1236-e1246

26. Fabricatore AN. Behavior therapy and cognitive-behavioral therapy of obesity: is there a difference? *J Am Diet Assoc.* 2007;107(1):92-99

27. Krebs NF, Jacobson MS; American Academy of Pediatrics Committee on Nutrition. Prevention of pediatric overweight and obesity. *Pediatrics.* 2003;112(2):424-430

28. McGuire S. US Department of Health and Human Services. The Surgeon General's Call to Action to Support Breastfeeding. US Department of Health and Human Services, Office of the Surgeon General. *Adv Nutr.* 2011;2(6):523-524

29. Jordan AB. Children's television viewing and childhood obesity. *Pediatr Ann.* 2010;39(9):569-573

30. Davis MM, Gance-Cleveland B, Hassink S, Johnson R, Paradis G, Resnicow K. Recommendations for prevention of childhood obesity. *Pediatrics.* 2007;120(suppl 4):S229-S253

31. Hammons AJ, Fiese BH. Is frequency of shared family meals related to the nutritional health of children and adolescents? *Pediatrics.* 2011;127(6):e1565-e1574

32. Spear BA, Barlow SE, Ervin C, et al. Recommendations for treatment of child and adolescent overweight and obesity. *Pediatrics.* 2007;120(suppl 4):S254-S288

33. US Department of Health and Human Services. Active adults. In: *2008 Physical Activity Guidelines for Americans.* Washington, DC: US Department of Health and Human Services; 2008:21-28. ODPHP publication U0036. http://health.gov/paguidelines/guidelines. Accessed August 16, 2016

34. American Academy of Pediatrics Council on Sports Medicine and Fitness, Council on School Health. Active healthy living: prevention of childhood obesity through increased physical activity. *Pediatrics.* 2006;117(5):1834-1842

PROMOTING HEALTHY WEIGHT

35. American Academy of Pediatrics Council on Communications and Media. Media and young minds. *Pediatrics.* 2016;138(5):e20162591

36. How to make a family media use plan. HealthyChildren.org Web site. https://www.healthychildren.org/English/family-life/Media/Pages/How-to-Make-a-Family-Media-Use-Plan.aspx. Updated October 21, 2016. Accessed December 14, 2016

37. American Academy of Pediatrics Council on Communications and Media. Media use in school-aged children and adolescents. *Pediatrics.* 2016;138(5):e20162592

38. Kohl HW III, Cook HD; Institute of Medicine. *Educating the Student Body: Taking Physical Activity and Physical Education to School.* Washington, DC: National Academies Press; 2013

39. Murray R, Ramstetter C; American Academy of Pediatrics Council on School Health. The crucial role of recess in school. *Pediatrics.* 2013;131(1):183-188

40. American Academy of Pediatrics Council on School Health, Committee on Nutrition. Snacks, sweetened beverages, added sugars, and schools. *Pediatrics.* 2015;135(3):575-583

41. Daniels SR, Arnett DK, Eckel RH, et al. Overweight in children and adolescents: pathophysiology, consequences, prevention, and treatment. *Circulation.* 2005;111(15):1999-2012

42. Fanburg J, ed. *5210 Pediatric Obesity Clinical Decision Support Chart.* 2nd ed. Elk Grove Village, IL: American Academy of Pediatrics; 2014

43. Estrada E, Eneli I, Hampl S, et al. Children's Hospital Association consensus statements for comorbidities of childhood obesity. *Child Obes.* 2014;10(4):304-317

44. Holt K, Wooldridge N, Story N, Sofka D. *Bright Futures: Nutrition.* 3rd ed. Elk Grove Village, IL: American Academy of Pediatrics; 2011

45. Mennella JA, Trabulsi JC. Complementary foods and flavor experiences: setting the foundation. *Ann Nutr Metab.* 2012;60(suppl 2):40-50

46. Daniels LA, Mallan KM, Nicholson JM, Battistutta D, Magarey A. Outcomes of an early feeding practices intervention to prevent childhood obesity. *Pediatrics.* 2013;132(1):e109-e118

47. Kaphingst K, Story M. Child care as an untapped setting for obesity prevention: state child care licensing regulation related to nutrition, physical activity, and media use for preschool-aged children in the United States. *Prev Chronic Dis.* 2009;6(1):A11

48. Neumark-Sztainer D. Preventing obesity and eating disorders in adolescents: what can health care providers do? *J Adolesc Health.* 2009;44(3):206-213

Promoting Healthy Nutrition

Infancy, childhood, and adolescence are marked by rapid physical growth and development, and every child's and adolescent's health and development depends on good nutrition. Any disruption in appropriate nutrient intake may have lasting effects on growth potential and developmental achievement. Physical growth, developmental requirements, nutrition needs, and feeding patterns vary significantly during each stage of growth and development.

The dramatic rise in pediatric overweight and obesity in recent years has increased health care professionals' and parents' level of attention to nutrition. Along with regular physical activity, a balanced and nutritious diet offered in a supportive feeding environment is essential to prevent pediatric overweight. Therefore, health care professionals are encouraged to review this Bright Futures theme in concert with the *Promoting Physical Activity and Promoting Healthy Weight themes.*

Key Food and Nutrition Considerations

Food and nutrition behaviors are influenced by myriad environmental and cultural forces. Health care professionals should keep these forces in mind as they work with patients and families. Four issues of particular importance are discussed here.

The Feeding Environment

The feeding and eating experience strongly affects an infant's, child's, and adolescent's physical, social, emotional, and cognitive development. The experience includes the foods selected and the environment within which food is offered. The relationship between the caregiver and the child reflects a dynamic process that is initiated during infancy and extends into adolescence.

In principle, the infant or child provides cues (expressing hunger) to the parent to begin the process. The caregiver responds by selecting and providing age-appropriate food. They continue to interact throughout the process until the infant or child provides satiety cues to the caregiver.

In reality, multiple issues affect the relationship. A host of psychosocial, economic, and other factors influence a parent's choice of foods and the style used to feed. Factors include how the caregiver was fed as a child and his or her current knowledge, skills, and attitudes. Caregivers have limited control over foods eaten away from home or prepared elsewhere to be consumed at home, among other

167

things. Adult interactions can be helpful or harmful as children try new foods, learn to self-regulate food intake, develop self-help skills, and fine-tune internal self-control over how much food to eat.

Recent evidence suggests decreasing quality in a child's diet with advancing age. Children aged 2 to 5 years are more likely to consume 3 meals a day, beginning with breakfast, while adolescent girls, young adult men, and those with lower incomes are least likely to have breakfast or consume 3 daily meals. Many young children consume recommended amounts of fruit and dairy, but that intake drops as they reach school age and beyond.[1] The reasons for this decline in diet quality are subjects for future study, but clinicians note that when children are young, parents and caregivers are highly motivated to provide healthy food and have significant control over what their children consume. With advancing age, however, children and adolescents increasingly make their own food choices and are influenced by the outside food environment.

Culture and Food

All people belong to some kind of cultural group. Culture influences the way people look at the world, how they interact with others, and how they expect others to behave. To meet the challenge of providing nutrition supervision to diverse populations, health care professionals must learn to respect and appreciate the variety of cultural traditions related to food and the wide variation in food practices within, among, and across cultural groups. Health care professionals also need to understand how their own cultures influence their attitudes and behaviors and the resulting implications for nutrition counseling. Sharing food experiences, asking questions, observing the food choices people make, and working with the community are important ways for health care professionals to learn about and appreciate the food and nutrition traditions of other cultures.[2]

Culture influences which foods people select to eat, how people prepare food, how they use seasonings, and how often they eat certain foods. These behaviors can differ from region to region and family to family, although some traditions exist across cultures. For example, staple, or core, foods form the foundation of the diet in all cultures. Staple foods, such as rice or beans, are typically bland, relatively inexpensive, easy to prepare, an important source of calories, and an indispensable part of the diet.

Acculturation, which is the adoption of the beliefs, values, attitudes, and behaviors of a dominant, or mainstream, culture, can be a significant influence on a person's food choices. Acculturation may involve altering traditional eating behaviors to make them similar to those of the dominant culture. These changes can be grouped into 3 categories: (1) the addition of new foods, (2) the substitution of foods, and (3) the rejection of foods. People add new foods for various reasons, including improved economic status and food availability (especially if the food is not readily available in the person's homeland). Substitution may occur because new foods are more convenient to prepare, more affordable, or better liked than traditional ones. Children and adolescents, in particular, may reject traditional foods because eating them makes them feel different from the mainstream.

Culture also influences nonnutritive aspects of food practices, and any nutritional information and guidance should take these preferences and practices into account. Some ethnic practices related to diet and nutrition may focus more on the food's texture, appearance, flavor, or aroma or on beliefs related to the complementary nature of the food items, rather than on specific nutritional value. Cultural flavor preferences may be adopted in utero as well as through breastfeeding and influence the dietary preferences for complementary foods when they are added at around 6 months of age.[3] For many people, certain foods are closely linked to strong feelings of being cared for and nurtured by their families or are a reflection of religious practices. People from virtually all cultures use food during celebrations.

In many cultures, people believe that food promotes health, cures disease, or has other medicinal qualities. In addition, many people believe foods can help maintain a balance in the body that is important to health. For example, many Chinese persons believe that health and disease are related to the balance between yin and yang forces in the body. Diseases caused by yin forces are treated with yang foods to restore balance, and vice versa. In Puerto Rico, foods are classified as hot or cold (which may not reflect the actual temperature or spiciness of foods), and people believe that maintaining a balance between these two types of foods is important to health.

Health care professionals can provide effective nutrition guidance by being sensitive to cultural beliefs that categorize foods in ways other than the Western scientific model, by exploring such beliefs, and by incorporating them into their guidance. When discussing their food choices, patients and their parents may respond by saying what they think the health care professional wants to hear. Health care professionals can encourage people to be more candid about their food choices by asking open-ended, nonjudgmental questions that reflect their knowledge of and sensitivity to these issues.

Two issues illustrate the challenges of providing nutrition supervision to people from diverse cultural backgrounds. The first, lactose intolerance, highlights the medical aspects involved. The second, attitudes about body weight, highlights the deep-seated emotional and attitudinal aspects that are often involved.

Lactose Intolerance

Lactose intolerance is common in people of non-European ancestry. When discussing calcium intake, health care professionals need to be sensitive to the fact that people may be lactose intolerant. People who are lactose intolerant may experience cramps and diarrhea when they eat moderate to large amounts of foods that contain lactose, such as milk and other dairy products. Children and adolescents may be able to avoid symptoms by consuming small servings of milk throughout the day, by consuming lactose-reduced milk, or by taking lactase tablets or drops with milk. Cheese and yogurt are often better tolerated than milk because they contain less lactose. For people who cannot tolerate any milk or dairy products, health care professionals can suggest a combination of other sources of calcium. A vitamin D supplement also may be needed.

Attitudes About Body Weight

People from different cultures can view body weight differently. Keeping a child from having underweight can be very important to people from cultures in which poverty or insufficient food supplies are common. Families may not recognize that their child has overweight according to body mass index (BMI) tables or may view excess weight as healthy. In these cases, the families may be offended if a health care professional refers to their child as having overweight or obesity. *(For more information on this topic, see the Promoting Healthy Weight theme.)*

Food Insecurity and Hunger

Hunger describes the personal sensation that results from a lack of food and is typically felt as unpleasant or painful. Involuntary hunger results from not being able to obtain enough food and excludes hunger related to voluntary dieting, religious fasting, or the personal choice to skip a meal.

Food insecurity for a family means limited or uncertain availability of nutritionally adequate and safe foods or uncertain ability to acquire appropriate foods in socially acceptable ways. In 2014, 19.2% of households with infants, children, and adolescents younger than 18 years were food insecure.[4]

Food insecurity may occur with or without hunger. At its most extreme, this problem is associated with hunger and is an indication of a serious nutritional problem and family predicament. Food insecurity without hunger is associated with increased nutritional risk. An important deleterious effect of food insecurity is that it forces people to buy and consume less expensive foods, which are often lower in nutritional value but more calorically dense than more expensive foods. As a result, the nutritional quality of the diet declines.[5] *(For more information on this topic, see the Promoting Healthy Weight theme.)*

The problems of food insecurity and hunger may be difficult to detect in the primary pediatric health care setting. Living with adult smokers is an independent risk factor for frequency and severity of food insecurity.[6] If disorders of growth, either underweight and overweight, are noted, health care professionals should consider food insecurity. Options for referral and community support are available for each developmental stage. For example, local lactation specialists or other knowledgeable health care professionals, such as doulas, promotoras, or home visitors, can provide follow-up care after a new mother is discharged from the hospital, and they can consult by phone or schedule visits to a hospital-based lactation clinic. Health care facilities, community health teams, and community hospitals also are sources of infant nutrition education. The US Department of Agriculture (USDA) Special Supplemental Nutrition Program for Women, Infants, and Children (WIC)[7] offers a food package for women who are pregnant or postpartum, women who are breastfeeding their infant, and infants and children up to 5 years of age. Health departments offer educational services through WIC and other programs in which public health nurses or nutritionists visit families at home. Additionally, early care and education programs, which include home visiting and child care, create opportunities to educate parents and families on nutrition, cooking, and healthy eating habits.

Another source of support for families experiencing food insecurity is programs such as the USDA Supplemental Nutrition Assistance Program (the program formerly known as Food Stamps).[8] A community food bank or pantry can provide additional food for families needing assistance. For young children, some child care settings are eligible for reimbursement from the USDA Child and Adult Care Food Program.[9] For school-aged children and for adolescents, community services expand to include free and reduced-cost school breakfast and lunch programs and, ideally, school food services that offer healthy and appealing food choices. For adolescents, some school programs focus on the importance of pre-conceptual nutrition to ensure good nutrition.

Partnerships With the Community

Partnerships among health care professionals, families, and communities are essential to ensure that infants and children have good nutrition and that parents receive guidance on infant and child nutrition and feeding. *(For more information on this topic, see the Promoting Lifelong Health for Families and Communities theme.)* Health care professionals can have a tremendous effect on decisions about feeding the family because they provide an opportunity for parents to discuss, reflect on, and decide on options that best suit their circumstances. As part of their guidance, health care professionals also can identify and refer parents to community resources that help at each stage of a child's development. Because of considerable media attention to the problem of overweight and obesity, the public has become increasingly aware of the importance of healthy eating and regular physical activity. Communities have responded by creating educational programs that provide nutritious school lunches, access to affordable nutritious foods, and safe neighborhood opportunities for play and exercise. Health care professionals can help families learn about and take advantage of these opportunities. These resources are particularly important for families with limited or no literacy skills and for those with limited English proficiency.

Essential Components of Nutrition

The following essential components of nutrition are useful constructs for discussing nutrition from birth through young adulthood:

- **Nutrition for appropriate growth.** Provide adequate energy and essential nutrients to ensure appropriate growth and prevent overweight or obesity.
- **Nutrition and development of feeding and eating skills.** Choose foods that provide essential nutrients and support the development of age-appropriate feeding and eating skills.
- **Healthy feeding and eating habits.** Establish a positive, nurturing environment and healthy patterns of feeding and eating to promote eating habits that are built on variety, balance, and moderation.
- **Healthy eating relationships.** Promote healthy adult-child feeding relationships and social and emotional development.
- **Nutrition for children and youth with special health care needs.** Recognize specific nutrient demands or supplemental needs for vitamins or minerals related to a child's special health condition and provide these nutritional components.

Promoting Nutritional Health: Preconception and the Prenatal Period

In deciding to become parents, a couple may examine many issues of lifestyle and health because they recognize that their nutrition and physical activity beliefs, habits, and practices not only affect their own health but will now also affect the health of their family and child. Obesity, smoking, alcohol consumption, and substance use affect the family as well as the individual. Women who are pregnant or who may become pregnant should be encouraged to follow a nutritious diet, abstain from alcohol, and take a daily prenatal vitamin and iron supplement to help ensure their health and that of a developing fetus. They also are encouraged to quit smoking during and after pregnancy and avoid all secondhand smoke exposure. Both active and maternal smoking and maternal secondhand tobacco smoke exposure have been shown to reduce birth weight. Many health care professionals recommend the continued use of prenatal vitamin supplements during lactation. Adequate intakes of certain nutrients, such as folic acid, omega-3 fatty acids, and choline, are important before conception as well as during lactation.

Folic Acid

Neural tube defects are among the most common birth defects contributing to infant mortality and serious disability. Women capable of becoming pregnant can substantially reduce the risk of having an infant with certain congenital malformations, including spina bifida, by taking appropriate amounts of folic acid before and during early pregnancy. Current guidelines indicate that all females capable of becoming pregnant take a daily multivitamin or multivitamin-mineral supplement containing 400 µg of synthetic folic acid (from fortified food or supplements) in addition to consuming foods rich in folate.[10-13] Women who have given birth previously to a child with a neural tube defect or women who have a history of insulin-dependent diabetes or a seizure disorder and are taking antimetabolites or antiepileptic drugs (eg, carbamazepine) require higher dosages of folate. Knowledge about appropriate folic acid dosages continues to evolve. Current recommendations are available from the Centers for Disease Control and Prevention (CDC).[12]

Omega-3 Fatty Acids and Choline

To guarantee a sufficient concentration of pre-formed docosahexaenoic acid (DHA) in her breast milk, the mother's diet should include an average daily intake of 200 to 300 mg of the omega-3 long-chain polyunsaturated fatty acid (PUFA) DHA.[14] One or two 3-oz servings of fish weekly will provide the necessary omega-3 long-chain PUFAs. The possible risk from intake of excessive mercury or other contaminants in fish is offset by the neurobehavioral benefits of adequate DHA intake. Predatory fish (eg, shark, king mackerel, tile fish, swordfish) are to be *avoided,* as they carry the highest heavy metal contamination risk. Salmon, herring, canned white tuna, and trout are *recommended* as very low-risk.[15] Additionally, the mother's diet should include 550 mg/day of choline because human milk is rich in choline and breastfeeding depletes the mother's tissue stores. Eggs, milk, chicken, beef, and pork are the biggest contributors of choline.[16]

Promoting Nutritional Health: Infancy—Birth Through 11 Months

Physical growth, developmental achievements, nutrition needs, and feeding patterns vary significantly in each stage of infancy. During the first 2 to 6 weeks of life, the infant primarily feeds, sleeps, and grows. The most rapid growth occurs in early infancy, between birth and 6 months of age. In middle infancy, from 6 to 9 months of age, and late infancy, from 9 to 12 months of age, rapid growth continues but at a slower pace. By late infancy, mastery of purposeful activity complements physical maturity, and loss of newborn reflexes allows the infant to progress from a diet of human milk or infant formula to feeding with an increasingly wide variety of flavors, textures, and foods.

Feeding practices and routines serve as the foundation for much of a child's and family's development, as parents build many important skills. These skills include identifying, assessing, and responding to infant cues, promoting reciprocity, and building the infant's feeding and pre-speech skills. When feeding their infant, parents clarify and strengthen their sense of what it means to be a parent. They gain a sense of responsibility by caring for an infant, experience frustration when they cannot easily interpret their infant's cues, and further develop their ability to negotiate and solve problems through their interactions with the infant.

Nutrition for Growth

The infant's diet must provide adequate energy and essential nutrients for appropriate growth. Conversely, growth is an important indicator of nutritional adequacy. Although newborns may lose up to 10% of their body weight in the first week of life, they usually regain their birth weight by 14 days after birth.[17] By the time they are 4 to 6 months of age, infants typically have doubled their birth weight, gaining about 4 to 7 oz per week. Infants typically triple their birth weight by 1 year of age, gaining about 2 to 3 oz per week (breastfed) and 3 to 5 oz per week (formula fed from 6–12 months of age).[18]

Infants grow approximately 1 in per month from birth to 6 months of age, but the rate of growth slows from 6 to 12 months of age when infants gain about a half an inch per month. Infants usually increase their length by 50% in the first year of life. Infant growth is properly assessed using the World Health Organization (WHO) Growth Charts for 0 to 2 years (Appendix A), as recommended by the American Academy of Pediatrics (AAP) and the CDC. The WHO charts are derived from a population of healthy breastfed infants.[18] They are conceptually prescriptive and prospective for desired growth, unlike the CDC birth to 2 charts, which are observational and often based on overweight populations and include a large number of formula-fed infants.

Infants who are fed on demand usually consume the amount they need to grow well. Breastfeeding initiation and duration are associated with a reduction in excess weight gain by age 3 years compared to formula feeding.[19] The significance of this difference to future growth or risk of overweight is uncertain. Infants' growth depends on nutrition, perinatal history, epigenetic and genetic factors (eg, parental height, genetic syndromes, disorders), and other physical factors.

Growth in head circumference up to 2 years of age is so closely related to growth in body length that head circumference measurements do not yield more information about an infant's nutritional status than do body length measures. After 2 years of age, head circumference grows so slowly that it is a poor indicator of nutritional status. However, in an older child, small head circumference may be a good indicator of malnutrition that occurred during the first 2 years. Head circumference, however, remains important in screening for microcephaly and macrocephaly because these abnormalities are not nutritional in origin.

Energy (Caloric) Needs

To meet growth demands, all infants require a high intake of calories and adequate intakes of fat, protein, carbohydrates, vitamins, and minerals. Human milk and infant formula provide 40% to 50% of energy from fat to meet the infant's growth and development demands. Fats should not be restricted in the first 2 years of life. Vitamin and mineral needs, with the exception of vitamin D, usually are supplied if the term infant is breastfed or if the infant receives an adequate volume of correctly prepared infant formula.

Vitamin and Mineral Supplements

A major concern in infancy is the adverse effect of early iron deficiency on psychomotor development. Iron deficiency can result in cognitive and motor deficits,[20] some of which may be prevented with iron supplementation.[21] A Cochrane Review

on the subject concluded there is no clear evidence that treating young children with anemia secondary to iron deficiency will improve psychomotor development within 30 days of therapy, but the effects of longer-term iron supplementation are not yet known.[22] Thus, prevention is extraordinarily important. During the first year of life, infants at highest risk of iron deficiency are those born prematurely, those fed infant formula that is not iron fortified, and those who are exclusively breastfed for more than 4 months without iron supplements. Term, healthy infants have enough iron stores for at least 4 months of life. Because human milk contains little iron, infants who receive only human milk are at an increasing risk for iron deficiency after 4 months of age.[15] Therefore, the AAP Committee on Nutrition recommends that oral iron drops (1 mg/kg/day) begin at 4 months of age and continue until iron- and zinc-rich complementary foods (baby meats and iron-fortified cereals) are introduced.[23]

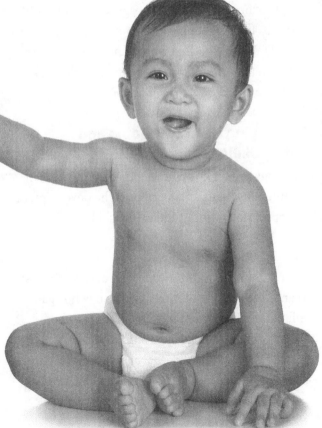

It may take a month or two following introduction of these foods for infants to consume sufficient iron from complementary foods alone. Red meat is a better source of iron than are iron-fortified cereals for older infants because a higher percentage of the iron in red meat is absorbed. Infants who receive at least 500 mL (17 oz) of iron-fortified infant formula per day do not need additional iron supplementation.

Vitamin D deficiency or insufficiency is now more prevalent in infants because of the decreased exposure to sunlight secondary to changes in lifestyle and use of topical sunscreens. The AAP recommends that all breastfed infants receive vitamin D supplementation (400 IU per day) beginning in the 2 months after birth.[24] Breastfed infants whose mothers are vegans or vitamin B_{12} deficient need supplements of vitamin B_{12}. Calcium intake is sufficient in infants who receive enough human milk or infant formula.

Fluoride supplementation is not indicated until after the eruption of teeth, which usually occurs at approximately 6 months of age. Beginning at 6 months, fluoride supplementation is recommended for infants and children who do not drink fluroridated water.[25] (For more information on this topic, see the Promoting Oral Health theme.)

Developing Healthy Feeding and Eating Skills

Feedings should be planned to provide all known essential nutrients and to support the development of appropriate feeding and eating skills.

Breastfeeding

Breastfeeding is recommended for at least the first year of life because of its benefits to newborn and infant nutrition, gastrointestinal function, host defense, neurodevelopment, and psychological well-being (Box 1). Maternal avoidance of highly allergenic foods during lactation is *not* recommended because it provides no proven benefit to the infants and children.

Immediately after delivery, early and frequent physical contact, rooming-in, and exclusion of commercial infant formula samples enhance the duration of breastfeeding. The AAP Section on Breastfeeding recommends exclusive breastfeeding for about 6 months to maximize its benefits.[15,26]

Because the decision about whether to breastfeed is often made before or early in pregnancy, the Prenatal Visit offers an important opportunity to promote exclusive breastfeeding. Women may have questions about breastfeeding and its nutritional adequacy, their ability to know if the infant is drinking enough human milk, the mother's ability to produce enough human milk to satisfy the infant's hunger, or whether the mother should breastfeed if she smokes or has an underlying health condition. Women also express concerns about their need to return to work or school within 6 to 8 weeks after the infant's birth, or the competing needs of other children and family members. To promote continued breastfeeding, health care professionals can inform women about breast pumping and proper storage and handling of human milk as an option for women returning to work and school. Prenatal and postpartum counseling can address these issues and also prolong the duration of breastfeeding.[27]

Parents also may raise concerns about maternal medication usage or maternal or infant illness and the advisability of breastfeeding. Decisions about the appropriateness of breastfeeding in these situations are best made on an individual basis with a health care professional. Under most circumstances, mothers can continue to breastfeed their infants or supply human milk if the infant is unable to feed directly at the breast, but a few contraindications to breastfeeding exist. Medications taken by the mother should be individually evaluated to determine whether they can be used safely when breastfeeding.[28] Few prescription and nonprescription medications are contraindicated for the mother who breastfeeds her infant.

Box 1

Benefits of Breastfeeding

Human milk is uniquely suited to the needs of the newborn and growing infant and provides many benefits for general health, growth, and development.[26]

Breastfeeding[15]

- Provides ideal nutrition and promotes the best possible growth and development
- Significantly decreases the incidence of diarrhea, lower respiratory tract infection, otitis media, bacteremia, bacterial meningitis, botulism, and urinary tract infection
- May be protective against inflammatory bowel disease, leukemias, and certain genotypes of type 1 diabetes mellitus
- Lowers the risk of obesity in some populations
- Promotes healthy neurologic development
- May reduce the incidence of atopic illness, such as allergy or eczema, in children at genetic risk[29]
- Promotes close mother-infant connection

Benefits to the Mother

- Breastfeeding increases levels of oxytocin, which results in less postpartum bleeding and more rapid uterine involution.
- Lactating women have an earlier return to prepregnancy weight, delayed resumption of ovulation with increased child spacing, improved postpartum bone remineralization, and reduced risk of ovarian cancer and premenopausal breast cancer.
- Lactation amenorrhea promotes the recovery of maternal iron stores depleted during pregnancy.
- Breastfeeding lowers the risk for maternal chronic diseases such as hypertension, type 2 diabetes, coronary artery disease, and some cancers.[30,31]

Benefits to the Family

- Breastfeeding has no associated costs and requires no equipment or preparation.
- It is easy to travel with a breastfed infant because no special equipment or supplies are necessary.

Benefits to the Community

- Breastfeeding reduces health care costs and employee absenteeism by reducing childhood illness.

Cultural factors may influence breastfeeding initiation and success. Parents need practical support for breastfeeding as well as culturally based information and guidance. A solid knowledge of the parents' culture and community will help health care professionals give parents the support, appropriate education, and guidance they need to be successful in breastfeeding their infant.

Formula Feeding

For infants who are not breastfed, iron-fortified infant formula is the recommended nutrition substitute during the first year of life. Cow's milk, goat's milk, soy beverages (not soy infant formula), and low-iron infant formulas should not be used during the first year of life. Reduced-fat (2%), low-fat (1%), fat-free (skim), and soy milk are not recommended for infants and children during the first 2 years of life.

Health care professionals should counsel parents to avoid propping the bottle or letting their infant self-feed. This precaution will minimize the risk for choking, ear infections, early childhood caries, insufficient intake, and the missed opportunities for enhancing the parent-child relationship. To prevent dental caries, parents should be instructed not to put the infant to bed with a bottle or sippy cup that contains milk, infant formula, juices, soda, or other sweetened beverages. *(For more information on this topic, see the Promoting Oral Health theme.)* Fruit juices are not needed during the first 6 months of life, but if they are given after 6 months, they should be given by cup, not a bottle. Caregivers should not add cereal or other foods to infant formula unless a health care professional has instructed them to do so.

Soy, protein hydrolysates, and amino acid infant formulas have been developed for infants who cannot tolerate milk protein or lactose. It is recommended that parents manage their infant's milk intolerance with guidance from their health care professional. Intolerance to cow's milk–based infant formulas, manifested by loose stools, spitting up, or vomiting, may prompt a change to soy infant formula, but little evidence supports this practice. Soy infant formulas may be recommended for a vegetarian lifestyle, transient lactase deficiency, and galactosemia. Soy infant formula should not be used for premature infants, cow's milk protein–induced enterocolitis, or the prevention of colic or allergy.[32]

Frequency and Amount of Feedings

Hunger cues for the newborn include rooting, sucking, and hand movements. In young infants, hunger cues may include hand-to-mouth movements and lip smacking. Smiling, cooing, or gazing at the parent during feeding can indicate that the infant wants more food. For older infants, hunger cues can include crying, excited arm and leg movements, opening mouth and moving forward as the spoon approaches, and swiping food toward the mouth. Crying is considered a late feeding cue and usually interferes with feeding as the infant becomes distressed and is less likely to eat well.

Infants can signal that they are full by becoming fussy during feeding, slowing the pace of eating, turning away, stopping sucking, or spitting out or refusing the nipple. Other satiety cues include refusing the spoon, batting the spoon away, and closing the mouth as the spoon approaches. As with all feeding interactions, parents should observe the infant's verbal and nonverbal cues and respond appropriately. If a food is rejected, parents should move on and try it again later rather than forcing the infant to eat or finish foods. It may take multiple exposures to a food before an infant is willing to recognize a new taste as part of her diet.

In the first months of life, breastfed infants must be fed a minimum of 8 to 12 times in 24 hours (ie, approximately every 2–3 hours). Parents should be taught to recognize and respond to early feeding cues. As infants grow older, they typically are satisfied by less frequent, larger feedings.

No recommendations exist for maximum volumes of infant formula at any one feeding, only for meeting total energy and fluid needs. Parents should offer 2 oz of infant formula every 2 to 3 hours in the first week of life. If the newborn still seems hungry, parents can provide more until the newborn indicates that she is full. As the newborn grows, a larger amount of infant formula is needed, and the newborn should feed until she indicates that she is full. Satiety cues in formula-fed newborns include turning away from the nipple, falling asleep, and spitting up milk. A newborn at the 50th percentile for weight will consume an average of 20 oz of infant formula per day; the amount of infant formula ranges from 16 to 24 oz per day.

When she begins to sleep for longer periods at night (4–5 hours at about 2 months of age), the formula-fed infant will still need to feed 6 to 8 times in 24 hours. A 4-month-old will consume an average of 31 oz of infant formula per day without complementary foods with a range of 26 to 36 oz per day. However, her intake will fluctuate from day to day and week to week. During growth spurts, intake volume increases but will fall back to lesser volumes when the growth spurt ends.

Infants 6 months and older generally consume 24 to 32 oz per day in addition to complementary foods. Over time, the increasing volume of complementary foods is accompanied by a decreasing volume of infant formula.

Introducing Complementary Foods

Complementary foods, commonly referred to as solids, include any foods or beverages besides human milk or infant formula. The AAP Committee on Nutrition states that complementary foods can be introduced in infants' diets at about 6 months of age and when the infant is developmentally ready.[33] During the second 6 months of life, complementary foods are an addition to, not a replacement for, human milk or infant formula.

Parents need practical guidance when they begin to introduce complementary foods, as they seek to determine the best time to start this exciting new phase. Infants differ in their readiness to accept complementary foods. Counseling parents on the normal progression of development of feeding and eating skills and the infant's related ability to safely eat will help them succeed in and enjoy the new experience.

Waiting until the infant is developmentally ready to begin eating complementary foods makes that process and the later transition to table foods easier. Signs that an infant is ready to begin semi-solid (pureed) foods include fading of the extrusion reflex (the tongue-thrust reflex that pushes

food out of the mouth) and elevating the tongue to move pureed food forward and backward in the mouth (which usually occurs between 4 and 6 months of age). An increased demand for breastfeeding that continues for a few days, is not affected by increased breastfeeding, and is unrelated to illness, teething, or changes in routine also may be a sign of readiness for complementary foods. At this stage, the infant sits self-supported by her arms and has good head and neck control. The infant can indicate her desire for food by opening her mouth and leaning forward and can indicate disinterest or satiety by leaning back and turning away.

When the infant is able to sit independently and tries to grasp foods with her palms, she is ready to progress to thicker pureed foods and soft, mashed foods without lumps. She also can begin to sip from a small cup. When the infant crawls and pulls to a standing position, she also begins to use her jaw and tongue to mash food, plays with a spoon at mealtime (but does not use it for self-feeding yet), and tries to hold a cup independently. At this stage, she is able to progress to ground or soft, mashed foods with small, soft, noticeable lumps (eg, finely chopped meat or poultry). At about 7 to 9 months of age, the infant learns to put objects in her mouth and will try to feed herself. At this age, the infant has developed a pincer grasp (the ability to pick up objects between thumb and forefinger). Any food the infant can pick up can be considered a finger food. Foods that dissolve easily, such as crackers or dry cereal, are good choices, but foods that can cause choking, such as popcorn, grapes, raw carrots, nuts, hard candies, and hot dogs, should be avoided.

Evidence for introducing complementary foods in a specific sequence or at any specific rate is not available. The general recommendation is that the first solid foods should be single-ingredient foods and should be introduced one at a time and no more frequently than every 3 days. The order in which solid foods are introduced is not critical as long as essential nutrients that complement human milk or infant formula are provided. Pureed meats and iron-fortified cereals provide many of these nutrients for both breastfed and formula-fed infants. After the infant has accepted these new foods, parents can gradually introduce other pureed foods or soft fruits and vegetables 2 to 3 times per day and allow her to control how much she eats. Parents also can offer store-bought or home-prepared baby food and soft table foods, such as mashed potatoes, bananas, or avocados. Breastfed infants are exposed to a variety of flavors through their mother's breast milk; thus, dietary variety is important not just for infants but for their mothers as well. Mixing cereal with human milk enhances acceptance of cereal by the breastfed infant.[34] Repeated exposures to foods enhances acceptance by both breastfed and formula-fed infants.[35]

A nutritious and balanced diet for the older infant includes appropriate amounts of human milk or infant formula and complementary foods to ensure intake of all essential nutrients and to foster

appropriate growth. By the end of the first year of life, the infant should be introduced to healthy foods, such as vegetables, fruits, and whole grains, as well as poultry, fish, and lean meats. Foods that are high in calories, saturated fats, and added sugars and low in essential nutrients, such as sweetened drinks, soda, chips, and french fries, should be avoided.

Parents should not give their infants soda and fruit drinks because of their high added sugar and calorie content and lack of nutrients. In addition, parents should give no more than 4 to 6 oz of 100% fruit juice daily to infants 6 months or older who can drink from a cup. Because many parents consider 100% fruit juice to be nutritious, they may not recognize the need to limit consumption. However, fruit juice is high in calories and sugar. Consuming large quantities can contribute to early childhood caries, pediatric overweight and obesity, and diarrhea. Fruit juice could be used as part of a meal; it should not be diluted with water and sipped throughout the day as a means to pacify an unhappy child.[36]

To establish habits of eating in moderation, infants should be allowed to stop eating at the earliest sign of unwillingness and not urged to consume more. Parents should allow the infant to control the amount of milk, infant formula, or complementary foods consumed according to her hunger and satiety cues. Breastfeeding can aid in establishing habits of eating in moderation because the breastfed infant has more control over the amount consumed at a feeding.[37] Parents who feed their infant using infant formula or human milk by bottle should be warned against encouraging the infant to finish the bottle when satiety cues are demonstrated.

Eating nutritious foods and avoiding foods that provide calories without nutrients help establish habits of eating in moderation. Furthermore,

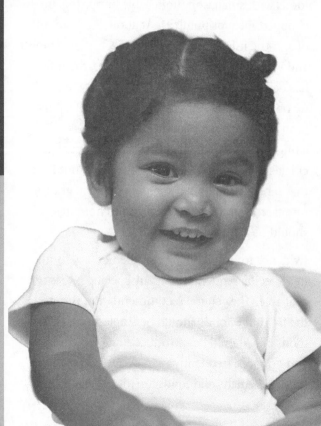

PROMOTING HEALTHY NUTRITION

establishing regular mealtimes and snack times and avoiding continuous feeding, or grazing, will help prevent overweight and underweight.

Handling Feeding and Eating Problems

Parents frequently have concerns and questions about infant feeding and eating issues, and an important aspect of health supervision during this developmental stage is helping parents distinguish normal infant feeding behaviors from feeding or eating problems.

Food Sensitivities and Allergies

Food allergy and hypersensitivity are forms of food intolerance characterized by reproducible symptoms with each exposure to the offending food and an abnormal immunologic reaction to the food. Symptoms and disorders such as irritability, hyperactivity, gastrointestinal discomfort, and asthma have been attributed to food allergies, but *true food allergies are not common.* Food hypersensitivity reactions occur in 2% to 8% of infants and children younger than 3 years. Food allergy can result in symptoms affecting the gastrointestinal tract (eg, vomiting, cramps, or diarrhea), skin (eg, eczema or hives), and respiratory tract (eg, asthma) or in generalized, life-threatening allergic reactions (ie, anaphylaxis). Hyperactivity is not a manifestation of food allergy.

The most common foods associated with allergic reactions in young children are cow's milk, eggs, peanuts, soy, and wheat. Approximately 2.5% of infants and children will experience an allergic reaction to cow's milk in the first 3 years of life, 1.3% will have a reaction to eggs, and 0.8% will have a reaction to peanuts. Tree nuts, fish, and shellfish become more common causes of food allergy in adolescence and adulthood.[38]

The American Academy of Allergy, Asthma & Immunology (AAAAI) has developed recommendations, based on current evidence and expert opinion, for the primary prevention of allergic disease through nutrition interventions. They endorse exclusive breastfeeding for at least 4 months and up to 6 months of age to reduce the incidence of atopic dermatitis, wheezing before 4 years of age, and cow's milk allergy but not food allergy in general.[39]

Additionally, the AAAAI endorses the introduction of complementary foods between 4 and 6 months of age, with recommendations for how and when to introduce the main allergenic foods (cow's milk, egg, soy, wheat, peanuts, tree nuts, fish, and shellfish). Importantly, they concluded that *delayed introduction* of solid foods, especially the highly allergenic foods, may *increase* the risk of food allergy or eczema.[39,40]

Once a few typical complementary foods (eg, pureed meat, infant cereal, yellow or orange vegetables [eg, sweet potato, carrots], fruits [eg, pears, bananas], green vegetables) are tolerated, foods considered to be potentially allergenic (eg, wheat, egg, fish, cow's milk in small amounts) may be introduced as complementary foods.

The infant should be given an initial taste of one of these foods *at home* rather than at day care or at a restaurant. Most reactions occur within a day or two in response to what is believed to be the initial ingestion. If there is no apparent reaction, the food can be introduced in gradually increasing amounts. Introduction of other new foods should continue if no adverse reactions occur.

Regurgitation, Spitting Up, and Gastroesophageal Reflux Disease

Regurgitation and spitting up are common concerns for parents. During the first year of life, particularly in the first few months, infants typically have episodes of vomiting or "wet burps" within the first 1 to 2 hours after feeding. Vomiting or wet burps are related to transient physiologic episodes of lowered esophageal sphincter tone with efflux of gastric contents into the esophagus. Spitting up often occurs because milk has been ingested too rapidly or as a reaction to overfeeding, inadequate burping, or improper feeding techniques (eg, bottle propped, bottle not adequately tipped up, or shaking infant formula too vigorously before feeding). Approximately half of infants younger than 3 months spit up or regurgitate 1 or 2 times a day, with the incidence peaking between 2 to 4 months of age. The frequency may increase again when the infant starts solid foods. Spitting up resolves itself in most children by 12 to 24 months of age.

Frequent spitting up or significant vomiting is classified as gastroesophageal reflux and usually is harmless in infants. The clinical manifestations of gastroesophageal reflux disease (GERD) include vomiting and associated poor weight gain, apparent discomfort with eating, esophagitis, and respiratory disorders.[41] The health care professional will need to differentiate these symptoms from pyloric stenosis in some young infants.

Providing a Nurturing and Healthy Feeding Environment

Infants need a nurturing environment and positive patterns of feeding and eating to promote healthy eating habits and build variety, balance, and moderation. In early infancy, feeding is crucial for developing a parent's responsiveness to an infant's cues of hunger and satiation. The close physical contact during feeding facilitates healthy social and emotional development.

During the first year, feeding the hungry infant helps her develop a sense of trust that her needs will be met. For optimum development, newborns should be fed as soon as possible when they express hunger. Children with special health care needs often have subtle cues that can be difficult for parents to interpret. Parents must be careful observers of the infant's behaviors, so they can respond to their infant's needs. As infants become more secure in their trust, they can wait longer for feeding. Infants should develop their feeding skills at their own rate. However, if significant delays

occur in the development of these skills or if delays are anticipated (eg, as in the case of some children with special health care needs), a health care professional should assess the infant.

The suck-and-pause sequence in breastfeeding or infant formula feeding and behaviors such as eye contact, open mouth, turning to the parent, and even turning away provide the foundation for the first communication between the infant and parents. Difficulties in early feeding elicit strong emotions in parents and can undermine parenting confidence and sense of competency. Thus, feeding difficulties must be addressed in a timely manner.

Over time, parents become more skilled at interpreting their infant's cues and increase their repertoire of successful responses to those cues. As they feed their infant, parents learn how their actions comfort and satisfy. Physical contact during breastfeeding or infant formula feeding strengthens the psychological bond between the parent and infant and enhances communication because it provides the infant with essential sensory stimulation, including skin and eye contact. A sense of caring and trust evolves, which lays the groundwork for communication patterns throughout life.

A healthy feeding relationship involves a division of responsibility between the parent and the infant. The parent sets an appropriate, safe, and nurturing feeding environment and provides appropriate, healthy foods. The infant decides when and how much to eat. In a healthy infant-parent feeding relationship, responsive parenting involves

- Responding early and appropriately to hunger and satiety cues
- Recognizing the infant's developmental abilities and feeding skills
- Balancing the infant's need for assistance with encouragement of self-feeding
- Allowing the infant to initiate and guide feeding interactions

Nutrition for Infants With Special Health Care Needs

Medical problems or other special health care needs can place the infant at nutritional risk. Because this is a time of high caloric need, health care professionals should consider referring the family for specialized medical and nutrition consultation.

Not all infants are able to easily develop the skills for feeding and eating. Approximately 25% of all children have some form of feeding problem, and 80% of children with a developmental disability have some form of feeding problem.[42] Feeding difficulties can lead to problems in the parent-child relationship, as well as growth problems, inadequate nutrition, and significant feeding problems later in childhood. It is recommended that health care professionals address the following common concerns expressed by parents:

- Refusing infant cereal and purees
- Difficulty transitioning to textures
- Gagging, choking, or vomiting with feeding
- Poor or inadequate food volume
- Poor or inadequate variety of foods, picky eating (eg, refusing to eat certain foods), or food jags (ie, favoring only 1 or 2 foods)
- Prolonged feeding time (>30 minutes)
- Respiratory symptoms after feeding

Infants with special health care needs are at increased risk of feeding complications, including failure to thrive, aspiration of food, and GERD. Parents of infants with special health care needs also may need extra emotional support and instruction about special techniques for positioning or special equipment. These accommodations can help overcome feeding problems and prevent suboptimal nutrition, poor weight gain, and growth deficiency.

Parents often blame themselves for their infant's feeding problem, yet the difficulty is typically related to the infant's oromotor developmental problem. Children with oromotor delay may retain primitive reflexes like the extrusion reflex and the tonic bite reflex. These behaviors can be mistakenly interpreted as food refusals. Thus, health care professionals should try to identify feeding challenges early and provide resources for evaluation, education, and support. Assessing and treating physical or behavioral feeding difficulties is best accomplished by an interdisciplinary team that may include a developmental and behavioral pediatrician, a dietitian, an occupational therapist, a speech pathologist, a nurse or nurse practitioner, a social worker, and a psychologist. Parents should learn the different philosophies, intervention strategies, and approaches of the different programs available, as well as their costs and outcomes, before they make a decision on the best approach for their child and family.

Low-birth-weight infants need additional iron after the first month of life (2 mg/kg/day) until they reach 1 year of age.[43] They also may need special food (eg, preterm discharge infant formulas with enhanced nutrients). Infants with sequelae of prematurity, chronic lung or reactive airway disease, short bowel syndrome, cholestasis, GERD, rickets, or chronic heart, kidney, or liver disease have medical and developmental factors that will affect their growth. They may require specialized feedings with nutritional supplements, including fortifiers, vitamins, and minerals. Medication use also may alter nutritional requirements.

Infants with special health care needs often need increased calories but may be limited by feeding issues. Because their immune systems may be compromised, most of these infants benefit from breastfeeding (or being fed expressed human milk). Parents may need to modify human milk or infant formula or adapt their feeding techniques to ensure that infants with the following conditions achieve adequate caloric intake:

- Prematurity and low birth weight
- Chronic respiratory or congenital heart disease

- Gastrointestinal tract disease
- Kidney disease
- Neurologic disorders
- Syndromes and genetic disorders affecting growth potential, such as cystic fibrosis

Promoting Nutritional Health: Early Childhood—1 Through 4 Years

Ensuring adequate nutrition during early childhood focuses on promoting normal growth by selecting appropriate amounts and kinds of foods and providing a supportive environment that allows the child to self-regulate food intake. Self-regulation of eating and its accompanying independence are major achievements during the early childhood years. Children continue their exposure to new tastes, textures, and eating experiences depending on their own developmental ability, cultural and family practices, and individual nutrient needs.

Nutrition for Growth

Most infants triple their birth weight within the first year of life and experience a significantly slower rate of weight gain after the first year, which results in a dramatic decrease in appetite and diminished food intake (Box 2). This diminished intake is compensated for by eating foods with increased caloric density. Health care professionals can alert parents to this change while plotting the child's height, weight, and BMI on the sex- and age-appropriate WHO or CDC Growth Charts (Appendixes A and B) to demonstrate expectations for healthy growth.

Monitoring growth measures by age also allows the health care professional to determine how the child compares with others of the same age and sex. These measures can be used to signal abnormal growth patterns. Linear growth is used to detect long-term undernutrition. Using weight-for-length until age 2 years, along with BMI growth charts after that, allows the health care professional to determine underweight and overweight or obesity and whether the child is maintaining his own growth trajectory. If the child has moved up or down 2 percentile lines on the growth chart since the previous visit, it is recommended that the health care professional question parents in detail about portion sizes, types of food served, and feeding frequency. Skinfold measurements for this age group are not used unless medically indicated and performed by an adequately trained technician.

Early childhood is the time to establish lifelong eating habits. Healthy eating includes 3 meals daily, beginning with breakfast, and 2 to 3 snacks. Because most children, adolescents, and adults in the United States consume too few vegetables, fruits, and whole grains and too little dairy, early

Box 2

Changes in Appetite in Early Childhood

The anticipated but sudden reduction in appetite is a common source of concern and anxiety to parents of infants soon after the first birthday. This parental concern affords a unique opportunity to educate parents about changing dietary needs.

Health care professionals can use this opportunity to emphasize that

- Reduced intake is normal.
- Picky eating more often reflects lack of hunger than a change in taste preferences.
- Encouraging a child to eat when he is not hungry leads to consumption of excess calories, an undesired outcome because obesity is a major nutrition problem.
- Offering multiple alternatives to a child who is not hungry is unnecessary and it rewards picky eating, potentially contributing to lifelong food biases.

childhood is the proper time to establish tastes and preferences, as well as healthy eating patterns. Refined grains, saturated fat, added sugars, and sodium are overconsumed throughout the age range, so care should be taken with introducing foods and beverages that are high in these components. Many young children do consume recommended amounts of fruit and dairy, a habit to be supported and maintained.

As additional table foods are offered, young children consume foods similar to those of the entire family. The Feeding Infant and Toddler Study suggests that, in general, young children are getting sufficient intakes of calcium.[44] Children in this age group using cow's milk or soy as a primary protein and calcium source should be encouraged to drink 16 to 32 oz (480–960 mL) of cow's milk or soy milk per day to receive adequate levels of these nutrients. Other products sold as "milk" (eg, almond milk, hemp milk) are generally lower in protein and have not been studied sufficiently to promote their use.

Even in early childhood, however, dietary preferences and patterns begin to be established, and, all too often, the reported amount of milk consumed decreases significantly, while the intake of juices, fruit drinks, and soda increases. The shift from milk to juice and soda lowers calcium intake and makes it more difficult for young children to attain the recommended calcium intake (Box 3). Fruit drinks and sodas are discouraged, and 100% fruit juice is recommended at no more than 4 to 6 oz daily.[36] Overuse may lead to excess energy intake, diarrhea, and dental caries. *(For more information on this topic, see the Promoting Healthy Weight and Promoting Oral Health themes.)*

A primary safety concern for young children during feeding is choking or inhalation of food. The following foods should be avoided at this age:

- Peanuts and other whole nuts
- Chewing gum
- Popcorn

Box 3

Dietary Reference Intakes for Calcium and Vitamin D[45]

Birth at Term Until 1 Year

- 200 mg calcium per day, birth–6 months
- 260 mg calcium per day, 7–12 months
- 400 IU vitamin D per day

Children Aged 1–3

- 500 mg calcium per day
- 400 IU of vitamin D per day

Children Aged 4–8

- 800 mg calcium per day
- 600 IU vitamin D per day

Children, Adolescents, and Young Adults Aged 9–18

- 1,300 mg calcium per day
- 600 IU vitamin D per day

Data derived from Ross AC, Taylor CL, Yaktine AL, Del Valle HB; Institute of Medicine Committee to Review Dietary Reference Intakes for Vitamin D, Calcium, Food and Nutrition Board. *Dietary Reference Intakes for Calcium and Vitamin D*. Washington DC: National Academies Press; 2011.

- Chips
- Round slices of hot dogs or sausages
- Raw carrot sticks
- Whole grapes and cherries
- Large pieces of raw vegetables or fruit
- Whole cherry or grape tomatoes
- Tough meat
- Hard candy

To limit the risk of choking, children should sit up while eating. Infants and children younger than 3 years should not eat without direct adult supervision, even if they are able to feed themselves. Parents should avoid feeding a young child while in a car because, if the child should begin to choke, pulling over to the side of the road in traffic to dislodge the food is difficult. Furthermore, feeding young children while driving contradicts the recommendation to feed children in appropriate locations.[46]

Because few data are available on nutrient adequacy for young children, the Institute of Medicine[46] extrapolated values from studies of infants and adults to establish Dietary Reference Intakes.[1,2] A clear translation of these nutrient intakes into specific food choices and portions for young children is not yet available. However, guidelines suggest offering appropriate nutritious foods spaced into 3 meals, along with 2 or 3 snacks per day.[2,21] For children older than 2 years, the *Dietary Guidelines for Americans* are the primary source of dietary guidance.[1] Other national health organizations also have developed nutrition policy statements to promote optimal health and reduce risk for obesity and chronic disease, and these statements can be used to guide food choices in children older than 2 years.[47–50]

All of these science-based nutrition guidelines recommend a diet that includes a variety of nutrient-dense foods and beverages from the major food groups and limits the intake of saturated and *trans* fats, added sugars, and salt. A basic premise is that nutrient needs should be met primarily by consuming a variety of foods that have beneficial effects on health. Supplementation with vitamins and minerals is not considered necessary when children are consuming the recommended amounts of healthy foods.[51] However, health care professionals should not assume that all young children are getting the nutrients they need.[52] A significant number of children in the United States live in households with insufficient healthy food.

Developing Healthy Feeding and Eating Skills

Young children often eat sporadically over one day or several days. Over a period of a week or so, their nutrient and energy intakes balance out. Food jags and picky eating are normal behaviors in young children. For most young children, these behaviors disappear before school age if parents continue to expose them to a variety of new and familiar foods.

As their manipulative skills mature, preschoolers also can successfully help in food preparation, which may help them accept new foods.

Unfortunately, some parents and other caregivers become discouraged and frustrated when their child seems to concentrate more on exploring food than eating it. This behavior reflects the emerging curiosity and independence associated with early childhood and is normal. Parents and caregivers can foster this newly found and often assertively expressed independence while still ensuring adequate nutrition by offering a well-balanced selection of foods and allowing children to choose the types and amounts of foods they want to eat. Parents and caregivers should encourage young children to explore food tastes and textures by repeating exposure to foods. Health care professionals can empower caregivers by letting them know that children will often begin to accept foods after 10 or more exposures to certain foods. Preparing a familiar-looking food in different ways can also increase acceptance of foods. Parents and other caregivers need to understand that recognizing the child's signals of hunger and fullness supports the child's innate ability to self-regulate energy intake and portion size. They also need to understand that a child does not have an innate ability to select only appropriate foods. Food choice remains the responsibility of the caregiver. Parents and other caregivers can be positive role models by practicing healthy eating behaviors themselves.

Mealtime provides opportunities for wonderful parent-child interactions. These opportunities exist for the toddler, who may be fed before the family meal, as well as for young children, who may participate in the family routine and sit at the table for a short time. Finger foods should be encouraged because they foster competence, mastery, and self-esteem. Even when the parent is doing the feeding, the child also should be given a spoon. The 12- to 15-month-old should be encouraged to use a spoon. When the toddler is finished eating, he should be allowed to leave the table and be placed where he can be supervised until the adults have finished their meal.

Nutrition for Children With Special Health Care Needs

Children with special health care needs generally follow similar developmental pathways as children without these challenges when they begin the process of self-feeding. However, the pace of development and the ultimate mastery of tasks will vary depending on the physical, emotional, or cognitive challenges facing the child. Attention to nutritional intake and physical activity is important.

The types of nutritional issues most common for children with special health care needs include feeding problems (eg, chewing and swallowing), slow growth, metabolic or gastrointestinal issues, and overweight or obesity. By age 15 months, children with autism spectrum disorder (ASD) demonstrate greater food selectivity compared to typically developing peers and demonstrate more challenging food-related behaviors as toddlers, even before diagnosis of ASD.[53] Sometimes, children with special health care needs require special feeding techniques, longer periods of time to feed, or special foods (both type and texture), infant formulas, and feeding approaches (eg, restriction of certain foods). The health care professional can identify these issues and refer the family, as needed, to a registered dietitian or interdisciplinary team for further assessment, intervention, and monitoring.

Promoting Nutritional Health: Middle Childhood—5 Though 10 Years

To achieve optimal growth and development, children need a variety of nutritious foods that provide sufficient—but not excessive—calories, protein, carbohydrates, fat, vitamins, and minerals. Recent data suggest that while many young children consume recommended amounts of fruit and dairy, the quality of dietary patterns drops in middle childhood and adolescence.[1] Even into middle childhood, a child needs 3 meals and 2 to 3 healthy snacks per day. As the child's ability to feed herself improves, she can help with meal planning and food preparation, and she can perform tasks related to mealtime. Performing these tasks enables the child to contribute to the family and can boost her self-esteem. The USDA MyPlate, which is based on the *Dietary Guidelines for Americans,* provides an easy reference on food intake and physical activity recommendations for children and adolescents 6 to 11 years.[54]

Nutrition for Growth

Middle childhood is characterized by a slow, steady rate of physical growth. Plotting the child's BMI allows the health care professional to note any percentile changes and provide early intervention as needed to prevent childhood underweight or overweight. During middle childhood, children gain an average of 7 lb in weight and 2½ in in height per year. The BMI gradually increases from its lowest point at 5 to 6 years of age. Additionally, during middle childhood, a child's body fat increases in preparation for the growth spurt. On average, the growth spurt and puberty begins for girls at ages 9 to 11 years (Tanner stages 2–3) and for boys at ages 10 to 12 years (Tanner stages 3–4). Children may become concerned about their appearance and body image and may eat less or go on diets for weight loss.

The health care professional can reassure the family about normal growth patterns while addressing the child's or family's weight concerns. Common nutrition concerns in middle childhood include

- Decreased consumption of milk and milk products
- Increased consumption of beverages high in added sugars
- Limited intake of fruit and vegetables

185

- High consumption of foods high in saturated fat, added sugars, refined grains, and sodium (primarily from snack foods)
- Rise of overweight and obesity
- Increase in body image concerns
- Effect of the media and advertising on nutritional intake

Calcium and Vitamin D

Calcium and vitamin D intake is a concern during middle childhood. These nutrients are critical for bone health, and a higher incidence of fractures is reported in children who do not get adequate amounts. Studies indicate that few children consume enough of either nutrient. Consumption of juice, soft drinks, or sports drinks often leads to reduced milk intake. Decreased outdoor activity, along with sunscreen use, also has resulted in reduced vitamin D absorption.

Nutrition recommendations for calcium change during middle childhood from 800 mg per day for children aged 4 to 8 years to 1,300 mg per day for children, adolescents, and young adults aged 9 to 18.[45] Health care professionals should encourage parents to provide several servings of low-fat or fat-free milk daily. One 8-oz glass of milk provides approximately 300 mg of calcium and 120 IU of vitamin D. For children who are unable to consume milk or dairy products, health care professionals can recommend the consumption of other calcium-rich foods, calcium-fortified products (eg, some orange juices

and breads), and soy milk foods and beverages that are similar to milk and dairy products in their content of calcium and vitamin D. Parents should be alert to the nutritional content of other products sold as "milk" (eg, almond milk, hemp milk) that may not provide equivalent calcium, vitamin D, or protein. A dietary supplement containing calcium and vitamin D may be recommended for children who do not consume enough of either through their diets.

Developing Healthy Eating Habits

Parents and other family members continue to have the most influence on children's eating behaviors and attitudes toward foods. They can be positive role models by practicing healthy eating behaviors themselves. The *2015–2020 Dietary Guidelines for Americans* explain that contemporary nutrient consumption patterns are of potential public health concern.[1]

- Vitamin D, calcium, potassium, and fiber are under-consumed.
- Iron is under-consumed in adolescent girls.
- Sodium is overconsumed by people of all ages.
- Saturated fats, added sugars, and refined grains are overconsumed.

Parents need to make sure that nutritious foods are available and decide when to serve them; however, children should decide how much of these foods to eat. During this period, when children may be missing several teeth, it can be difficult for them to chew certain foods (eg, meat). Offering foods that are easy to chew can alleviate this problem. Responsive feeding remains important during middle childhood as a means of reinforcing awareness of hunger and satiety cues.

Health care professionals should try to determine whether families have access to and can afford nutritious foods. They also should discuss families' perceptions of which foods are nutritious and their cultural beliefs about foods. Families should eat together in a pleasant environment (without the television and other media distractions), allowing time for social interaction. Participation in regular family meals is positively associated with appropriate intakes of energy, protein, calcium, and many micronutrients and can reinforce the development of healthy eating patterns.[55]

During middle childhood, mealtimes take on social significance, and children become increasingly influenced by outside sources (eg, their peers and the media) regarding eating behaviors and attitudes toward foods. In addition, they eat a growing number of meals away from home and may have expanding options for consuming nonnutritious foods. Their willingness to eat certain foods and to participate in nutrition programs (eg, School Breakfast Program and National School Lunch Program) may be based on what their friends are doing. However, some children can have difficulty adapting to school meals. This difficulty can result from the foods being different from those at home, the foods not conforming to cultural and religious practices, or children having less time to eat than they are accustomed to, eating at different times than accustomed, or having difficulty serving their own food.

Nutrition for Children With Special Health Care Needs

Children with special health care needs can have significant nutritional challenges that can lead to underweight or overweight. These challenges can be the result of behavioral disturbances or of children needing assistance with feeding. Some children may require gastrostomy tubes and fundoplications. Medications also can affect appetite, leading to weight loss or weight gain. When weight gain is desired, nutritious high-calorie foods should be served rather than calorie-dense foods with little nutritional value. Overweight and obesity are risks

when physical activity is limited by a special health care need. In addition, children may be making food choices at school, and parents may need help in guiding them to make healthy choices, depending on their particular needs. Health care professionals should be aware of these challenges and be prepared to seek assistance in monitoring and facilitating appropriate nutrition. When a child has a special dietary need, it should be shared with school personnel and included on her Individualized Education Program, if one is in effect. This will allow the school to provide any special foods that may be needed.

Promoting Nutritional Health: Adolescence—11 Through 21 Years

Adolescence is one of the most dynamic periods of human development. The increased rate of growth that occurs during these years is second only to that occurring in the first year of life. Nutrition and physical activity can affect adolescents' energy levels and influence growth and body composition, and the changes associated with puberty can influence adolescents' satisfaction with their appearance. Health supervision visits provide an opportunity for health care professionals to discuss healthy eating and physical activity behaviors with adolescents and their parents. *(For more information on this topic, see the Promoting Healthy Weight and the Promoting Physical Activity themes.)*

Nutrition for Growth

The adolescent's diet should follow the *2015–2020 Dietary Guidelines for Americans*[1] and complementary recommendations from national health organizations.[49,54] These recommendations emphasize eating healthy foods such as vegetables, fruits, whole-grain products (eg, cereals, bread, or crackers), low-fat or nonfat milk and dairy products (eg, cheese, cottage cheese, and unsweetened yogurt), and lean meats, fish, chicken, eggs, beans, and nuts and limiting or avoiding foods high in saturated fat, added sugars, sodium, and refined grains. They also emphasize balancing calories consumed from foods and beverages with calories expended in normal body functions and through physical activity.[49]

Nutrient needs should be met by consuming a variety of healthy foods. In certain cases, fortified foods and dietary supplements may be useful sources of one or more nutrients that otherwise might not be consumed in the adequate amounts. However, although they are recommended in some cases, dietary supplements cannot replace a healthy diet.

For many adolescents, particularly girls and those from families with low incomes, intake of certain vitamins (ie, folate and vitamins A, B$_6$, and E) and minerals (ie, iron, calcium, magnesium, and zinc) is inadequate. Box 4 provides current

recommendations for folate, iron, and calcium, which are nutrients of particular concern for adolescents because they are often under-consumed.[33]

Adolescents of both sexes and all income and racial and ethnic groups often consume excess amounts of total fat, saturated fat, and added sugars. Other nutrition-related concerns for adolescents include low intakes of vegetables, fruits, whole-grain products, and low-fat and nonfat milk and other dairy products.[56] These dietary patterns constitute a significant risk factor for obesity and other health conditions.[2,56] Reducing the consumption of high-fat foods as well as beverages and foods with added sugars will lower the caloric content of the diet without compromising its nutrient adequacy.[1]

Box 4

Current Recommendations for Selected Nutrients[33]

Folate

The IOM recommends that, to reduce the risk of giving birth to an infant with neural tube defects, female adolescents who are capable of becoming pregnant should take 400 µg of synthetic folic acid per day from fortified foods, a supplement, or both in addition to consuming foods rich in folate.[1,46]

Iron

The body's need for iron increases dramatically during adolescence, primarily because of rapid growth. Adolescent boys require increased amounts of iron to manufacture myoglobin for expanding muscle mass and hemoglobin for expansion of blood volume. Although adolescent girls generally have less muscular development than adolescent boys, they have a greater risk for iron-deficiency anemia because of blood lost through menstruation. Iron-deficiency anemia in adolescents may be caused by inadequate dietary intake of iron, which results from low-calorie and extremely restrictive diets, periods of accelerated iron demand, and increased iron losses. The DRIs for iron are[2]

- Girls and boys 9–13 years of age: 8 mg iron per day
- Females 14–18 years: 15 mg iron per day
- Women 19–21 years: 18 mg iron per day
- Males 14–18 years: 11 mg iron per day
- Men 19 and 21 years: 8 mg iron per day

Calcium

Adequate calcium intake is essential for peak bone mass development during adolescence, a period when 45% of the total permanent adult skeleton is formed. Calcium requirements increase with the growth of lean body mass and the skeleton. Therefore, requirements are greater during puberty and adolescence than in childhood or adulthood. The current calcium DRIs for children and adolescents are[1]

- Children, adolescents, and young adults 9–18 years of age: 1,300 mg calcium per day
- Young adults 19–21 years: 1,000 mg calcium per day

Abbreviations: DRI, Dietary Reference Intake; IOM, Institute of Medicine.

PROMOTING HEALTHY NUTRITION

Only 22% of adolescents report eating fruit 3 or more times per day, only 15% report eating vegetables 3 or more times per day, and only 15% report drinking 3 or more glasses of milk per day. In addition, 11% of adolescents report drinking soda 3 or more times a day, only 37% report eating breakfast every day, 29% describe themselves as having slight or substantial overweight, 46% report trying to lose weight, and 12% report not eating for 24 hours or more to lose weight or to keep from gaining weight.[57] Common nutrition concerns during adolescence include

- Increase in overweight and obesity
- Increase in eating disorders and body image concerns
- Prevalence of iron-deficiency anemia in girls
- Prevalence of hyperlipidemia and type 2 diabetes
- Food insecurity among adolescents from families with low incomes[2]

Assessing the Adolescent Diet

Evaluating the dietary intake of an adolescent is a fundamental component of health supervision. It is useful for health care professionals to gather quantitative and qualitative data about foods and beverages consumed (both common and unusual), eating patterns, attitudes about foods and eating, and other issues, such as cultural and religious patterns and taboos associated with food.

Developing Healthy Eating Habits

Developing an identity and becoming an independent young adult are central to adolescence. Adolescents may use foods to establish individuality and to express their identity. They usually are interested in new foods, including those from different cultures and ethnic groups, and may adopt certain eating behaviors (eg, vegetarianism) to explore various lifestyles or to show concern for the environment. Parents can have a major influence on adolescents' eating behaviors by providing a variety of healthy foods at home and by making family mealtimes a priority.[58] Parents also can be positive role models by practicing healthy eating behaviors themselves.

As adolescents strive for independence, they begin to spend large amounts of time outside the home. Parents can encourage adolescents to choose nutritious foods when eating away from home.[59] Many adolescents walk or drive to neighborhood stores and fast-food restaurants and purchase foods with their own money. This situation can be especially problematic for adolescents from families with low incomes or adolescents who live in neighborhoods with many fast-food restaurants and no grocery or other stores that sell affordable, nutritious foods.

Although eating together as a family is a challenge for many adolescents and their families who are coping with school demands, after-school activities, and work schedules, having frequent family meals can promote the development of healthy eating patterns that may continue into adulthood and can protect against the inadequate dietary intake reported by many adolescents.[56,58,60] Having meals together is positively associated with intake of vegetables, fruits, grains, and milk and dairy products rich in calcium and negatively associated with soda consumption. Frequency of family meals also is positively associated with more appropriate intake of energy, protein, iron, folate, fiber, and vitamins A, C, E, and B_6.[60]

Body Image and Eating Disorders

The physical changes that are associated with puberty can affect adolescents' satisfaction with their appearance. For some adolescent boys, the increased height, weight, and muscular development that come with physical maturation can lead to a positive body image. However, for many adolescents, puberty-related changes (in adolescent girls in particular, the normal increase in body fat) may result in weight concerns. The social pressure to be thin and the stigma of having overweight can lead to unhealthy eating behaviors and a poor body image.[61] Adolescents may attempt to lose weight or avoid gaining weight by eating smaller amounts of food, foods with fewer calories, or foods low in fat. They also may forego eating for many hours; engage in excessive physical activity; take diet pills, powders, or liquids without a physician's advice; use illegal "street" drugs (eg, methamphetamines); and vomit or take laxatives. Fad diets that recommend unusual and, sometimes, inadequate or unbalanced dietary patterns promise the loss of several pounds in a short period of time. In addition, the lack of evidence about their efficacy and safety in adolescents make such regimens a poor choice for adolescents who want to lose weight and who may underestimate the health risks associated with them.[62]

Unhealthy eating behaviors and preoccupation with body image can lead to life-threatening eating disorders (eg, anorexia nervosa, bulimia nervosa, binge-eating disorder). Although eating disorders are more prevalent among adolescent girls (prevalence is 1%–2%) than among adolescent boys, they occur in both sexes across socioeconomic and racial and ethnic groups and are even seen in children and young adolescents (10–12 years of age).[63] Major medical complications of eating disorders include cardiac arrhythmia, dehydration and electrolyte imbalances, delayed growth and development, endocrine disturbances (eg, menstrual dysfunction or hypothermia), gastrointestinal problems, oral health problems (eg, enamel demineralization or salivary dysfunction), osteopenia, osteoporosis, and protein and calorie malnutrition and its consequences. In 2009, the mortality rate for anorexia nervosa was 4.0%; for bulimia, 3.9%; and for eating disorders not otherwise specified, 5.2%.[64] Death may be caused by cardiac arrhythmia, acute cardiovascular failure, gastric hemorrhaging, or suicide. Bulimia nervosa can damage teeth and cause enlargement of the parotid gland.

Athletics and Performance-Enhancing Substances

Inadequate nutritional intake and unsafe weight control methods can adversely affect performance and endurance, jeopardize health, and undermine the benefits of training. Health supervision includes the promotion of healthy eating and weight management strategies to enhance performance and endurance while ensuring optimal growth and development.

The AAP recommends against the use of performance-enhancing substances (eg, supplements, ergogenic aids [eg, amphetamines, creatine, and steroids]) for athletic or other purposes.[65] Performance-enhancing substances may pose a significant health risk to adolescents. Supplements and amphetamines do not contribute positively to athletic performance. Health care professionals can stress the importance of seeking accurate information so young athletes and their parents can make informed choices.

Nutrition for Adolescents With Special Health Care Needs

As with younger age groups, adolescents with special health care needs are at increased risk for nutrition-related health problems.[66]

- Physical disabilities can affect their capacity to consume, digest, or absorb nutrients.
- Long-term medications or metabolic disturbances can lead to biochemical imbalances.
- Psychological stress that results from a chronic condition or physical disorder can affect appetite and food intake.
- Environmental factors, often controlled by parents or other caregivers, may influence access to and acceptance of food.

The energy and nutrient requirements of adolescents with special health care needs have been reviewed.[2] The adolescent's diagnosis, medical status, individual metabolic rate, and activity level are used to determine a desired energy level to be established and achieved. The adolescent is subsequently monitored to (1) ensure adequate nutrition for growth, development, and health and (2) make adjustments for periods of stress and illness.

References

1. US Department of Health and Human Services, US Department of Agriculture. *2015-2020 Dietary Guidelines for Americans.* 8th ed. 2015. http://health.gov/dietaryguidelines/2015/guidelines. Accessed September 15, 2016

2. Holt K, Wooldridge N, Story N, Sofka D. *Bright Futures: Nutrition.* 3rd ed. Elk Grove Village, IL: American Academy of Pediatrics; 2011

3. Mennella JA. Ontogeny of taste preferences: basic biology and implications for health. *Am J Clin Nutr.* 2014;99(3):704S-711S

4. Coleman-Jensen A, Rabbitt MP, Gregory C, Singh A. *Household Food Security in the United States in 2014.* Washington, DC: US Department of Agriculture, Economic Research Service; 2015. Publication ERR-194. http://www.ers.usda.gov/media/1896841/err194.pdf. Accessed September 17, 2016

5. Widome R, Neumark-Sztainer D, Hannan PJ, Haines J, Story M. Eating when there is not enough to eat: eating behaviors and perceptions of food among food-insecure youths. *Am J Public Health.* 2009;99(5):822-828

6. Cutler-Triggs C, Fryer GE, Miyoshi TJ, Weitzman M. Increased rates and severity of child and adult food insecurity in households with adult smokers. *Arch Pediatr Adolesc Med.* 2008;162(11):1056-1062

7. US Department of Agriculture, Food Nutrition Service. Women, Infants, and Children (WIC) Web site. http://www.fns.usda.gov/wic/women-infants-and-children-wic. Accessed September 17, 2016

8. US Department of Agriculture, Food and Nutrition Service. Supplemental Nutrtion Assistant Program (SNAP) Web site. http://www.fns.usda.gov/snap/supplemental-nutrition-assistance-program-snap. Accessed September 17, 2016

9. US Department of Agriculture, Food and Nutrition Service. Child and Adult Care Food Program (CACFP): Child Day Care Centers. http://www.fns.usda.gov/cacfp/child-day-care-centers. Updated January 27, 2014. Accessed September 17, 2016

10. Bailey LB, Rampersaud GC, Kauwell GP. Folic acid supplements and fortification affect the risk for neural tube defects, vascular disease and cancer: evolving science. *J Nutr.* 2003;133(6):1961S-1968S

11. Centers for Disease Control and Prevention. Recommendations for the use of folic acid to reduce the number of cases of spina bifida and other neural tube defects. *MMWR Recomm Rep.* 1992;41(RR-14):1-7

12. Facts about folic acid. Centers for Disease Control and Prevention Web site. http://www.cdc.gov/ncbddd/folicacid/about.html. Updated December 24, 2014. Accessed September 17, 2016

13. Lumley J, Watson L, Watson M, Bower C. Periconceptional supplementation with folate and/or multivitamins for preventing neural tube defects. *Cochrane Database Syst Rev.* 2001;(3):CD001056

14. Carlson SE. Docosahexaenoic acid supplementation in pregnancy and lactation. *Am J Clin Nutr.* 2009;89(2):678S-684S

15. American Academy of Pediatrics Section on Breastfeeding. Breastfeeding and the use of human milk. *Pediatrics.* 2012;129(3):e827-e841

16. Zeisel SH, da Costa KA. Choline: an essential nutrient for public health. *Nutr Rev.* 2009;67(11):615-623

17. Crossland DS, Richmond S, Hudson M, Smith K, Abu-Harb M. Weight change in the term baby in the first 2 weeks of life. *Acta Pædiatr.* 2008;97(4):425-429

18. WHO Multicentre Growth Reference Study Group. *WHO Child Growth Standards: Growth Velocity Based on Weight, Length, and Head Circumference: Methods and Development.* Geneva, Switzerland: World Health Organization; 2009. http://www.who.int/childgrowth/standards/velocity/technical_report/en. Accessed September 17, 2016

19. Griffiths LJ, Smeeth L, Hawkins SS, Cole TJ, Dezateux C. Effects of infant feeding practice on weight gain from birth to 3 years. *Arch Dis Child.* 2009;94(8):577-582

20. Lozoff B, Jimenez E, Hagen J, Mollen E, Wolf AW. Poorer behavioral and developmental outcome more than 10 years after treatment for iron deficiency in infancy. *Pediatrics.* 2000;105(4):E51

21. American Academy of Pediatrics Committe on Nutrition. Iron. In: Kleinman RE, Greer FR, eds. *Pediatric Nutrition: Policy of the American Academy of Pediatrics.* 7th ed. Elk Grove Village, IL: American Academy of Pediatrics; 2014:449-466

22. Wang B, Zhan S, Gong T, Lee L. Iron therapy for improving psychomotor development and cognitive function in children under the age of three with iron deficiency anaemia. *Cochrane Database Syst Rev.* 2013;(6):CD001444

23. Baker RD, Greer FR; American Academy of Pediatrics Committee on Nutrition. Diagnosis and prevention of iron deficiency and iron-deficiency anemia in infants and young children (0-3 years of age). *Pediatrics.* 2010;126(5):1040-1050

24. Wagner CL, Greer FR; American Academy of Pediatrics Section on Breastfeeding, Committee on Nutrition. Prevention of rickets and vitamin D deficiency in infants, children, and adolescents. *Pediatrics.* 2008;122(5):1142-1152

25. Clark MB, Slayton RL; American Academy of Pediatrics Section on Oral Health. Fluoride use in caries prevention in the primary care setting. *Pediatrics.* 2014;134(3):626-633

26. Kramer MS, Kakuma R. Optimal duration of exclusive breastfeeding. *Cochrane Database Syst Rev.* 2012;(8):CD003517

27. Overfield ML, Ryan CA, Spangler A, Tully MR. *Clinical Guidelines for the Establishment of Exclusive Breastfeeding.* Raleigh, NC: International Lactation Consultant Association; 2005. http://www.breastcrawl.org/pdf/ilca-clinical-guidelines-2005.pdf. Accessed September 17, 2016

28. Hale TW, Rowe HE. *Medications and Mothers' Milk 2014.* 16th ed. Plano, TX: Hale Publishing; 2014

29. Greer FR, Sicherer SH, Burks AW; American Academy of Pediatrics Committee on Nutrition, Section on Allergy and Immunology. Effects of early nutritional interventions on the development of atopic disease in infants and children: the role of maternal dietary restriction, breastfeeding, timing of introduction of complementary foods, and hydrolyzed formulas. *Pediatrics.* 2008;121(1):183-191

30. Schwarz EB, Ray RM, Stuebe AM, et al. Duration of lactation and risk factors for maternal cardiovascular disease. *Obstet Gynecol.* 2009;113(5):974-982

31. Collaborative Group on Hormonal Factors in Breast Cancer. Breast cancer and breastfeeding: collaborative reanalysis of individual data from 47 epidemiological studies in 30 countries, including 50302 women with breast cancer and 96973 women without the disease. *Lancet.* 2002;360(9328):187-195

32. Bhatia J, Greer F; American Academy of Pediatrics Committee on Nutrition. Use of soy protein-based formulas in infant feeding. *Pediatrics.* 2008;121(5):1062-1068

33. Kleinman RE, Greer FR; American Academy of Pediatrics Committe on Nutrition. *Pediatric Nutrition: Policy of the American Academy of Pediatrics.* 7th ed. Elk Grove Village, IL: American Academy of Pediatrics; 2014

34. Mennella JA, Beauchamp GK. Mothers' milk enhances the acceptance of cereal during weaning. *Pediatr Res.* 1997;41(2):188-192

35. Forestell CA, Mennella JA. Early determinants of fruit and vegetable acceptance. *Pediatrics.* 2007;120(6):1247-1254

36. American Academy of Pediatrics Committee on Nutrition. The use and misuse of fruit juice in pediatrics. *Pediatrics.* 2001;107(5):1210-1213

37. Li R, Fein SB, Grummer-Strawn LM. Do infants fed from bottles lack self-regulation of milk intake compared with directly breastfed infants? *Pediatrics.* 2010;125(6):e1386-e1393

38. Sampson HA. Update on food allergy. *J Allergy Clin Immunol.* 2004;113(5):805-820

39. Fleischer DM, Spergel JM, Assa'ad AH, Pongracic JA. Primary prevention of allergic disease through nutritional interventions. *J Allergy Clin Immunol Pract.* 2013;1(1):29-36

40. Boyce JA, Assa'ad A, Burks AW, et al. Guidelines for the Diagnosis and Management of Food Allergy in the United States: summary of the NIAID-sponsored expert panel report. *J Am Diet Assoc.* 2011;111(1):17-27

41. Rerksuppaphol S, Barnes G. Guidelines for evaluation and treatment of gastroesophageal reflux in infants and children: recommendations of the North American Society for Pediatric Gastroenterology and Nutrition. *J Pediatr Gastroenterol Nutr.* 2002;35(4):583

42. Manikam R, Perman JA. Pediatric feeding disorders. *J Clin Gastroenterol.* 2000;30(1):34-46

43. Mills RJ, Davies MW. Enteral iron supplementation in preterm and low birth weight infants. *Cochrane Database Syst Rev.* 2012;(3):CD005095

44. Devaney B, Ziegler P, Pac S, Karwe V, Barr SI. Nutrient intakes of infants and toddlers. *J Am Diet Assoc.* 2004;104(1 suppl 1):s14-s21

45. Ross AC, Taylor CL, Yaktine AL, Del Valle HB; Institute of Medicine Committee to Review Dietary Reference Intakes for Vitamin D, Calcium, Food and Nutrition Board. *Dietary Reference Intakes for Calcium and Vitamin D.* Washington DC: National Academies Press; 2011

46. Institute of Medicine Standing Committee on the Scientific Evaluation of Dietary Reference Intakes. *Dietary Reference Intakes for Thiamin, Riboflavin, Niacin, Vitamin B$_6$, Folate, Vitamin B$_{12}$, Pantothenic Acid, Biotin, and Choline.* Washington, DC: National Academy Press; 1998

47. Gidding SS, Dennison BA, Birch LL, et al. Dietary recommendations for children and adolescents: a guide for practitioners: consensus statement from the American Heart Association. *Circulation.* 2005;112(13):2061-2075

48. Daniels SR, Arnett DK, Eckel RH, et al. Overweight in children and adolescents: pathophysiology, consequences, prevention, and treatment. *Circulation.* 2005;111(15):1999-2012

49. Krebs NF, Jacobson MS; American Academy of Pediatrics Committee on Nutrition. Prevention of pediatric overweight and obesity. *Pediatrics.* 2003;112(2):424-430

50. Slawson DL, Fitzgerald N, Morgan KT. Position of the Academy of Nutrition and Dietetics: the role of nutrition in health promotion and chronic disease prevention. *J Acad Nutr Diet.* 2013;113(7):972-979

51. Fox MK, Reidy K, Novak T, Ziegler P. Sources of energy and nutrients in the diets of infants and toddlers. *J Am Diet Assoc.* 2006;106(1 suppl 1):S28-S42

52. Fox MK, Pac S, Devaney B, Jankowski L. Feeding infants and toddlers study: what foods are infants and toddlers eating? *J Am Diet Assoc.* 2004;104(1 suppl 1):S22-S30

53. Emond A, Emmett P, Steer C, Golding J. Feeding symptoms, dietary patterns, and growth in young children with autism spectrum disorders. *Pediatrics.* 2010:126(2):e337-e342

54. US Department of Agriculture. ChooseMyPlate.gov Web site. http://www.choosemyplate.gov. Accessed September 17, 2016

55. Neumark-Sztainer D, Hannan PJ, Story M, Croll J, Perry C. Family meal patterns: associations with sociodemographic characteristics and improved dietary intake among adolescents. *J Am Diet Assoc.* 2003;103(3):317-322

56. Munoz KA, Krebs-Smith SM, Ballard-Barbash R, Cleveland LE. Food intakes of US children and adolescents compared with recommendations [published correction appears in *Pediatrics.* 1998;101(5):952-953]. *Pediatrics.* 1997;100(3 pt 1):323-329

57. Eaton DK, Kann L, Kinchen S, et al. Youth risk behavior surveillance—United States, 2011. *MMWR Surveill Summ.* 2012;61(4):1-162

58. Neumark-Sztainer D, Story M, Perry C, Casey MA. Factors influencing food choices of adolescents: findings from focus-group discussions with adolescents. *J Am Diet Assoc.* 1999;99(8):929-937

59. Savage JS, Fisher JO, Birch LL. Parental influence on eating behavior: conception to adolescence. *J Law Med Ethics.* 2007;35(1):22-34

60. Larson NI, Neumark-Sztainer D, Hannan PJ, Story M. Family meals during adolescence are associated with higher diet quality and healthful meal patterns during young adulthood. *J Am Diet Assoc.* 2007;107(9):1502-1510

61. Kleinman RE, Greer FR; American Academy of Pediatrics Committe on Nutrition. Fast foods, organic foods, fad diets, and herbs, herbals, and botanicals. In: Kleinman RE, Greer FR, eds. *Pediatric Nutrition: Policy of the American Academy of Pediatrics.* 7th ed. Elk Grove Village, IL: American Academy of Pediatrics; 2014:299-356

62. Neumark-Sztainer D. Preventing obesity and eating disorders in adolescents: what can health care providers do? *J Adolesc Health.* 2009;44(3):206-213

63. Swanson SA, Crow SJ, Le Grange D, Swendsen J, Merikangas KR. Prevalence and correlates of eating disorders in adolescents. Results from the national comorbidity survey replication adolescent supplement. *Arch Gen Psychiatry.* 2011;68(7):714-723

64. Crow SJ, Peterson CB, Swanson SA, et al. Increased mortality in bulimia nervosa and other eating disorders. *Am J Psychiatry.* 2009;166(12):1342-1346

65. Gomez J; American Academy of Pediatrics Committee on Sports Medicine and Fitness. Use of performance-enhancing substances. *Pediatrics.* 2005;115(4):1103-1106

66. Kleinman RE, Greer FR; American Academy of Pediatrics Committe on Nutrition. Nutritional support for children with developmental disabilities. In: Kleinman RE, Greer FR, eds. *Pediatric Nutrition: Policy of the American Academy of Pediatrics.* 7th ed. Elk Grove Village, IL: American Academy of Pediatrics; 2014:883-906

PROMOTING HEALTHY NUTRITION

Promoting Physical Activity

Participating in physical activity is an essential component of a healthy lifestyle and ideally begins in infancy and extends throughout adulthood. Regular physical activity increases lean body mass, muscle, and bone strength and promotes physical health. It fosters psychological well-being, can increase self-esteem and capacity for learning, and can help children and adolescents handle stress. Parents should emphasize physical activity, beginning early in a child's life.

The dramatic rise in pediatric overweight and obesity in recent years has increased attention to the importance of physical activity. Along with a balanced and nutritious diet, regular physical activity is essential to preventing pediatric overweight. Therefore, health care professionals are encouraged to review this Bright Futures theme in concert with the *Promoting Healthy Nutrition and Promoting Healthy Weight themes.*

A number of groups have released physical activity guidelines. The *Physical Activity Guidelines for Americans,* which include guidance for children and adolescents aged 6 to 17 years, were released in 2008.[1] These guidelines recommend that children and adolescents engage in 60 minutes or more of physical activity daily. In 2009, the National Association for Sport and Physical Education released physical activity guidelines for infants and children younger than 6.[2] More recent reviews have found evidence to support physical activity interventions across a variety of settings important to children and youth, including early care and education, schools, and communities.[3]

Other health guidelines support these physical activity recommendations. For example, the US Department of Health and Human Services and US Department of Agriculture *2015–2020 Dietary Guidelines for Americans*[4] emphasize adopting healthy eating habits and maintaining a healthy body weight by balancing calories from foods and beverages with calories expended (physical activity).

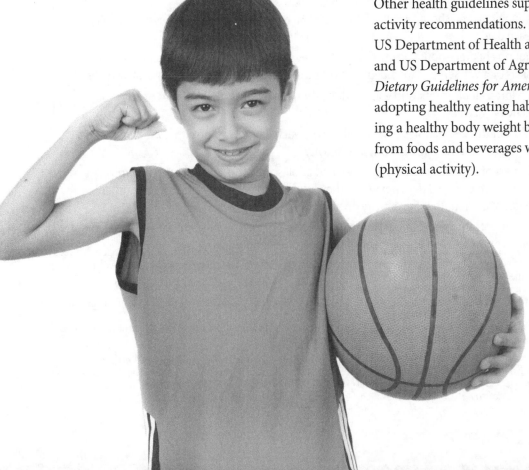

Table 1 summarizes the physical activity guidelines for infants, children, and adolescents from birth through age 21 years. It is important to note that children do not usually need formal muscle-strengthening programs, such as lifting weights. Instead, children strengthen their muscles when they engage in activities such as running or biking, gymnastics, playing on a jungle gym, or climbing trees.

Table 1

Physical Activity Guidelines for Infants, Children, and Adolescents[1,2]	
Infancy (birth–11 months)	• Infants should interact with caregivers in daily physical activities that are dedicated to exploring movement and the environment. • Caregivers should place infants in settings that encourage and stimulate movement experiences and active play for short periods of time several times a day. • Infants' physical activity should promote skill development in movement. • Infants should have supervised "tummy time" on a daily basis while awake. Tummy time should last as long as the infant shows enjoyment.[5]
Early childhood (1–4 years)	• Toddlers aged 1–3 years should engage in at least 60 minutes and up to several hours per day of unstructured[a] physical activity. They should not be sedentary for >60 minutes at a time except when sleeping. • At least 30 minutes should be structured physical activity[b] each day. • Toddlers should be given ample opportunities to develop movement skills that will serve as the building blocks for motor skill and bone development. • Young children aged 3–5 years should engage in at least 60 minutes and up to several hours of unstructured physical activity[a] each day. They should not be sedentary for >60 minutes at a time except when sleeping. • Young children should accumulate at least 60 minutes of structured physical activity[b] each day. • Young children should be encouraged to develop competence in fundamental motor skills that will serve as the building blocks for future motor skills and physical activity.
Middle childhood, adolescence, and young adulthood (5–21 years)	• Children, adolescents, and young adults should engage in ≥60 minutes of physical activity each day. • Most of the ≥60 minutes of physical activity each day should be either moderate[c]- or vigorous[d]-intensity aerobic physical activity. • As part of their daily activity, children and adolescents should engage in vigorous activity on at least 3 days per week. They also should engage in muscle-strengthening and bone-strengthening activity on at least 3 days per week. • It is important to encourage young people to participate in physical activities that are appropriate for their age, are enjoyable, and offer variety.

[a] Unstructured physical activity is sometimes called "free time" or "self-selected free play." It is activity that children start by themselves. It happens when children explore the world around them.
[b] Structured physical activity is planned and intentionally directed by an adult.
[c] Moderate activity is activity that makes children's and adolescents' hearts beat faster than normal, makes them breathe harder than normal, and makes them sweat. They should be able to talk but not sing.
[d] Vigorous activity is activity that makes children's and adolescents' hearts beat much faster than normal and makes them breathe much harder than normal. Children and adolescents should be able to speak only in short sentences.

From US Department of Health and Human Services. Active children and adolescents. In: 2008 *Physical Activity Guidelines for Americans*. Washington, DC: US Dept of Health and Human Services; 2008:15-21. ODPHP publication U0036. http://health.gov/paguidelines/guidelines. Accessed September 16, 2016; and adapted with permission from National Association for Sport and Physical Education. *Active Start: A Statement of Physical Activity Guidelines for Children Birth to Five Years*. Reston, VA: National Association for Sport and Physical Education; 2009.

Physical Inactivity: A Growing Problem for Children and Adolescents

For children and adolescents today, spending time in sedentary activities is increasingly common. Many ride in a car or bus to school rather than walk or bike, many schools are reducing or eliminating physical education classes and time for recess, many parents are afraid to let their children play outside, and labor-saving devices abound. Screens—televisions (TVs), computers, and handheld devices—are everywhere and screen time is an important component of daily life.

Screen time takes up a remarkable portion of children's and adolescent's lives, and new types of media are becoming increasingly popular. Parental awareness and assessment of screen time should encourage a balance that includes adequate time for physical activity. The American Academy of Pediatrics (AAP) recommends that infants and children younger than 18 months have no screen time and that children aged 18 months through 4 years limit screen time to no more than 1 hour per day.[6] For school-aged children and adolescents, parents can consider making a family media use plan, which can help them balance the child's needs for physical activity, sleep, school activities, and unplugged time against time available for media (**www.HealthyChildren.org/MediaUsePlan**).[7]

In an environment that encourages inactivity, being physically active must be a lifelong, conscious decision. Health care professionals can do much to support children, adolescents, and families in this daily commitment by explaining why physical activity is important to overall health, providing information about community physical activity resources, and being physically active themselves.

Promoting Physical Activity in Children and Adolescents With Special Health Care Needs

Children and adolescents with special health care needs should be encouraged to participate in physical activity, according to their ability and health status, as appropriate. Participating in physical activity can make their activities of daily living easier, can improve their health status, and ultimately can reduce morbidity from secondary conditions during adulthood. Health care professionals should help parents, children, and adolescents select appropriate activities and duration by considering the child's or adolescent's needs and concerns, cognitive abilities, and social skills, as well as implement adaptations that will enable the child or adolescent to have a positive experience. (*For more information on this topic, see the Promoting Health for Children and Youth With Special Health Care Needs theme.*)

Opportunities for physical activity for children and adolescents with special health care needs are mandated by the Individuals with Disabilities Act.[8] Physical activity is an essential component in the child's or adolescent's Individualized Education Program at school. It also is an essential component in the care plan for home services for children older than 3 years and in the Individualized Family Service Plan for infants and children birth to age 3.[7] Many organizations (eg, American Physical Therapy Association, Disabled Sports USA, and National Sports Center for the Disabled) provide information on appropriate physical activities and potential adaptations for specific conditions and disabilities. State and federal laws often require programs to address these issues and include children with special needs. Programs such as Special Olympics also can encourage children and adolescents with special heath care needs to become involved with physical activity.[9] Infants and young children who have significant physical or cognitive impairments are usually enrolled in early intervention programs in which physical activity takes place as part of the daily routine. Alternatively, they are in preschool or child care settings in which physical movement activities are adapted to their particular needs, if necessary.

Physical Activity and Sports

Preventing Heat-Related Illness and Sickling

Adequate fluid intake and preventing dehydration are critical for children's and adolescents' health. The risk of dehydration becomes greater with increased heat, humidity, intensity or duration of physical activity, body surface area, and sweating.[10] It is no longer believed that children are at greater risk of dehydration and heat-related illness than adults.[11]

Heat-related illness can be critical and sometimes life-threatening. It is important for health care professionals, coaches, parents, and adolescents to be able to recognize the signs and symptoms of heat-related illness and to know the recommendations for treating it.

The AAP councils on sports medicine and fitness and on school health recommend that sufficient and appropriate fluid be readily available and consumed at regular intervals before, during, and after physical activity. Assuming normal hydration at the beginning of sports activity, children aged 9 to 12 years require 100 to 250 mL (3–8 oz) *every 20 minutes*. Both adolescent girls and boys require up to 1.0 to 1.5 L (34–50 oz) *per hour* to minimize sweating-induced body-water deficits.[11]

Sickle cell trait (SCT) also can pose a grave risk for some children and adolescents. During intense bouts of physical activity participation, sickle cells can accumulate and block blood vessels, causing

explosive rhabdomyolysis that can lead to death. Sickling can begin after 2 to 5 minutes of extreme exertion and can reach life-threatening levels soon thereafter if the child or adolescent struggles on or is urged on by coaches despite warning signs. Sickling collapse is an intensity syndrome that differs from other common causes of collapse. Tailored precautions can prevent sickling collapse and can enable children or adolescents with SCT to thrive (Box 1).[12] In addition to SCT, other risk factors to heat illness include obesity, diabetes mellitus, cardiovascular disease, and recent or concomitant illness.

Table 2 reviews the 3 types of heat-related illness as well as exertional sickling.

Ensuring Adequate Nutrition

To perform optimally in sports, children and adolescents need to consume adequate protein and a diet high in carbohydrates: whole grains, pasta, vegetables, fruits, and low-fat milk products. Moderate amounts of sugar also may help to meet carbohydrate needs. Inadequate carbohydrate intake may be associated with fatigue, weight loss or inability to gain weight, and decreased performance.

Box 1

Managing Sickle Cell Trait in Athletic Settings[13]

- Any child or adolescent with SCT who develops symptoms of cramping, pain, weakness, fatigue, or shortness of breath should stop exercising immediately.
- Any child or adolescent with SCT should avoid timed serial sprints and sustained exertions for >2–3 minutes without a break.
- Preventive measures are encouraged, including decreasing exercise intensity, slower buildup of conditioning by allowing for frequent rest and recovery periods, and increasing opportunities for hydration.

Abbreviation: SCT, sickle cell trait.

PROMOTING PHYSICAL ACTIVITY

196

Table 2

Heat-Related Illness: Signs, Symptoms, and Treatment[12,14]		
Condition	**Signs and Symptoms**	**Treatment**
Heat cramps	• Disabling muscle cramps • Thirst • Rapid heart rate • Normal body temperature • Alertness • Normal blood pressure	• Give child or adolescent 4–8 oz of cold water every 10–15 minutes. • Make sure child or adolescent avoids caffeine. • Move child or adolescent to a cool place. • Remove as much clothing and equipment as possible. • Provide passive stretching. • Apply ice massage to cramping muscles.
Heat exhaustion	• Sweating • Dizziness • Headache • Light-headedness • Clammy skin • Flushed face • Shallow breathing • Nausea • Body temperature of 100.4°F–104°F • Normal mental activity	• Give child or adolescent 16 oz of cold water for each pound of weight lost. • Move child or adolescent to a cool place. • Remove as much clothing and equipment as possible. • Cool child or adolescent (eg, with ice packs, ice bags, immersion in ice water).
Heat stroke	• Shock • Collapse • Body temperature >104°F • Delirium • Hallucinations • Loss of consciousness • Seizures • Inability to walk	• Call 911 for emergency medical treatment. • Cool child or adolescent (eg, with ice packs, ice bags, immersion in ice water). • Administer intravenous fluids.
Exertional sickling (with SCT)	• Muscle weakness exceeds pain. • May slump to ground because of weakness. • Rapid tachypnea. • Rectal temperature <103°F. • May occur quickly and without warning. • Muscles appear normal. • Quicker recovery compared to heat cramps.	• Call 911 for emergency medical treatment. • Provide supplemental oxygen by face mask. • Cool child or adolescent if necessary. • Prepare for CPR. • Tell hospital to expect "exertional rhabdomyolysis."

Abbreviations: CPR, cardiopulmonary resuscitation; SCT, sickle cell trait.

For children and adolescents who train intensively (eg, for those competing at the national or international level), the recommended carbohydrate intake is 60% to 70% of total calories consumed; those who train moderately do not need more than the acceptable macronutrient distribution range of 45% to 65% of calories from carbohydrates, as recommended by the Institute of Medicine.[15] The amount of carbohydrates required depends on the child's or adolescent's sex, weight, energy expenditure, level of physical activity, and type of sport performed, as well as on environmental factors.[16]

Meals Before and After Physical Activity or Competitions

Consuming a light meal high in complex carbohydrates (eg, rice, pasta, bread) and ample caffeine-free beverages (eg, fruit juice, water) is recommended 2 to 4 hours before an event to prevent hunger, provide energy, ensure gastric emptying, and prevent respiratory and cardiac stress. During physical activities involving several events, energy can be obtained by consuming sports drinks or unsweetened fruit juice diluted to a half strength with water up to 1 hour before physical activity. If events are 1 to 3 hours apart, carbohydrate snacks (eg, cereal bars, sports bars, crackers, fruit, whole-wheat bread, bagels) or liquid meals are recommended. After intense physical activity, it is important to replace muscle and liver glycogen stores by consuming carbohydrates within 2 hours. Drinking beverages containing carbohydrates should be encouraged if foods are not well tolerated or not available within 2 hours after physical activity. Drinking low-fat chocolate milk after prolonged vigorous activity helps with muscle recovery and has many of the nutrients of most commercial recovery drinks, including high-quality protein and key electrolytes, such as calcium, potassium, sodium, and magnesium. It is readily available and affordable and accepted by children and adolescents. It has been shown to improve muscle recovery comparable to other commercial carbohydrate drinks.[17]

Preventing Injury

Preventing injury in children and adolescents during physical activity is a responsibility shared by parents, physical education teachers, coaches, recreation program staff, and children and adolescents themselves. The practices listed in Box 2 have been shown to help prevent physical activity injury.

Conducting Pre-participation Physical Evaluation

A pre-participation physical evaluation as part of the yearly Bright Futures Health Supervision Visit is recommended to promote the health and safety of the athlete in training and competition. Annual or preseason evaluation of the athlete provides the medical background for athletes and parents to make physical activity decisions with the athlete's physician or the team physician. Pre-participation physical evaluation components and technique have been developed by a collaboration of sports physicians caring for children and adolescents.[18]

Box 2

Preventing Physical Activity Injury

- Stretch before participating in physical activity, and cool down afterward with a period of walking or stretching.
- Use appropriate safety equipment in low-, moderate-, and high-risk sports, as required by the sport. This equipment includes mouth guards, helmets, shin guards, elbow pads and knee pads, and eye protection. The use of sports eye safety goggles should be emphasized for children with impaired vision or blindness in one eye. *(For more information on this topic, see the Promoting Safety and Injury Prevention theme.)*
- Limit duration of specific, repetitive physical activities that require repeated use of the same muscles (eg, pitching, running).
- Set an appropriate pace when beginning an activity, and be aware of early symptoms of injury (eg, increase in muscle soreness, bone or joint pain, excessive fatigue, decrease in performance). Children and adolescents who experience any of these symptoms should decrease participation in physical activity until symptoms diminish or, if the injury is severe, cease participation temporarily.

Promoting Physical Activity: Infancy— Birth Through 11 Months

The first year of life is marked by dramatic changes in the amount and type of physical activity the infant displays. Motor skill development begins with involuntary reflexes. These reflexes recede as the infant gains voluntary control over her body. Infants usually acquire motor skills in a similar order, but the rate at which they acquire the skills varies.

Health care professionals may offer parents valuable guidance at each visit for the infant's next developmental steps to help parents plan safe, educational, and appropriate physical activities (see Table 1). Infants need consistent, lively, and developmentally appropriate physical activities. Without adequate physical stimulation, infants adopt more sedentary behaviors and tend to roll over, crawl, and walk later than those who enjoy physical activity with a parent or other caregiver.

Part of the infant's day should be spent with a parent who provides both systematic and spontaneous opportunities for active play and physical activity. Parents or caregivers can help the infant be active through floor play, "tummy time," and all daily routines, such as diapering, dressing and bathing, gently pulling to a sitting position, rolling over, lifting arms over head, pulling to a standing position, and helping lift a foot for a sock. Games such as pat-a-cake, peekaboo, and "How big is the baby?" all encourage the infant's active movement.

Giving infants freedom of movement encourages them to explore their environments and learn about their surroundings. Playpens, swings, and infant seats may be appropriate at certain times, but parents should be encouraged to let the infant move around freely with close supervision. Health care professionals can counsel parents to avoid using infant walkers, jumpers, or a car safety seat as positioning devices in the home. It is important to be aware that some parents—such as those who live in shelters or substandard housing—feel it is unsafe for their infant to explore. Health care professionals can help parents living in these environments identify appropriate activities so their infant can meet daily physical activity recommendations.

Health care professionals should caution parents not to use TV or other media to entertain or educate fussy or bored infants during the first years of life. At this stage of development, TVs, computers, and digital devices are not appropriate tools for these purposes. The AAP recommends that children at this age have no screen time.[6]

Promoting Physical Activity: Early Childhood—1 Through 4 Years

A primary reason for promoting physical activity during early childhood is to help young children master basic motor skills.[19] Most children develop gross motor skills in a typical sequence: walking, marching, galloping, hopping, running, traveling around obstacles, and skipping.[19] As a child progresses through infancy into early childhood, the child's strength and flexibility increases, and he is better able to control his head and neck. In addition, all gross motor skills improve. Most children master fine motor skills (manipulation) and spatial relationships during early childhood. Eye-hand and eye-foot coordination, balance, and depth perception typically develop during this period as well. Physical activity can promote mastery of these skills, all of which are important developmental milestones. In addition, physical activity can improve physical and mental health and is fun for children.

Component activities that build on each other include gross motor activity (large movement skills), stability activity, manipulative (small movement or fine motor skills) activity, and rhythm activity.[19] Some activities, such as dancing, combine several of these components. Movement concepts include learning about where and how the body moves, the effort it takes to move the body (eg, time, force), and the relationship of the body to what is around it. Structured play contributes to stability, flexibility, and stamina.

Engaging young children in structured and unstructured play promotes joy of movement, a sense of control, and the ability to navigate the body through space. The most prevalent form of physical activity in early childhood is unstructured play. Simply playing outside—walking, running, climbing, and exploring the environment—is an important opportunity for physical activity. Structured play, which includes developmentally appropriate forms of physical activity, such as dancing or simple games, allows parents to help children master specific motor skills in a safe and supervised manner.

Physical activity in early childhood also has other benefits. An Iowa study of young children showed that physical activity contributes to optimal bone development.[20] Other research has shown that adolescents who had the highest levels of activity in early childhood had lower accretion of body fat compared with those who had lower levels of physical activity during early childhood. Unstructured play and structured play during early childhood can help prevent pediatric overweight[21] and also appear to increase self-esteem and reduce symptoms of depression and anxiety during early childhood.[21]

Promoting Physical Activity: Middle Childhood—5 Through 10 Years

As children grow and develop, their motor skills increase, giving them an opportunity to participate in a wider variety of physical activities. Children may try many different physical activities and choose one or more in which they are particularly

interested. When children have multiple options for physical activity available in the community, they can be encouraged to express their preferences, develop competencies, and find activities that fit their skills and interests and promote fitness throughout life.

During middle childhood, parents strongly influence a child's physical activity level. Parents should encourage their child to be physically active. Parents who participate in physical activity with their child (eg, walking, dancing, biking, hiking, playing outside, participating in sports such as basketball or baseball) demonstrate the importance of regular physical activity and show their child that physical activity can be fun. Other family members, peers, teachers, and media figures also can encourage children to be physically active.

Children are motivated to participate in physical activity by having fun, by feeling competent, and through variety. Feelings of failure, embarrassment, and boredom, as well as rigid structure, discourage participation. Table 3 shows age-appropriate activities in which children should be engaged and skills to be developed during middle childhood. There should be less emphasis on competition and more on skill development and learning rules and strategy.

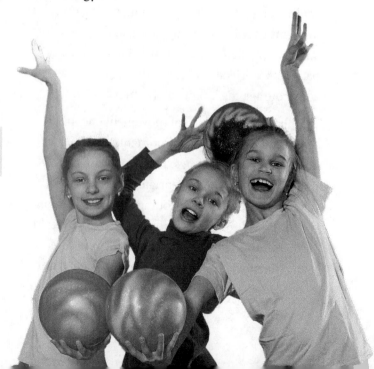

Table 3

Age-Appropriate Physical Activities		
Age, years	**Motor Skills Being Developed**	**Appropriate Physical Activities**
5–6	Fundamental (eg, running, galloping, jumping, hopping, skipping, throwing, catching, striking, or kicking)	• Activities that focus on having fun and developing motor skills rather than on competition • Simple activities that require little instruction • Repetitive activities that do not require complex motor and cognitive skills
7–9	Fundamental transitional (eg, throwing for distance or throwing for accuracy)	• Activities that focus on having fun and developing motor skills rather than on competition • Activities with flexible rules • Activities that require little instruction • Activities that do not require complex motor and cognitive skills
10–11	Transitional complex (eg, playing basketball, soccer)	• Activities that continue to focus on having fun and developing motor skills • Activities that require entry-level complex motor and cognitive skills • Activities that continue to emphasize motor skill development but begin to incorporate instruction on strategy and teamwork

Parents should be cautioned against relying exclusively on schools to provide adequate physical activity for their child. Pressures on school budgets have had the consequence of reducing or eliminating physical education curricula and thus students' opportunities for physical activity.[22] Additionally, indoor and outdoor recesses have been curtailed in many school systems. However, recess can serve as an important break from the rigors of concentrated academic challenge and can improve cognitive, social, emotional, and physical health.[23] Recess is a complement to a physical education program.

Promoting Physical Activity: Adolescence —11 Through 21 Years

Participating in regular physical activity helps adolescents develop skills and pastimes they can enjoy throughout their lives. Adolescents who participate in physical activity increase muscle and bone strength and lean muscle mass. In addition, they may have less body fat and may be better able to maintain a healthy body weight. Physical activity also can reduce symptoms of depression and anxiety and improve overall mood.[1,21] Weight-bearing physical activity contributes to building greater bone density in adolescence and helps maintain peak bone density in adulthood.[24]

Some adolescents are aware of diseases that affect their family or community (eg, overweight, diabetes, cardiovascular disease). This awareness may make them receptive to actions that may reduce risks of these diseases. Health care professionals can consider explaining to adolescents the link between participating in physical activity and reduced risk of diseases that negatively affect their families and perhaps many people within their communities.

Adolescents have numerous options for regular physical activity. Competitive sports appeal to some; others enjoy noncompetitive activities that provide variety and opportunities for socialization. Meeting the recommended 60 minutes or more per day can be done through sustained periods of physical activity or multiple short periods (eg, at least 10 minutes) at various times during the day. Even adolescents who are heavily scheduled with school, extracurricular activities, and part-time jobs can be physically active through short periods of moderate-intensity activity. The accumulated total is the important variable for overall health and calorie burning.

Social and peer influences can positively or negatively affect participation in physical activity. The best physical activities are those that adolescents enjoy. In some communities, the lack of safe places for recreation necessitates creative alternatives for participating in physical activity (eg, using the steps at school or in apartment complexes).

During early adolescence, girls and boys can participate in competitive sports together. However, with the onset of puberty, weight and strength differences between girls and boys rapidly become great enough to pose a safety concern. Coed activities should be limited to non-collision sports.

Adolescents participating in competitive sports and other physical activities can be vulnerable to misinformation and unsafe practices that promise enhanced performance. Pressure to compete can lead them to experiment with ergogenic aids or performance-enhancing substances. These enhancements all lack efficacy and many are dangerous.

References

1. US Department of Health and Human Services. Active children and adolescents. In: *2008 Physical Activity Guidelines for Americans.* Washington, DC: US Department of Health and Human Services; 2008:15-21. ODPHP publication U0036. http://health.gov/paguidelines/guidelines. Accessed September 16, 2016

2. National Association for Sport and Physical Education. *Active Start: A Statement of Physical Activity Guidelines for Children Birth to Five Years.* Reston, VA: National Association for Sport and Physical Education; 2009

3. President's Council on Fitness, Sports & Nutrition. *Physical Activity Guidelines for Americans Midcourse Report: Strategies to Increase Physical Activity Among Youth.* Washington, DC: US Department of Health and Human Services; 2012. http://health.gov/paguidelines/midcourse/pag-mid-course-report-final.pdf. Accessed September 16, 2016

4. US Department of Health and Human Services, US Department of Agriculture. *Dietary Guidelines for Americans 2015–2020 Dietary Guidelines for Americans.* 8th ed. http://health.gov/dietaryguidelines/2015/guidelines. Accessed September 15, 2016

5. American Academy of Pediatrics Task Force on Sudden Infant Death Syndrome. SIDS and other sleep-related infant deaths: updated 2016 recommendations for a safe infant sleeping environment. *Pediatrics.* 2016;138(5):e20162938

6. American Academy of Pediatrics Council on Communications and Media. Media and young minds. *Pediatrics.* 2016;138(5): e20162591

7. American Academy of Pediatrics Council on Communications and Media. Media use in school-aged children and adolescents. *Pediatrics.* 2016;138(5):e20162592

8. Office of Special Education and Rehabilitative Services, Office of Special Education Programs. *Creating Equal Opportunities for Children and Youth with Disabilities to Participate in Physical Education and Extracurricular Athletics.* Washington, DC: US Department of Education; 2011. https://www2.ed.gov/policy/speced/guid/idea/equal-pe.pdf. Accessed September 16, 2016

9. Special Olympics Web site. http://www.specialolympics.org. Accessed September 16, 2016

10. Sawka MN, Burke LM, Eichner ER, et al; American College of Sports Medicine. American College of Sports Medicine position stand. Exercise and fluid replacement. *Med Sci Sports Exerc.* 2007;39(2):377-390

11. Bergeron MF, Devore C, Rice SG; American Academy of Pediatrics Council on Sports Medicine and Fitness, Council on School Health. Climatic heat stress and exercising children and adolescents. *Pediatrics.* 2011;128(3):e741-e747

12. Eichner ER. Sickle cell considerations in athletes. *Clin Sports Med.* 2011;30(3):537-549

13. Anderson S, Eichner ER. Consensus statement: sickle cell trait and the athlete. National Athletic Trainers' Association Web site. https://www.nata.org/sites/default/files/sicklecelltraitandtheathlete.pdf. Accessed September 16, 2016

14. Howe AS, Boden BP. Heat-related illness in athletes. *Am J Sports Med.* 2007;35(8):1384-1395

15. Institute of Medicine. Dietary reference intakes for macronutrients. National Academies of Science, Engineering, and Medicine Web site. http://www.nationalacademies.org/hmd/Activities/Nutrition/DRIMacronutrients.aspx. Accessed September 16, 2016

16. Rodriguez NR, DiMarco NM, Langley S. Position of the American Dietetic Association, Dietitians of Canada, and the American College of Sports Medicine: nutrition and athletic performance. *J Am Diet Assoc.* 2009;109(3):509-527

17. Thomas K, Morris P, Stevenson E. Improved endurance capacity following chocolate milk consumption compared with 2 commercially available sport drinks. *Appl Physiol Nutr Metab.* 2009;34(1):78-82

18. Bernhardt DT, Roberts WO, eds. *PPE: Preparticipation Physical Evaluation.* 4th ed. Elk Grove Village, IL: American Academy of Pediatrics; 2010

19. Sanders SW. *Active for Life: Developmentally Appropriate Movement Programs for Young Children.* Washington, DC: National Association for the Education of Young Children; 2002

20. Janz KF, Burns TL, Torner JC, et al. Physical activity and bone measures in young children: the Iowa Bone Development Study. *Pediatrics.* 2001;107(6):1387-1393

21. Davis MM, Gance-Cleveland B, Hassink S, Johnson R, Paradis G, Resnicow K. Recommendations for prevention of childhood obesity. *Pediatrics.* 2007;120(suppl 4):S229-S253

22. Kohl HW III, Cook HD; Institute of Medicine. *Educating the Student Body: Taking Physical Activity and Physical Education to School.* Washington, DC: National Academies Press; 2013

23. Murray R, Ramstetter C; American Academy of Pediatrics Council on School Health. The crucial role of recess in school. *Pediatrics.* 2013;131(1):183-188

24. Hind K, Burrows M. Weight-bearing exercise and bone mineral accrual in children and adolescents: a review of controlled trials. *Bone.* 2007;40(1):14-27

Promoting Oral Health

Oral health is critically important to the overall health and well-being of infants, children, and adolescents. It covers a range of health promotion and disease prevention concerns, including dental caries; periodontal (gums) health; proper development and alignment of facial bones, jaws, and teeth; other oral diseases and conditions; and trauma or injury to the mouth and teeth. Oral health is an important issue requiring continued health supervision from the health care professional.

Childhood caries is a preventable and transmissible infectious disease caused by bacteria (eg, *Streptococcus mutans* or *Streptococcus sobrinus*) that form plaque on the surface of teeth. The bacteria interact with sugar in foods and beverages, turning them into acids that dissolve tooth enamel, causing caries. Caries is one of the most common chronic diseases in children—5 times more common than asthma.[1] Left untreated, pain and infection caused by dental caries can lead to problems in eating, speaking, and learning.[2] Twenty-three percent of children aged 2 to 5 years and 56% of children aged 6 to 8 have caries, and many school hours are lost each year because of dental problems related to caries.[3]

Dental caries is a complex disease with individual-, family-, and community-level influences.[4] Several population groups are particularly vulnerable to caries. For example, children and youth with special health care needs are at increased risk. National surveys also have demonstrated that children in low- and moderate-income households are more likely to have caries and more decayed teeth than are children from more affluent households. Even within income levels, children of color are more likely to have caries than are white children.[1] Thus, sociodemographic status should be viewed as an initial indicator of risk.

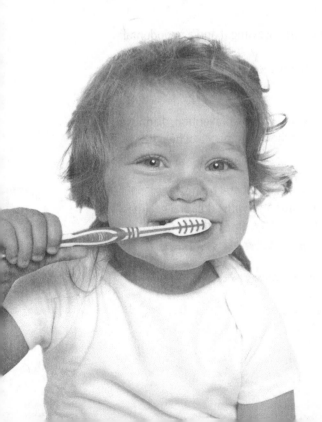
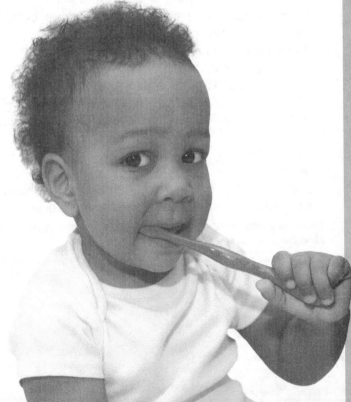

Health care professionals can teach children, adolescents, and their families about oral hygiene, healthy diet and feeding practices, optimal exposure to fluoride, and timely referral to a dentist (see Box 1 for useful resources). Health care professionals also often provide the initial response for oral trauma. They should keep in mind that the differential diagnosis for oral trauma includes intentional injury.[5]

The Importance of a Dental Home

The dental home is the ongoing relationship between the dentist and the patient, includes all aspects of oral health, and is delivered in a comprehensive, continuously accessible, coordinated, and family-centered way (Box 2).[8]

Three dental organizations (the American Dental Association, the Academy of General Dentistry,

---

Box 1

Oral Health Resources

Bright Futures in Practice: Oral Health Pocket Guide (2016) provides a structured and comprehensive approach to oral health anticipatory guidance for the health care professional.[6] The Health Resources and Services Administration National Maternal and Child Oral Health Resource Center (**www.mchoralhealth.org**) also provides many valuable tools and resources for health care professionals.[7] Additional information is available at the AAP Web site (**www.aap.org**).

Abbreviation: AAP, American Academy of Pediatrics.

Box 2

Responsibilities of the Dental Home[9]

According to the AAPD, the dental home should provide

- Comprehensive oral health care, including acute care and preventive services, in accordance with AAPD periodicity schedules.
- Comprehensive assessment for oral diseases and conditions.
- An individualized preventive dental health program based on a caries risk assessment and a periodontal disease risk assessment.
- Anticipatory guidance about growth and development issues (ie, teething, thumb- or finger-sucking behaviors, or pacifier habits).
- A plan for responding to acute dental trauma.
- Information about proper care of the child's teeth and gingivae. This would include prevention, diagnosis, and treatment of disease of the supporting and surrounding tissues and the maintenance of health, function, and esthetics of those structures and tissues.
- Dietary counseling.
- Referrals to dental specialists when care cannot directly be provided within the dental home.
- Education regarding future referral to a dentist knowledgeable and comfortable with adult oral health issues for continuing oral health care. Referral at an age determined by patient, parent, and pediatric dentist.

Abbreviation: AAPD, American Academy of Pediatric Dentistry.

Reproduced with permission from American Academy of Pediatric Dentistry Council on Clinical Affairs. Policy on the dental home. *Pediatr Dent.* 2015;37(6)(Reference Manual):24-25.

and the American Academy of Pediatric Dentistry [AAPD]) are united in encouraging parents to establish a dental home for their child no later than 12 months of age.[9] As children and adolescents mature into adulthood, a dental home also can ensure that they receive oral health education and counseling, preventive and early intervention measures, and treatment, including treatment for periodontal care, orthodontic services, trauma, and other conditions.

Efforts to establish a dental home offer an opportunity for partnerships and foster a connection with the community. A partnership among health care professionals in primary care, dental health, public health, early care and education (including child care and home visiting), and school settings can help ensure access to a dental home for each child during the early childhood, middle childhood, and adolescent years.

Fluoride

Fluoride plays a key role in preventing and controlling caries. Fluoride helps reduce the loss of minerals from tooth enamel (demineralization) and promotes the replacement of minerals (remineralization) in dental enamel that has been damaged by acids produced by bacteria in plaque. Regular and frequent exposure to small amounts of fluoride is the best way to protect the teeth against caries. This exposure can be readily accomplished through drinking water that has been optimally fluoridated[10] and brushing with fluoride toothpaste twice daily.[11]

Fluoride supplementation typically is not needed in the first 6 months of life. Children who do not drink fluoridated water should begin taking fluoride supplements (ie, drops or chewable tablets) at 6 months of age.[12] Parents can purchase bottled water that contains fluoride, as an alternative to fluoride supplements. Evidence reviewed by the US Preventive Services Task Force (USPSTF) found

oral fluoride supplementation effective at reducing caries incidence.[13,14]

Additional types of fluoride may be used as a primary preventive measure and, generally, are recommended for infants, children, and adolescents who are deemed to be at high risk of caries. Research has shown that the primary caries prevention effects of fluoride result from its topical contact with enamel and through its antibacterial actions.[12] The USPSTF also found new evidence to support the effectiveness of fluoride varnish in infants and children, starting at first primary tooth eruption through age 5.[13,14]

Even if indicated, additional or combination of fluoride intake should be used judiciously in children to minimize the risk of fluorosis from the overexposure to fluoride. Fluoride varnish is not a risk factor for fluorosis. Fluorosis can come from swallowing too much toothpaste that contains fluoride, drinking water with higher than recommended fluoride levels, and taking fluoride supplements when other sources of fluoride are available.[15] To prevent fluorosis, if noncommunity water sources, such as wells and other natural sources, are the primary water sources, they must be tested before parents are advised to supplement with fluoride.[16]

For all children and adolescents, optimal fluoride levels in drinking water combined with fluoride-containing preparations, such as toothpastes, gels, varnishes, and rinses, have significantly reduced dental decay, but caries risk remains high during childhood.[3,14] Children and adolescents at high risk of caries should be risk assessed and evaluated for topical fluoride beyond that provided by water supply and a fluoridated toothpaste.

Fluoridated toothpaste also is recommended for all children from the time the first tooth erupts. Children's teeth should be brushed with fluoride toothpaste twice a day, after breakfast and before bed. Use a soft toothbrush made for young children. Infants and children younger than 3 years should use a small smear (ie, no larger than a grain of rice); children aged 3 to 6 should use a pea-sized amount of toothpaste (Figure 1).[17]

Children and Youth With Special Health Care Needs

Children with special health care needs present a unique set of concerns for oral health because they are particularly prone to developing caries. Because dental care for these children is often difficult and sometimes risky, the health care professional should refer the child to a dentist as early as possible for vigilant preventive oral health care, which may alleviate the need for future surgical intervention.

Oral diseases also may have a direct and devastating effect on the general health of children with certain systemic or developmental problems or conditions. Children with compromised immunity or certain cardiac, kidney, or liver conditions may be especially vulnerable to the effects of oral diseases. Children with cognitive disabilities or developmental or neuromuscular conditions who do not have the ability to understand and assume responsibility for or adhere to preventive oral health practices may be at higher risk for complications or systemic infections from oral diseases.[18]

Children and youth with special health care needs may require more help with their oral self-care routines (ie, brushing and flossing) than other children. Health care professionals should advise parents or caregivers to supervise and intervene as needed to help their children with brushing and flossing if their special needs prevent them from doing a thorough job. As with all other children, the child with special needs should begin dental care in the first year and visit the dentist every 6 months or more frequently, as needed.

Adolescents with special health care needs may face difficulties because of their physical condition, malformations, medicines, or nutrition. They

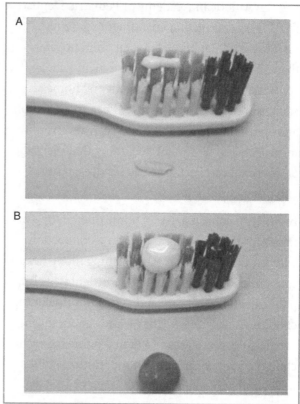

Figure 1: Recommended Amounts of Toothpaste

Reproduced with permission from Lewis CW. Fluoride and dental caries prevention in children. *Pediatr Rev.* 2014;35(3). Figure 5.

should receive regular dental care and be encouraged to take as much responsibility as possible for their own oral hygiene.[18,19]

Promoting Oral Health: Infancy—Birth Through 11 Months

Even though a infant's teeth do not begin to appear until the middle of this developmental period, oral health is still a concern because caries can develop during the first year of life. Exclusive breastfeeding has been associated with a reduction in malocclusion.[20]

Oral Hygiene and Feeding Practices That Promote Oral Health

Even before the baby's birth, parents and other caregivers should make sure their own mouths are as healthy as possible to reduce transmission of caries-causing harmful bacteria from their saliva to the newborn's mouth.[21] Health care professionals should educate family members in the following ways to promote the adult's oral health and prevent the transmission of caries-causing bacteria from adult to infant:

- Practice good oral hygiene and seek oral health care.
- Do not share utensils, cups, spoons, or toothbrushes with the infant.
- Do not put the child's pacifiers in their own mouths. Clean pacifiers with mild soap and water.
- Consult with an oral health professional about the use of xylitol gum or lozenges (if the adult's oral health is a concern). This gum may have a positive effect on oral health by decreasing the bacterial load in an adult's mouth.[22,23]

The primary teeth begin to erupt at different ages during the first year of life. An infant is susceptible to tooth decay as soon as the first teeth come into his oral cavity if he has a sufficient bacterial load already present in his mouth and prolonged exposure to sugars. Chalky white areas on the teeth are the first sign of dental decay. Both inadequate oral hygiene and inappropriate feeding practices that expose teeth to natural or refined sugars for prolonged periods contribute to the development of early childhood caries. Health care professionals should educate parents in the following ways to keep teeth clean and remove plaque:

- Minimize exposure to natural or refined sugars in the infant's mouth.
  - Avoid frequent exposure to foods that can lead to dental caries.
  - Hold the infant while feeding. Never prop a bottle (ie, use pillows or any other object to hold a bottle in the infant's mouth).
  - Do not allow the infant to fall asleep with a bottle that contains milk, formula, juice, or other sweetened liquid.
  - Avoid dipping pacifiers in any sweetened liquid, sugars, or syrups.[16]

- For infants and children younger than 3 years, brush the teeth with a small smear (ie, no larger than a grain of rice) of fluoride toothpaste twice a day (after breakfast and before bed). The child should not spit out the toothpaste or rinse with water. The small amount of toothpaste that remains in his mouth helps prevent dental caries.[11,17]

To help prevent early childhood caries, parents also should take advantage of this developmental stage to establish lifelong nutritious eating patterns for the family that emphasize consumption of vegetables, fruits, whole grains, lean meats, and dairy products and that minimize consumptions of foods and beverages containing added sugars. (*For more information on this topic, see the Promoting Healthy Nutrition theme.*)

Oral Health Risk Assessment

Since 2003, the American Academy of Pediatrics (AAP) has recommended that health care professionals conduct an oral health risk assessment when an infant is 6 months of age.[24] In 2012, the AAP refined the risk factors and developed an Oral Health Risk Assessment Tool for caries risk determination (Figure 2).[6,25] This assessment consists of the health care professional asking parents about their and the child's oral health practices and examining the child's mouth to assess the risk of caries. Fluoride varnish may be applied in the primary care medical home every 6 months, beginning when the first tooth erupts until age 5 years.

The AAP recognizes that, even today, some children live in communities that lack pediatric dentists or general dentists who are able to see infants and young children. Therefore, health care professionals who care for these children may have to continue to perform periodic oral health risk assessments even after 6 to 12 months of age. These assessments allow health care professionals to identify children at the highest risk of oral health

Patient Name:_____ Date of Birth:_____ Date:_____

Visit: ☐ 6 month ☐ 9 month ☐ 12 month ☐ 15 month ☐ 18 month ☐ 24 month ☐ 30 month ☐ 3 year
☐ 4 year ☐ 5 year ☐ 6 year ☐ Other_____

RISK FACTORS	PROTECTIVE FACTORS	CLINICAL FINDINGS
⚠ Mother or primary caregiver had active decay in the past 12 months ☐ Yes ☐ No	● Existing dental home ☐ Yes ☐ No ● Drinks fluoridated water or takes fluoride supplements ☐ Yes ☐ No ● Fluoride varnish in the last 6 months ☐ Yes ☐ No ● Has teeth brushed twice daily ☐ Yes ☐ No	⚠ White spots or visible decalcifications in the past 12 months ☐ Yes ☐ No ⚠ Obvious decay ☐ Yes ☐ No ⚠ Restorations (fillings) present ☐ Yes ☐ No
● Mother or primary caregiver does not have a dentist ☐ Yes ☐ No		
● Continual bottle/sippy cup use with fluid other than water ☐ Yes ☐ No ● Frequent snacking ☐ Yes ☐ No ● Special health care needs ☐ Yes ☐ No ● Medicaid eligible ☐ Yes ☐ No		● Visible plaque accumulation ☐ Yes ☐ No ● Gingivitis (swollen/bleeding gums) ☐ Yes ☐ No ● Teeth present ☐ Yes ☐ No ● Healthy teeth ☐ Yes ☐ No

ASSESSMENT/PLAN

Caries Risk:
☐ Low ☐ High

Completed:
☐ Anticipatory Guidance
☐ Fluoride Varnish
☐ Dental Referral

Self Management Goals:

☐ Regular dental visits	☐ Wean off bottle	☐ Healthy snacks
☐ Dental treatment for parents	☐ Less/No juice	☐ Less/No junk food or candy
☐ Brush twice daily	☐ Only water in sippy cup	☐ No soda
☐ Use fluoride toothpaste	☐ Drink tap water	☐ Xylitol

Figure 2: Oral Health Risk Assessment Tool[25]

Reproduced with permission from Oral Health Risk Assessment Tool. American Academy of Pediatrics Children's Oral Health Web site. http://www2.aap.org/oralhealth/docs/RiskAssessmentTool.pdf. Accessed November 20, 2016.

problems so they can be referred to whatever limited resources are available.[26-29] In addition, public health professionals often assist health care professionals and families to link to a dental home.

Promoting Oral Health: Early Childhood—1 Through 4 Years

The key oral health priorities of this developmental stage are the same as those of infancy—namely, preventing caries and developing healthy oral hygiene habits. Early childhood also is a good time for parents, caregivers, and health care professionals to build positive dietary habits as they introduce new foods and the child establishes taste preferences. Parents may have questions during this period about pacifiers and thumb- and finger-sucking behaviors that are related to teeth and jaw alignment.

Oral Hygiene, Fluoride, and Feeding Practices That Promote Oral Health

Parents and caregivers can do much to prevent the development of caries and promote overall oral health during this period. As noted earlier, caries is an infectious disease, and parents should make sure their oral hygiene and diet meet the standards outlined here. Health care professionals should educate the family and caregivers in the following ways to promote the adult's oral health and prevent transmission of bacteria from the adult to the child:

- Practice good oral hygiene and seek oral health care.
- Do not share utensils, cups, spoons, or toothbrushes with the child.
- Do not put the child's pacifiers in their own mouths. Clean pacifiers with mild soap and water.
- Consult with an oral health care professional about the use of gum or lozenges containing xylitol (if the adult's oral health is a concern).

Health care professionals also should educate parents about ways to keep their child's teeth clean and ensure sufficient fluoride intake.

- Brush children's teeth with fluoride toothpaste twice daily as soon as teeth erupt. Because young children do not have the manual dexterity to brush their teeth well until they are able to tie their own shoes (usually around age 7 or 8 years), an adult should brush or help children brush their teeth. For children younger than 3, brush the teeth with a small smear (ie, no larger than a grain of rice) of fluoride toothpaste twice a day (after breakfast and before bed). The child should not spit out the toothpaste or rinse with water. The small amount of toothpaste that remains in her mouth helps prevent dental caries.[11,17]

    For children aged 3 to 6, brush the teeth with no more than a pea-sized amount of fluoride toothpaste twice a day (after breakfast and before bed). The child should spit out the toothpaste after brushing but not rinse her mouth with water. The small amount of toothpaste that remains in her mouth helps prevent tooth decay. Children can be taught to floss if recommended by the dental professional.

- Make sure the child drinks fluoridated water or takes prescribed fluoride supplements.

Early childhood is a time in which children are exposed to new tastes, textures, and eating experiences. It is an important opportunity for parents and caregivers to firmly establish healthful eating patterns for the child and her family. These patterns should emphasize consumption of vegetables, fruits, whole grains, lean meats, and dairy products and minimize consumptions of foods and beverages containing added sugars. (For more information on this topic, see the Promoting Healthy Nutrition theme.)

Oral Health Risk Assessment

As recommended by the AAPD, by 12 months of age, a child should be seen by a dentist every 6 months or according to a schedule recommended by the dentist, based on the child's individual needs and susceptibility to disease.[30] If a dental home is unavailable, the primary care professional should apply topical fluoride varnish to patients every 6 months. As noted by the AAP, in the absence of a dental home program that is able to see a child between the ages of 1 and 4, the primary care professional should continue to perform oral health risk assessments. The AAPD also recommends that health care professionals use the AAP Oral Health Risk Assessment Tool (see Figure 2).

Other Oral Health Issues

The health care professional should be prepared to discuss the use of pacifiers and thumb- or finger sucking. Finger sucking often fills an emotional need, but it can lead to malocclusion, including anterior open bite (top teeth do not overlap the bottom teeth) and excess overjet (top teeth protrude relative to the bottom teeth). The intensity, duration, and nature of the sucking habit can be used to predict the amount of harm that can occur. Positive reinforcement, including a reward system or reminder system, is the most effective way to discourage finger sucking.

Promoting Oral Health: Middle Childhood—5 Through 10 Years

During the early part of middle childhood, a child loses his first tooth, and the first permanent teeth (maxillary and mandibular incisors and first molars) start to erupt. By the end of middle childhood, many of the permanent teeth have erupted. For the child, these are exciting signs of getting older. Middle childhood also is a good time for parents and caregivers to reinforce oral hygiene, optimal fluoride exposure, proper protection to avoid oral traumatic injuries, and the positive dietary habits they pursued in early childhood.

The history and physical examination performed by the health care professional should include oral health and, as necessary, an oral health risk assessment (see Figure 2). The child should see the dentist every 6 months or according to a schedule recommended by the dentist, based on the child's individual needs and susceptibility to disease. When the permanent molars erupt, the dentist should evaluate the child's teeth to determine the need for sealants that protect the teeth from caries.

The key oral health issues for this developmental stage are preventing caries and gingivitis and ensuring proper development of the mouth and jaw. Reducing the risk of injury or trauma to the mouth and teeth and avoiding risky behaviors that negatively affect oral health also are important.

Oral Hygiene, Fluoride, and Nutrition Practices That Promote Oral Health

Health care professionals should educate parents in the following ways to help their child keep his teeth clean and remove plaque:

- Helping with, and supervising, the brushing of their child's teeth at least twice a day for 2 minutes and flossing once a day before bedtime.

- Using a pea-sized amount of fluoridated toothpaste to clean the child's teeth. The child should spit out the toothpaste after brushing but not rinse his mouth with water. The small amount of toothpaste that remains in his mouth helps prevent tooth decay.[11,17]
- Make sure the child drinks fluoridated water. Children who do not drink fluoridated water and are at high risk of caries should take prescribed fluoride supplements.

As children begin school and expand their horizons beyond the immediate circle of home and family, they are increasingly exposed to eating habits and foods that put them at increased risk of caries. Media, especially television (TV), likely play a role in this increasing risk. Studies of the content of TV programming show that advertisements directed at children are heavily weighted toward foods high in added sugars, such as sweetened breakfast cereals, fruit juice, soft drinks, snacks, and candy.[31]

Parents continue to have the most influence on their children's eating behaviors and attitudes toward food. To the extent possible, parents should make sure that nutritious foods are available to their children, and they should continue to emphasize healthful eating patterns. It is important to avoid the frequent consumption of sugar-sweetened beverages and snacks. *(For more information on this topic, see the Promoting Healthy Nutrition theme.)*

Other Oral Health Issues

Finger or other sucking habits sometimes continue into middle childhood. These habits should be stopped when the permanent teeth begin to erupt. As the child begins to grow, the mouth grows, and the child should be evaluated by a dentist if malocclusion is seen.

Some children begin using tobacco during middle childhood. Therefore, the child should be encouraged not to smoke or use smokeless tobacco because smoking increases the risk of periodontal disease and oral cancer and poses substantial risks to overall health.

As children mature and begin to play with increased strength and vigor, in free play and organized sports, the risk of injury to the mouth increases. The child and parent should know what to do in the event of an emergency, especially if a tooth is visibly broken (chipped or fractured), displaced (luxated), or knocked completely out of the socket (avulsed). In these cases, the child should be referred to a dentist immediately. An avulsed permanent tooth needs to be reimplanted as quickly as possible, but an avulsed primary tooth should not be reimplanted, because it likely would cause damage to developing permanent teeth.[5]

Mouth guards worn during sports and other athletics greatly reduce the severity of unintentional trauma to individual teeth by distributing the forces of impact to all of the teeth and jaws. Custom adaptations range from softening a generic plastic mouth guard in boiling water and biting into it to register a custom bite to fabricating a guard on a custom mold. Both types work well to prevent oral trauma; they differ only in cost and comfort. The protection afforded by any type of guard mandates use in both organized and leisure-time sports activity.

Promoting Oral Health: Adolescence—11 Through 21 Years

Adolescence is characterized by the loss of the remaining primary teeth and complete eruption of all the permanent teeth, including the third molars or wisdom teeth in late adolescence. Growth spurts of the facial bones occur early and then taper off as adolescence progresses. The end result is a fully established bite.

Several oral health issues from earlier developmental stages continue to be important in adolescence. For example, vigilant oral hygiene and positive dietary habits can strengthen a sound foundation

for adult oral health by preventing destructive periodontal disease and dental caries. Avoiding traumatic injury to the mouth is another continuing priority. Other issues are new. For example, adolescence brings increased susceptibility to irreversible periodontal or gum disease that may be related to hormonal and immunologic changes. A comprehensive oral hygiene regimen of brushing and flossing combined with regular professional care can manage this response.

Oral Hygiene, Fluoride, and Nutrition Practices That Promote Oral Health

The adolescent should be responsible for her own preventive oral health care and should have an established dental home. She should see the dentist every 6 months or according to a schedule recommended by the dentist, based on individual needs and susceptibility to disease. The dental professional also may consider diet analysis, topical fluoride applications, antimicrobial regimens, and dental sealants for high-risk patients or those with significant dental disease.[1,3,32,33]

Although preventive therapy has resulted in increased numbers of adolescents with healthy teeth, caries is still common in adolescents and untreated caries is higher among adolescents and young adults aged 16 to 19 years compared with adolescents aged 12 to 15.[3]

Adolescents' risk of caries may be increased by

- Susceptible tooth surfaces caused by immature enamel in newly erupted permanent teeth.
- Indifference to oral hygiene, which allows plaque to accumulate and mature.
- Frequent and unregulated exposure to high quantities of sugars, a feature of many adolescent diets, which provides the perfect medium for caries to develop.[34]
- Frequent consumption of acidic drinks, such as juices, and acid-producing drinks, such as sugar-sweetened beverages, which can directly erode the enamel.[35]

PROMOTING ORAL HEALTH

- Eating disorders, such as bulimia, which can result in a characteristic erosion of the dental enamel by repeated exposure of the teeth to gastric acids.
- Use of certain drugs, specifically methamphetamine, which has a detrimental effect on oral health. Methamphetamine use is associated with rampant decay that is attributed to some combination of the acidic nature of the drug, decreased saliva, tooth grinding and clenching, poor oral hygiene, and drug-induced cravings for high-calorie carbonated beverages.[36]

Health care professionals should educate adolescents to keep their teeth clean and remove plaque by following a comprehensive, daily home care regimen, including a minimum of twice-daily brushing with fluoride toothpaste and once-daily flossing. It is recommended that the adolescent spit out the toothpaste but not rinse with water. This regimen should be customized to each patient according to risk factors. Adolescents also should follow nutritious eating patterns that include only modest consumption of foods and beverages high in added sugars and should drink fluoridated water. *(For more information on this topic, see the Promoting Healthy Nutrition theme.)* If necessary, prescribed fluoride supplements until the age of 16 years are appropriate.[37]

Other Oral Health Issues

Adolescence is a period of experimentation and making choices. Added freedom and extension of boundaries are characteristic of appropriate supervision, but certain behaviors can lead to oral health problems. Substance use, including tobacco and drugs, can affect soft and hard tissues of the oral cavity and is linked to oral cancer.[38] Oral piercing can cause local and systemic infection, tooth fracture, and hemorrhage. Sexual behaviors can lead to infectious and traumatic consequences to the mouth. The health care professional should

ontinue to counsel the adolescent about these non-dietary behavioral factors that affect oral health.

Periodontal Conditions

Evidence suggests that irreversible tissue damage from periodontal disease begins in late adolescence and early adulthood. Early diagnosis, prevention, and treatment can, in most cases, prevent irreversible damage to the periodontal structures in adulthood.[39] Preventing this damage obviates the need for dental restorations, which require lifelong care and monitoring.

Traumatic Injury to the Mouth

Adolescents' risk of traumatic injury to the mouth may be increased by

- High-risk behaviors that may involve trauma to the head and neck
- Driving crashes
- Injuries that occur because of participating in organized and leisure-time sports
- Family or peer violence

Health care professionals should make sure that parents and adolescents know what to do and who to call if an injury occurs and a tooth is fractured or avulsed.

Orthodontics

Genetically related abnormal development, premature primary tooth loss or extraction, or thumb- or finger sucking all can result in significant crowding and malalignment of the teeth, which can adversely affect oral health, function, and aesthetics. Preventing premature tooth loss early in life has a significant effect on minimizing space loss and the resultant crowding in adolescence.

References

1. Dye BA, Li X, Beltrán-Aguilar ED. Selected oral health indicators in the United States, 2005-2008. *NCHS Data Brief*. 2012;(96):1-8. http://www.cdc.gov/nchs/data/databriefs/db96.pdf. Accessed September 14, 2016

2. Jackson SL, Vann WF Jr, Kotch JB, Pahel BT, Lee JY. Impact of poor oral health on children's school attendance and performance. *Am J Public Health*. 2011;101(10):1900-1906

3. Dye BA, Thornton-Evans G, Li X, Iafolla TJ. Dental caries and sealant prevalence in children and adolescents in the United States, 2011-2012. *NCHS Data Brief*. 2015;(191):1-8. http://www.cdc.gov/nchs/data/databriefs/db191.pdf. Accessed September 17, 2016

4. Fisher-Owens SA, Gansky SA, Platt LJ, et al. Influences on children's oral health: a conceptual model. *Pediatrics*. 2007;120(3):e510-e520

5. Keels MA; American Academy of Pediatrics Section on Oral Health. Management of dental trauma in a primary care setting. *Pediatrics*. 2014;133(2):e466-e476

6. Casamassimo PS, Holt KA, eds. *Bright Futures: Oral Health–Pocket Guide*. 3rd ed. Washington, DC: National Maternal and Child Oral Health Resource Center; 2016

7. National Maternal and Child Oral Health Resource Center Web site. http://www.mchoralhealth.org. Accessed September 17, 2016

8. American Academy of Pediatrics Children's Oral Health Web site. http://www2.aap.org/commpeds/dochs/oralhealth/index.html. Accessed September 17, 2016

9. American Academy of Pediatric Dentistry Council on Clinical Affairs. Policy on the dental home. *Pediatr Dent*. 2015;37(6)(Reference Manual):24-25

10. US Department of Health and Human Services Federal Panel on Community Water Fluoridation. U.S. Public Health Service recommendation for fluoride concentration in drinking water for the prevention of dental caries. *Public Health Rep*. 2015;130(4):318-331

11. American Dental Association Council on Scientific Affairs. Fluoride toothpaste use for young children. *J Am Dent Assoc*. 2014;145(2):190-191

12. Clark MB, Slayton RL; American Academy of Pediatrics Section on Oral Health. Fluoride use in caries prevention in the primary care setting. *Pediatrics*. 2014;134(3):626-633

13. Chou R, Cantor A, Zakher B, Mitchell JP, Pappas M. Preventing dental caries in children <5 years: systematic review updating USPSTF Recommendation. *Pediatrics*. 2013;132(2):332-350

14. Moyer VA; US Preventive Services Task Force. Prevention of dental caries in children from birth through age 5 years: US Preventive Services Task Force recommendation statement. *Pediatrics*. 2014;133(6):1102-1111

15. Levy SM, Broffitt B, Marshall TA, Eichenberger-Gilmore JM, Warren JJ. Associations between fluorosis of permanent incisors and fluoride intake from infant formula, other dietary sources and dentifrice during early childhood. *J Am Dent Assoc*. 2010;141(10):1190-1201

16. American Academy of Pediatrics Committe on Nutrition. Kleinman RE, Greer FR, eds. *Pediatric Nutrition: Policy of the American Academy of Pediatrics*. 7th ed. Elk Grove Village, IL: American Academy of Pediatrics; 2014

17. Wright JT, Hanson N, Ristic H, Whall CW, Estrich CG, Zentz RR. Fluoride toothpaste efficacy and safety in children younger than 6 years: a systematic review. *J Am Dent Assoc*. 2014;145(2):182-189

18. American Academy of Pediatric Dentistry Council on Clinical Affairs. Guideline on management of dental patients with special health care needs. *Pediatr Dent*. 2015;37(6)(Reference Manual):166-171

19. Norwood KW Jr, Slayton RL; American Academy of Pediatrics Council on Children With Disabilities, Section on Oral Health. Oral health care for children with developmental disabilities. *Pediatrics*. 2013;131(3):614-619

20. Peres KG, Cascaes AM, Peres MA, et al. Exclusive breastfeeding and risk of dental malocclusion. *Pediatrics*. 2015;136(1):e60-e67

21. Weintraub JA, Prakash P, Shain SG, Laccabue M, Gansky SA. Mothers' caries increases odds of children's caries. *J Dent Res*. 2010;89(9):954-958

22. Laitala ML, Alanen P, Isokangas P, Söderling E, Pienihäkkinen K. Long-term effects of maternal prevention on children's dental decay and need for restorative treatment. *Community Dent Oral Epidemiol*. 2013;41(6):534-540

23. Riley P, Moore D, Sharif MO, Ahmed F, Worthington HV. Xylitol-containing products for preventing dental caries in children and adults. *Cochrane Database Syst Rev*. 2015;(3):CD010743

24. Hale KJ; American Academy of Pediatrics Section on Pediatric Dentistry. Oral health risk assessment timing and establishment of the dental home. *Pediatrics*. 2003;111(5 pt 1):1113-1116

25. Oral Health Risk Assessment Tool. American Academy of Pediatrics Children's Oral Health Web site. http://www2.aap.org/oralhealth/docs/RiskAssessmentTool.pdf. Accessed September 17, 2016

26. Stearns SC, Rozier R, Kranz AM, Pahel BT, Quiñonez RB. Cost-effectiveness of preventive oral health care in medical offices for young Medicaid enrollees. *Arch Pediatr Adolesc Med*. 2012;166(10):945-951

27. Pahel BT, Rozier RG, Stearns SC, Quiñonez RB. Effectiveness of preventive dental treatments by physicians for young Medicaid enrollees. *Pediatrics*. 2011;127(3):e682-e689

Bright Futures Guidelines for Health Supervision of Infants, Children, and Adolescents

PROMOTING ORAL HEALTH

28. Rozier RG, Stearns SC, Pahel BT, Quinonez RB, Park J. How a North Carolina program boosted preventive oral health services for low-income children. *Health Aff (Millwood)*. 2010;29(12):2278-2285

29. Rozier RG, Slade GD, Zeldin LP, Wang H. Parents' satisfaction with preventive dental care for young children provided by nondental primary care providers. *Pediatr Dent*. 2005;27(4):313-322

30. American Academy of Pediatric Dentistry Clinical Affairs Committee. Guideline on periodicity of examination, preventative dental services, anticipatory guidance/counseling, and oral treatent for infants, children, and adolescents. *Pediatr Dent*. 2015;37(6)(Reference Manual):123-130

31. Galbraith-Emami S, Lobstein T. The impact of initiatives to limit the advertising of food and beverage products to children: a systematic review. *Obes Rev*. 2013;14(12):960-974

32. Dye BA, Li X, Thornton-Evans G. Oral health disparities as determined by selected Healthy People 2020 Oral Health Objectives for the United States, 2009-2010. *NCHS Data Brief*. 2012;(104):1-8. http://www.cdc.gov/nchs/data/databriefs/db104.pdf. Accessed September 17, 2016

33. Dye BA, Tan S, Smith V, et al. Trends in oral health status: United States, 1988-1994 and 1999-2004. *Vital Health Stat 11*. 2007;(248):1-92. http://www.cdc.gov/nchs/data/series/sr_11/sr11_248.pdf. Accessed September 17, 2016

34. Moynihan PJ, Kelly SA. Effect on caries of restricting sugars intake: systematic review to inform WHO guidelines. *J Dent Res*. 2014;93(1):8-18

35. American Academy of Pediatric Dentistry Clinical Affairs Committee. Policy on dietary recommendations for infants, children, and adolescents. *Pediatr Dent*. 2015;37(6)(Reference Manual):56-58

36. American Dental Association Division of Communications, Division of Scientific Affairs. For the dental patient ... methamphetamine use and oral health. *J Am Dent Assoc*. 2005;136(10):1491

37. American Academy on Pediatric Dentistry Liaison with Other Groups Committee. Guideline on fluoride therapy. *Pediatr Dent*. 2015;37(6)(Reference Manual):176-179

38. Petti S. Lifestyle risk factors for oral cancer. *Oral Oncol*. 2009;45(4-5):340-350

39. American Academy of Pediatric Dentistry, American Academy of Periodontology Research Science and Therapy Committee. Periodontal diseases of children and adolescents. *Pediatr Dent*. 2015;37(6)(Reference Manual):352-360

Promoting Healthy Sexual Development and Sexuality

Family members have different perspectives on how sexuality should be discussed with children and adolescents, such as who should be involved in those discussions and how much young people need to know and at what age. With respect for different individual and cultural values, health care professionals can address this important component of healthy development by incorporating sexuality education that includes gender identity development into health supervision from early childhood through adolescence.[1] In the supportive environment of the medical home, health care professionals can provide personalized information, confidential screening of risk status, health promotion, and counseling for the child and adolescent. Developmentally appropriate, accurate resources that are related to sex education and healthy sexuality provide parents with factual information and encouragement as they educate and guide their growing child.

Health care professionals also should acknowledge and discuss the healthy sexual feelings that all children and adolescents have, including children with special health care needs. Families of children with special health care needs may require additional counseling around sexual development issues to ensure a healthy understanding of their child's pubertal and sexual development.[2]

Promoting Healthy Sexual Development and Sexuality: Infancy—Birth Through 11 Months

Nurturing the development of the biological and physical foundations of healthy intimacy is an important goal that begins in infancy. These foundations require the ability to be comfortable and safe in a close physical relationship with another person. Intimacy begins in the parent's arms with good parent-child reciprocity, response to cues, management of states of arousal such as pain and hunger, and establishment of regular cycles of excitement and relaxation (waking up and falling asleep). The infant needs to have the sense that he is valued, loved, and important for who he is.

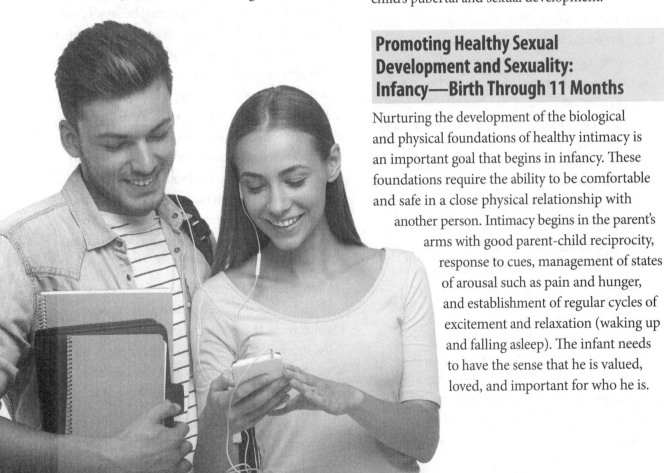

Parents often ask how to handle their infant's sexual behavior, such as genital touching, as the infant becomes aware of his own genitalia. This issue can be addressed as typical behavior with parents during the 6 and 9 Month Visits, perhaps when discussing bathing or diapering. Parents can be encouraged to practice proper naming of their infant's genitalia (eg, penis and vulva) during diapering and bathing. Doing so may facilitate future discussion between parents and their children about sexuality.

Promoting Healthy Sexual Development and Sexuality: Early Childhood—1 Through 4 Years

Sexual exploration is a normal, universal, and healthy part of early childhood development. At this age, children show interest in their own, as well as others', "private" areas, and they become aware of gender differences. Their curiosity can be shown in behaviors such as playing doctor with their peers, undressing during play activities, trying to watch people when they are nude, and physically touching their parents' body parts (eg, their mother's breasts). In early childhood, children also are exposed to social norms and learn boundaries regarding sexual behaviors. All people maintain personal boundaries, both physical and emotional, and young children first learn personal boundaries in their families. Issues related to the timing, settings (eg, public versus private), and spectrum of sexual behaviors can best be discussed in the context of trusting relationships and open communication between the parent and the child.[3]

The most common sexuality issues for this age group are related to bathing and showering, toileting, modesty, privacy, masturbation, and sexual play. Uninhibited verbal references to sexual organs and elimination are common at this age. Masturbation is frequently a concern for parents but is normal behavior unless it becomes excessive. A variety of behaviors can be seen, such as posturing, tightening of thighs, sexual arousal, and handling of genitals. Gently setting limits on such activities when they are done in the presence of nonfamily members or in public, without harsh reaction to or shaming of the child, helps the child grasp socially acceptable behavior. Parent experiences, as well as cultural, religious, and family norms, influence parents' responses to their children's sexual behavior.

Sexual play between same-age peers usually is lighthearted and voluntary in nature, often serving as a source of humor for toddlers. This behavior usually diminishes when children are requested to stop and limits are set. Because of the potential relationship between child sexual abuse and sexual behavior, some sexual behaviors in children can create uncertainty for the health care professional. Consequently, it is important to understand normative sexual childhood activities. The less frequent and more concerning sexual behaviors are intrusive, such as inserting objects into the vagina or anus or aggressive sexual actions. Health care professionals should be able to distinguish healthy and natural from concerning and distressing sexual behaviors They should provide reassurance about normal activities, provide developmentally appropriate parameters for identifying problem behaviors, and encourage family discussions regarding sexual behavior issues.[4] Exposure to media should be age appropriate to reduce the likelihood that undesirable sexual references and language will arise.

Children become aware of the differences in genitals as well as how boys and girls express themselves to the outside world through gender roles, hairstyles, and fashion. Fantasy play with gender expression is common at this age, and many children will explore the clothing or roles of the other gender.

Parental acceptance of their child regardless of how she identifies her gender is important for the child's mental health and adjustment (Box 1). The sex (female or male) of most newborns and infants is known prenatally or immediately at birth, but some endocrinologic and genetic conditions may result in ambiguity of the external genitalia, making sex assignment difficult initially. Gender identity, however, is a gradual process that is based on an internal conviction of belonging to a gender. Gender identity is distinct from gender role, which refers to "behaviors, attitudes, and personality traits a society designates as masculine or feminine."

Some children may identify with a different gender from their sex assigned at birth (ie, transgender). Evidence of gender nonconformity is often apparent in early childhood, as early as 2 years of age; for others, it does not occur until later in adolescence or even during adulthood.[5] For children who establish a transgender identity, the main factor associated with persistence into adolescence and adulthood is the intensity of their gender nonconformity in childhood. For others, gender nonconformity may change over the years or disappear altogether.[5]

Children whose developing gender identity is at odds with their assigned birth sex may show distress when identity or expression is restricted. For the health care professional, the principal task is to recognize the child's current status and to provide the parents with the best strategies to support their child. Families may benefit from supportive mental health professionals, especially those trained in gender issues, who can help guide a child's self-exploration.

Promoting Healthy Sexual Development and Sexuality: Middle Childhood—5 Through 10 Years

Middle childhood is the time to begin providing accurate sexual information for children and give them opportunities to explore, question, and assess their own and their family's attitudes toward gender, sexuality, and human relationships. At this age, the changes of puberty also can be addressed.

Box 1

Definitions of Terms Related to Sex and Gender[5,a]

Gender: Behavioral, cultural, and psychological characteristics associated with femaleness or maleness.

Sex: Physical attributes that characterize maleness and femaleness (eg, the genitalia).

Gender identity: Person's internal sense of being male, female, or somewhere else on the gender spectrum.

Gender role: Behaviors, attitudes, and personality traits a society designates as masculine or feminine.

Gender expression: The way a person outwardly communicates gender. A person's gender expression may or may not be consistent with internal gender identity.

Gender dysphoria: A clinical symptom characterized by a sense of alienation to some or all of the physical characteristics or social roles of one's assigned gender.

Gender nonconforming people: Persons with behaviors, appearances, or identities that are incongruent with those culturally assigned to their birth sex. Gender nonconforming individuals may refer to themselves as transgender, gender queer, gender fluid, gender creative, gender independent, or non-cisgender.

Transgender: This term can be synonymous with gender nonconforming. Some use this term to refer to individuals with gender identities that are the opposite of their assigned gender.

[a] This box is not all-inclusive of the terminology used in the medical community or gender nonconformity community.

Adapted with permission from Vance SR Jr, Ehrensaft D, Rosenthal SM. Psychological and medical care of gender nonconforming youth. *Pediatrics.* 2014;134(6):1184-1192.

Health care professionals should perform a sexual maturity rating beginning at age 7 years because of many reports of increasingly early pubertal onset. It is appropriate to ask a child aged 7 to 8 if he has ever heard the word *puberty* and help him describe what it means: "Puberty is the time when your body grows, matures, and changes." Health care professionals should address upcoming stages of sexual development as part of their anticipatory guidance because children and their parents can be reluctant to ask questions about normal physical development or the differences noted in their child's development compared with that of the child's peers. Normal pubertal development varies widely in the US population, and racial and ethnic differences are now observed (eg, African American girls and Mexican American girls have been shown to have a higher rate of early-onset puberty than do white girls).[6]

Concepts of family, friendship, and other human relationships are core components of healthy sexuality. Children should learn to express love and intimacy in appropriate ways and to avoid manipulative or exploitative relationships. Empathy and respect for another's feelings also is an essential component of a healthy relationship, facilitated through effective communication skills. Kissing, hugging, and touching are understood within the norms of the child and family's culture. Children need to understand their rights and responsibilities for their own bodies (eg, privacy and hygiene) and the importance of communicating fears and concerns with trusted adults. Children should know that no other child or adult has the right to tell them to keep secrets from either parent, especially when someone is touching their body inappropriately. Parents should give their child permission to tell them about any uncomfortable or threatening experiences, reassuring the child that he will be believed and will not be in trouble for telling.

In middle childhood, children should appreciate wide variations in body shapes and sizes and acquire pride in their own body and gender. Children this age can and should understand that their bodies will change as they grow older. They should learn the differences between male and female genitalia and the correct name and specific function of each body part. They also can learn that some body parts can feel good when touched, it is normal to be curious about one's body, and not all exploratory behaviors are appropriate in every place and time. The age at which to teach about sexual intercourse and reproduction depends on the parents' assessment of the child's need for this information, his developmental level, and parental readiness. Over time, parents might include a discussion of human immunodeficiency virus (HIV) infection and other sexually transmitted infections (STIs), including an explanation of their causes (eg, viruses and bacteria, respectively) and general modes of transmission. For many children, this topic is more appropriate during early adolescence.

Children's exposure to elements of sexuality from their peers, families of their peers, and the media (eg, news stories, advertisements, television programs, video games, and pornography on the Internet) can influence them to make choices that may not be healthy, safe, or consistent with family values. It is important to review Internet safety with children and parents as children's online time and experiences increase during middle childhood. *(For more information on this topic, see the Promoting the Healthy and Safe Use of Social Media theme.)* Health care professionals can encourage parents to talk with their children about these issues and suggest resources to help open these discussions and conduct them comfortably.[7,8]

Middle childhood also is a good age to open discussions with children about gender roles they see in the media and the world around them and to support healthy development of their own sense of self as a developing male or female, including discussion of how gender roles have changed over time and what constitutes healthy emotional relationships for both genders. For children who have been persistently gender nonconforming, puberty can be a distressing age as their body goes through changes that may not feel right to them. Current best practice focuses on supporting the child's journey and affirming the child's gender identity. No evidence exists that professionals can change a child's internal sense of gender identity. Referral to a specialist who can further explore the gender nonconformity can be considered. Guidance from a knowledgeable mental health professional also can be considered because distress accompanying pubertal change can be associated with mental health concerns.[9]

Promoting Healthy Sexual Development and Sexuality: Adolescence—11 Through 21 Years

Experiences with romantic relationships, exploration of sexual roles, and self-awareness of sexual orientation commonly occur during adolescence. Decisions that are associated with sexual development in the adolescent years often have important implications for health and education, as well as current and future relationships.

Key Data and Statistics

Several existing databases provide important and useful information related to adolescent sexual behaviors in addition to many other aspects of health.

Parent and Adolescent Sexual Decision-making

A national survey of adolescents and young adults aged 12 to 19 years conducted by the National Campaign to Prevent Teen and Unplanned Pregnancy[10] showed that

- Adolescents and young adults aged 12 to 19 continue to report that parents (38%) are the greatest influence regarding sexual decision-making and values, more than peers (22%), media (9%), siblings (6%), religious

leaders (6%), teachers and educators (4%), or "someone else" (10%).

- Eighty-seven percent of adolescents and 93% of parents believe that it is important for teens to be given a strong message that they should not have sex before completing high school.

- Nearly 87% of adolescents agree that "it would be easier for adolescents to postpone sexual activity and avoid adolescent pregnancy if they were able to have more open, honest conversation about these topics with their parents."

A separate report further outlined various factors that influence adolescents' decisions related to abstinence, safe sexual behaviors, and teen pregnancy.[11] Among the protective factors were living in a 2-parent household; high level of parental education; family connectedness, with active parental monitoring and supervision; and open parent-adolescent communication about sex and contraception before the initiation of sex. Other protective factors that influence delayed initiation of sex include strong community support, connectedness to schools and faith communities, high academic achievement, and strong personal values or religious beliefs.

Percentage of Youth Who Report Having Had Sexual Intercourse

The Youth Risk Behavior Survey (YRBS), conducted by the Centers for Disease Control and Prevention (CDC), is a national paper-based survey conducted every other year with more than 13,000 youth in grades 6 to 12.[12] Data from the 2013 survey show that

- Thirty percent reported having had sexual intercourse by the spring semester of grade 9.
- Of those surveyed, 46.8% reported ever having had sex.
- Thirty-four percent reported having had sexual intercourse during the 3 months before the survey.

In a smaller 12-site YRBS survey, which assessed the sex of sexual contacts, 2.5% (0.7%–3.9%) of youth reported sex with the same sex and 3.3% (1.9%–4.9%) reported sexual contact with both sexes.[13]

Onset of Intercourse

- According to YRBS 2013 data, the percentage of adolescents, both girls and boys, who have had sexual intercourse, including nonconsensual sex, before age 13 years has decreased from 10.2% in 1991 to 5.6% in 2013. A higher percentage of boys (8.3%) are sexually active before age 13 as compared to females (3.1%).[12]

- Among sexually experienced adolescents and young adults aged 12 to 19 years, 67% of females and 53% of males who participated in a survey by the National Campaign to Prevent Teen and Unplanned Pregnancy reported that they wished they had waited longer before initiating sexual intercourse.[10]

Contraception

- Data from the 2013 YRBS show that of students who were currently sexually active, 59% reported they or their partner used a condom at last intercourse and 25% reported they or their partner used other birth control methods to prevent pregnancy before last sexual intercourse. Methods included pills (19%), intrauterine device (IUD) or implant (1.6%), or an injectable, patch, or birth control ring (4.7%).[12]

- The CDC National Center of Health Statistics also conducts the National Survey of Family Growth (NSFG), which includes face-to-face interviews with adolescents and adults aged 15 to 19 years.[14,15] Data from the 2011–2013 NSFG survey show that 79% of females and 84% of males used a contraceptive method at first sexual intercourse. This was especially true of males aged 17 to 19 years, in which contraception use was more than 90%. This survey also found that the use of emergency contraception by female teenagers and adults aged 15

to 19 who had sexual intercourse at least once has increased over the past decade, from 8% in 2002 to 22% in 2011–2013.[15]

Pregnancy Rates

- According to the National Vital Statistics Report, the adolescent pregnancy rate among those aged 15 to 19 years declined substantially between 1990 and 2008.[16] Since 2008, the rate has dropped 15%, from 67.8 per 1,000 to 57.4.[17]

Sexually Transmitted Infections

- Approximately 20 million new STIs occur each year; 50% occur among adolescents and young adults aged 15 to 24 years.[18] Common STIs include human papillomavirus (HPV) infection, trichomoniasis, chlamydial infection, herpes simplex virus infection, and gonorrhea.

- Young female adolescents are particularly vulnerable to acquisition of STIs and are prone to complications, such as pelvic inflammatory disease. They also have much higher rates of gonorrhea and chlamydial infection than do older women.[19] The high prevalence is the result of behavioral, biological, social, and epidemiologic factors, including high-risk sexual partners, inconsistent lack of condoms, lack of immunity from previous infections, sexual violence, lack of access to confidential care, and lack of screening.

- In 2010, 26% of new HIV infections were reported to occur in those aged 13 to 24 years. Young males who have sex with males are at an increased risk of acquiring HIV infection, and approximately 72% of new HIV infections among youth occurred in that group.[20]

Role of the Health Care Professional

Clinical care for adolescents and young adults is commonly related to concerns about sexual development, contraception, STIs, and pregnancy. Healthy sexuality is an important component of a healthy, happy life, and clinical encounters for acute care, health maintenance visits, or sports physical examinations all provide opportunities to teach adolescents and their families about sexuality. Health care professionals can discuss sexual maturation, sexual attraction, family or cultural values, communication, monitoring and guidance patterns for the family, personal goals, informed sexual decision-making, and safety.

The American Academy of Pediatrics (AAP) policy statement "Sexuality Education for Children and Adolescents"[1] advises health care professionals to integrate sexuality education into the longitudinal relationship they develop through their care experiences with the preadolescent, the adolescent, and the family. Confidential, culturally sensitive, and nonjudgmental counseling and care are important to all youth. Historically, sexual and reproductive health services have been designed for female adolescents. New guidance describes how to structure services specifically for male adolescents as well.[21] Adolescents with special health care needs and their families can benefit from knowledgeable, personalized anticipatory guidance.[22] Education about normal puberty and sexuality can be augmented with information that is germane to adolescents with physical differences, especially those that directly affect sexual functioning, as well as youth with cognitive delays.[23,24] The risk of sexual exploitation and the protection of youth are always critical.[23,24]

Parents and health care professionals should be partners with youth in supporting healthy adolescent development and decision-making, as the reward is long-term. Although parents of most adolescents are concerned and available, health care professionals also should offer appropriate care to adolescents whose parents are absent or disengaged.

Health care professionals can acknowledge the appeal of sex and the normalcy of sexual interest with their adolescent patients and also share the advantages of delaying sexual involvement, suggest skills for refusing sexual advances, provide information about drug and alcohol risks, and express encouragement for healthy decisions. The risks of date rape should be emphasized. In addition, the health care professional can discuss poor decision-making under the influence of alcohol or cognition-altering drugs. Adolescents with and without sexual experience may welcome support for avoiding sex until later in their lives. Information about contraception, emergency contraception, and STI prevention should be offered to all sexually active adolescents and those who plan to become sexually active.[25,26] Each contraceptive method has instructions for correct use, effectiveness for preventing pregnancy, potential adverse effects, and long-term consequences. Inconsistent or incorrect use of contraceptives contribute to the incidence of unintended pregnancy. Long-acting reversible contraception (LARC), delivered through IUDs and subdermal implants, are safe for adolescents[25,27-29] and are the most effective reversible contraceptive methods. Health care professionals are encouraged to counsel adolescents on contraception, discussing the most effective contraceptive methods (ie, LARC methods) first. Adolescents also may be counseled on emergency contraception to prevent pregnancy after intercourse.[30] Many teens who self-identify as gay, lesbian, or bisexual may have sexual encounters that may not be predicted by their orientation, and conversation about birth control is important.[14,31,32] It is important to screen youth for risks related to the sexual activities in which they participate and the body parts they possess (ie, ensuring pregnancy protection for a transgender boy who has a uterus). It is important to remain nonjudgmental and allow autonomy for adolescents when they are making decisions about their preferred method of birth control.

Adolescents should be reminded that hormonal contraception and IUDs do not protect against

STIs, and they should be encouraged to use dual protection. The latex condom is the only method available to prevent the spread of HIV and can reduce the risks of other STIs, including chlamydial infection, gonorrhea, and trichomoniasis.[33] Condoms also can reduce the risk of genital herpes, syphilis, and HPV infection when the infected areas are covered or protected by the condom.

Caring for Youth Who Are Lesbian, Gay, Bisexual, Transgender, Questioning, or Gender Nonconforming

The development of a sexual identity is important in adolescence. Health care professionals should be sensitive to the full spectrum of sexual behaviors and gender identities. Youth express a variety of sexual orientation or gender identity differences. According to the AAP clinical report "Sexual Orientation and Adolescents," "sexual orientation refers to an individual's pattern of physical and emotional arousal toward other persons."[34] Some youth may be aware of this attraction to people of the same sex before or early in adolescence, but other youth may not recognize same-sex attractions until later in adolescence or adulthood. Although sexual orientation is stable over time for many people, it may be fluid for some individuals, especially during adolescence.[35,36]

Studies document resilience and positive outcomes for lesbian, gay, bisexual, transgender, or questioning (LGBTQ) youth associated with supportive families, teachers, and gay-straight alliances at school.[37,38] It has been demonstrated that family acceptance has the strongest overall influence on positive health outcomes for youth

who are LGBTQ.[39] Absent family acceptance or lacking community supports, LGBTQ youth are at risk of isolation, abuse or bullying, depression, and suicide.[32] Care needs to be confidential, but with the youth's permission, health care professionals can explore the family's values and attitudes so they can address the youth's sexual orientation or questioning status in ways that respect the family's values and meet the adolescent's need for support, acceptance, and competent health care. Health care professionals can provide accurate information and answer parent and youth questions about what supports healthy development for youth who are LGBTQ and what does not.[10,31] They also can identify experienced and knowledgeable mental health professionals for youth with mental health concerns and provide referrals for specialty consultation about puberty blockers and hormone therapy when requested or indicated. Some adolescents may feel alone, especially if their family is not supportive or if they live in a community that does not have an active support system for LGBTQ youth.

Health care professionals should be prepared to support the LGBTQ youth and the family when immediate parental acceptance is not given. This can be done in various

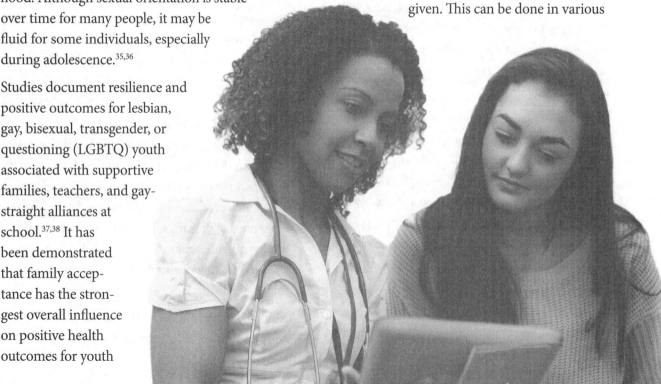

ways. For example, the health care professional can encourage parents to seek support and encourage them to have an open and nonjudgmental dialogue with their adolescent. The health care professional's goals for these youth are the same as for all adolescents—to assess for risks behaviors and to promote healthy development, social and emotional well-being, and optimal physical health. Supportive, quality health care for adolescents means that adolescents are welcomed as individuals, regardless of social status, gender identity or expression, disability, religion, sexual orientation, ethnic background, or country of origin. The health care professional must be prepared to discuss sensitive personal issues, including sexual orientation and gender identity.[31,40]

Clinic personnel and practice materials can convey a nonjudgmental and safe environment for care and confidentiality for adolescents who self-identify as LGBTQ.[41] However, self-identified youth are only a small percentage of LGBTQ youth. Health care professionals who provide care to adolescents are caring for some who have not disclosed their gender identity or sexual orientation. Professional development, course work, or other modalities may be necessary to ensure that health care professionals can provide comprehensive health care and quality care to all adolescents. Health care professionals should learn about local LGBTQ centers and programs in their communities and should be able to provide online national resources.[42] If the health care professional cannot ensure a supportive environment for these adolescents because of personal feelings or other barriers, the adolescent should be referred to another practice or clinic with appropriate services.[31]

As with all other patients, the adolescent should be assured that confidentiality will be protected and also should be told of the conditions under which it can be broken. *(See also the Introduction to the Bright Futures Health Supervision Visits section.)* In situations of serious concern, the health care professional should help the adolescent discuss the issue with parents or family and, if necessary, obtain additional services with mental health professionals or other health care professionals. The health care professional also should offer advice to guide these adolescents in avoiding sexual and other health risk behaviors. A focus on youth access to accurate and complete information and support for healthy decision-making is key for all youth who are transitioning to adulthood.

References

1. American Academy of Pediatrics Committee on Psychosocial Aspects of Child Family Health, Committee on Adolescence. Sexuality education for children and adolescents. *Pediatrics.* 2001;108(2):498-502

2. Sexual development and behavior in children: information for parents and caregivers. National Child Traumatic Stress Network Web site. http://nctsn.org/nctsn_assets/pdfs/caring/sexualdevelopmentandbehavior.pdf. Accessed September 17, 2016

3. Kellogg ND; American Academy of Pediatrics Committee on Child Abuse and Neglect. Clinical report—the evaluation of sexual behaviors in children. *Pediatrics.* 2009;124(3):992-998

4. Kellogg N, ed. *Preventing Sexual Violence: An Educational Toolkit for Health Care Professionals.* Elk Grove Village, IL: American Academy of Pediatrics; 2010

5. Vance SR Jr, Ehrensaft D, Rosenthal SM. Psychological and medical care of gender nonconforming youth. *Pediatrics.* 2014;134(6):1184-1192

6. Rosenfield RL, Lipton RB, Drum ML. Thelarche, pubarche, and menarche attainment in children with normal and elevated body mass index. *Pediatrics.* 2009;123(1):84-88

7. Levine SB. Facilitating parent-child communication about sexuality. *Pediatr Rev.* 2011;32(3):129-130

8. Ginsburg KR, Kinsman SB. Talking to your child about sex. American Academy of Pediatrics Web site. http://www.healthychildren.org/English/ages-stages/gradeschool/puberty/Pages/Talking-to-Your-Child-About-Sex.aspx. Accessed September 17, 2016

9. Substance Abuse and Mental Health Services Administration. *Ending Conversion Therapy: Supporting and Affirming LGBTQ Youth.* Rockville, MD: Substance Abuse and Mental Health Services Administration; 2015. HHS publication (SMA) 15-4928. https://store.samhsa.gov/shin/content/SMA15-4928/SMA15-4928.pdf. Accessed September 17, 2016

10. Albert B. *With One Voice 2012: America's Adults and Teens Sound Off About Teen Pregnancy.* Washington, DC: National Campaign to Prevent Teen and Unplanned Pregnancy; 2012. https://thenationalcampaign.org/sites/default/files/resource-primary-download/wov_2012.pdf. Accessed September 17, 2016

11. Kirby D, Lepore G. *Sexual Risk and Protective Factors: Factors Affecting Teen Sexual Behavior, Pregnancy, Childbearing and Sexually Transmitted Disease: Which Are Important? Which Can You Change?* Washington, DC: National Campaign to Prevent Teen and Unplanned Pregnancy; 2007. https://thenationalcampaign.org/sites/default/files/resource-primary-download/protective_factors_full.pdf. Accessed September 17, 2016

12. Kann L, Kinchen S, Shanklin SL, et al. Youth risk behavior surveillance—United States, 2013 [published correction appears in *MMWR Surveill Summ.* 2014;63(26):576]. *MMWR Surveill Summ.* 2014;63(4):1-168

13. Kann L, Olsen EO, McManus T, et al. Sexual identity, sex of sexual contacts, and health-risk behaviors among students in grades 9-12: youth risk behavior surveillance, selected sites, United States, 2001-2009. *MMWR Surveill Summ.* 2011;60(7):1-133

14. National Survey of Family Growth. Key statistics from the National Survey of Family Growth. Centers for Disease Control and Prevention Web site. http://www.cdc.gov/nchs/nsfg/key_statistics/t.htm#teenagers. Accessed September 17, 2016

15. Martinez GM, Abma JC. Sexual activity, contraceptive use, and childbearing of teenagers aged 15–19 in the United States. *NCHS Data Brief.* 2015;(209):1-8

16. Ventura SJ, Curtin SC, Abma JC, Henshaw SK. Estimated pregnancy rates and rates of pregnancy outcomes for the United States, 1990-2008. *Natl Vital Stat Rep.* 2012;60(7):1-21

17. Kost K, Henshaw S. U.S. teenage pregnancies, births and abortions, 2010: national and state trends by age, race and ethnicity. Guttmacher Institute Web site. https://www.guttmacher.org/pubs/USTPtrends10.pdf. Published May 2014. Accessed September 17, 2016

18. CDC fact sheet: incidence, prevalence, and cost of sexually transmitted infections in the United States. Centers for Disease Control and Prevention Web site. http://www.cdc.gov/std/stats/STI-Estimates-Fact-Sheet-Feb-2013.pdf. Accessed September 17, 2016

19. Shrier LA. Sexually transmitted infections: chlamydia, gonorrhea, pelvic inflammatory disease and syphilis. In: Emans SJH, Laufer MR, eds. *Emans, Laufer, Goldstein's Pediatric & Adolescent Gynecology.* 6th ed. Philadelphia, PA: Wolters Kluwer/Lippincott Williams & Wilkins; 2012:325-348

20. National Center for HIV/AIDS, Viral Hepatitis Sexual Transmitted Diseases and Tuberculosis Prevention, Division of HIV/AIDS Prevention. HIV among youth. Centers for Disease Control and Prevention Web site. http://www.cdc.gov/hiv/group/age/youth. Updated April 8, 2016. Accessed September 17, 2016

21. Marcell AV, Wibbelsman C, Seigel WM; American Academy of Pediatrics Committee on Adolescence. Male adolescent sexual and reproductive health care. *Pediatrics.* 2011;128(6):e1658-e1676

22. American College of Obstetricians and Gynecologists Committee on Health Care for Underserved Women. Access to reproductive health care for women with disabilities. In: American College of Obstetricians and Gynecologists. *Special Issues in Women's Health.* Washington, DC: American College of Obstetricians and Gynecologists; 2005:39-59

23. Murphy NA, Elias ER; American Academy of Pediatrics Council on Children With Disabilities. Sexuality of children and adolescents with developmental disabilities. *Pediatrics.* 2006;118(1):398-403

24. Interactive site for clinicians serving women with disabilities. American Congress of Obstetricians and Gynecologists Web site. http://www.acog.org/About-ACOG/ACOG-Departments/Women-with-Disabilities/Interactive-site-for-clinicians-serving-women-with-disabilities. Accessed September 17, 2016

25. Ott MA, Sucato GS; American Academy of Pediatrics Committee on Adolescence. Contraception for adolescents. *Pediatrics.* 2014;134(4):e1257- e1281

26. Gavin L, Moskosky S, Carter M, et al. Providing quality family planning services: recommendations of CDC and the U.S. Office of Population Affairs. *MMWR Recomm Summ.* 2014;63(RR-04):1-54

27. Centers for Disease Control and Prevention. U.S. medical eligibility criteria for contraceptive use, 2010. *MMWR Recomm Rep.* 2010;59(RR-4):1-86

PROMOTING HEALTHY SEXUAL DEVELOPMENT AND SEXUALITY

28. Centers for Disease Control and Prevention. U.S. selected practice recommendations for contraceptive use, 2013: adapted from the World Health Organization selected practice recommendations for contraceptive use, 2nd edition. *MMWR Recomm Rep.* 2013;62(RR-05):1-60

29. American College of Obstetricians and Gynecologists Committee on Adolescent Health Care Long-Acting Reversible Contraception Working Group. Committee opinion no. 539: adolescents and long-acting reversible contraception; implants and intrauterine devices. *Obstet Gynecol.* 2012;120(4):983-988

30. American Academy of Pediatrics Committee on Adolescence. Emergency contraception. *Pediatrics.* 2012;130(6):1174-1182

31. Levine DA; American Academy of Pediatrics Committee on Adolescence. Office-based care for lesbian, gay, bisexual, transgender, and questioning youth. *Pediatrics.* 2013;132(1):e297-e313

32. Goodenow C, Szalacha LA, Robin LE, Westheimer K. Dimensions of sexual orientation and HIV-related risk among adolescent females: evidence from a statewide survey. *Am J Public Health.* 2008;98(6):1051-1058

33. Condom fact sheet in brief. Centers for Disease Control and Prevention Web site. http://www.cdc.gov/condomeffectiveness/brief.html. Accessed September 17, 2016

34. Frankowski BL; American Academy of Pediatrics Committee on Adolescence. Sexual orientation and adolescents. *Pediatrics.* 2004;113(6):1827-1832

35. Katz-Wise SL. Sexual fluidity in young adult women and men: associations with sexual orientation and sexual identity development. *Psychol Sex.* 2015;6(2):189-208

36. Ott MQ, Corliss HL, Wypij D, Rosario M, Austin SB. Stability and change in self-reported sexual orientation identity in young people: application of mobility metrics. *Arch Sex Behav.* 2011;40(3):519-532

37. Cohn TJ, Hastings SL. Resilience among rural lesbian youth. *J Lesbian Stud.* 2010;14(1):71-79

38. Russell ST, Muraco A, Subramaniam A, Laub C. Youth empowerment and high school gay-straight alliances. *J Youth Adolesc.* 2009;38(7):891-903

39. Snapp SD, Watson RJ, Russell ST, Diaz RM, Ryan C. Social support networks for LGBT young adults: low cost strategies for positive adjustment. *Fam Relat.* 2015;64(3):420-430

40. Spack NP, Edwards-Leeper L, Feldman HA, et al. Children and adolescents with gender identity disorder referred to a pediatric medical center. *Pediatrics.* 2012;129(3):418-425

41. American College of Obstetricians and Gynecologists Committee on Health Care for Underserved Women. ACOG Committee Opinion No. 525: Health care for lesbians and bisexual women. *Obstet Gynecol.* 2012;119(5):1077-1080

42. PFLAG: parents, families, friends, and allies united with LGBTQ people to move equality forward! PFLAG Web site. http://community.pflag.org. Accessed September 17, 2016

PROMOTING HEALTHY SEXUAL
DEVELOPMENT AND SEXUALITY

Promoting the Healthy and Safe Use of Social Media

Social media use is a topic that affects every stage of health supervision, from before birth to adulthood. Health care professionals should understand the benefits and risks involved with social media use in the families they serve. This theme explores various types of social media use that a health care professional should be prepared to discuss with families during all preventive visits, from the prenatal period through young adulthood. Social media are the latest representation of all media and have an ever-increasing effect on communication, interpersonal relations, development, and health. Traditional media, such as television (TV), movies, and games, are discussed in Bright Futures Health Supervision Visits.

Social media are Web sites or applications that allow users to create and share content and to interact with other users. There are numerous types of social media sites and applications, and more are always being developed. Through social media, people share information about themselves, share links to content, create written content (eg, blogs), upload video or audio content, comment on content, engage in conversations around topics, play games, organize events or movements, and otherwise connect with other people.

Although many parents are comfortable with social media and use it regularly, they may not fully understand all of its capabilities and uses—and they may not understand the effect it can have on their children. Used properly, social media can provide children and families with positive social networks, social support, and opportunities for learning. For patients and families struggling with chronic health problems, social media can provide education, the ability to connect with others who share the same struggles, and access to helpful resources.

At the same time, however, social media use has some risks. Many of the risks associated with social media are not so much inherent to social media itself as they are related to the ability of social media to amplify and make public the actions of children and youth. Other risks of social media are related to technology use itself (eg, distraction or sleep problems). It is important for parents to become social media literate so they understand these risks and benefits of social

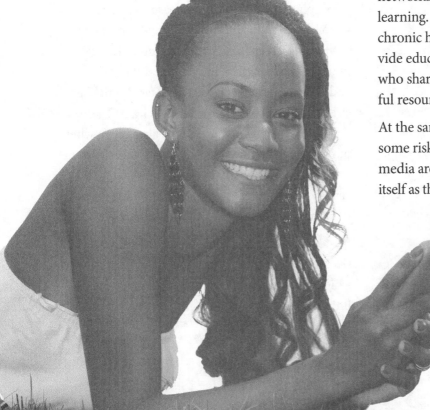

media and so they can guide their children and make the best decisions for their families. Health care professionals can serve an important role for families and children as an educator about social media and a supportive resource if problems or challenges arise.

Information Quality

Social media exposes children and youth to all sorts of information—some of which may be inaccurate or biased. Parents should help their children and teens look critically at information they find and help them be able to assess its source and biases.[1] Critical thinking skills are particularly important with health information. Health care professionals should be ready to provide youth and families with trusted health resources. Studies show that most adults who use the Internet have looked up health information online—and many people self-diagnose without ever talking with a health care professional.[2] For adolescents, who may be reluctant to talk with their parents or health care professionals about reproductive or other health concerns, social media and other Internet sources may be a natural place to go for information. Vetted resources provided by their health care professional may be helpful.

Distraction and Displacement

Increasingly, people of all ages are becoming distracted by their devices. This can have devastating consequences if done while driving, biking, or walking. Parents need to talk with their children and youth about being sure that their device use never puts them in any physical danger.

Distraction by social media can affect school success as well. Families should set expectations and rules about social media use during school and homework time.[3] Many software programs can temporarily block access to Web sites and

social media platforms. These, along with moving the cell phone or other portable screen device to another room, may help youth who have difficulty fighting the distractions of social media.

Social media can distract from and displace social interactions. Conversations with families about establishing cell phone–free zones or media-free zones, such as at the dinner table and during family gatherings, can increase their awareness of their child's media use and help them formulate ways to ensure that the child does not replace face-to-face encounters and activities with social media and maintains ample off-line social interactions.

Social media use also can displace other healthy and important activities, such as exercise, reading, or hobbies. Parents should be aware of how much time their child is spending online and encourage adequate exercise and other off-line activities.

Sleep

Computer and device use can interfere with sleep. Youth may stay up later than they should using them, and the light emitted from the devices themselves may delay melatonin release and increase sleep latency.[4] This may be a particular problem with small screens, such as those found in cell phones. The content is interactive and inviting, and the screen is held close to the face, which may strengthen the effect of the emitted light. These devices also can generate audible alerts even when put aside, which may wake up or attract resting youth. Studies show that youth who sleep with a cell phone or tablet nearby sleep less and less well than those who do not.[5]

Inadequate sleep has been associated with daytime sleepiness, school difficulties, increased injuries, a higher risk of mental health problems, possible immune dysfunction, and a higher risk of future cardiovascular disease.[6]

Role Modeling

Finally, children typically pay more attention to what parents do than to what they say—and this is true of social media use as well. Parents should be cognizant of their own social media habits and postings and consider whether they are setting the best example for their children as positive mentors and guides. Reflective modeling of using media as a tool for good purposes is important for children at any age. Open communications should be encouraged between parents and children to mitigate risks and to provide resources and support in case of cyberbullying or other online challenges.

Promoting the Healthy and Safe Use of Social Media: The Prenatal Period and Infancy—Birth Through 11 Months

Social media can be a great tool for parents to find and share parenting tips and resources and create a virtual support network. Health care professionals can talk with parents about what sites (including blogs and birth groups) they are using for networking and finding information about pregnancy, birth, parenting, and their new baby. Although these social media sites and tools can be useful, it is a good idea for parents to discuss the health information and advice they obtain with a health care professional to be sure that the information is accurate and applicable to (and a good idea for) them. It is also important for health care professionals to discuss with parents how to be critical consumers of information, especially health information, and to carefully assess the source before believing or following it. A list of useful and reliable sites and applications can be a valuable resource for parents.

The American Academy of Pediatrics (AAP) **HealthyChildren.org** Web site is one resource for parents (Twitter: @healthychildren).[7] Parents of hospitalized infants or infants with special health care needs may be more likely to seek out virtual networks for support and information. Health care professionals can provide them with trusted and vetted resources.

Promoting the Healthy and Safe Use of Social Media: Early Childhood— 1 Through 4 Years

Social media offer many beneficial opportunities for families with young children. Parents may find it useful to connect with and learn from other parents, and young children may benefit from talking online with grandparents or family members who live far away. However, social media also can present challenges, including exposure to excessive screen time for young children instead of focused adult-child interactions, which enhance language and social development, or exposure to inappropriate content when they watch their parents use social media. Remind them that device use before bedtime may interfere with sleep, and the AAP recommends that TVs not be in children's bedrooms. The AAP encourages all screens, including tablets, be turned off at least 1 hour before bedtime.[8] Encourage parents to reflect on and monitor the content that their child may be exposed to and to consider how their own social media and device use may affect not just the time they spend interacting with their child but the quality of those interactions. Be sure to ask parents to include tablet computers, phones, and other digital devices when adding up overall screen time for their child. Starting healthy media habits now is important because they are considerably harder to change when children are older. Parents' use of interactive media has the potential to distract from parent-child interactions. Parental media use usually involves work, errands, and social or other content requiring significant information processing, which makes it hard to balance attention between devices and their child.[9,10] Health care professionals can suggest that parents consider making a family media use plan (Box 1).

Box 1

Family Media Use Plan[11,12]

A family media use plan is an online tool on media use and screen time that all family members can fill out together. Take into account not only the quantity but the quality and location of media use. Consider TVs, phones, tablets, and computers, as well as social media use. Rules should be followed by parents as well as children. This kind of plan can help parents and children balance the child's needs for physical activity, sleep, school activities, and unplugged time against time available for media. It can also help families preserve special face-to-face time during routines, such as meals, playtime, and bedtime. Families may even want to designate some parts of the home as media-free.

Once a plan is established, families can revisit it periodically. This not only reinforces the plan's importance to the family but gives all members a chance to discuss how it should be updated to reflect the family's changing media use.

The AAP has information and resources to help parents learn about media use in childhood and ways to manage their children's media exposure (see **www.HealthyChildren.org/MediaUsePlan**).

Abbreviations: AAP, American Academy of Pediatrics; TV, television.

Promoting the Healthy and Safe Use of Social Media: Middle Childhood— 5 Through 10 Years

Pediatric health care professionals should emphasize to parents the importance of monitoring and offering guidance as their children interact with social media, just as they would with any other format of social contact. As children in middle childhood begin to use social media, health care professionals can help parents recognize the integral role that social media play in our lives and help their child use social media to build positive social networks. For children who have disabilities or those who may be socially marginalized, social media may provide an invaluable opportunity to develop and engage in friendships and obtain support.

At the same time, parents have a responsibility to help their children use social media in healthy and safe ways. Beginning in middle childhood, health care professionals can encourage parents to

- **Talk with their children about platforms and applications, and choose with them the ones best suited to their children's ages,**

temperaments, and abilities. Talking with children about which social media sites and applications their friends are using can provide useful information for parents in guiding their own children's use. Although it can be almost impossible to know everything a child is doing on social media, setting up usernames and passwords together can help spur discussions and build good social media habits as children get started online.

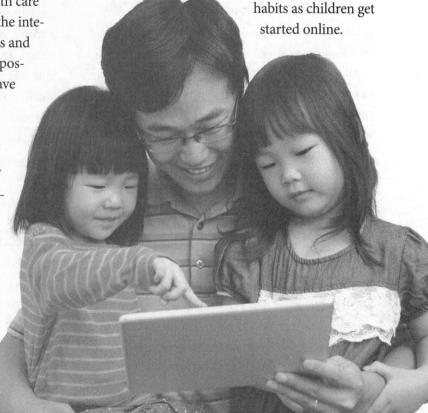

232

- **Help them understand how content can be misunderstood—and hurtful.** This is a hard lesson for people to learn at any age, but the earlier parents and children start talking about it, the better. Starting these conversations early and checking in often can help prevent children from becoming cyberbullied or the perpetrator of cyberbullying. Parents should help their children learn to be kind and thoughtful in what they say and do on social media—and teach them to tell a parent or other trusted adult if they or anyone else is hurt or scared by social media content.
- **Help them understand that nothing is truly private.** Although children should use all the privacy settings possible (parents should talk with them about this, as well as help them set them up if needed), it is impossible to keep everything private. Through screen shots and other technology, anything they post anywhere can potentially be shared. A useful guiding principle is that if there is any person in the world they would not want to see something they post, they should not post it.
- **Help them be safe.** Although online predation is actually rare, it is best that children not give out information that would allow a stranger to find them (eg, address, phone number, school). Parents should tell children to check with a parent before interacting online with anyone they do not know off-line.

Promoting the Healthy and Safe Use of Social Media: Adolescence— 11 Through 21 Years

As children grow into adolescence, social media use generally increases and becomes more sophisticated. Parents' role in helping adolescents use social media responsibly becomes all the more important. Parents should regularly talk with their adolescents about their social media use. Monitoring an adolescent's use of social media can be difficult, especially given that more and more youth access the Internet using their phone.[13] This means that discussion is key. The more that families create a culture of open communication about social media, the more opportunities they will have to guide their adolescent's use now and in the future.

Health care professionals can encourage parents to continue the guidance they provided during their child's earlier years, particularly with conversations about safety and privacy. Although research shows[14] that adolescents do think about privacy and take steps to protect theirs, it is still important to talk with them about it, especially because research suggests youth rely on parents for advice about privacy.[15]

Continued conversations about how content on social media can be hurtful, directly and indirectly, also are important. Parents should talk with their adolescents about standing up for anyone who is being hurt by social media content, about not passing on any possible hurtful content, and about alerting a parent, guidance counselor, or other helping adult if someone is being hurt, threatened, or bullied using social media.

Parents also can help their adolescents understand that anything they put on social media can stay there forever—and may be found by admissions officials or future employers. This "digital footprint" may have unintended consequences and should be created thoughtfully and carefully. In addition, adolescents should be particularly careful about any sexual content they post. It could be misinterpreted or become an unwanted part of their digital footprint or may be considered pornography and have legal repercussions.

References

1. Gasser U, Cortesi S, Malik M, Lee A. Youth and digital media: from credibility to information quality. The Berkman Center for Internet & Society at Harvard University. http://papers.ssrn.com/sol3/papers.cfm?abstract_id=2005272. Published 2012. Accessed November 11, 2016

2. Fox S, Duggan M. Health online 2013. Pew Research Center Web site. http://www.pewinternet.org/files/old-media/Files/Reports/PIP_HealthOnline.pdf. Published January 15, 2013. Accessed November 11, 2016

3. Radesky JS, Schumacher J, Zuckerman B. Mobile and interactive media use by young children: the good, the bad, and the unknown. *Pediatrics*. 2015;135(1):1-3

4. Chang AM, Aeschbach D, Duffy JF, Czeisler CA. Evening use of light-emitting eReaders negatively affects sleep, circadian timing, and next-morning alertness. *Proc Natl Acad Sci U S A*. 2015;112(4):1232-1237

5. Falbe J, Davison KK, Franckle RL, et al. Sleep duration, restfulness, and screens in the sleep environment. *Pediatrics*. 2015;135(2):e367-e375

6. American Academy of Pediatrics Adolescent Sleep Working Group, Committee on Adolescence, Council on School Health. School start times for adolescents. *Pediatrics*. 2014;134(3):642-649

7. American Academy of Pediatrics. HealthyChildren.org Web site. https://healthychildren.org. Accessed November 11, 2016

8. American Academy of Pediatrics Council on Communications and Media. Media and young minds. *Pediatrics*. 2016;138(5):20162591

9. Radesky J, Miller AL, Rosenblum KL, Appugliese D, Kaciroti N, Lumeng JC. Maternal mobile device use during a structured parent-child interaction task. *Acad Pediatr*. 2015;15(2):238-244

10. Radesky JS, Kistin CJ, Zuckerman B, et al. Patterns of mobile device use by caregivers and children during meals in fast food restaurants. *Pediatrics*. 2014;133(4):e843-e849

11. How to make a family media use plan. HealthyChildren.org Web site. https://www.healthychildren.org/English/family-life/Media/Pages/How-to-Make-a-Family-Media-Use-Plan.aspx. Updated October 21, 2016. Accessed November 11, 2016

12. American Academy of Pediatrics Council on Communications and Media. Media use in school-aged children and adolescents. *Pediatrics*. 2016;138(5):e20162592

13. Madden M, Lenhart A, Duggan M, Cortesi S, Gasser U. Teens and technology 2013. Pew Research Center Web site. http://www.pewinternet.org/files/old-media/Files/Reports/2013/PIP_TeensandTechnology2013.pdf. Published March 13, 2013. Accessed November 11, 2016

14. Madden M, Lenhart A, Cortesi S, Gasser U. Teens and mobile apps privacy. Pew Research Center Web site. http://www.pewinternet.org/files/old-media/Files/Reports/2013/PIP_Teens%20and%20Mobile%20Apps%20Privacy.pdf. Published August 22, 2013. Accessed November 11, 2016

15. Madden M, Lenhart A, Cortesi S, Gasser U, Smith A. Where teens seek online privacy advice. Pew Research Center Web site. http://www.pewinternet.org/files/old-media/Files/Reports/2013/PIP_TeensandPrivacyAdvice.pdf. Published August 15, 2013. Accessed November 11, 2016

Promoting Safety and Injury Prevention

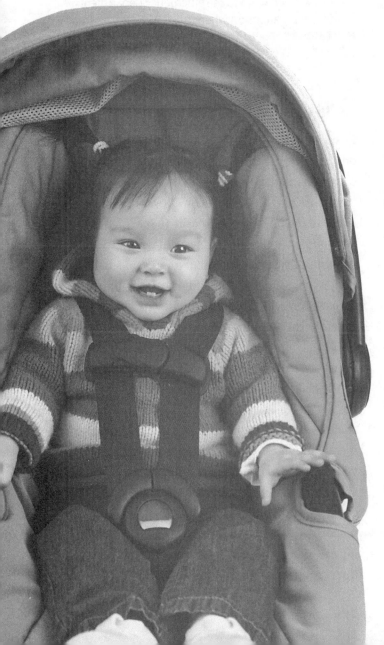

Ensuring a child remains safe from harm or injury during the long journey from infancy through adolescence is a task that requires the participation of parents and the many other adults who care for and help raise children. It also, of course, requires the participation of the children themselves. Health care professionals have long recognized the importance of safety and injury prevention counseling as a tool to help educate and motivate

parents in keeping their children safe. Many professional societies have bolstered these efforts by recommending guidance to prevent injuries.[1-3]

Safety and injury prevention is a topic area that covers a wide array of issues for infants, children, and adolescents. These issues can be grouped into 2 general categories.

- **Unintentional injury** continues to be the leading cause of death and morbidity among children older than 1 year, adolescents, and young adults. Serious unintentional injuries result from myriad causes, including motor vehicle crashes, falls, burns, poisoning, drowning, firearms, recreational activities, prescription or other drug overdose, and sports. Unintentional injuries take an enormous financial, emotional, and social toll on children and adolescents, their families, and society as a whole. Although the word *accident* is familiar, the word *injury* is preferred because it connotes the medical consequences of events that are both predictable and preventable. The causes of unintentional injury–related illness and death vary according to a child's age, sex, race, environment, geographic region, and socioeconomic status and depend on developmental abilities, exposure to potential hazards, and parental perceptions of a child's abilities and the injury risk. Younger children, boys, Native Americans and Alaska Natives, adolescents, and children who live in poverty are affected at disproportionately higher rates than are other children and adolescents.[4,5]

- **Intentional injury,** which results from behaviors that are designed to hurt oneself or others, is a multifaceted social problem and a major health hazard for children and youth. Homicide and suicide are particularly important for the health care professional to consider because their frequency increases as children grow older. In addition, in infants and very young children, intentional injury is a leading cause of morbidity and mortality. Intentional injuries cover a wide array of mechanisms, and the effect on children is great, no matter whether the violence is directly experienced or is witnessed. The association of early childhood exposure to violence and subsequent violent behaviors has been established.[6-9] The prevention of violence in all its forms therefore follows a developmental trajectory, beginning with infancy. To provide appropriate guidance and counseling, health care professionals need to be alert to the possible presence of violence in a family or to the effects of a violent environment on a child, which may include seemingly unrelated physical concerns.

Guidance on interventions and strategies to ensure safety and prevent injuries target 3 domains: (1) the development and age of the child, (2) the environment in which the safety concern or injury takes place, and (3) the circumstances surrounding the event. The health supervision visit provides a venue to assess the parents' and the child's current safety strategies, encourage and praise their positive behaviors, provide guidance about potential risks, and recommend community interventions that promote safety.[10]

The health supervision visit also is a good venue in which to review emergency and disaster preparedness measures (Box 1). Information on handling emergencies, how to access local emergency care systems, and CPR and first aid can be made available to all parents. Information on disaster preparedness includes knowing the risks and hazards in the area, making a plan, preparing a kit of emergency supplies, and getting involved in community readiness efforts.[11]

Box 1

Emergency Preparedness Suggestions for Parents

Health care professionals can suggest that parents

- Complete an American Heart Association or American Red Cross first aid and CPR program.
- Have a first aid kit and know local emergency telephone numbers and Web sites. The number for the **national Poison Help line** is **800-222-1222.** The FEMA preparedness planning Web site is **www.ready.gov/ make-a-plan.**
- Know when to call a health care professional (counsel parents to call whenever they are not sure what to do).
- Know when to go to the emergency department (counsel parents on when to call **911**).

Abbreviation: FEMA, Federal Emergency Management Agency.

Child Development and Safety

Ensuring safety and preventing injuries must be an ongoing priority for parents as their children progress from infancy through adolescence. However, the nature of their efforts evolves over time. Safety issues in infancy relate primarily to the infant's environment and interactions with parents. Parents must modify the environment to prevent suffocation, motor vehicle–related injuries, falls, burns, choking, drowning, poisoning, violence, and other hazards. They also must maintain active supervision, which means focused attention and intentional observation of children at all times. As a young child's independence emerges and mobility rapidly increases, new safety and injury prevention challenges arise and necessitate further environmental modifications, or childproofing. Parents of young children often underestimate the level of the child's motor skill development (eg, age of ability to climb) and overestimate their cognitive and sensory skills (eg, assessing the speed of an oncoming car or being able to learn from past mistakes). Integrating injury prevention counseling with developmental and behavioral discussions when talking with the family can be an effective method of delivering this important information.

The middle childhood years are a period during which safety challenges at home begin to be augmented by those outside the home (eg, at school, in sports, and with friends). During middle childhood, increasing independence allows the child to broaden his world beyond that of the immediate family. This requires good decision-making skills to stay safe and reduce the risk of injury. During adolescence, decision-making about safety shifts to choices the adolescent makes about his activities, behavior, and environment.

Parents have an important role to play in keeping their children and adolescents safe through maintaining open lines of communication, balancing strong support with clear limits, and monitoring closely. Strong support and close monitoring by parents have been linked with positive outcomes in children regardless of race, ethnicity, family structure, education, income, or sex.[12,13] Health care professionals can help parents foster openness, encourage communication with their child, and address concerns when they arise.

When a risky behavior is identified, counseling can be directed toward helping the parent and child with strategies to reduce or avoid the risk, such as using appropriate protective gear (eg, seat belts, helmets, hearing protection, and sports equipment), not riding in a car or boat with someone who has been drinking alcohol, locking up prescription drugs, and ensuring that firearms are inaccessible to children and adolescents, especially those with suspected depression or other mental health concerns. Parents should be alert to unusual changes in behavior, such as sleep disturbances, withdrawal, aggression, sudden isolation from peer groups, or the need for unusual or extreme privacy, which can indicate mental or behavioral health problems that need to be addressed. *(For more*

information on this topic, see the Promoting Mental Health theme.) Risk-reduction counseling is most likely to be effective when it is used in a repetitive, multi-setting approach, rather than being isolated in the medical office.[14] Partnering with the parent and sharing strategies for how to promote positive youth development, address strengths, and reduce risk-taking behaviors is an important collaborative approach as parents gradually decrease their supervisory responsibilities and help their child transition to young adulthood.[2] *(For more information on this topic, see the Promoting Lifelong Health for Families and Communities theme.)*

Families and Culture in Safety and Injury Prevention

Parents often feel challenged as they try to set priorities among the many health and safety messages that are given to them by the medical community. For some families, these messages may conflict with their cultural or personal beliefs and may result in parents disregarding the health and safety recommendations on topics such as safe infant sleep or the safe storage of firearms. In addition, certain culturally derived medical or alternative health practices may place children at risk of injury. Cultural or gender roles, in which women are not able to tell men in the household what to do, may limit women's ability to enact a safety measure. In some communities, cultural beliefs dictate that the mother or parents are not the primary decision-makers or caregivers for their young children. Acknowledging the influential roles that older women (eg, grandmothers or mothers-in-law) and other elders and spiritual leaders play in guiding child care practices is key to the effective delivery of safety, injury prevention, and health promotion messages. Health care professionals should be sensitive to these cultural perspectives and alert to any potential health and safety issues that may influence the child and family.

The health care professional has the dual role of helping families set priorities among health and safety messages in the context of the child's health, developmental age, and family circumstances, as well as helping families carry out these recommendations within their own cultural framework. The health care professional also should recognize when health and safety information is ineffective because of cultural differences in beliefs about the care of the child. A familiarity with local community public health services and state and local resources is critical to tailoring information and care recommendations to best suit the needs of the child and family. Rather than giving a parent or child an absolute requirement, the health care professional might consider where an appropriate adaptation or modification can be made to accommodate cultural and family circumstances.

Economic realities often affect parents' ability to alter their home to create a safer environment for their child. Children who live in poverty often live in substandard, crowded homes in unsafe neighborhoods. They may be homeless and may be exposed to environmental pollution, such as lead and carbon monoxide. Their parents often experience poor health, economic stresses, and discrimination. These families are least able to make the changes they want and need in their homes and communities. *(For more information on this topic, see the Promoting Family Support theme.)* Health care professionals should be aware of housing codes that govern safety issues (eg, hot water, window guards, carbon monoxide and smoke alarms, and lead paint) and of tenant codes, which require landlords to install or allow the installation of safety devices, require certain upkeep, and protect the tenants from injury. Access to legal services for families who live in poverty has brought improvements to child health and safety. Low-income families, who are least likely to be able to afford injury prevention devices, may require assistance to overcome cost barriers. Community-based injury prevention interventions are effective and are models of community partnership.[15,16] These programs can address cultural beliefs, income barriers, and community norms to help families implement safety interventions, especially those that have been shown to reduce injuries (eg, car safety seats, bike helmets, firearm locks, smoke alarms, and window guards). Community-based interventions are more likely to be successful at reducing injuries if they are integrated into and tailored to the community and involve community stakeholders.[17,18] Trials of community programs that involve home visits to distribute free smoke alarms have reported large increases in smoke alarm ownership and decreases in fire-related injuries.[19]

Safety Considerations for Children and Youth With Special Health Care Needs

Children with special health care needs may have unique needs for safety and injury prevention. Parental supervision must be focused on the developmental level and physical capabilities of the child. To ensure a safe environment, parents of children with special health care needs may have to seek alternative safety equipment, such as specially designed car safety seats or additional door locks to protect children who may wander at night, such as children with autism spectrum disorder. Providing information or resources may improve the quality of life for families, as in the case, for example, of a family that may not be able to travel together without such equipment.[20] Increasing parents' awareness of the potential added complexity of creating a safe environment for their child with special health care needs and guiding parents toward local and national resources are ways that the health care professional can help parents provide a safe environment.

Many children with special health care needs encounter new safety challenges as they enter school and begin to deal with the community at large. They often are vulnerable and at risk of being bullied or abused. They also may have an increased risk of maltreatment, including child neglect and physical or sexual abuse, including by professionals in schools and other institutions. Because they may rely heavily on caregivers for their physical needs and hygiene, their mental or physical limitation may impair their ability to defend themselves. Health care professionals can discuss appropriate caregiving, highlight risks for abuse, discuss the potential of bullying, and encourage parents to establish monitoring systems at home, in the community, and at school to protect their child. Planning for children with special health care needs requires understanding and anticipating the child's limitations and needs, with designated roles for family members and referral to additional community resources to ensure safety.

Parents of children with special health care needs may want to consider developing a disaster plan that includes lists of medications, food and supplies, equipment, and contact information for health care professionals that are part of their care team.[21] The plan also can include the use of an Emergency Information Form,[22] advanced registration for special needs shelters and evacuation plans, and extra medications and supplies.

Safety and Injury Prevention Counseling in the Bright Futures Health Supervision Visit

Anticipatory guidance for safety is an integral part of the medical care of all children. Counseling needs to be directed to the parent as the role model for the child's behavior and as the person who is most capable of modifying the child's environment. Counseling about some of the more effective safety and injury prevention interventions, such as using car safety seats and seat belts, spans infancy through adolescence, while other issues, such as bicycle safety, are developmentally and age specific.

Evidence from several systematic reviews confirms that injury prevention guidance is effective and beneficial. Because families seek the trusted opinion of pediatric health care professionals, these professionals can deliver important preventive messages that are intended to alter risky behaviors.[23,24] Bass et al[25] found that positive effects from injury prevention counseling included improved knowledge, improved safety behaviors, and decreased numbers of injuries involving motor vehicles and nonmotorized vehicles. However, Barkin et al found that parents can retain only a limited number of topics.[26] Thus, Bright Futures injury prevention topics are distributed across visits so that each visit has no more than 4 to 5 safety-related topics for the health care professional to discuss.

DiGuiseppi and Roberts[27] systematically reviewed 22 randomized controlled trials to examine the effect on child safety practices and unintentional injuries of interventions delivered in the clinical setting. The results indicate that some, but not all, safety practices are increased after counseling or other interventions in this setting. Specifically, guidance about car safety seats for young children, smoke alarms, and maintenance of a safe hot water temperature was more likely to be followed after interventions in the clinical setting than was guidance on other issues. Clinical interventions were most effective when they combined an array of health education materials and behavior change strategies, such as counseling, demonstrations, the provision of subsidized safety devices, and reinforcement.

The effectiveness of counseling can be improved if a health care professional knows the risks specific to the local population. For example, if the major cause of morbidity in the local population is drowning, counseling about active supervision around water is appropriate. In a farming community, counseling about the risk of agricultural injury and farming equipment safety can be especially pertinent. This advice also applies to counseling regarding the common recreational activities in a professional's geographic area (eg, all-terrain vehicle riding, snowmobiling, personal watercraft). Particularly for adolescents, common occupational hazards should be discussed and use of protective equipment (eg, safety glasses, protective ear covers) should be encouraged. Local injury data can be obtained from state or local departments of health, and statewide fatality data are available online.[28] It is therefore expected that the health care professional will adapt the safety anticipatory guidance to meet the needs of the child, family, and community on the basis of a sound knowledge of the local causes, risks of injury in the child's environment, and the assessed and expressed needs of the child and family.

TIPP (The Injury Prevention Program[3]), developed by the American Academy of Pediatrics (AAP), is a developmentally based, multifaceted counseling program that allows the health care professional to use safety surveys at strategic visits and counsel parents on unintentional injury prevention topics delineated as areas of specific risk. Parents can complete TIPP surveys, which are distributed by office staff, in a few minutes. According to information from the surveys, health care professionals can use different parts of TIPP to individualize and supplement their anticipatory guidance with counseling and handouts that are appropriate for the child's age and community. In an effort to better tailor anticipatory guidance, primary care practices have used kiosk systems to help delineate specific injury risks that families might have in the home.

Four safety topics that deal with ways to reduce or prevent violence have particularly strong research evidence and lend themselves to pediatric anticipatory guidance.

- Using constructive disciplining techniques and alternatives to corporal punishment[29-31] (For more information on this topic, see the Promoting Family Support and Promoting Healthy Development themes.)
- Promoting factors associated with psychological resilience among adolescents[32-35] (For more information on this topic, see the Promoting Mental Health and Promoting Lifelong Health for Families and Communities themes.)
- Preventing bullying[36-40] (For more information on this topic, see the Promoting Mental Health theme.)
- Preventing firearm injury[41-43] (For more information on this topic, see the Safety priority in selected visits.)

Since its peak in the mid-1990s, the epidemic of fatal youth violence has steadily declined. Many segments of society, in addition to the health care system, have contributed to this reduction.[44,45] Programs with proven effectiveness are described by the University of Colorado Center for the Study and Prevention of Violence (**www.blueprintsprograms.com**).[46] Information about a wide variety of violence prevention programs, ranging from public service announcements to school curricula, also is available through the Centers for Disease Control and Prevention (CDC) program STRYVE (Striving To Reduce Youth Violence Everywhere).[47]

Surveys and focus groups have demonstrated that parents want to discuss community violence with their child's health care professional.[48] Pediatricians also have expressed enduring interest in violence prevention counseling, although many feel inadequately trained to do so.[49] Few published studies directly address the effectiveness of health care professional counseling in violence prevention. However, the strong supporting research evidence provides a rationale for incorporating violence prevention into routine clinical practice.[1]

Connected Kids: Safe, Strong, Secure, also developed by the AAP, takes an asset-based approach to violence prevention anticipatory guidance.[2] Recommended counseling topics for each health supervision visit discuss the child's development, the parent's feelings and reactions to the child's development and behavior, and specific practical suggestions on how to encourage healthy social, emotional, and physical growth in an environment of support and open communication. Counseling can be supplemented by the use of Connected Kids brochures for parents and their children.

Each Bright Futures Visit has established safety priorities for discussion, and sample questions are provided in the Anticipatory Guidance sections. The priorities and sample questions in each visit that are relevant to safety are specifically linked to the counseling guidelines in TIPP (for Infancy, Early Childhood, and Middle Childhood Visits) and Connected Kids (for all visits), making it easy for the health care professional to incorporate these tools in a Bright Futures practice. In addition, the *Bright Futures Tool and Resource Kit* includes many other resources that may assist the health care professional.

Safe Use of the Internet, Social Media, and Texting

Many children and youth use the Internet, social media, and mobile devices in their daily lives to chat, text message, play games, and conduct searches. *(For more information on this topic, see the Promoting the Healthy and Safe Use of Social Media theme.)* Internet safety and etiquette is important to discuss to help prevent children and youth from being involved with or becoming the victim of bullying, abuse, scams, or stalking. Families should be aware that all information and actions taken online should be considered permanent and can be traced. For example, commercial companies trace actions of online users for research and design to improve their products and services marketed to the public, but others trace this same information for harmful purposes.

Information in the form of public or private postings on social media or online communication through texting or chatting, whether sent or received, can be categorized into online safety issues, including (1) sexual solicitation, (2) harassment, (3) exposure to inappropriate content, and (4) youth-generated problematic content.[50,51] Surveys of youth have demonstrated that the proportion of youth Internet users aged 10 to 17 years who reported being harassed online almost doubled between 2000 and 2010, from 6% to 11%.[52] Rates of unwanted exposure, as in being harassed or solicited online or abused off-line, appear to be higher among youth who are older or who have depression.[38]

Although, at present, no information is available about the effectiveness of Internet safety programs, these programs can offer parents and institutions some guard against the harms of using the

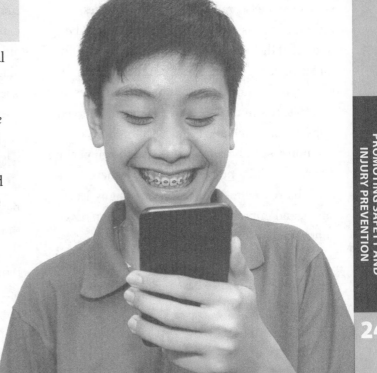

Internet. Parents and health care professionals should have frank discussions on the safety, benefits, and harms of using the Internet and social media. Although data are lacking to support specific policies, basic interventions that promote safe use of the Internet are recommended. Schools can employ programs that teach skills in negotiating peer conflict and managing anger issues online and off-line. These anti-bullying and social and emotional learning programs target relational and verbal harassment behaviors and may involve role-playing and discussion exercises to assist identifying and practicing pro-social skills relevant to their youth peer culture. Schools also can ensure that their bullying and harassment policies address online harassment and cyberbullying incidents. Children and youth should be encouraged to disclose to an adult, including parents, school staff, and other adults, if they are bullied or abused on the Internet.

The Health Care Professional as a Community Advocate for Safety

The clinical setting may not be suitable for carrying out the entire range of information, modeling, resources, and reinforcement that are required to change safety practices. For some families, the effectiveness of clinical interventions can be boosted if they are delivered in concert with efforts that involve representatives from the community to overcome language and cultural differences. For example, community-based educational interventions that have included clinical counseling as one component of a broader effort have shown positive effects on childhood bicycle helmet ownership and use.[53] Bicycle helmet education campaigns, legislation, and improvements in helmet design have contributed to a reduction of fatalities.[54]

Health care professionals can consider participating in fun, community-based safety activities and can work with community partners to increase public awareness about safety issues and provide prevention education. In most communities, it is possible to partner with agencies such as fire departments and Emergency Medical Services for Children departments, state and local Safe Kids coalitions (**www.safekids.org**),[55] and public health programs that work directly with families of young children. In addition, health care professionals often provide leadership for effective safety and injury prevention programs and legislation through advocacy activities and testimony at public hearings. On an individual patient level, health care professionals always should be aware of their role as mandated reporters for suspected child abuse and neglect and risk of harm, including health and safety risks.

Promoting Safety and Injury Prevention: The Prenatal Period

Safety and injury prevention begins in the prenatal period. Preparing for the arrival of an infant should include the purchase of an approved car safety seat and working with a Child Passenger Safety Technician to learn how to install it, as well as purchasing a crib that meets current safety standards. Car seat loaner programs are available in many communities. Prospective parents also can be encouraged to take an infant CPR and first aid class, get a first aid kit, check or install smoke alarms, and place the national Poison Help line telephone number (**800-222-1222**) on all their telephones and in their mobile phone contact lists.

Promoting Safety and Injury Prevention: Infancy—Birth Through 11 Months

Promoting safety and preventing injuries is a continuing task for parents during the first year of their child's life. Injury prevention for the infant requires careful integration of awareness of developmental skills, as they are rapidly acquired, and the active supervision and interventions necessary to ensure the infant's safety. Parents commonly underestimate their infant's motor skills while overestimating their infant's cognitive skills and judgment. Counseling in the primary care setting is important to help parents understand the correct timing of the development of these skills so that they can focus their safety interventions most appropriately.

Although suffocation and motor vehicle crashes are the most common causes of unintentional injury and death during this age, the infant also is at risk of other injuries, including falls, fires and burns, poisoning, choking, animal bites, and drowning. Each of these tragedies is preventable, and appropriate counseling can provide parents with the knowledge and strategies for reducing the likelihood that these injuries will occur. Vulnerable infants who are exposed to maternal substance use, secondhand smoke, malnutrition, lack of caregiver supervision, or caregiver neglect also are at increased risk of morbidity or death. The importance of establishing good habits begins in infancy, and parents can be counseled about the positive value of their own behavior as a role model for their child.

Sudden Infant Death

Sudden unexpected infant death (SUID) describes certain types of infant mortality, including sudden infant death syndrome (SIDS). After autopsy, case review, and death scene investigation, a SUID may be determined to be caused by asphyxiation, suffocation, parental overlie, infection, or other medical causes. The diagnosis of SIDS is reserved for unexpected and unexplained deaths that occur in infants younger than 1 year.[56] Although SIDS is the leading cause of death in infancy beyond the neonatal period, rates of sleep-related infant deaths, such as accidental suffocation and strangulation in bed (known as ASSB), are on the rise. Leading causes of this form of sudden infant death include suffocation by soft bedding, overlay (when another person rolls on top of or against the infant), wedging

or entrapment (when an infant gets trapped between 2 objects, such as the mattress and a wall), and strangulation (when something presses on or wraps around the infant's head and neck, blocking the airway).

A robust body of evidence indicates that the risk of SIDS and other sleep-related infant deaths is reduced when infants sleep on their backs and in their parents' room but not in their parents' bed.[56] Pacifiers have been linked with a lower risk of SIDS. It is recommended that infants be placed for sleep with a pacifier. For breastfed infants, this can be started after breastfeeding is well established (usually by 3–4 weeks of age). A pacifier can be started in formula-fed infants soon after birth. It should not be forced if the infant refuses. It also should not be reinserted once the infant is asleep.

The following independent risk factors for SUID, including SIDS, have been identified:

- Young maternal age
- Maternal smoking during pregnancy
- Inadequate prenatal care
- Exposure to secondhand cigarette smoke
- Low birth weight or premature birth
- Male gender
- An overheated infant
- Prone sleep position for infant
- Infant sleeping on a soft surface
- Bedding (eg, pillows, blankets, bumper pads, stuffed toys) in the infant sleep area
- Infant sleeping on a couch, a sofa, or other cushioned surface
- Bed sharing (infant sleeping with parent or other adult)

Other sleep-related infant deaths, such as those caused by unintentional suffocation or asphyxia, have similar risk factors. Several of these risk factors are under parental control during infancy. Personal experience and beliefs significantly influence a family's acceptance of specific messages regarding infant sleep position and sleep location.

The health care professional should learn the family's views about infant sleep, room sharing, and bed sharing to appropriately tailor sleep-related death prevention and risk reduction counseling. (See Box 2.)

Room Sharing and No Bed Sharing

Parent and infant sleeping practices are influenced by custom and family traditions.[58] It is important to work with families to ensure safe sleep practices while still being culturally sensitive.

Room sharing, defined as an infant sleeping in the parents' room in a separate sleep space, is a common practice in many cultures worldwide. In many cultures, sharing a room is viewed as a part of the parents' overall commitment to their children's well-being. *Evidence shows that room sharing is associated with a reduced risk of sudden infant death, and it is recommended that babies sleep in their parents' room for at least the first 6 months of life but not in their parents' bed.*[57] It should be noted that the case-control studies

Box 2
Reducing Sudden Unexpected Infant Death Risks

In 2016, the AAP Task Force on Sudden Infant Death Syndrome reviewed the evidence and compiled the following recommendations to reduce the risk of sleep-related infant deaths[57]:

- Do not smoke during pregnancy. Avoid alcohol and drugs during and after pregnancy.
- Breastfeeding is recommended and is associated with a reduced risk of SIDS. If breastfeeding occurs in the mother's bed, the infant should be returned to her separate sleep place when the mother is drowsy or ready for sleep.
- Supine sleep position is safest for every sleep; side sleeping is associated with increased risk and is not advised.
- A separate but nearby sleep environment is safest for the infant ("in your room but not in your bed"). The infant's crib or bassinet can be placed immediately next to the parents' bed.
- Parents or other caregivers should not share a bed with their infant; accumulating evidence reveals increased risk of SUID for infants who share a bed with others.
  - The risk is further increased if parents smoke, use drugs or alcohol, or take medications that cause drowsiness or fatigue or induce a deep sleep.
  - Parents should never sleep with their infants on a sofa or couch.
  - There is no evidence that devices claiming to make bed sharing "safe" reduce the risk of SIDS. They are not to be recommended.
  - Provide separate sleep areas for twins and other multiples.
- A pacifier should be offered for naps and night sleep.
- Use a firm sleep surface. Avoid placing soft objects and loose bedding in cribs, bassinets, and playpens. Bumper pads are not recommended.
- Do not allow smoking in the child's environment.
- Avoid overheating the infant; do not over-bundle the infant or set the room temperature too high.
- Do not use home cardiorespiratory monitors as a strategy to reduce the risk of SIDS.
- No evidence is available to recommend swaddling as a strategy to reduce SIDS risk. *(For more information on swaddling, see the Prenatal, First Week, and 1 Month Visits.)*
- Infants should be fully immunized according to AAP and CDC recommended immunization schedules. No evidence exists that links immunizations to SIDS.
- Health care providers, staff in newborn nurseries and NICUs, and child care providers should endorse and model the SIDS risk reduction recommendations from birth.
- Media and manufacturers should follow safe sleep guidelines in their messaging and advertising.

Abbreviations: AAP, American Academy of Pediatrics; CDC, Centers for Disease Control and Prevention; NICU, neonatal intensive care unit; SIDS, sudden infant death syndrome; SUID, sudden unexpected infant death.

regarding room sharing do not provide data or information regarding when it is safe for infants to move out of their parents' room. Previous recommendations used the 6 month recommendation, and other considerations led to the *at least 6 months* recommendation: 90% of SIDS occurs during the first 6 months of life,[56] the highest risk of death with bed sharing is in the first 3 months of life, and it may be difficult to establish good sleep habits in older infants if they are sleeping in the parents' bedroom.[57]

Sleep practices in which parents and infants share a bed also are common in many cultures. Bed sharing can take the form of mother, father, and infant together in the same bed, to mother and infant together with father sleeping elsewhere, to all family members in the same bed. Advocates of this practice claim that bed sharing facilitates breastfeeding, promotes parent-infant attachment, and allows parents to quickly comfort a fussy infant. *However, bed sharing is to be discouraged.* It is associated with a higher frequency of infant death that can be caused by overlying by a parent, sibling, or other adult sharing the bed; wedging or entrapment of the infant between the mattress and another object; head entrapment in bed railings; and suffocation on water beds or because of clothing or bedding causing oral-nasal obstruction.[59] Parent movement also may push the infant out of the bed.

Sleep Position

Despite more than 20 years of recommendations, at least 25% of infants,[60] overall, continue to be placed in the prone or side position for sleep, and 23% of white[61] and 43% of black infants[62] still sleep on their side or in the prone position. These percentages have become stable over the past 10 years as the progress made by the Back to Sleep campaign has plateaued.[63] The prone sleep position used more often by African American families[24] and in friend and family care settings is a contributing

factor to disparate SIDS rates. Side lying, an alternative sleep position that is practiced by many families who are concerned about using the prone position, statistically carries the same degree of increased risk of SIDS as the prone position, largely because of the significant probability that the infant will roll from the side position to the prone position during sleep.[56] The risk of death caused by SIDS is approximately 8 times higher for infants who are placed for sleep on their side or in the prone position.[56]

Promoting Safety and Injury Prevention: Early Childhood—1 Through 4 Years

Young children are especially vulnerable to many of the preventable injuries because their physical abilities exceed their capacities to understand the consequences of their actions. They are extraordinary mimics, but their understanding of cause and effect is not as developed as their motor skills. Gradually, between the ages of 1 and 4 years, children develop a sense of themselves as people who can make things happen. However, at this age, young children are likely to see only their part in the action. A 2-year-old whose ball rolls into the road will think only about retrieving the ball, not about the danger of being hit by a motor vehicle. Parents and other caregivers of young children must provide active supervision. They should establish and consistently enforce safety rules, recognizing that this is done to establish a foundation for following rules because young children do not have the cognitive capacity to understand the rule, take action, and avoid the hazard. Water safety is critical at these ages, when the ability to swim safely is not developed. Parents and other caregivers should be aware of potential hazards in their home, including common household chemicals (eg, dishwasher detergent, pesticides), medications, heavy objects (eg, televisions [TVs]), furniture tip-overs, and family or neighborhood pets, and should create a safe environment that will allow the young child to have the freedom he needs to explore. Creating a safe environment involves storing potentially harmful items out of sight and out of reach of children. Medicines in purses, cupboards, and on shelves are common sources of potentially harmful items. Choking hazards include small toy parts, plastic bags, and certain foods, such as peanuts, popcorn, raw carrots, uncut hotdogs or grapes, and hard candy. Educational materials are available as part of the PROTECT initiative in partnership with the CDC (**www.cdc.gov/MedicationSafety/protect/ protect_Initiative.html**).[64]

Parents can teach their child about personal safety at an early age. Parents should train their child how to approach authority figures (eg, teachers, police, and salesclerks) and ask them for help in the event he becomes lost or temporarily separated from his parents. Health care professionals also can play an important role in preventing and identifying child sexual abuse, particularly because they are mandated reporters. It is important to have discussions with families and caregivers about healthy sexual development and sexuality to assess for any problems and concerns. Providers should be able to talk with parents and caregivers about concerns and should be aware of problems signs. *(For more information on this topic, see the Promoting Healthy Sexuality and Sexual Development theme.)*

A child aged 1 to 4 years also does not fully understand that his actions can have harmful consequences for himself or for others, and parental guidance is therefore necessary to shape aggressive behaviors. Longitudinal observations have suggested that childhood aggression peaks around age 17 months and, with adult guidance, most children learn to regulate these tendencies before school age.[65]

Promoting Safety and Injury Prevention: Middle Childhood—5 Through 10 Years

Middle childhood is a time of intellectual and physical growth and development, when children become more independent. The controls and monitoring that parents provided during the early childhood years change as children get older. As children go to school, participate in activities away from home, and engage in more complex and potentially dangerous physical and social activities, they need to develop good judgment and other skills to function safely in their expanding environment. Safety promotion and injury prevention are central aspects of the child's education.

Preventing or lessening the effects of violence also is an ongoing concern for many children during the middle childhood years, especially those living in families or communities in which violence is prevalent. Television and other media violence[66] also may have serious effects during this period, as children spend increasing amounts of time away from home or out of the active supervision of a parent and have increased opportunities to watch TV.

School and Community Safety
During this time, children begin transitioning from complete dependence on their parents to developing their own strategies and decision-making skills for ensuring their own safety. Nowhere is this more apparent than when children

are out of the home and functioning independently in their community. The process of going to school, on errands, to a friend's house, or to a music lesson, scout meeting, or team practice can present challenges to the young child who is negotiating her environment. Walking or taking the bus, going with groups of other children, and meeting new adults all have the potential to increase social skills and respect for others, as well as the potential to place the child in danger. This developmental stage is the time when children acquire essential interpersonal skills, including conflict resolution. School-based conflict resolution and skill-building programs have been shown to be effective.[67]

The health care professional should encourage parents to know their child's activities, daily whereabouts, and friends. Good communication between parent and child is essential to the child's safety. Lessons that were introduced in early childhood, such as pedestrian safety (eg, retrieving a ball from the street), pet safety, dealing with authority figures, and appropriate touching by others, should continue as needed. This information does not need to be communicated specifically as a safeguard against abduction or abuse but can be taught as developmental achievements in the growing child.[68] The message to parents is that they should actively teach their children about safe behaviors but not generate unnecessary fear or overly restrict freedom and independence.

Children this age should never be left at home alone but increasingly will be spending time away from home at school, friends' homes, or organized activities. Parents should make sure the child has information about her home, including address, telephone number, parents' cell phone numbers, and keys to the home, and a backup contact person if the parents are not available. Parents should insist that the child check in with her family. Health care professionals also can partner with child care centers, schools, after-school programs, and municipalities to enhance public awareness

and modify physical environments. Speed bumps, crosswalks, the passage and enforcement of school zone speed limits, and school bus safety laws can create a safer environment for child pedestrians.

Peer pressure also emerges during this period. Children need to be encouraged to develop a sense of their own identity and locus of control and be taught strategies for dealing with inappropriate peer pressure or behavior. Health care professionals can use anticipatory guidance to address these issues with parents and encourage them to discuss these issues with their child. By discussing these issues openly, the health care professional is modeling safe behavior and is encouraging the parent and child to communicate.

Bullying

Bullying is a social phenomenon in which a larger or more powerful child repeatedly attacks (physically or emotionally) a smaller or weaker child.[37,69,70] Cyberbullying is bullying that uses the Internet or electronic devices to spread written or photographic mean-spirited messages about a person. *(For more information on this topic, see the Promoting Mental Health theme.)* Children can be identified as bullies, being bullied, or bystanders; they may both be a bully and be bullied. In some cases, they may be all three. Effective bullying prevention programs have been demonstrated for use in the schools, and all rely on direct measures by school administration and the mobilization of bystanders to protect the children being bullied and identify bullying behavior as socially intolerable. Physician counseling of individual patients begins with the recognition of bullying as a potential cause of psychosomatic concerns and may include both individual counseling and referral of parents to effective bullying prevention resources. It is important to recognize that bullying behavior is often rooted in stressful or traumatic experiences.[71] Bullies, themselves, are at high risk of long-term adverse consequences and often need behavioral counseling and other interventions to help them interact more positively with their peers.

Play, Sports, and Physical Activity

Physical activities play an important role in a child's life during this age, and participation in team and individual sports can consume considerable amounts of time. Although the overall health effect is usually positive, children need to learn and follow safety rules for their protection and the protection of others. *(For more information on this topic, see the Promoting Physical Activity theme.)* Parents also should be encouraged to model safe behaviors, such as wearing bicycle helmets and sports protective gear. Children should follow traffic rules and safety guides concerning bicycle riding, skating, skiing, and other similar activities. The use of protective gear, such as helmets, eye protection, mouth and wrist guards, and personal floatation devices or personal protective devices, is not negotiable and should be used at all times by everyone.

Promoting Safety and Injury Prevention: Adolescence—11 Through 21 Years

In caring for the adolescent patient, the approach to injury prevention shifts from parental control to the adolescent himself. Anticipatory guidance can now be directed to the adolescent, with a focus on encouraging behaviors that promote safety. Injury and violence are major causes of morbidity and mortality among adolescents. Although the leading causes of death of adolescents and young adults aged 11 to 21 years vary by race and age, the top 3 causes consistently are motor vehicle crash injury, homicide, and suicide.[72] Although serious injuries and death are more common among boys, reports of violence among girls are

increasing.[73] Dropping out of school, using drugs, and getting in physical fights place adolescents at increased risk of severe injury or death. Protective factors, such as connectedness with school and adults, are associated with reduced violence in youth.[44] Health care professionals can recognize and encourage protective factors in youth as a strategy to promote safety and reduce injuries.

Driving

Learning to drive is a privilege and considered a rite of passage for many adolescents. It is a reflection of their growing independence and maturity. Adapted equipment and special driving techniques make it possible for many youth with special health care needs to drive. Health care professionals can encourage parents to be initially involved with their adolescent's driver's education by doing practice driving sessions together and by establishing rules that foster safe, responsible driving behaviors. Parents should enforce and model safe driving habits, including wearing seat belts at all times, not using cell phones or texting while driving, and not driving under the influence of drugs or alcohol. State laws regarding mobile device and seat belt use are becoming more common. Once the adolescent receives his license,

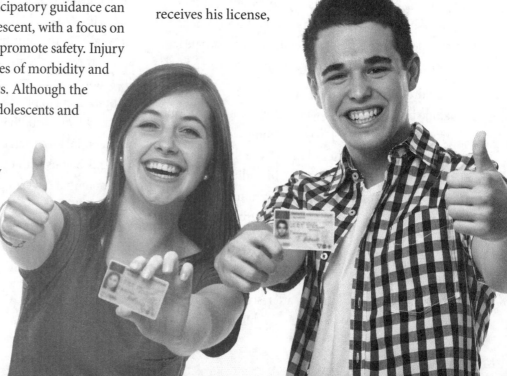

parents should continue to monitor his driving skills and habits to ensure that safe behaviors persist. Current research suggests that severe motor vehicle crashes involving inexperienced drivers are associated with (1) other teens in the car, (2) driving at night, and (3) distractions, such as using a cell phone, texting, e-mailing, using the Internet, or adjusting devices such as a radio, mapping device, music player, or mobile phone. Comprehensive graduated driver licensing (GDL) programs enacted in many states have been shown to reduce fatal crashes.[74] Parents should familiarize themselves with the provisions of the GDL law in their state and require their adolescent to adhere to the law, whether as a driver or as a passenger of a newly licensed teen driver. However, parents should know that state GDL laws do not include all the provisions recommended by the AAP. Health care professionals can support parents in setting rules and limits that reflect best practice, which is likely stricter than state GDL requirements. This can be accomplished with the use of a parent-teen driving agreement tool; such tools are available on **HealthyChildren.org,**[75] through the CDC,[76] and from motor vehicle insurance companies.

Preventing Distracted Driving

In 2013, the National Safety Council estimated that 21% (1.2 million) of all motor vehicle crashes involved the use of cell phones, with 6% caused by texting while driving.[77] At a speed of 55 mph, a driver who turns his eyes to a phone for 5 seconds will travel more than the length of a football field without looking at the road.[78] Adolescents are more likely than older drivers to talk or text on a cell phone while driving.[78]

Other potential distractions posed by mobile devices include viewing or posting to social media platforms, interacting with a GPS mapping application, playing electronic games, and reading electronic books or Web sites. Although the increased risk associated with such activities is not yet well described, any manipulation of a mobile device while driving is a distraction and likely increases the risk of a crash.

Though little data exist to demonstrate efficacy, strategies to decrease distracted driving include legislation, enforcement, pledges, and the use of technology to block mobile device functionality while in a moving vehicle. States and municipalities increasingly are enacting bans on the use of mobile devices by drivers. Use of technology, such as in-car cameras and anti-texting applications for smartphones, may help prevent texting and driving. Given that teens are more likely to use safety belts and helmets if their parents do, it is reasonable to deduce that teens may be positively influenced by parents who demonstrate undistracted driving behaviors. Parents and adolescents can be encouraged to discuss the topic of distracted driving and to use a text-free-driving pledge. Resources available to prevent distracted driving are available at **www.distraction.gov.**[79]

Violence

Violence and exposure to violence increase the risk of homicide, aggressive behavior, and psychological sequelae, including post-traumatic stress disorders.[6,80-85] It has been estimated that each year approximately 8.2 million children have been exposed to intimate partner violence (IPV).[83] Childhood exposure to IPV seems to increase the likelihood of risky behaviors later in adolescence and adulthood.[86] Additionally, children who witness IPV are at increased risk of adverse behavioral and mental health issues.[80,83]

Sexual and dating assaults are a leading cause of violence-related injury in adolescence.[28,87] In the 2013 Youth Risk Behavior Survey, among high school students reporting having dated in the prior 12 months, 10.3% report physical dating violence and 10.4% report sexual dating violence, with a higher prevalence among girls.[87] Adolescents who report a history of experiencing dating violence are more likely to experience negative health consequences and engage in serious risk behaviors.[88] Comprehensive IPV interventions conducted by teachers in schools in combination with community activities have been effective in preventing IPV perpetration and abuse among adolescents.[89] Screening for violence exposure can identify those who need further intervention.

Certain youth subcultures may experience comparatively greater violence, including injury, abuse, and rape. Teens who use drugs, report having been in more than 4 fights in the past year, are failing in school, or have dropped out of school are at substantially increased risk of serious violence-related injury.[90,91] Studies have found abuse, substance use, and sexual risk behaviors among gay youth to be significantly higher than among their heterosexual peers.[92] Homicide is consistently the leading cause of death for male African American adolescents.[93]

Suicide

Suicide is the third leading cause of death for adolescents, and a 2013 survey found that suicidal ideation is reported by more than one-sixth of high school students.[87] Medications, knives, automobiles, and firearms are all readily available to most adolescents, representing ubiquitous opportunities for depressed youth to harm themselves. *(For more information on these topics, see the Promoting Mental Health theme.)*

Gangs

The 2012 National Youth Gang Survey (NYGS) estimates there are 30,000 active gangs and 850,000 gang members throughout 3,100 jurisdictions in the United States.[94] The 2012 NYGS results reveal that more than one-third of the jurisdictions that city (populations of ≥2,500) and county law enforcement agencies serve experienced gang problems between 2005 and 2012.[95] This number translates to an estimated 3,100 jurisdictions with gang problems across the United States. The prevalence of

youth gang membership varies according to the city but is higher in larger cities and those with a history of gang activity. Risk factors for gang involvement include prior and early involvement in delinquency, especially violence involvement; poor parental supervision and monitoring; low academic achievement and attachment to school; association with peers who are delinquent; and criminogenic neighborhoods with drug use and youth who are in trouble.[96] *(For more information on this topic, see the Promoting Lifelong Health for Families and Communities theme.)* Health care professionals should be alert to these risk factors and should screen for gang exposure. The National Youth Gang Center has resources for gang prevention, intervention, and suppression.[97]

Sports

Pre-participation sports physical examinations, which are directed at identifying the few adolescents for whom a sport would be dangerous, provide a unique opportunity for health care professionals to counsel adolescents and their parents on preventing sports injury and violence (eg, intentional fouls during contact sports, hazing, brawling) and promoting general health. Generally, sports participation should be encouraged because of the physical, emotional, and social benefits. *(For more information on this topic, see the Promoting Physical Activity theme.)*

Some medical conditions warrant a limitation in sports or require further evaluation before participating. An AAP policy statement from the Council on Sports Medicine and Fitness provides a detailed review of medical issues that limit participation.[98] Some youth with special health care needs may have condition-specific restrictions on their activity and may require alternative or adapted activities that are safe and appropriate. If a heart murmur is innocent (eg, it does not indicate heart disease), full participation is permitted,[98] but other cardiac disorders may require further evaluation. The presence of significant hypertension without heart disease or organ damage should not limit participation, but the adolescent's blood pressure should be measured at the heath care professional's office every 2 months. Adolescents with severe hypertension should be restricted from isometric activities (eg, weight lifting) and competitive sports until their hypertension is under control and they have no end-organ damage.[99] Any temporary suspension from sports participation because of a medical condition (eg, concussion or surgery) should be reinforced by the health care professional, and adolescents and parents should be made aware of the importance in adhering to all recommendations as to when to resume sport activities.

Health care professionals should advise adolescents to use appropriate protective gear (eg, helmets, eye protection, knee and elbow pads, personal floatation devices or personal protective devices, mouth and wrist guards, and athletic supporter with cup) during recreational and organized sports activities and focus on overall strengthening and conditioning as well as training for their specific sport as key ways to prevent injury and maintain fitness.

Performance-enhancing substances, including anabolic steroids, are an important topic for discussion, and adolescents should not use them. Health care professionals also can encourage parents to be cautious about allowing their adolescents to participate in highly competitive sports until they are physically and emotionally mature enough and to ensure that such programs are properly certified and staffed by qualified trainers and coaches.

The use of sports and energy drinks by adolescents is another issue that health care professionals can address during a pre-participation examination. As stated in an AAP policy statement, these drinks "…are a large and growing beverage industry now marketed to children and adolescents for a variety of uses.… Sports drinks are different products than energy drinks…[they] are flavored beverages that often contain carbohydrates, minerals, electrolytes (eg, sodium, potassium, calcium, magnesium), and sometimes vitamins or other nutrients. Although the term 'energy' can be perceived to imply calories, energy drinks typically contain stimulants, such as caffeine and guarana, with varying amounts of carbohydrate, protein, amino acids, vitamins, sodium, and other minerals." Energy drinks pose potential health risks primarily because of stimulant content. They are not appropriate for children and adolescents and should never be consumed. "Sports drinks are appropriate when there is a need for rapid replenishment of carbohydrates and/or electrolytes in combination with water during periods of prolonged, vigorous sports participation or intense physical activity."[100] *(For more information on this topics, see the Promoting Physical Activity theme.)*

Recent new knowledge on sports injuries has focused greater attention on 2 issues: concussions and the injuries resulting from cheerleading. Clinicians should be aware of recommendations from the AAP and should address these issues during pre-participation sports examinations.

- **Concussion.** Although the collision sports of football and boys' lacrosse have the highest number of concussions and football the highest concussion rate (0.6 per 1,000), concussion occurs in all other sports and has been observed in girls' sports at rates similar to or higher than those of boys' sports. Girls' soccer produces the most concussions among girl athletes and has the second highest incidence rate (0.35 per 1,000) of all sports.[101] As of 2014, all 50 states had enacted laws on concussion awareness and management of young athletes.[102] Parents, coaches, and athletic trainers can ensure that return-to-play guidelines are followed and that the student-athlete is provided sufficient time for recovery from any injury before resuming the sport.[103]

- **Cheerleading.** Over the past 30 years, cheerleading has increased dramatically in popularity and has evolved from leading the crowd in cheers at sporting events into a competitive, year-round sport involving complex acrobatic stunts and tumbling. Consequently, cheerleading injuries have steadily increased over the years in both number and severity. Sprains and strains to the lower extremities are the most common injuries. Although the overall injury rate remains relatively low, cheerleading has accounted for approximately 66% of all catastrophic injuries in high school girl athletes over the past 25 years. Cheerleaders should have a pre-participation physical examination before participating in a cheerleading program and should have access to appropriate strength and conditioning programs.[104]

References

1. American Academy of Pediatrics Committee on Injury, Violence, and Poison Prevention. Role of the pediatrician in youth violence prevention. *Pediatrics.* 2009;124(1):393-402

2. Spivak H, Sege R, Flanigan E, Licenziato V. *Connected Kids: Safe, Strong, Secure Clinical Guide.* Elk Grove Village, IL: American Academy of Pediatrics; 2006. https://www2.aap.org/connectedkids/ClinicalGuide.pdf. Accessed October 5, 2016

3. American Academy of Pediatrics. TIPP: The Injury Prevention Program patient education handouts. http://patiented.solutions.aap.org/handout-collection.aspx?categoryid=32033. Accessed October 5, 2016

4. Brownell MD, Derksen SA, Jutte DP, Roos NP, Ekuma O, Yallop L. Socio-economic inequities in children's injury rates: has the gradient changed over time? *Can J Public Health.* 2010;101(suppl 3):S28-S31

5. Borse NN, Gilchrist J, Dellinger AM, Rudd RA, Ballesteros MF, Sleet DA. *CDC Childhood Injury Report: Patterns of Unintentional Injuries among 0-19 Year Olds in the United States, 2000-2006.* Atlanta, GA: Centers for Disease Control and Prevention; 2008:3. http://www.cdc.gov/safechild/images/CDC-ChildhoodInjury.pdf. Accessed October 5, 2016

6. Miller E, Breslau J, Chung WJ, Green JG, McLaughlin KA, Kessler RC. Adverse childhood experiences and risk of physical violence in adolescent dating relationships. *J Epidemiol Community Health.* 2011;65(11):1006-1013

7. Falb KL, McCauley HL, Decker MR, Gupta J, Raj A, Silverman JG. School bullying perpetration and other childhood risk factors as predictors of adult intimate partner violence perpetration. *Arch Pediatr Adolesc Med.* 2011;165(10):890-894

8. Black DS, Sussman S, Unger JB. A further look at the intergenerational transmission of violence: witnessing interparental violence in emerging adulthood. *J Interpers Violence.* 2010;25(6):1022-1042

9. Adverse Childhood Experiences (ACEs). Center for Disease Control and Prevention Web site. http://www.cdc.gov/violenceprevention/acestudy. Updated April 1, 2016. Accessed October 5, 2016

10. Maternal and Child Health Bureau. *Basic Emergency Lifesaving Skills (BELS): A Framework for Teaching Emergency Lifesaving Skills to Children and Adolescents.* Newton, MA: Children's Safety Network, Education Development Center Inc; 1999. http://www.nmschoolhealthmanual.org/forms/sectionVIII/BELSBook.pdf. Accessed October 5, 2016

11. Steps to Prepare Your Family for Disasters. HealthyChildren.org Web site. https://www.healthychildren.org/English/safety-prevention/at-home/Pages/Getting-Your-Family-Prepared-for-a-Disaster.aspx. Accessed November 16, 2016

12. Amato PR, Fowler F. Parenting practices, child adjustment, and family diversity. *J Marriage Fam.* 2002;64(3):703-716

13. Hoskins DH. Consequences of parenting on adolescent outcomes. *Societies.* 2014;4(3):506-531

14. Haegerich TM, Dahlberg LL, Simon TR, et al. Prevention of injury and violence in the USA. *Lancet.* 2014;384(9937):64-74

15. Falcone RA Jr, Edmunds P, Lee E, et al. Volunteer driven home safety intervention results in significant reduction in pediatric injuries: a model for community based injury reduction. *J Pediatr Surg.* 2016;51(7):1162-1169

16. Nauta J, van Mechelen W, Otten RH, Verhagen EA. A systematic review on the effectiveness of school and community-based injury prevention programmes on risk behaviour and injury risk in 8-12 year old children. *J Sci Med Sport.* 2014;17(2):165-172

17. Nilsen P. What makes community based injury prevention work? In search of evidence of effectiveness. *Inj Prev.* 2004;10(5):268-274

18. Ingram JC, Deave T, Towner E, Errington G, Kay B, Kendrick D. Identifying facilitators and barriers for home injury prevention interventions for pre-school children: a systematic review of the quantitative literature. *Health Educ Res.* 2012;27(2):258-268

19. DiGuiseppi C, Higgins JP. Interventions for promoting smoke alarm ownership and function. *Cochrane Database Syst Rev.* 2001;(2):CD002246

20. Automotive Safety Program: Special Needs Transportation. Prevention.org Web site. http://www.preventinjury.org/Special-Needs-Transportation. Accessed October 5, 2016

21. American Academy of Pediatrics. Children and Disasters: Children and Youth with Special Needs. American Academy of Pediatrics Web site. https://www.aap.org/en-us/advocacy-and-policy/aap-health-initiatives/Children-and-Disasters/Pages/CYWSN.aspx. Accessed November 16, 2016

22. Emergency Information Form for Children with Special Heath Care Needs. American College of Physicians Web site. http://www.acep.org/content.aspx?id=26276. Accessed October 5, 2016

23. Barkin SL, Finch SA, Ip EH, et al. Is office-based counseling about media use, timeouts, and firearm storage effective? Results from a cluster-randomized, controlled trial. *Pediatrics.* 2008;122(1):e15-e25

24. Colson ER, Willinger M, Rybin D, et al. Trends and factors associated with infant bed sharing, 1993-2010: The National Infant Sleep Position Study. *JAMA Pediatr.* 2013;167(11):1032-1037

25. Bass JL, Christoffel KK, Widome M, et al. Childhood injury prevention counseling in primary care settings: a critical review of the literature. *Pediatrics.* 1993;92(4):544-550

26. Barkin SL, Scheindlin B, Brown C, Ip E, Finch S, Wasserman RC. Anticipatory guidance topics: are more better? *Ambul Pediatr.* 2005;5(6):372-376

27. DiGuiseppi C, Roberts IG. Individual-level injury prevention strategies in the clinical setting. *Future Child.* 2000;10(1):53-82

28. WISQARS Leading Causes of Nonfatal Injury Reports. Centers for Disease Control and Prevention Web site. http://www.cdc.gov/injury/wisqars/nonfatal.html. Accessed October 5, 2016

29. Sege RD, Hatmaker-Flanigan E, De Vos E, Levin-Goodman R, Spivak H. Anticipatory guidance and violence prevention: results from family and pediatrician focus groups. *Pediatrics.* 2006;117(2):455-463

30. Afifi TO, Mota N, MacMillan HL, Sareen J. Harsh physical punishment in childhood and adult physical health. *Pediatrics.* 2013;132(2):e333-e340

31. MacKenzie MJ, Nicklas E, Waldfogel J, Brooks-Gunn J. Spanking and child development across the first decade of life. *Pediatrics.* 2013;132(5):e1118-e1125

32. Murphey DA, Lamonda KH, Carney JK, Duncan P. Relationships of a brief measure of youth assets to health-promoting and risk behaviors. *J Adolesc Health*. 2004; 34(3):184-191

33. Frankowski BL, Brendtro LK, Van Bockern S, Duncan PM. Strength-based interviewing: the circle of courage. In: Ginsburg KR, Kinsman SB, eds. *Reaching Teens: Strength-Based Communication Strategies to Build Resilience and Support Healthy Adolescent Development*. Elk Grove Village, IL: American Academy of Pediatrics; 2014:237-242

34. Harper Browne C. *Youth Thrive: Advancing Healthy Adolescent Development and Well-Being*. Washington, DC: Center for the Study of Social Policy; 2014. http://www.cssp.org/reform/child-welfare/youth-thrive/2014/Youth-Thrive_Advancing-Healthy-Adolescent-Development-and-Well-Being.pdf. Accessed November 16, 2016

35. Duke NN, Borowsky IW. Youth violence prevention and safety: opportunities for health care providers. *Pediatr Clin North Am*. 2015;62(5):1137-1158

36. PSA: Take a Stand. Lend a Hand. Stop Bullying Now! US Department of Defense Education Activity Web site. http://www.dodea.edu/StopBullying/stopbullyingvideo1.cfm. Accessed October 5, 2016

37. Olweus Bullying Prevention Program. The Olweus Program Web site. http://www.clemson.edu/olweus/index.html. Accessed October 5, 2016

38. Selkie EM, Fales JL, Moreno MA. Cyberbullying prevalence among US middle and high school-aged adolescents: a systematic review and quality assessment. *J Adolesc Health*. 2016;58(2):125-133

39. Beckman L, Svensson M. The cost-effectiveness of the Olweus Bullying Prevention Program: results from a modelling study. *J Adolesc*. 2015;45:127-137

40. Hatzenbuehler ML, Schwab-Reese L, Ranapurwala SI, Hertz MF, Ramirez MR. Associations between antibullying policies and bullying in 25 states. *JAMA Pediatr*. 2015;169(10):e152411

41. Albright TL, Burge SK. Improving firearm storage habits: impact of brief office counseling by family physicians. *J Am Board Fam Pract*. 2003;16(1):40-46

42. Xuan Z, Hemenway D. State gun law environment and youth gun carrying in the United States. *JAMA Pediatr*. 2015;169(11):1024-1031

43. Crossen EJ, Lewis B, Hoffman BD. Preventing gun injuries in children. *Pediatr Rev*. 2015;36(2):43-51

44. Fagan AA, Catalano RF. What works in youth violence prevention: a review of the literature. *Res Soc Work Pract*. 2013;23(2):141-156

45. Sood AB, Berkowitz SJ. Prevention of youth violence: a public health approach. *Child Adolesc Psychiatr Clin N Am*. 2016;25(2):243-256

46. University of Colorado. Blueprints for Healthy Youth Development Web site. http://www.blueprintsprograms.com. Accessed November 20, 2016

47. NSVRC: National Sexual Violence Resource Center Web site. http://www.nsvrc.org. Accessed October 5, 2016

48. Kogan MD, Schuster MA, Yu SM, et al. Routine assessment of family and community health risks: parent views and what they receive. *Pediatrics*. 2004;113(6 suppl):1934-1943

49. Trowbridge MJ, Sege RD, Olson L, O'Connor K, Flaherty E, Spivak H. Intentional injury management and prevention in pediatric practice: results from 1998 and 2003 American Academy of Pediatrics Periodic Surveys. *Pediatrics*. 2005;116(4):996-1000

50. Schrock A, Boyd D; Research Advisory Board Report for the Internet Safety Technical Task Force. Online threats to youth: solicitation, harassment, and problematic content. Berkman Center for Internet & Society, Harvard University, Web site. http://cyber.law.harvard.edu/sites/cyber.law.harvard.edu/files/RAB_Lit_Review_121808_0.pdf. Accessed October 5, 2016

51. Jones LM, Mitchell KJ, Finkelhor D. Trends in youth internet victimization: findings from three youth internet safety surveys 2000-2010. *J Adolesc Health*. 2012;50(2):179-186

52. Jones LM, Mitchell KJ, Finkelhor D. Online harassment in context: trends from three youth internet safety surveys (2000, 2005, 2010). *Psychol Violence*. 2013;3(1):53-69

53. Baeseman ZJ, Corden TE. A social-ecologic framework for improving bicycle helmet use by children. *WMJ*. 2014; 113(2):49-51

54. Meehan WP III, Lee LK, Fischer CM, Mannix RC. Bicycle helmet laws are associated with a lower fatality rate from bicycle-motor vehicle collisions. *J Pediatr*. 2013;163(3):726-729

55. Safe Kids Worldwide Web site. http://www.safekids.org. Accessed October 5, 2016

56. Moon RY; American Academy of Pediatrics Task Force on Sudden Infant Death Syndrome. SIDS and other sleep-related infant death: evidence base for 2016 updated recommendations for a safe infant sleeping environment. *Pediatrics*. 2016;138(5):e2016940

57. American Academy of Pediatrics Task Force on Sudden Infant Death Syndrome. SIDS and other sleep-related infant deaths: updated 2016 recommendations for a safe infant sleeping environment. *Pediatrics*. 2016;138(5):e2016938

58. Owens JA. Sleep in children: cross-cultural perspectives. *Sleep Biol Rhythms*. 2004;2(3):165-173

59. Shapiro-Mendoza CK, Colson ER, Willinger M, Rybin DV, Camperlengo L, Corwin MJ. Trends in infant bedding use: National Infant Sleep Position Study, 1993-2010. *Pediatrics*. 2015;135(1):10-17

60. The usual position in which mothers place their babies to sleep: data from the national NISP telephone survey for years 1992-2010. Slone Epidemiology Center, Boston University, Web site. http://slone-web2.bu.edu/ChimeNisp/Tables_in_PDF/NISP%201992-2010%20The%20usual%20sleep%20position.pdf. Accessed October 5, 2016

61. The usual position in which mothers place their babies to sleep: data from the national NISP telephone survey for years 1992 - 2010. Mother's race/ethnicity - White. http://slone-web2.bu.edu/ChimeNisp/Tables_in_PDF/NISP%201992-2010%20The%20usual%20sleep%20position%20(whites).pdf. Accessed October 5, 2016

62. The usual position in which mothers place their babies to sleep: data from the national NISP telephone survey for years 1992-2010. Mother's race/ethnicity - Black. http://slone-web2.bu.edu/ChimeNisp/Tables_in_PDF/NISP%201992-2010%20The%20usual%20sleep%20position%20(blacks).pdf. Accessed October 5, 2016

63. Colson ER, Rybin D, Smith LA, Colton T, Lister G, Corwin MJ. Trends and factors associated with infant sleeping position: The National Infant Sleep Position Study, 1993-2007. *Arch Pediatr Adolesc Med*. 2009;163(12):1122-1128

64. The PROTECT Initiative: Advancing Children's Medication Safety. Centers for Disease Control and Prevention Web site. http://www.cdc.gov/MedicationSafety/protect/protect_Initiative.html. Updated July 17, 2012. Accessed October 5, 2016

65. Tremblay RE, Nagin DS, Seguin JR, et al. Physical aggression during early childhood: trajectories and predictors. *Pediatrics.* 2004;114(1):e43-e50

66. American Academy of Pediatrics Council on Communications and Media. Media violence. *Pediatrics.* 2009;124(5):1495-1503

67. Multisite Violence Prevention Project. The Multisite Violence Prevention Project: impact of a universal school-based violence prevention program on social-cognitive outcomes. *Prev Sci.* 2008;9(4):231-244

68. Howard BJ, Broughton DD; American Academy of Pediatrics Committee on Psychosocial Aspects of Child and Family Health. The pediatrician's role in the prevention of missing children. *Pediatrics.* 2004;114(4):1100-1105

69. US Department of Health and Human Services. StopBullying. gov Web site. http://www.stopbullying.gov/index.html. Accessed October 5, 2016

70. Institute of Medicine, National Research Council. *Building Capacity to Reduce Bullying Workshop Summary.* Washington, DC: National Academies Press; 2014

71. Support the Kids Involved. StopBullying.gov Web site. http:// www.stopbullying.gov/respond/support-kids-involved/index. html. Accessed October 5, 2016

72. WISQARS Leading Causes of Death. Centers for Disease Control and Prevention Web site. http://www.cdc.gov/injury/ wisqars/leading_causes_death.html. Updated December 18, 2015. Accessed October 5, 2016

73. Zahn MA, Brumbaugh S, Steffensmeier D, et al. *Girls Study Group: Understanding and Responding to Girls' Delinquency: Violence by Teenage Girls: Trends and Context.* Washington, DC: US Department of Justice, Office of Juvenile Justice and Delinquency Prevention; 2008. https://www.ncjrs.gov/pdffiles1/ ojjdp/218905.pdf. Accessed October 5, 2016

74. Russell KF, Vandermeer B, Hartling L. Graduated driver licensing for reducing motor vehicle crashes among young drivers. *Cochrane Database Syst Rev.* 2011(10):CD003300

75. Ages & Stages: Parent-Teen Driving Agreement. HealthyChildren.org Web site. https://www.healthychildren. org/English/ages-stages/teen/safety/Pages/Teen-Driving- Agreement.aspx. Updated November 21, 2015. Accessed October 5, 2016

76. Parent-Teen Driving Agreement. Centers for Disease Control and Prevention Web site. http://www.cdc.gov/parentsarethekey/ agreement/index.html. Updated September 22, 2015. Accessed October 5, 2016

77. Cell Phone Distracted Driving. National Safety Council Web site. http://www.nsc.org/learn/NSC-Initiatives/Pages/distracted- driving-problem-of-cell-phone-distracted-driving.aspx. Accessed November 16, 2016

78. National Highway Traffic Safety Administration. Distracted Driving Facts and Statisitics. http://www.distraction.gov/ stats-research-laws/facts-and-statistics.html. Accessed October 5, 2016

79. National Highway Traffic Safety Administration. Distraction. gov Web site. http://www.distraction.gov. Accessed October 5, 2016

80. Holt S, Buckley H, Whelan S. The impact of exposure to domestic violence on children and young people: A review of the literature. *Child Abuse Negl.* 2008;32(8):797-810

81. Turner HA, Finkelhor D, Ormrod R. The effect of lifetime victimization on the mental health of children and adolescents. *Soc Sci Med.* 2006;62(1):13-27

82. Fowler PJ, Tompsett CJ, Braciszewski JM, Jacques-Tiura AJ, Baltes BB. Community violence: a meta-analysis on the effect of exposure and mental health outcomes of children and adolescents. *Dev Psychopathol.* 2009;21(1):227-259

83. Hamby S, Finkelhor D, Turner H, Ormrod R. Children's exposure to intimate partner violence and other family violence. *Juvenile Justice Bulletin.* 2011:1-12. http://www.ncjrs. gov/pdffiles1/ojjdp/232272.pdf. Accessed October 5, 2016

84. Eriksson L, Mazerolle P. A cycle of violence? Examining family- of-origin violence, attitudes, and intimate partner violence perpetration. *J Interpers Violence.* 2015;30(6):945-964

85. Garner AS, Shonkoff JP; American Academy of Pediatrics Committee on Psychosocial Aspects of Child and Family Health; Committee on Early Childhood, Adoption, and Dependent Care; Section on Developmental Behavioral Pediatrics. Early childhood adversity, toxic stress, and the role of the pediatrician: translating developmental science into lifelong health. *Pediatrics.* 2012;129(1):e224-e231

86. Bair-Merritt MH, Blackstone M, Feudtner C. Physical health outcomes of childhood exposure to intimate partner violence: a systematic review. *Pediatrics.* 2006;117(2):e278-e290

87. Kann L, Kinchen S, Shanklin S, et al. Youth risk behavior surveillance—United States, 2013 [published correction appears in *MMWR Surveill Summ.* 2014;63(26):576]. *MMWR Surveill Summ.* 2014;63(4):1-168

88. Exner-Cortens D, Eckenrode J, Rothman E. Longitudinal associations between teen dating violence victimization and adverse health outcomes. *Pediatrics.* 2013;131(1):71-78

89. De Koker P, Mathews C, Zuch M, Bastien S, Mason-Jones AJ. A systematic review of interventions for preventing adolescent intimate partner violence. *J Adolesc Health.* 2014;54(1):3-13

90. Borowsky IW, Ireland M. Predictors of future fight-related injury among adolescents. *Pediatrics.* 2004;113(3):530-536

91. Sege R, Stringham P, Short S, Griffith J. Ten years after: examination of adolescent screening questions that predict future violence-related injury. *J Adolesc Health.* 1999;24(6): 395-402

92. Levine DA; American Academy of Pediatrics Committee on Adolescence. Office-based care for lesbian, gay, bisexual, transgender, and questioning youth. *Pediatrics.* 2013;132(1): e297-e313

93. Heron M. Deaths: leading causes for 2010. *Natl Vital Stat Rep.* 2013;62(6):1-96

94. National Youth Gang Survey Analysis: Measuring the Extent of Gang Problems. National Gang Center Web site. https:// www.nationalgangcenter.gov/Survey-Analysis/Measuring- the-Extent-of-Gang-Problems. Accessed October 5, 2016

95. National Youth Gang Survey Analysis: Prevalence of Gang Problems. National Gang Center Web site. https://www. nationalgangcenter.gov/survey-analysis/prevalence-of-gang- problems. Accessed November 16, 2016

96. O'Brien K, Daffern M, Chu CM, Thomas SDM. Youth gang affiliation, violence, and criminal activities: a review of motivational, risk, and protective factors. *Aggress Violent Behav.* 2013;18(4):417-425

97. National Gang Center Web site. https://www. nationalgangcenter.gov. Accessed October 5, 2016

98. Rice SG; American Academy of Pediatrics Council on Sports Medicine and Fitness. Medical conditions affecting sports participation. *Pediatrics.* 2008;121(4):841-848

PROMOTING SAFETY AND INJURY PREVENTION

99. McCambridge TM, Benjamin HJ, Brenner JS, et al; American Academy of Pediatrics Council on Sports Medicine and Fitness. Athletic participation by children and adolescents who have systemic hypertension. *Pediatrics.* 2010;125(6):1287-1294

100. American Academy of Pediatrics Committee on Nutrition, Council on Sports Medicine and Fitness. Sports drinks and energy drinks for children and adolescents: are they appropriate? *Pediatrics.* 2011;127(6):1182-1189

101. Lincoln AE, Caswell SV, Almquist JL, Dunn RE, Norris JB, Hinton RY. Trends in concussion incidence in high school sports: a prospective 11-year study. *Am J Sports Med.* 2011;39(5):958-963

102. Frollo J. See where your state stands on concussion law. USA Football Web site. http://usafootball.com/blog/health-and-safety/see-where-your-state-stands-concussion-law. Updated April 21, 2013. Accessed October 5, 2016

103. HEADS UP: Managing Return to Activities. Centers for Disease Control and Prevention Web site. http://www.cdc.gov/headsup/providers/return_to_activities.html. Updated February 8, 2016. Accessed October 5, 2016

104. LaBella CR, Mjaanes J; American Academy of Pediatrics Council on Sports Medicine and Fitness. Cheerleading injuries: epidemiology and recommendations for prevention [published correction appears in *Pediatrics.* 2013;131(2):362]. *Pediatrics.* 2012;130(5):966-971

Bright Futures Health Supervision Visits

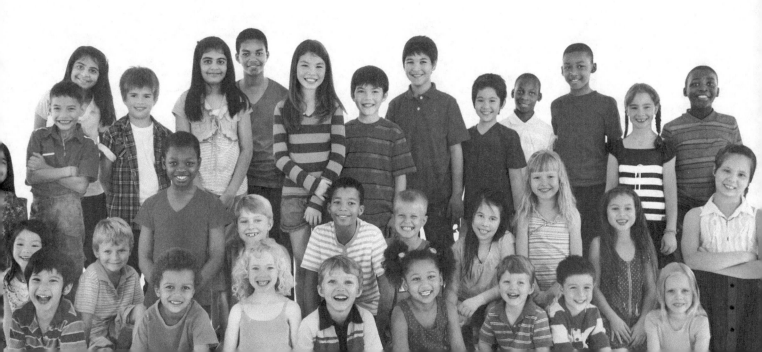

Introduction to the Bright Futures Health Supervision Visits

Health supervision visits are an important opportunity to assess the health and function of a family and child. *Bright Futures: Guidelines for Health Supervision of Infants, Children, and Adolescents* exists "to improve the health and well-being of all children" by improving a practice's clinical health promotion and disease prevention efforts and the organizational processes necessary to meet this goal.

This fourth edition of the *Guidelines* follows the *Bright Futures/American Academy of Pediatrics (AAP) Recommendations for Preventive Pediatric Health Care,* commonly referred to as the *Periodicity Schedule,* which provides an up-to-date summary of the "what to do" in primary care practice today. The *Guidelines* seek to describe "how to do" this work efficiently.

Certainly, no health care professional has the time to do every possible Bright Futures intervention discussed for a particular age visit. How, then, can health care professionals choose what is most important for one child and family at this time in this community? Experienced health care professionals often say that a visit is made up of many "to dos"—things we *must* do, things we *need* to do, and things we *want* to do.

Families bring an agenda, and we *must* address these needs in the visit if we are to be successful. An overlap generally exists between what the family needs us to discuss and what we feel is important to discuss; thus, creating a shared agenda is essential to the visit's success. Helping parents enumerate their concerns and questions is an efficient and effective way of establishing this shared agenda. Using parent and patient Previsit

Questionnaires, such as those provided in the *Bright Futures Tool and Resource Kit,* enhances visit efficiency by identifying concerns at the beginning of the visit.

Certainly, we *need* to do things for which evidence of effectiveness exists. We also may *need* to provide other services that we consider essential to that particular child's health and well-being, such as those defined by professional guidelines or state mandates.

What about the things that we *want* to do? We bring a personal view to health based on our training and experience, our knowledge of our unique community and its needs, and our desires to adhere to guidelines from the AAP, American Academy of Family Physicians (AAFP), National Association of Pediatric Nurse Practitioners (NAPNAP), the American Academy of Pediatric Dentistry, the American Dietetic Association, or others. Often, the interventions we *want* to include relate to disease prevention and health promotion. Elucidation and enumeration of a child's and family's strengths is an important undertaking and a good example of what many experienced health care professionals *want* to do.

Accommodating all the *musts, needs,* and *wants* sounds like a pretty big task and an extremely long visit, unless a health care professional tailors the visit and possible interventions to *one* child and family in the community. Not everything needs to be done at every visit. The specifics covered during the physical examination, screenings, and anticipatory guidance will evolve over a sequence of visits during an age range. The time frame for providing health supervision is not just one visit. Actually, it occurs over a child's development and may be provided by a variety of health care professionals in a variety of settings.

The following sections explore these ideas in further detail through a discussion of the content of the health supervision visit, the timing of the visit, and the structure of the visit. We also recognize both the importance and relative paucity of evidence supporting many components of the visit, and describe how supporting evidence is represented in the *Guidelines*.

The Content of the Visit

A visit is composed of many potential interventions or health care professional activities with the patient. Interventions include obtaining a medical history, administering questionnaires or screening tools, performing a physical examination, entering into discussion, and providing anticipatory guidance.

Some interventions, such as assessing growth and development, occur at all visits. But how do we capture the elements of disease prevention and health promotion that are important to an individual child? And, when we find these elements, how are the best interventions chosen so that the best outcomes can be sought?

Many health care professionals see *one* child health visit as *one* encounter, a view encouraged by third-party payers. Unlike sick care visits, which aim to remedy a particular malady, the health supervision visit seeks many unique outcomes, often related only in their shared goal of the child's health. Multiple desired outcomes inevitably drive many separate interventions within the one encounter of the visit. Would it not be better conceptualized as a visit of multiple encounters?

This question can be answered by considering 4 components of the health supervision encounter—disease detection, disease prevention, health promotion, and anticipatory guidance. Disease detection is the easiest to describe. Every professional in child health care has been trained in the disease model, in the care of children who are sick. However, the desired outcomes of the health supervision visit are broader than just detecting disease and they involve very different actions in the same encounter. Failure to recognize their inherent incongruence will lead to incongruent practice, with frustrations and compromised outcomes. The tone and content of disease detection should be remarkably different from that employed in discussing health-promoting behaviors.

Disease Detection

Surveillance and Screening

Child health care professionals generally report 2 techniques of disease detection over time—surveillance and screening. Dworkin discussed surveillance and screening in the context of child development, and defined developmental surveillance as "a flexible, continuous process whereby knowledgeable professionals perform skilled observations of children during the provision of health care. The components of surveillance include eliciting and attending to parental concerns, obtaining a relevant developmental history, making accurate and informative observations of children, and sharing opinions and concerns with other relevant professionals."[1]

Screening, on the other hand, is a formal process that employs a standardized tool to detect a particular disease state. Screening can be for all patients or for only some. Universal screening is performed on all patients at certain ages. Selective screening is performed on patients for whom a risk assessment suggests concern. For example, Bright Futures recommends universal screening of 1-year-olds for anemia with a hemoglobin or hematocrit test. But, for a 2-year-old, anemia risk assessment includes dietary history, family history, and knowledge of socioeconomic risk factors. Determination of an increased risk would lead to hemoglobin or hematocrit screening.

Both surveillance and screening are essential elements of the disease-detection functions of the health supervision visit in helping determine how the characteristics of an individual child compare with characteristics of other children. Through ongoing assessment, the developmental trajectory of an individual child can be plotted and compared, just as height and weight are plotted and compared. This edition of Bright Futures will broaden the health care professional's detection skills by including or suggesting appropriate screening and assessment tools, found in the *Bright Futures Tool and Resource Kit,* according to a child's age or clinical presentation. Screening tools alone, however, are not sufficient. Health care professionals should couple screening with careful attention to parental concerns and insights (particularly during crucial developmental stages). This is particularly important for families who may have a child or youth with special health care needs, as this combination of screening and careful attention is more likely to successfully identify these special health care needs early and allow the health care professional to provide quality follow-up and intervention.

Surveillance and screening for developmental disorders has been reviewed.[2] Traditionally, health care professionals have used surveillance to assess development according to knowledge of the child over time and knowledge of child development milestones. It is held to be useful, but is certainly dependent on the health care professional, and has been shown to detect less than 30% of problems. Screening at select times, using a structured developmental assessment tool, increases the

identification rate with sensitivities and specificities of 90% or higher.[2]

Tools for surveillance and screening have been reviewed[2] and effective tools can be found in both the private and public domain. Screening tools vary by condition, by population screened, and in the scope of the conditions assessed. Sensitivity and specificity may vary within the same tool for related though different conditions assessed. Commonly used proprietary tools for use in the primary care setting include the *Ages and Stages Questionnaires (ASQ)*[3] and the *Parents' Evaluation of Developmental Status (PEDStest).*[4] The *Survey of Well-being of Young Children (SWYC)*[5] and *Modified Checklist for Autism in Toddlers, Revised with Follow-Up,*[6] are screening tools in the public domain.

The *SWYC* uses brief questionnaires to assess 3 domains of children's developmental and emotional functioning—the Developmental Domain, the Behavioral/Emotional Domain, and the Family Context for socioeconomic risk assessment. The *SWYC* specifically assesses developmental milestones and notes red flags of developmental concern for clinicians. The Behavioral/Emotional assessment includes Parents' Observations of Social Interaction, a 7-item screening instrument for autism spectrum disorder.

The *ASQ* and *PEDStest* also assess social-emotional function, but do not include socioeconomic screening. Other tests are available and may be appropriate alternatives.

All screening tools should be administered at least as frequently as the times noted in the *Periodicity Schedule.* Some practices will elect to employ a screening tool at additional health supervision visits, although payment for screening may be limited to the recommended visits. The screening tools described always may be used as an assessment for a developmental concern identified with routine surveillance.

The Physical Examination

The authors of this fourth edition of the *Guidelines* suggest that each visit include a complete physical examination, with particular focus on certain aspects at each visit. Experienced health care professionals will simultaneously champion the complete examination on the basis of their discovery of a previously asymptomatic neuroblastoma or murmur of aortic stenosis and point out the rarity of detecting significant pathology. Although the burden of suffering of these disease processes may be great, health analysts correctly question the cost-effectiveness of this approach to disease detection—many normals must be assessed to detect one abnormal. Despite these doubts, we believe that, in current practice in the care of children and adolescents, the complete physical examination does comprise "best care." We acknowledge that, in certain situations, portions of the examination may be appropriately omitted (eg, an examination of the genitalia or when a specialist has recently assessed an organ system).

Disease Prevention

The second essential component of the child health encounter—disease prevention—includes both primary prevention activities applied to a whole population and secondary prevention activities aimed at patients with specific risk factors. An example of a successful primary prevention is the recommendation that all infants be placed on their back for sleep and not sleep in bed with their parents to reduce the risk of sudden unexplained infant death. "Back to sleep," like immunizations, is an essential disease prevention activity for the care of the infant. Bright Futures can assist the child and adolescent health care professional to individualize additional disease prevention strategies to the community and to the specific child and family.

The *Guidelines* are an appropriate compendium of both primary and secondary prevention topics, again noted by age and stage of development. However, a compendium such as ours cannot, by itself, drive an encounter. Where evidence exists for specific disease prevention activities at a particular age, it has been incorporated into the guidance for that encounter. The Bright Futures expert panels have used clinical guidelines and other sources of evidence to feature 5 priorities for each visit as particularly high in value to the clinical visit for health care professionals to consider. *(For more information on this topic, see the Evidence and Rationale chapter.)*

Health Promotion

Health promotion activities constitute the third component of the encounter. These actions distinguish health supervision from other work that health care professionals do with children and families. Other encounters with the health care system focus on disease detection and, often, on disease prevention, but it is health promotion activities that focus the visit on *wellness*.

Social Determinants of Health

This fourth edition of the *Guidelines* includes a new health promotion theme, *Promoting Lifelong Health for Families and Communities*. What are now referred to as social determinants of health are social factors that affect children and families. These factors have driven Bright Futures, beginning with the planning of the first edition of the *Guidelines*. Reflecting a growing body of neuroscience on social determinants of health and a greater focus on this issue by the public health community and the AAP, this fourth edition highlights social determinants of health to reflect the importance of a broad view of health promotion. Contemporary health supervision looks beyond the office encounter to assess and address the family's risks, and strengths and protective factors, through intensified efforts in health promotion to focus on family, community, and social factors, that affect health, both positively and negatively. Although social factors are not new issues for health care professionals who care for children, adolescents, and families, new science underpins their importance and provides evidence for effective interventions. If we are to intervene to address risks and bolster strengths and protective factors, we must know the problem. And to know the problem, we must have effective screening techniques.

Brief and standardized screening tools now exist for prenatal alcohol exposure, parental depression, food insecurity, and adverse family experiences. These screens are included in selected visits according to age of the child and timing of risk. Certain screening is included in the previsit screening tools for these visits, and additional social determinants of health questions are found in the Anticipatory Guidance section of the visits.

The *Guidelines* intentionally include some repetition in these questions. Experienced health care professionals recognize that sensitive topics typically require that patient and family trust be established before affected individuals are likely or able to speak up. To avoid causing upset to families by questioning about sensitive and private topics, such as family violence, alcohol and drug use, and similar risks, screening about these topics can begin with an introductory statement, such as, "I ask all patients standard health questions to understand factors that may affect the health of their child and their health." Perhaps the patient becomes more comfortable *with the health care professional's comfort with the topic.*

Health promotion activities add new opportunities to the encounter. They shift the focus from disease to assets and strengths, on what the family does well and how health care professionals can help them do even better. The skilled health care professional uses these strengths to help the family build assets.

Anticipatory Guidance

Brazelton described the process of anticipatory guidance as one in which child health care professionals assess emerging issues that a child and family face and give advice that is developmentally consistent.[7] For anticipatory guidance to be effective, it must be *timely* (ie, delivered at the right age), *appropriate* to the child and family in their community, and *relevant,* so that key recommendations are adopted by the family. This is an opportunity to broach important safety topics, help the family address relationship issues, access community services, and engage with the extended family, school, neighborhood, and faith communities. Again, the health care professional must prioritize and select. But how? Bright Futures provides techniques to assist the health care professional in designing effective and time-efficient child health supervision interventions.

The Anticipatory Guidance section of each visit does not simply tell clinicians what to do, but suggests how to do it. Sample questions and suggested talking points are provided for the health care professional to use and adapt to the individual patient and family. The wording was provided by expert panel members from their own clinical experience and from that of colleagues. Health care professionals are encouraged to model this approach in developing their own anticipatory guidance discussions.

Children and Youth With Special Health Care Needs

The care of children and youth with special health care needs requires a dual approach consisting of both (1) screening and ongoing assessment to identify the special health care needs and (2) health supervision and anticipatory guidance.

An essential task of a Bright Futures Visit is to identify children with special health care needs. Ongoing surveillance over sequential Bright Futures Visits, careful attention to parental concerns, and screening allow practitioners to find and diagnose these children. Screening may be structured and generalized to be applicable for all children or it can be specific to address concerns in one child.

Bright Futures emphasizes that children and youth with special health care needs are, of course, children, and they have health care needs like all their peers. Their special health care needs, while important, do not negate their needs for health supervision, identification of strengths, and anticipatory guidance. Immunizations, nutrition and physical activity, screening for vision and hearing, school adjustment, and vehicle or firearm safety are only a few of the topics that are important to the health of every child and youth. Sufficient time and attention to identifying and reinforcing youth strengths and their healthy emotional development are key. Through ongoing assessment, the developmental trajectory of an individual child can be plotted and compared, just as height and weight are plotted and compared, and the process of providing care is normalized.

Child and adolescent health care professionals, who couple clinical observation with careful attention to parental concerns and insights, particularly during crucial developmental stages, competently serve children and youth with special health care needs. The Bright Futures Visits support that goal.

The Timing of the Visit

Health supervision visits usually are scheduled as a longer encounter than a sick visit. Data from an AAP survey of pediatricians found that the average length of a preventive care visit, including all care by all personnel, ranges from 28 to 30 minutes,

depending on the age of the patient. Pediatricians personally spend an average of 17 to 20 minutes with patients and parents, depending on the patient's age.[8] The complexity of family questions is often a determinant in visit duration, as are the needs of the child that are anticipated before the visit or detected during the visit. The pressures of practice cost and the day's queue of patients may limit the time available.

Experienced health care professionals see the Bright Futures Visit as an opportunity, but most also report a genuine tension as they seek to accomplish so much in so little time. Resolving this tension is important to the success of the visit and is key to family and health care professional satisfaction. This edition of the *Guidelines* provides solutions to improve clinical and organizational processes in health supervision care. Using the Bright Futures materials, health care professionals who work with office or clinic staff can create effective encounters that meet their goals of disease detection, disease prevention, health promotion, and anticipatory guidance (Box 1).

We chose 15 to 18 minutes as the target time for the face-to-face encounter of the health care professional and the patient. This time does not include screening time for the patient, which may include parent questionnaires, developmental screenings, and professional nursing time with the patient. Consequently, the patient's time of encounter will exceed that of the health care professionals.

Employing Evidence

Satisfactory studies on preventive health issues in children are uncommon. Few studies have evaluated the effectiveness of components of the physical examination, for example. Absent evidence does not demonstrate a lack of usefulness, however. The lack of evidence of effectiveness most often simply reflects the lack of study. This edition

Box 1

The *Bright Futures Tool and Resource Kit*

The *Bright Futures Tool and Resource Kit* provides forms and tools for health care professionals, patients, and families to complete before, during, or after health supervision visits. Practitioners can use or adapt these materials to meet the needs of their individual practice setting and to ensure they are following the recommendations presented in the *Bright Futures: Guidelines for Health Supervision of Infants, Children, and Adolescents* when delivering care to patients. Core tools include

- Previsit Questionnaires
- Visit Documentation Forms
- Patient/Parent Education Handouts

Clinicians who participated in quality improvement projects using Bright Futures measures found that the Previsit Questionnaires, documentation forms, and patient handouts in the *Guidelines* were most commonly used in their practices. Supplemental tools and additional patient education materials also are included in the *Bright Futures Tool and Resource Kit.*

---

of the *Guidelines* relies on a range of sources to ensure that relevant evidence and expert opinion are included in the construct of every Bright Futures encounter. *(For more information on this topic, see the Evidence and Rationale chapter.)*

Components of the Bright Futures Visit

Bright Futures views the relationship of parents and pediatric health care professionals as a partnership, consistent with the "medical home" philosophy. The *Guidelines* support the care of children and youth in their families, in their personal cultures, and in their community.

Bright Futures practitioners recognize the importance of a family's strengths in caring for their children. We seek to identify strengths in each encounter, and move the focus of the health supervision visit away from the disease detection model toward a strength-based approach to health promotion and disease prevention. Each visit is an essential opportunity to help a family recognize their strengths and protective factors to enhance their health.

The remainder of this section describes the health supervision visit as presented in the *Guidelines* and illustrated in Box 2.

A. Context

For each visit, the Bright Futures expert panels begin with a description of children at the age of the visit, their developmental milieu, their family development, and their environment. This information reminds health care professionals of key developmental tasks and milestones for that age. Contextual discussions describe expected growth and development over time and set the stage for the priorities and tasks that follow. It is intended to assist the health care professional in focusing on the unique qualities of a child this age, as opposed to their near-age peers.

B. Priorities for the Visit

For the visit to be successful, the needs and agenda of the family must be addressed. Thus, the Bright Futures expert panels note that "the first priority is to address the concerns of the parents and the child/adolescent and parent."

Box 2

Bright Futures Health Supervision Visit Outline, Using a Strength-Based Approach

A. Context

B. Priorities for the Visit
  - The first priority is to attend to the concerns of the parents.
  - The Bright Futures expert panel has given priority to 5 additional topics for discussion in each visit.

C. Health Supervision
  - C1. History
    - General Questions
    - Past Medical History
    - Family History
    - Social History
  - C2. Surveillance of Development
  - C3. Review of Systems
  - C4. Observation of Parent-Child/Youth Interaction
  - C5. Physical Examination
    - Assessment of Growth
      ▸ <2 years: weight, length, head circumference, and weight-for-length
      ▸ ≥2 years: weight, height, and BMI
    - Listing of particular components of the examination that are important for the child at each age visit
  - C6. Screening
    - Universal Screening
    - Selective Screening
      ▸ Risk Assessment
      ▸ Action if Risk Assessment Positive (+)
  - C7. Immunizations

D. Anticipatory Guidance
  - Information for the health care professional
  - Health promotion questions for the 5 priorities for the visit
  - Anticipatory guidance for the parent and child

Abbreviation: BMI, body mass index.

Each Bright Futures expert panel has enumerated 5 additional priorities for each visit. These priorities and their component elements assist the health care professional to focus the visit on the most important priorities for a child this age. The priorities are drawn from relevant literature, expert opinion, and the rich conversation of expert panel members. They are offered as a representation of current practice in the care for children of each age. Given the multiple sources of the priorities and the guidance contained within them, it must be noted that although evidence for an intervention strengthens the health care professional's knowledge of child health supervision and assists in setting priorities and managing time, a lack of evidence does not imply lower priority, lack of value, or irrelevance.

C. Health Supervision

C1. History

In each Bright Futures Visit, the history component begins with the following guidance:

- "Interval history may be obtained according to the concerns of the family and the health care professional's preference or style of practice."

266

History that is relevant to the age-specific health supervision encounter is determined to assess strengths, accomplish surveillance, and enhance the health care professional's understanding of the child and family and to guide their work together. Past Medical History and pertinent Family History are important elements of the initial and interval history. Some visits also include relevant Social History questions.

The Bright Futures expert panels also suggest questions that can encourage an in-depth discussion about certain priorities for this visit.

C2. Surveillance of Development

Developmental surveillance occurs with each clinical encounter with the infant, child, and adolescent, and these observations are central to health supervision for children. Surveillance is the observation over time by experienced eyes of a child's acquisition of developmental milestones. To assist health care professionals in their observations, each Bright Futures Visit includes a rich discussion of developmental nuance for that age.

As children grow older, developmental *milestones* are replaced with developmental *tasks*. For older children and adolescents, developmental tasks assume a central position in this assessment. Developmental tasks of middle childhood and adolescence, such as connection to family and peers and autonomy, are described in the *Promoting Lifelong Health for Families and Communities theme.*

C3. Review of Systems

A standard, brief review of systems is an effective method of ensuring that significant problems are addressed.

C4. Observation of Parent-Child/Youth Interaction

Health supervision activities always involve observation of the parent-child interaction. Often accomplished without formal thought, this assessment provides context for the work of the visit.

C5. Physical Examination

The physical examination is the cornerstone of any pediatric evaluation. It is the one portion of the evaluation that only a licensed child health care professional can perform. Molded by a thoughtful acquisition of medical history, a complete physical examination is included as part of every visit. The physical examination must be comprehensive, yet also focus on specific assessments that are appropriate to the child's or adolescent's age, developmental attainment, and needs, which are discerned from the patient history. This portion of each Bright Futures Visit opens with the following guidance:

- "A complete physical examination is included as part of every health supervision visit."

In the context of a complete physical examination, the experienced health care professional incorporates certain specific components that are necessary to the examination of a child of a specific age or stage of development. To set this stage, the following statement also is made in each visit:

- "When performing a physical examination, the health care professional's attention is directed to the following components of the examination that are important for a child/youth this age:"

Most children in the United States are healthy and have normal physical examinations. Regardless of health status, for all children, each visit's examination will be different, will demonstrate growth and maturation, and will provide the opportunity for discussion of the physical changes associated with healthy development.

No evidence-based data exist to indicate that a complete physical examination dramatically improves health care outcomes. However, evidence does demonstrate the importance of key elements of the complete physical examination at different ages. *(For more information on this topic, see the Evidence and Rationale chapter.)* In addition, there are numerous reasons why the examination may be in the best interests of the child and family. Most important is the possibility that a silent or subtle illness could be identified. Furthermore, the examination provides an opportunity for the child health care professional to model respect for the child, to educate both the child and the parents about the child and her body and growth, and to acknowledge the child's individuality. One study of well child care found the importance of this reassurance to parents regarding their parenting and their child's health.[9]

The health supervision examination should be unhurried, with adequate uninterrupted time set aside for questions and discussion by parents and the child. Ensuring privacy can help the parents and the child address a variety of issues in a comfortable and non-pressured setting. Beginning in middle childhood and by adolescence, policies related to privacy and confidentiality must be established and reviewed for the child and family (Box 3). Children are reminded that we want them to begin to make their own good health decisions, that good decisions require good information, and that our questions are aimed at really getting

to know them better. Children and adolescents are always encouraged to discuss any concerns with their parents, the adults who know them best and, in most families, the people who can best help them find answers and solve problems. But, if patients of any age prefer to discuss concerns privately with their health care professional, they should be supported and allowed to do so.

The practice's or clinic's policies regarding privacy should be shared and discussed with parents and children by the 7 or 8 Year Visit. At this time, it is appropriate to offer the option of part of the visit without the parent present. Most health care professionals will always excuse the parent from part of the visit by the 12 Year Visit. In some health care systems, time alone with the health care professional is a quality-control measure for adolescent care. It is useful to frame confidentiality and privacy as part of the child's increasing self-reliance and a standard part of the visit.

The physical examination always should include an assessment of growth.

- Younger than 2 years: weight, length, head circumference, and weight-for-length
- 2 years and older: weight, height, and body mass index (BMI)[10]

Measurements should be plotted on the World Health Organization (WHO) Growth Charts for birth to age 18 months (Appendix A), and beginning at age 2 years on the Centers for Disease Control and Prevention (CDC) growth

---

Box 3

Privacy, Confidentiality, and the Bright Futures Health Supervision Visit

Practices may want to establish formal confidentiality policies. Parents are important participants in these policies. A sample confidentiality statement addressed to youth could look as follows:

"Our discussions with you are private. We hope you will feel free to talk openly with us about yourself and your health. Information is not shared with other people without your permission unless we are concerned that someone is in danger."

From Jack Mayer, MD, MPH, Rainbow Pediatrics, Middlebury, VT.

and BMI-for-age charts (Appendix B). Growth charts permit the evaluation of appropriate changes in growth over time. Deviations from normed percentiles require further investigation or anticipatory guidance. *(For more information on this topic, see the Promoting Healthy Weight theme.)*

Children and youth with special health care needs have chronic physical, developmental, behavioral, or emotional conditions that may affect their growth. Growth may be further affected by illness, medication use, congenital anomalies, and impaired motor skills. Assessment of growth is a key component of care for children and youth with special health care needs, and use of age-appropriate WHO or CDC growth charts, especially weight and height charts, for early detection of growth trends is important. The CDC also has evaluated reference growth charts for some children with special health care needs, including trisomy 21, achondroplasia, Prader-Willi syndrome, Turner syndrome, and Williams syndrome. Use of these specialized charts may be considered for affected children. Important limitations of these charts are the small sample sizes on which these charts are based, the lack of BMI data, and the risk of underestimating the child's growth potential. It is recommended that these charts be used in conjunction with the standard-reference WHO or CDC growth and BMI-for-age charts. The child's growth then can be assessed against that of the general population of children and can be monitored more accurately for inadequate growth or overweight. These CDC charts and guidance regarding their use are available at **www.cdc.gov/growthcharts.**[11]

Body mass index should be calculated at each visit beginning at age 2 years, when the measurement of height replaces the measurement of length. *(For more information on this topic, see the Promoting Healthy Weight theme.)* At earlier visits, when length is measured, the weight-for-length should be plotted on the WHO Growth Chart. Weight-for-length and BMI charting can improve recognition of an underweight or overweight problem, prompt health care professional concerns, and enhance guidance about techniques to promote a healthy weight (Table 1).[12] Review of growth charts with the parent and child is an important component to the discussion of growth and development at each visit.

The US Preventive Services Task Force recommends screening for overweight in children older than age 6 years,[13] and Bright Futures recommends plotting BMI growth curves. Some populations, such as Native Americans, Mexican Americans, Asian and Pacific Islanders, and non-Hispanic blacks, are at a greater risk of developing overweight than are whites. Following BMI curves in these groups may offer long-term benefits.

Table 1

Interpreting Body Mass Index		
Growth Indicator	**Anthropometric Indexes**	**Percentile Cutoff**
Underweight	Low BMI for age and sex	<5th percentile
Healthy	Normal BMI for age and sex	≥5th percentile but <85th percentile
Overweight	High BMI for age and sex	≥85th percentile but <95th percentile
Obese	High BMI for age and sex	≥95th percentile

Abbreviation: BMI, body mass index.

Source: Centers for Disease Control and Prevention; Division of Nutrition, Physical Activity, and Obesity; National Center for Chronic Disease Prevention and Health Promotion. About Children & Teen BMI. http://www.cdc.gov/healthyweight/assessing/bmi/childrens_ bmi/about_ childrens_bmi.html. Updated May 15, 2015. Accessed September 18, 2016.

C6. Screening

A. Universal Screening

B. Selective Screening
- Risk Assessment
- Action if Risk Assessment Positive (+)

Recommended screening occurs at each Bright Futures Visit. Certain screening is universal—it is applied to each child at that visit. Other screening is selective and occurs only if a risk assessment is positive. For example, 1-year-olds are universally screened for elevated blood lead levels in most states, but only those children whose parents have concerns are selectively screened with a hearing test. Where specific screening tools or tests are indicated, they are noted in the visit.

Screening recommendations are derived from the *Recommendations for Preventive Pediatric Health Care (Periodicity Schedule).*[14] Screening tasks were chosen on the basis of available evidence or on expert opinion statements from the Maternal and Child Health Bureau, CDC, AAP, AAFP, NAPNAP, and others. Broad consultation was obtained to achieve consensus.

C7. Immunizations

Assessing the completeness of a child's or adolescent's immunizations is a key element of preventive health services. The value of immunizations in avoiding preventable diseases and disease complications is an important discussion for providers to have with parents. Often, parental anxiety and misinformation regarding immunization must be addressed.

Bright Futures uses the following sources for up-to-date immunization schedules:

- The CDC National Immunization Program, **www.cdc.gov/vaccines.**[15] This source is listed in each Bright Futures Visit.

- American Academy of Pediatrics Red Book, **http://redbook.solutions.aap.org,** is recommended as an additional source of information for the health care professional.

Both sources include professionals' and parents' guides, address evidence behind immunizations, and discuss myths regarding immunization. The CDC-INFO Contact Center, a toll-free number to request information on immunization (**800-CDC-INFO**), is an additional resource.

D. Anticipatory Guidance

The Bright Futures expert panels have provided extensive detail for anticipatory guidance activities.

For each visit, anticipatory guidance is organized by the visit's 5 priorities and their component elements. Within each priority, the anticipatory guidance begins with a brief description for the health care professional. This provides a developmental context for the sample questions and guidance that follow, and it may highlight aspects of a topic that are of particular importance for discussion. The sample questions and anticipatory guidance points provide a possible script for discussion and help frame a relevant conversation with the family and child. Many questions are framed as Ask the Parent. Throughout Bright Futures, the term *parent* encompasses all types of caregivers who care for and raise children, including grandparents, other kin, or guardians. Health care professionals are encouraged to adjust and enhance the questions and guidance as needed.

Examining Children and Adolescents at Each Stage: Useful Information to Make the Visit Go Smoothly

Infancy

The health care professional should examine the infant in front of the parents so that the parents can ask questions and the health care professional can comment on the physical findings. This is a wonderful opportunity to evaluate parent-infant interactions. During the examination, the health care professional can reinforce positive interactions between infant and parents as well as provide guidance for dealing with upcoming changes in infant development. The neurodevelopmental assessment is an ideal opportunity to discuss developmental milestones. The health care professional can incorporate anticipatory guidance regarding developmental stimulation and injury prevention in a developmental context.

The health care professional can speak about sounds, light, touch (both light and firm), body movement, and position (proprioceptive and vestibular input), while stressing that every baby is unique. The parents need to understand the individual aspects of their baby, which will enable them to comfort and support his development. Approaching the baby's development this way helps parents recognize those very important qualities of the caretaking environment. Demonstrating ways to interact with the infant helps give parents a sense of confidence in making changes to best fit their infant.[16]

Early Childhood

Successfully accomplishing an accurate physical examination of a young child requires both skill and art. An ordered approach to the child as a whole and to each individual organ system reduces the likelihood of missing a problem. Younger children need close contact with a parent to reduce anxiety and to ease performance of the examination, whereas older children may take the lead in guiding the health care professional through the examination. Box 4 summarizes some calming techniques to improve cooperation in children aged 1 to 4 years.

Middle Childhood

Middle childhood includes many important milestones for children—learning to read and write, developing important relationships outside the family with friends and teachers, and, for some, the onset of puberty. This is a period of time when lifelong habits that can influence health promotion and disease prevention become established.

The identification of learning barriers and mental health problems are important issues in this age group. Close monitoring of physical health and development are essential for preventive care and the early identification of neurodevelopmental and mental health problems.

In middle childhood, children are developing a growing consciousness about their bodies and may feel uncomfortable without an examination gown or a curtain around the examination table. The child's privacy should be respected.

Adolescence

Adolescence is often thought of as the healthiest age group in the human lifespan. The infectious diseases and developmental issues that constitute most visits to health care professionals during the childhood years are much less common during adolescence, and the chronic illnesses of adulthood are not yet an issue for most adolescents.

Box 4

Calming Techniques to Improve Physical Examination Accuracy in 1- to 4-Year-Olds

Preparation: Encourage parents to read stories about health checkups or health visits before the appointment.

Parent contact: The child sits or lies in the parent's lap or is held chest-to-chest by the parent.

Distraction
Auditory: Gentle, relaxed, reassuring constant banter from the examiner or parent, singing or music, or nonsense buzzing noises or whispering.
Manual: The child holds a tongue blade in each hand or feels the stethoscope head, holds jingling keys, or brings dolls or toys to the appointment.
Visual: The otoscope is shown to the child while lighting the examiner's palm, then the child's, before the ear examination; or the examiner puts the otoscope into his or her own ear declaring, "See! It's okay! Just a flashlight. Do you have a flashlight at home?"

Demonstration: A doll or stuffed animal is examined before the patient, or the child's shoe is "listened" to with the stethoscope before listening to the patient.

Recruitment: Request the child's help in holding the stethoscope head or tongue blade; "blowing out" the otoscope light; or while listening to the chest, asking the child to blow on a piece of tissue held in front of the mouth to encourage deep breathing.

Comfort Measures
Avoid fear-inducing actions: Avoid direct looks into the eyes of a young toddler until the eyes are examined; delay invasive portions of the examination (eg, otoscopy) until last; or examine toes or fingers first.
Provide pleasant office surroundings: Books, toys, and pictures or drawings on the walls.

Despite their relatively good health, adolescents have significant physical issues that require attention on preventive health visits. The significant growth and major hormonal changes that mark the adolescent years, for example, make it necessary to follow growth parameters, including height, weight, and sexual maturity rating,[17] to ensure that they are proceeding appropriately and to watch for the development of possible problems (eg, scoliosis, myopia, or acne) that accompany changes in growth and hormonal milieu.

Other medical issues are related to adolescent health-risk behaviors. Because 46.8% of adolescents report ever having sex,[18] and with a pregnancy rate of 57.4 per 1,000, among female

adolescents aged 15 to 19 years, managing sexuality-related issues, including contraception and sexually transmitted infections (STIs), is an important component of adolescent health care.[19] The CDC estimates that 20 million new STIs occur each year, of which 50% occur among adolescents and young adults aged 15 to 24 years.[20]

The health care professional also can help prevent the onset of diseases in adulthood, particularly cardiovascular disease and malignancies. Factors associated with the onset of cardiovascular disease in adults (eg, overweight, hypertension, hyperlipidemia, and cigarette smoking) may have antecedents in the adolescent age group. Screening for these cardiovascular risk factors is increasingly important.

INTRODUCTION TO THE BRIGHT FUTURES HEALTH SUPERVISION VISITS

With rising levels of overweight and obesity in all age groups, the association between overweight and adult-onset diabetes mellitus in adolescents also has become a major concern. Human papillomavirus immunization and counseling about sun protection and tobacco use also are important interventions to prevent future malignancies.

School-Based Health Clinics

School-based health clinics, which are on-site integrated health services in the schools, are an increasingly prevalent model for delivery of adolescent health care. Referrals for supplementary services are made available to health care professionals and community agencies and mental health centers.

The school-based health center may be the only medical home for some youth. School-based health centers can be especially effective in ensuring immunizations, promoting sports safety, and providing access for students with special health care needs. All services and programs should work to improve communication between school and home so that parents stay involved in their

adolescents' lives away from home and learn effective strategies to deal with some of the challenges that their children face.

Health care professionals may use Bright Futures for health promotion in schools to help adolescents establish good health habits and avoid those that can lead to morbidity and mortality. Health promotion curricula can include family life education and social skills training, as well as information on pregnancy prevention, abstinence, conflict resolution, healthy nutrition and physical activity practices, and avoidance of unhealthy habits, such as the use of tobacco products, alcohol, or other drugs. Referrals to appropriate, culturally respectful, and accessible community resources also help adolescents learn about and address mental health concerns, nutrition and physical health, and sexual health issues. When young people decide to seek assistance beyond their family, these resources should provide appropriate confidential counseling and support to them in making healthy choices while encouraging good communication with parents and family.

References

1. Dworkin PH. Detection of behavioral, developmental, and psychosocial problems in pediatric primary care practice. *Curr Opin Pediatr.* 1993;5(5):531-536
2. American Academy of Pediatrics Council on Children With Disabilities, Section on Developmental Behavioral Pediatrics, Bright Futures Steering Committee, Medical Home Initiatives for Children With Special Needs Project Advisory Committee. Identifying infants and young children with developmental disorders in the medical home: an algorithm for developmental surveillance and screening. *Pediatrics.* 2006;118(1):405-420
3. Paul H. Brookes Publishing Company. *Ages and Stages Questionnaires.* http://agesandstages.com. Accessed September 20, 2016
4. Glascoe FP. PEDStest.com Web site. http://www.pedstest.com/default.aspx. Accessed September 20, 2016
5. Floating Hospital for Children at Tufts Medical Center. *Survey of Well-being of Young Children.* https://sites.google.com/site/swyc2016/home. Accessed September 20, 2016
6. Robins D, Fein D, Barton M. M-Chat.org Web site. https://m-chat.org. Accessed September 20, 2016
7. Brazelton TB. Symposium on behavioral pediatrics. Anticipatory guidance. *Pediatr Clin North Am.* 1975;22(3):533-544
8. American Academy of Pediatrics Division of Health Policy Research. Periodic Survey of Fellows #56: Pediatricians' Provision of Preventative Care and Use of Health Supervision Guidelines: Executive Summary. Elk Grove Village, IL: American Academy of Pediatrics; 2004. https://www.aap.org/en-us/professional-resources/Research/Pages/PS56_Executive_Summary_PediatriciansProvisionofPreventiveCareandUseofHealthSupervisionGuidelines.aspx. Accessed September 20, 2016
9. Radecki L, Olson LM, Frintner MP, Tanner JL, Stein MT. What do families want from well-child care? Including parents in the rethinking discussion. *Pediatrics.* 2009;124(3):858-865
10. Accurately Weighing and Measuring: Technique. University of Washington Web site. http://depts.washington.edu/growth/module5/text/contents.htm. Accessed September 20, 2016
11. National Center for Health Statistics. Growth Charts. Centers for Disease Control and Prevention Web site. http://www.cdc.gov/GrowthCharts. Accessed September 20, 2016
12. Perrin EM, Flower KB, Ammerman AS. Body mass index charts: useful yet underused. *J Pediatr.* 2004;144(4):455-460
13. US Preventive Services Task Force. Screening for obesity in children and adolescents: US Preventive Services Task Force recommendation statement. *Pediatrics.* 2010;125(2):361-367

INTRODUCTION TO THE BRIGHT
FUTURES HEALTH SUPERVISION VISITS

14. American Academy of Pediatrics. Periodicity Schedule. American Academy of Pediatrics Web site. http://www.aap.org/periodicityschedule. Accessed August 8, 2016

15. Vaccines and Immunizations. Centers for Disease Control and Prevention Web site. http://www.cdc.gov/vaccines. Accessed September 20, 2016

16. Medina J. *Brain Rules for Baby: How to Raise a Smart and Happy Child from Zero to Five.* 2nd ed. Seattle, WA: Pear Press; 2014

17. Rosen DS. Physiologic growth and development during adolescence. *Pediatr Rev.* 2004;25(6):194-200

18. Kann L, Kinchen S, Shanklin SL, et al. Youth risk behavior surveillance—United States, 2013 [published correction appears in *MMWR Surveill Summ.* 2014;63(26):576]. *MMWR Surveill Summ.* 2014;63(4):1-168

19. Martinez GM, Abma JC. Sexual activity, contraceptive use, and childbearing of teenagers aged 15-19 in the United States. *NCHS Data Brief.* 2015;(209):1-8

20. CDC Fact Sheet-Incidence, Prevalence, and Cost of Sexually Transmitted Infections in the United States. Centers for Disease Control and Prevention Web site. http://www.cdc.gov/std/stats/STI-Estimates-Fact-Sheet-Feb-2013.pdf. Published February 2013. Accessed September 20, 2016

Evidence and Rationale

Health supervision is a complex and comprehensive package of services that takes place over each child's lifetime. It includes recommended preventive interventions, such as counseling or screening, and addresses the particular needs of each child in the context of family and community. Pediatric health care professionals have a unique opportunity to assess the health and developmental trajectory of children over time because of the frequent visits for both well-child and sick care. Monitoring a child's health over time (known as surveillance) is an important and complementary process of defined periodic assessment using standardized screening tools.

The *Bright Futures/AAP Recommendations for Preventive Pediatric Health Care (Periodicity Schedule)* are the standard for child preventive services. The *Bright Futures Guidelines,* 4th Edition, provide, evidence-informed guidance for implementing the recommendations included in the *Periodicity Schedule.* The *Bright Futures Guidelines* also describe other preventive care services that are likely to be beneficial but that are not supported by the same degree of evidence. In these instances, the *Guidelines* provide a rationale for the recommended preventive service and guidance to help pediatric health care professionals implement the service. We encourage pediatric health care professionals to also adopt these recommendations, for they were developed by expert panels with extensive feedback from families and the general public. Understanding the value of any specific preventive care service for children and their families is challenging because the intended outcomes may not develop for many years and may be difficult to measure. In addition, individual preventive services are not provided in isolation but are additive. For example, recommendations about how to have a stimulating but safe environment can be based on a developmental assessment and at the same time incorporate anticipatory guidance promoting early literacy.

Evidence regarding the overall benefit and feasibility of providing preventive services in the primary care setting continues to be central to the recommendations for child health supervision in the *Bright Futures Guidelines.* We continue to emphasize that lack of evidence does not mean a lack of effectiveness. However, we also recognize the importance of demonstrating the value of the services that are central to pediatric care and for ensuring that the potential benefit of each recommended preventive service is balanced against potential harm (eg, labeling, overdiagnosis, opportunity cost). Filling the evidence gaps is highly desirable, and additional research is strongly encouraged.[1] However, it is not necessarily in the best interests of children's health for many of the specific interventions to stop until the evidence base is adequate. We believe that it is central to the practice of pediatric preventive care for health care professionals to understand the current state of the evidence, and we hope that they will participate in the important work necessary to improve the evidence base.

The *Periodicity Schedule* is reserved for preventive services with the highest degree of supporting evidence. Included are the Grade A and Grade B recommendations made by the US Preventive Services Task Force (USPSTF), the community-based recommendations endorsed by the Centers for Disease Control and Prevention (CDC) Community Guide, and other preventive care services endorsed by the American Academy of Pediatrics (AAP) Executive Committee and Board of Directors. All of these services are based on a high degree of certainty of net benefit to children and their families. The *Periodicity Schedule* is continually reviewed and updated between editions of the *Bright Futures Guidelines* in a process directed by the Bright Futures Steering Committee and the AAP Committee on Practice and

Ambulatory Medicine. Deciding which preventive services should be included in the *Periodicity Schedule* is a complex task because of the incomplete evidence base regarding benefits and harms of preventive care services. The committees are fully committed to using a clearly defined and fully transparent process that weighs benefits, risk, and uncertainties of preventive services when making recommendations for updates to the *Periodicity Schedule*.

Updates to Recommended Preventive Services Since the *Bright Futures Guidelines*, 3rd Edition

The following preventive services are new to the *Bright Futures Guidelines,* 4th Edition. Other preventive services contained in the *Periodicity Schedule* have been modified to be in step with new recommendations. A more detailed summary of changes can be found on the *Periodicity Schedule* at **www.aap.org/periodicityschedule.**

- Universal prepubertal cholesterol screening (in addition to the existing universal cholesterol screening in late adolescence)
- Universal depression screening for adolescents
- Universal human immunodeficiency virus (HIV) screening in middle/late adolescence
- Universal maternal depression screening
- Universal newborn critical congenital heart disease screening
- Universal newborn bilirubin screening
- Oral health (universal fluoride varnish for ages 6 months through 5 years, in addition to universal fluoride supplementation for ages 6 months to 16 years)
- Universal adolescent hearing screening

This following preventive service has been deleted from the *Periodicity Schedule:*

- Annual pelvic examinations for cervical dysplasia for sexually active adolescent and young adult females before age 21 years

Evidence Summaries and Rationale Tables

Bright Futures and its partners strive to ensure that, to the greatest extent possible, children receive health promotion and preventive services that are comprehensive, evidence based, and evidence informed and that reflect the knowledge and experience of the health care professionals from many disciplines who work together to ensure best outcomes in childhood and throughout the life course.

The remainder of this chapter presents the components of the *Periodicity Schedule* included in the fourth edition of the *Bright Futures Guidelines.* Each component begins with text that summarizes the supporting evidence. This summary is followed by tables that provide evidence citations, the rationale for the screening tasks, techniques, and risk assessment questions used in the *Guidelines.* The components are presented alphabetically by topic, unlike the *Periodicity Schedule,* which follows a different order.

Anemia

The USPSTF has concluded that current evidence is insufficient to recommend for or against screening for iron deficiency anemia in infants and children between 6 and 24 months of age (I Statement).[2]

Screening for anemia has limited accuracy for iron deficiency. Treatment of iron deficiency anemia shows improvement in iron deficiency but not necessarily in developmental outcomes. Evidence suggests some harm caused by increased incidence of iron poisoning when iron-containing medications are kept in the home. No high-quality studies were found regarding screening adolescents for anemia.

Because iron deficiency is associated with many and sometimes subtle detrimental effects, the AAP recommends iron supplementation or fortification in infants. They also recommend that all infants at age 12 months be screened for anemia by determining hemoglobin concentration.

Anemia: Universal	
Bright Futures Visits	**12 Month**
Citation	American Academy of Pediatrics Committee on Nutrition. Iron. In: Kleinman RE, Greer FR, eds. *Pediatric Nutrition: Policy of the American Academy of Pediatrics.* 7th ed. Elk Grove Village, IL: American Academy of Pediatrics; 2014:449-466 (p 462)

EVIDENCE AND RATIONALE

Anemia: Selective	
Bright Futures Visits	**4, 15, 18 Month; 2, 2½ Year, Annually Beginning With 3 Year**
Risk assessment	**4 Month Visit** • Prematurity • Low birth weight • Use of low-iron formula or infants not receiving iron-fortified formula • Early introduction of cow's milk **15, 18 Month; 2, 2½, 3, 4, 5 Year Visits** • At risk of iron deficiency because of special health needs • Low-iron diet (eg, nonmeat diet) • Environmental factors (eg, poverty, limited access to food)
Citation	American Academy of Pediatrics Committee on Nutrition. Iron. In: Kleinman RE, Greer FR, eds. *Pediatric Nutrition: Policy of the American Academy of Pediatrics.* 7th ed. Elk Grove Village, IL: American Academy of Pediatrics; 2014:449-466 (p 457)
Risk assessment	**6 through 10 Year Visits** • Children who consume a strict vegetarian diet and are not receiving an iron supplement • Environmental factors (eg, poverty, limited access to food)
Citation	American Academy of Pediatrics Committee on Nutrition. Iron. In: Kleinman RE, Greer FR, eds. *Pediatric Nutrition: Policy of the American Academy of Pediatrics.* 7th ed. Elk Grove Village, IL: American Academy of Pediatrics; 2014:449-466 (p 460)
Risk assessment	**Adolescents (11 through 21 Year Visits)** • Starting in adolescence, screen all nonpregnant females for anemia every 5 to 10 years throughout their childbearing years during routine health examinations. • Annually screen for anemia in females having risk factors for iron deficiency (eg, extensive menstrual or other blood loss, low iron intake, or a previous diagnosis of iron deficiency anemia). • Environmental factors (eg, poverty, limited access to food)
Citation	American Academy of Pediatrics Committee on Nutrition. Iron. In: Kleinman RE, Greer FR, eds. *Pediatric Nutrition: Policy of the American Academy of Pediatrics.* 7th ed. Elk Grove Village, IL: American Academy of Pediatrics; 2014:449-466 (p 460)

EVIDENCE AND RATIONALE

Autism Spectrum Disorder

The AAP has recommended administering an autism spectrum disorder (ASD)–specific screening tool at the 18 Month and 2 Year health supervision visits in addition to a general developmental screening tool. The USPSTF has concluded that current evidence is insufficient to recommend for or against screening for ASD in young children when no concerns of ASD have been raised by their parents or no clinical suspicion exists (I Statement).[3] Although the USPSTF found that screening can accurately identify children with ASD, it found a lack of evidence regarding the benefit of treatment for otherwise asymptomatic individuals.

Autism Spectrum Disorder: Universal	
Bright Futures Visits	18 Month, 2 Year
Citation	American Academy of Pediatrics Council on Children with Disabilities, Section on Developmental Behavioral Pediatrics, Bright Futures Steering Committee and Medical Home Initiatives for Children With Special Needs Project Advisory Committee. Identifying infants and young children with developmental disorders in the medical home: an algorithm for developmental surveillance and screening. *Pediatrics.* 2006;118(1):405-420

Blood Pressure

Bright Futures Guidelines includes blood pressure screening as a vital sign for all visits beginning with the 3 Year Visit. The USPSTF recommends screening for high blood pressure beginning at 18 years of age (Grade A).[4]

In babies and children younger than 3 years, blood pressure is a selective screening with risk assessment questions drawn from the National High Blood Pressure Working Group on High Blood Pressure in Children and Adolescents, cited in the next table. The USPSTF has concluded that current evidence is insufficient to recommend for or against blood pressure screening in children and adolescents younger than 18 years (I Statement).[5]

Blood Pressure: Selective	
Bright Futures Visits	**All Visits <3 Years** (This screening becomes a component of the annual physical examination at the 3 Year Visit.)
Risk assessment	• History of prematurity, very low birth weight, or other neonatal complication requiring intensive care • Congenital heart disease (repaired or non-repaired) • Recurrent urinary tract infections, hematuria, or proteinuria • Known kidney disease or urological malformations • Family history of congenital kidney disease • Solid-organ transplant • Malignancy or bone marrow transplant • Treatment with drugs known to raise blood pressure • Other systemic illnesses associated with hypertension (eg, neurofibromatosis, tuberous sclerosis) • Evidence of increased elevated intracranial pressure
Citation	National High Blood Pressure Education Program Working Group on High Blood Pressure in Children and Adolescents. The fourth report on the diagnosis, evaluation, and treatment of high blood pressure in children and adolescents. *Pediatrics.* 2004;114(2 suppl 4th report):555-576 (p 556)

Cervical Dysplasia

The USPSTF recommends *against* cervical dysplasia screening (Grade D)[6] for females younger than 21 years.

The USPSTF recommends cytology screening for cancer for women aged 21 to 65 (Grade A). Cervical dysplasia screening is recommended at the 21 Year Visit.

Cervical Dysplasia: Universal	
Bright Futures Visits	**21 Year**
US Preventive Services Task Force	Moyer VA; US Preventive Services Task Force. Screening for cervical cancer: US Preventive Services Task Force recommendation statement. *Ann Intern Med.* 2012;156(12):880-891

Depression: Adolescent

The USPSTF recommends screening for major depressive disorder in adolescents and adults aged 12 to 18 years (Grade B) and for the general adult population (Grade B). The USPSTF further notes, "screening should be implemented with adequate systems in place to assure accurate diagnosis, effective treatment, and appropriate follow-up."[7]

The USPSTF has concluded that current evidence is insufficient to recommend for or against screening for major depressive disorder in children younger than 12 years (I Statement).[7]

The USPSTF has concluded that current evidence is insufficient to recommend for or against screening for suicide risk in adolescents or adults (I Statement).[8]

Depression: Universal	
Bright Futures Visits	**Adolescents (12 Through 21 Year)**
US Preventive Services Task Force	Siu AL; US Preventive Services Task Force. Screening for depression in children and adolescents: US Preventive Services Task Force recommendation statement. *Pediatrics*. 2016;137(3):1-8
	Siu AL, Bibbins-Domingo K, Grossman DC, et al; US Preventive Services Task Force. Screening for depression in adults: US Preventive Services Task Force recommendation statement. *JAMA*. 2016;315(4):380-387

Depression: Maternal

The USPSTF recommends screening for depression in the general adult population, including pregnant and postpartum women (Grade B). The USPSTF further notes, "screening should be implemented with adequate systems in place to assure accurate diagnosis, effective treatment, and appropriate follow-up."[9] The AAP has suggested screening up to 6 months of age.

Maternal Depression: Universal	
Bright Futures Visits	**1, 2, 4, 6 Month**
US Preventive Services Task Force	Siu AL; US Preventive Services Task Force. Screening for depression in adults: US Preventive Services Task Force recommendation statement. *JAMA*. 2016;315(4):380-387
Citation	Earls MF; American Academy of Pediatrics Psychosocial Aspects of Child and Family Health. Incorporating recognition and management of perinatal and postpartum depression into pediatric practice. *Pediatrics*. 2010;126(5):1032-1039

EVIDENCE AND RATIONALE

Development

Consensus exists within the AAP and with others regarding the value of early detection and intervention for developmental delays, including gross motor, fine motor, communication, and social development. Surveillance, even by experienced parents and pediatric health care professionals, can miss cases. Therefore, in 2006 the AAP recommended developmental screening at specific ages in addition to surveillance at each preventive care visit.

All children, most of whom will not have identifiable risks or whose development appears to be proceeding typically, should receive periodic developmental screening using a standardized test. In the absence of established risk factors or parental or provider concerns, a general developmental screening, including neuromotor screening, is recommended at the 9 Month, 18 Month, and 2½ Year Visits.

These recommended ages for developmental screening are suggested only as a starting point for children who appear to be developing normally. Surveillance should continue throughout childhood, and screenings should be conducted anytime concerns are raised by parents, child health professionals, or others involved in the care of the child.

Speech and Language

The USPSTF has concluded that current evidence is insufficient to recommend for or against the routine use of brief, formal screening instruments in primary care to detect speech and language delay in babies and children up to age 5 years (I Statement).[10]

Uncertainty exists on the accuracy of tests available to screen specifically for speech or language delay or disorders and the outcomes for children identified specifically through screening.

Bright Futures does not recommend screening specifically for speech or language delay or disorders but instead recommends broadband developmental screening as well as surveillance over time to evaluate the developmental trajectory of the child. This approach can identify speech and language delay or disorders, as well as other developmental problems.

Gross Motor and Other Development Screening at 4 Years of Age

Bright Futures does not recommend screening at 4 years of age. No new strong evidence has been published since the AAP 2006 statement. Motor development evaluation at 4 years of age has been reviewed and is a suggested component of the physical examination at this visit.[11]

Development: Universal	
Bright Futures Visits	9, 18 Month; 2½ Year
Citations	American Academy of Pediatrics Council on Children With Disabilities, Section on Developmental Behavioral Pediatrics, Bright Futures Steering Committee and Medical Home Initiatives for Children With Special Needs Project Advisory Committee. Identifying infants and young children with developmental disorders in the medical home: an algorithm for developmental surveillance and screening. *Pediatrics.* 2006;118(1):405-420 (pp 409, 414)
	AAP publications retired and reaffirmed. *Pediatrics.* 2010;125(2):e444-e445
	AAP publications reaffirmed or retired. *Pediatrics.* 2014;134(5):e1520-e1520

Dyslipidemia

The Expert Panel on Integrated Guidelines for Cardiovascular Health and Risk Reduction in Children and Adolescents of the National Heart, Lung, and Blood Institute and the AAP found sufficient evidence to support universal prepubertal cholesterol screening. A fasting lipoprotein profile (total cholesterol, low-density lipoprotein cholesterol, high-density lipoprotein cholesterol, and triglyceride) should be obtained before pubertal onset and in late adolescence. Screening should be considered for younger children when a history of familial hypercholesterolemia has been identified.

The USPSTF has concluded that current evidence is insufficient to recommend for or against lipid screening from infancy to age 20 years (I Statement).[12]

Dyslipidemia: Universal	
Bright Futures Visits	**Once Between 9 and 11 Year; Once Between 17 and 21 Year**
Citation	National Heart, Lung, and Blood Institute. Expert Panel on Integrated Guidelines for Cardiovascular Health and Risk Reduction in Children and Adolescents: summary report. *Pediatrics.* 2011;128(suppl 5):S213-S256

Dyslipidemia: Selective	
Bright Futures Visits	**2, 4, 6, 8 Year**
Risk assessment	Measure fasting lipid profile (FLP) twice. Average the results if • Parent, grandparent, aunt or uncle, or sibling with myocardial infarction (MI); angina; stroke; or coronary artery bypass graft (CABG)/stent/angioplasty at <55 years in males and <65 years in females. • Parent with total cholesterol ≥240 mg/dL or known dyslipidemia. • Patient has diabetes, hypertension, or body mass index (BMI) ≥95th percentile or smokes cigarettes. • Patient has a moderate- or high-risk medical condition.
Bright Futures Visits	**12 Through 16 Year**
Risk assessment	Measure FLP twice. Average the results if new knowledge of • Parent, grandparent, aunt or uncle, or sibling with MI, angina, stroke, CABG/stent/angioplasty, or sudden death at <55 years in males and <65 years in females. • Parent with total cholesterol ≥240 mg/dL or known dyslipidemia. • Patient has diabetes, hypertension, or BMI ≥85th percentile or smokes cigarettes. • Patient has a moderate- or high-risk medical condition.
Citation	National Heart, Lung, and Blood Institute. Expert Panel on Integrated Guidelines for Cardiovascular Health and Risk Reduction in Children and Adolescents: summary report. *Pediatrics.* 2011;128(suppl 5):S213-S256

Hearing

Strong evidence shows that newborn hearing screening leads to earlier identification and treatment of babies with hearing loss. The AAP supports the 1994 statement of the Joint Committee on Infant Hearing, which endorses the goal of universal detection of hearing loss in babies before 3 months of age, with appropriate intervention no later than 6 months of age.[13] Universal detection of infant hearing loss requires universal screening of all infants. Newborn hearing screening is mandated in most states.

No high-quality studies were found on hearing screening for older children or adolescents. In spite of the rising incidence of hearing loss, presumably related to environmental or headphone and earbud acoustic trauma, hearing screening questions used in the primary care setting do not identify adolescents at risk of hearing loss. For these reasons, universal hearing screening is recommended once during the Early Adolescence, the Middle Adolescence, and the Late Adolescence Visits. Screening in these age groups may be enhanced by including 6,000 and 8,000 Hz high frequencies in the screening audiogram. In addition to screening, counseling on the risk of hearing loss caused by environmental exposures may be considered.

Hearing: Universal	
Bright Futures Visits	**Newborn, First Week; 1, 2 Month**
Citation	American Academy of Pediatrics Task Force on Newborn and Infant Hearing. Newborn and infant hearing loss: detection and intervention. *Pediatrics.* 1999;103(2):527-530
Bright Futures Visits	**4, 5, 6, 8, 10 Year**
Citation	Harlor AD Jr, Bower C. Hearing assessment in infants and children: recommendations beyond neonatal screening. *Pediatrics.* 2009;124(4):1252-1263
Bright Futures Visits	**Once During the Early, the Middle, and the Late Adolescence Visits**
Citation	Sekhar DL, Zalewski TR, Beiler JS, et al. The sensitivity of adolescent hearing screens significantly improves by adding high frequencies. *J Adolesc Health.* 2016;59(3):362-364

Hearing: Selective	
Bright Futures Visits	**4, 6, 9, 12, 15, 18 Month; 2, 2½ Year**
Risk assessment	• Caregiver concern[a] regarding hearing, speech, language or developmental delay. • Family history[a] of permanent childhood hearing loss. • Neonatal intensive care of >5 days or any of the following regardless of length of stay: extracorporeal membrane oxygenation, assisted ventilation, exposure to ototoxic medications (gentamycin and tobramycin) or loop diuretics (furosemide/Lasix), and hyperbilirubinemia that requires exchange transfusion. • In utero infections such as cytomegalovirus,[a] herpes, rubella, syphilis, and toxoplasmosis. • Craniofacial anomalies, including those involving the pinna, ear canal, ear tags, ear pits, and temporal bone anomalies.

continued

Hearing: Selective *(continued)*	
Bright Futures Visits	**4, 6, 9, 12, 15, 18 Month; 2, 2½ Year**
Risk assessment *(continued)*	• Physical findings, such as white forelock, associated with a syndrome known to include a sensorineural or permanent conductive hearing loss. • Syndromes associated with hearing loss or progressive or late-onset hearing loss,[a] such as neurofibromatosis, osteopetrosis, and Usher syndrome. Other frequently identified syndromes include Waardenburg, Alport, Pendred, and Jervell and Lange-Nielson. • Neurodegenerative disorders,[a] such as Hunter syndrome, or sensory motor neuropathies, such as Friedreich ataxia and Charcot-Marie-Tooth disease. • Culture-positive postnatal infections associated with sensorineural hearing loss,[a] including confirmed bacterial and viral (especially herpesvirus and varicella-zoster virus) meningitis. • Head trauma, especially basal skull or temporal bone fracture[a] requiring hospitalization. • Chemotherapy.[a] The Joint Committee on Infant Hearing recognizes that an optimal surveillance and screening program within the medical home would include • At each visit consistent with the *Periodicity Schedule,* infants should be monitored for auditory skills, middle ear status, and developmental milestones (surveillance). Concerns elicited during surveillance should be followed by administration of a validated global developmental screening tool. A validated global developmental screening tool is administered at 9, 18, and 24 to 30 months or, if there is physician or parental concern about hearing or language, sooner. • If an infant does not pass the speech-language portion of the global screening in the medical home or if there is physician or caregiver concern about hearing or spoken-language development, the child should be referred immediately for further evaluation by an audiologist and a speech-language pathologist for a speech and language evaluation with validated tools. • A careful assessment of middle ear status (using pneumatic otoscopy, tympanometry or both) should be completed at all well-child visits, and children with persistent middle ear effusion (≥3 months) should be referred for otologic evaluation. • Once hearing loss is diagnosed in an infant, siblings who are at increased risk of having hearing loss should be referred for audiological evaluation. • All infants with a risk indicator for hearing loss, regardless of surveillance findings, should be referred for an audiological assessment at least once by 24 to 30 months of age. Children with risk indicators that are highly associated with delayed-onset hearing loss, such as having received extracorporeal membrane oxygenation or having cytomegalovirus infection, should have more frequent audiological assessments. • All infants for whom the family has significant concerns regarding hearing or communication should be promptly referred for an audiological and speech-language assessment. [a] Risk indicators that are of greater concern for delayed onset hearing loss.

EVIDENCE AND RATIONALE

continued

Hearing: Selective *(continued)*	
Bright Futures Visits	4, 6, 9, 12, 15, 18 Month; 2, 2½ Year
Citation	American Academy of Pediatrics Joint Committee on Infant Hearing. Year 2007 position statement: principles and guidelines for early hearing detection and intervention programs. *Pediatrics.* 2007;120(4):898-921
Bright Futures Visits	3, 7, 9 Year
Risk assessment	Parental concern
Citation	At this time, no studies provide validated screening questions for this age group.

Human Immunodeficiency Virus

The USPSTF recommends screening for HIV infection in adolescents and adults aged 15 to 65 years. Screening of younger and older persons at increased risk is also recommended (Grade A). Youth at increased risk of HIV infection, including those who are sexually active, participate in injected drug use, or are being tested for other sexually transmitted infections (STIs), should be tested for HIV and reassessed annually. Bright Futures recommendations follow the USPSTF and call for HIV screening once between the ages of 15 and 18 years, making every effort to preserve confidentiality of the adolescent.

Human Immunodeficiency Virus: Universal	
Bright Futures Visits	Once Between 15 and 18 Year
US Preventive Services Task Force	Moyer VA; US Preventive Services Task Force. Screening for HIV: US Preventive Services Task Force recommendation statement. *Ann Intern Med.* 2013;159(1):51-60

EVIDENCE AND RATIONALE

Human Immunodeficiency Virus: Selective	
Bright Futures Visits	**Adolescents (11 Through 21 Year)**
Risk assessment	• Males who have sex with males • Active injection drug users • Males and females having unprotected vaginal or anal intercourse • Males and females having sexual partners who are human immunodeficiency virus (HIV) infected, bisexual, or injection drug users • Males and females who exchange sex for drugs or money • Males and females who have acquired or request testing for other sexually transmitted infections Patients may request HIV testing in the absence of reported risk factors. To further clarify, the US Preventive Services Task Force notes "that these categories are not mutually exclusive, the degree of sexual risk is on a continuum, and individuals may not be aware of their sexual partners' risk factors for HIV infection. For patients younger than 15 years and older than 65 years, it would be reasonable for clinicians to consider HIV risk factors among individual patients, especially those with new sexual partners. However, clinicians should bear in mind that adolescent and adult patients may be reluctant to disclose having HIV risk factors, even when asked."
Citation	Moyer VA; US Preventive Services Task Force. Screening for HIV: US Preventive Services Task Force recommendation statement. *Ann Intern Med.* 2013;159(1):51-60 (p 53)

EVIDENCE AND RATIONALE

Lead

The USPSTF has concluded that current evidence is insufficient to recommend for or against routine screening for elevated lead levels for asymptomatic children between ages 1 and 5 years who are at increased risk (I Statement).[14]

The USPSTF recommends *against* routine screening for elevated lead levels for asymptomatic children between ages 1 and 5 who are at average risk (Grade D).

Controlled trials demonstrate no neurodevelopmental benefit from interventions to decrease blood lead levels in asymptomatic children. However, lead screening is mandated in many states because of high prevalence of elevated blood lead levels, older housing stock, or Medicaid requirements. Identification might help decrease ongoing exposure and may be of benefit to other children in the same environment.

Bright Futures recommends blood lead screening at the 12 Month Visit. It may be considered again at the 2 Year Visit when blood lead levels peak. The AAP recommends targeted screening of children 12 to 24 months of age for elevated blood lead level concentrations "who live in communities or census block groups with >25% of housing built before 1960 or a prevalence of children's blood concentrations >5 ug/dL (>50 ppb) of >5%."

Elevated Blood Lead Levels: Universal

Bright Futures Visits	12 Month (High Prevalence Area or Medicaid); 2 Year (High Prevalence Area or Medicaid)
Citations	American Academy of Pediatrics Council on Environmental Health. Prevention of children lead toxicity. *Pediatrics*. 2016;138(1):e20161493 Advisory Committee on Childhood Lead Poisoning Prevention of the Centers for Disease Control and Prevention. *Low Level Lead Exposure Harms Children: A Renewed Call for Primary Prevention*. Atlanta, GA; 2012. http://www.cdc.gov/nceh/lead/ACCLPP/Final_Document_030712.pdf. Accessed November 22, 2016

Lead: Selective

Bright Futures Visits	6, 9 Month; 12 Month (Low Prevalence, Not on Medicaid); 18 Month; 2 Year (Low Prevalence, Not on Medicaid); 3, 4, 5, 6 Year
Risk assessment	Does your child live in or visit a home or child care facility with an identified lead hazard or a home built before 1960 that is in poor repair or was renovated in the past 6 months?
Citation	American Academy of Pediatrics Council on Environmental Health. Prevention of childhood lead toxicity. *Pediatrics*. 2016;138(1):e20161493
Risk assessment	Local health care professionals should work with state, county, or local health authorities to develop sensitive, customized questions appropriate to the housing and hazards encountered locally.
Citation	Advisory Committee on Childhood Lead Poisoning Prevention of the Centers for Disease Control and Prevention. *Low Level Lead Exposure Harms Children: A Renewed Call for Primary Prevention*. Atlanta, GA; 2012. http://www.cdc.gov/nceh/lead/ACCLPP/Final_Document_030712.pdf. Accessed November 22, 2016
Risk assessment	The Centers for Disease Control and Prevention recommends blood lead testing for all refugee children who are 6 months to 16 years of age upon entering the United States. Repeated blood lead level testing of all refugee children who are 6 months to 6 years of age 3 to 6 months after they are placed in permanent residences should be considered a "medical necessity," regardless of initial test results.
Citation	Advisory Committee on Childhood Lead Poisoning Prevention of the Centers for Disease Control and Prevention. *Low Level Lead Exposure Harms Children: A Renewed Call for Primary Prevention*. Atlanta, GA; 2012. http://www.cdc.gov/nceh/lead/ACCLPP/Final_Document_030712.pdf. Accessed November 22, 2016

Newborn: Bilirubin

The AAP recommends universal assessment of bilirubin level in infants with gestational age of 35 weeks or greater, using either measurement of total serum bilirubin or transcutaneous bilirubin, with standardized management and follow-up based on the bilirubin level, gestational age, and other risk factors for the development of hyperbilirubinemia.

It is important to critically consider the initial bilirubin level and individual child risk factors to avoid missing cases but also to avoid overtreatment and overdiagnosis.

This recommendation was based primarily on expert opinion and the development of nomograms regarding age-based changes in bilirubin levels. The goal of this assessment is to prevent the development of chronic bilirubin encephalopathy or kernicterus. As kernicterus is a rare event, evaluating the direct linkage between screening and changes in the incidence of kernicterus is difficult. However, the indirect linkage between bilirubin levels and kernicterus and the treatment effect of phototherapy was considered strong enough to support this recommendation. Timely identification could also decrease the need for exchange transfusion, which can be associated with significant morbidity.

Bilirubin: Universal	
Bright Futures Visits	**Newborn**
Citation	Maisels MJ, Bhutani VK, Bogen D, Newman TB, Stark AR, Watchko JF. Hyperbilirubinemia in the newborn infant ≥35 weeks' gestation: an update with clarifications. *Pediatrics.* 2009;124(4):1193-1198

Newborn: Blood

Newborn screening is an essential public health responsibility that is critical for improving the health outcomes of affected children. Participation by pediatric health care professionals is necessary to ensure that testing and any indicated follow-up are completed in a timely fashion. Because of state-by-state variation, it is important for health care professionals know which conditions are included in the panel in the state in which a child was born.

Because the conditions that are included in newborn screening are mandated at the state level, Bright Futures did not summarize the evidence supporting this testing.

Newborn Blood: Universal	
Bright Futures Visits	**Newborn, First Week; 1, 2 Month**
Citation	American College of Medical Genetics Newborn Screening Expert Group. Newborn screening: toward a uniform screening panel and system—executive summary. *Pediatrics.* 2006;117(5 pt 2):S296-S307 (p S298)

Newborn: Critical Congenital Heart Disease

A significant body of evidence suggests that early detection of critical congenital heart disease through pulse-oximetry monitoring is an effective strategy for reducing morbidity and mortality rates in young children. In some states, this screening is mandated as a component of newborn screening. Health care professionals should be aware of state-specific reporting requirements.

Critical Congenital Heart Disease: Universal	
Bright Futures Visits	**Newborn**
Citations	Kemper AR, Mahle WT, Martin GR, et al. Strategies for implementing screening for critical congenital heart disease. *Pediatrics.* 2011;128(5):e1259-e1267
	Mahle WT, Martin GR, Beekman RH III, Morrow WR; American Academy of Pediatrics Section on Cardiology and Cardiac Surgery Executive Committee. Endorsement of Health and Human Services recommendation for pulse oximetry screening for critical congenital heart disease. *Pediatrics.* 2012;129(1):190-192

Oral Health

No high-quality studies were found that examined accuracy by the primary care health professional in identifying children who displayed one or more risk indicators for oral disease.

Referral by the primary care physician or health care professional has been recommended, based on risk assessment, as early as 6 months of age, 6 months after the first tooth erupts, and no later than 12 months of age.

Fluoride Dental Varnish

Strong evidence shows that providing fluoride varnishing in the primary care setting for children younger than 5 years as part of a comprehensive approach to preventing caries is beneficial.

The USPSTF recommends that primary health care professionals apply fluoride varnish to the primary teeth of all infants and children from the time of primary tooth eruption through age 5 years (Grade B). The USPSTF found that the "optimum frequency of fluoride varnishing is not known." Three good- and fair-quality trials assessed by the USPSTF compared varnishing every 6 months versus no varnishing.

A recent Cochrane Review evaluated the effect of fluoride varnish in children and adolescents.[15] Of the 21 trials that were identified, 8 included children aged 1 to 5 years. Across all studies, use of fluoride varnish on primary dentition was associated with approximately a 37% reduction in decayed, missing, and filled tooth surfaces. This report did not identify the optimum frequency of varnishing. No important adverse events were reported. However, the review identified that this might be a limitation in the quality of reporting.

The AAP recommends that fluoride varnish be applied to the teeth of all infants and children at least once every 6 months and every 3 months for children at elevated caries risk, starting when the first tooth erupts and until establishment of a dental home. This was based on the recommendations from the American Academy of Pediatric Dentistry to apply fluoride to high-risk children. Some health insurers, including some state Medicaid programs, limit the application to every 6 months.

Fluoride Supplementation

The USPSTF recommends "that primary care clinicians prescribe oral fluoride supplementation starting at 6 months of age for children whose water supply is deficient in fluoride" (Grade B).

Systemic fluoride intake through optimal fluoridation of drinking water or professionally prescribed supplements is recommended to at least age 16 years or the eruption of the second permanent molars, whichever comes first.

Oral Health Risk Assessment: Universal	
Bright Futures Visits	**6, 9 Month**
Citations	American Academy of Pediatric Dentistry Council on Clinical Affairs. Policy on the dental home. *Reference Manual.* 2015;37(6):24-25. http://www.aapd.org/media/Policies_Guidelines/P_DentalHome.pdf. Accessed August 8, 2016
	Casamassimo P, Holt K, eds. *Bright Futures in Practice: Oral Health—Pocket Guide.* 3rd ed. Washington, DC: National Maternal and Child Oral Health Resource Center; 2016

EVIDENCE AND RATIONALE

Fluoride Dental Varnishing: Universal (in the absence of a dental home)

Bright Futures Visits	6 Month Through 5 Year
US Preventive Services Task Force	Moyer VA; US Preventive Services Task Force. Prevention of dental caries in children from birth through age 5 years: US Preventive Services Task Force recommendation statement. *Pediatrics.* 2014;133(6):1102-1111
Citations	Marinho VC, Worthington HV, Walsh T, Clarkson JE. Fluoride varnishes for preventing dental carries in children and adolescents. *Cochrane Database Syst Rev.* 2013;(7):CD002279
	Clark MB, Slayton RL; American Academy of Pediatrics Section on Oral Health. Fluoride use in caries prevention in the primary care setting. *Pediatrics.* 2014;134(3):626-633
	Achembong LN, Kranz AM, Rozier RG. Office-based preventive dental program and statewide trends in dental caries. *Pediatrics.* 2014;133(4):e827-e834

Oral Health (Dental Home): Selective

Bright Futures Visits	12, 18 Month; 2, 2½, 3, 4, 5, 6 Year
Risk assessment	Referral by the primary care physician or health care professional has been recommended, based on risk assessment, as early as 6 months of age, 6 months after the first tooth erupts, and no later than 12 months of age.
Citations	American Academy of Pediatric Dentistry Council on Clinical Affairs. Policy on the dental home. *Reference Manual.* 2015;37(6):24-25. http://www.aapd.org/media/Policies_Guidelines/P_DentalHome.pdf. Accessed August 8, 2016
	Casamassimo P, Holt K, eds. *Bright Futures in Practice: Oral Health—Pocket Guide.* 3rd ed. Washington, DC: National Maternal and Child Oral Health Resource Center; 2016

Oral Health (Fluoride Supplementation): Selective

Bright Futures Visits	6, 9, 12, 18 Month; 2, 2½, 3, 4, 5, 6 to 16 Years
Risk assessment	The US Preventive Services Task Force recommends that primary care clinicians prescribe oral fluoride supplementation at currently recommended doses to preschool children >6 months whose primary water source is deficient in fluoride.
Citation	US Preventive Services Task Force. *Prevention of Dental Caries in Preschool Children: Recommendations and Rationale.* Rockville, MD. Agency for Healthcare Research and Quality; 2004. http://www.ahrq.gov/clinic/3rduspstf/dentalchild/dentchrs.htm. Accessed August 8, 2016
Risk assessment	Systemic fluoride intake through optimal fluoridation of drinking water or professionally prescribed supplements is recommended to 16 years of age or the eruption of the second permanent molars, whichever comes first.
Citations	American Academy of Pediatric Dentistry Clinical Affairs Committee. Clinical guideline on adolescent oral health care. *Reference Manual.* 2015;37(6):151-158. http://www.aapd.org/media/policies_guidelines/g_adoleshealth.pdf. Accessed August 8, 2016
	Moyer VA. Prevention of dental caries in children from birth through age 5 years: US Preventive Services Task Force recommendation statement. *Pediatrics.* 2014;133(6):1102-1111

Scoliosis

Bright Futures includes examination of the back for scoliosis or other abnormality for all Adolescence Visits; a scoliometer may be employed to avoid overidentification. The AAP has endorsed the American Academy of Orthopedic Surgeons and Scoliosis Research Society recommendation to screen for scoliosis.[16,17]

The USPSTF recommends *against* routine screening for scoliosis (Grade D).[18]

Sexually Transmitted Infections

Prenatal Screening

Screening pregnant women for hepatitis B, HIV, syphilis, chlamydia, and gonorrhea can have direct health benefits later for the child.

The USPSTF recommends that all pregnant women be screened for hepatitis B (Grade A), HIV (Grade A), and syphilis (Grade A). Each of these infections requires urgent treatment of the newborn.

The USPSTF recommendation for chlamydia and gonorrhea screening of pregnant women is the same as for nonpregnant women. The USPSTF recommends that females younger than 25 years and those engaging in high-risk sexual behaviors be screened for chlamydia (Grade B) and gonorrhea (Grade B). Although the USPSTF does not recommend routine screening for chlamydia in pregnant women who are older than 25 and not at increased risk, it notes that individual circumstances may support screening.

The USPSTF has concluded that current evidence is insufficient to recommend for or against screening for gonorrhea in pregnant women who are not at increased risk (I Statement).[19]

Screening Adolescents for *Chlamydia trachomatis*

Chlamydia is the most common STI in the United States, and many of those infected are asymptomatic. In females, untreated chlamydial infection can lead to infertility. Furthermore, infants may develop serious illness if chlamydial infection is acquired through vertical transmission. In adolescent and adult males, chlamydia rarely leads to significant illness. Of course, infected adolescent and adult males can be important vectors for transmission.

The USPSTF recommends screening for chlamydial infection in all sexually active, nonpregnant females 24 years and younger (Grade B).

The USPSTF has concluded that current evidence is insufficient to recommend for or against screening for chlamydial infection in men (I Statement).[19]

The *Periodicity Schedule* calls for screening of adolescents for STIs according to the recommendations in the current edition of the AAP *Red Book: Report of the Committee on Infectious Diseases.*

Screening Adolescents for *Neisseria gonorrhea*

The USPSTF recommends screening for gonorrheal infection in all sexually active, nonpregnant females 24 years and younger (Grade B).

The USPSTF has concluded that current evidence is insufficient to recommend for or against screening for gonorrheal infection in men (I Statement).[19] Asymptomatic infection is less common in males than in females.

Males who have sex with males or who have other STIs are at increased risk.

Screening Adolescents for Syphilis

The USPSTF strongly recommends that clinicians screen persons at increased risk for syphilis infection (Grade A).

The USPSTF does not recommend routine screening of asymptomatic persons who are not at increased risk for syphilis infection (Grade D).

Chlamydia: Selective	
Bright Futures Visits	**Adolescents (11 Through 21 Year)**
Risk assessment	The US Preventive Services Task Force strongly recommends that clinicians routinely screen all sexually active females ≤25 years and other asymptomatic females at increased risk for infection for chlamydial infection.
US Preventive Services Task Force	LeFevre ML; US Preventive Services Task Force. Screening for chlamydia and gonorrhea: US Preventive Services Task Force recommendation statement. *Ann Intern Med.* 2014;161(12):902-910
Risk assessment	The American Academy of Pediatrics recommends that sexually active males who have sex with females may be considered for annual screening in settings with high prevalence rates. • Jails or juvenile corrections facilities • National job training programs • Sexually transmitted infection clinics • High school-based clinics • Adolescent clinics for patients who have a history of multiple partners Sexually active males who have sex with males (MSM) should be screened annually for rectal and urethral chlamydia. MSM at high risk should be screened every 3 to 6 months. • Multiple or anonymous sex partners • Sex in conjunction with illicit drug use • Sex with partners who participate in these activities
Citation	American Academy of Pediatrics Committee on Adolescence, Society for Adolescent Health and Medicine. Screening for nonviral sexually transmitted infections in adolescents and young adults. *Pediatrics.* 2014;134(1):e302-e311

EVIDENCE AND RATIONALE

Gonorrhea: Selective

Bright Futures Visits	Adolescents (11 Through 21 Year)
Risk assessment	The US Preventive Services Task Force recommends that clinicians screen all sexually active females, including those who are pregnant, for gonorrheal infection if they are at increased risk for infection (ie, if they are young or have other individual or population risk factors).
US Preventive Services Task Force	LeFevre ML; US Preventive Services Task Force. Screening for chlamydia and gonorrhea: US Preventive Services Task Force recommendation statement. *Ann Intern Med.* 2014;161(12):902-910
Risk assessment	The American Academy of Pediatrics recommends that sexually active males who have sex with females (known as MSF) may be considered for annual screening on the basis of individual and population risk factors, such as disparities by race and neighborhood. Sexually active males who have sex with males (MSM) should be screened annually for rectal and urethral gonorrhea. MSM at high risk should be screened every 3 to 6 months. • Multiple or anonymous sex partners • Sex in conjunction with illicit drug use • Sex with partners who participate in these activities
Citation	American Academy of Pediatrics Committee on Adolescence, Society of Adolescent Health and Medicine. Screening for nonviral sexually transmitted infections in adolescents and young adults. *Pediatrics.* 2014;134(1):e302-e311

Syphilis: Selective

Bright Futures Visits	Adolescents (11 Through 21 Year)
Risk assessment	• Males who have sex with males and engage in high-risk sexual behavior • Persons living with human immunodeficiency virus • Commercial sex workers • Persons who exchange sex for drugs • Those in adult correctional facilities
US Preventive Services Task Force	US Preventive Services Task Force. Screening for syphilis infection in nonpregnant adults and adolescents: US Preventive Services Task Force recommendation statement. *JAMA.* 2016;315(21):2321-2327
Citation	American Academy of Pediatrics Committee on Adolescence, Society of Adolescent Health and Medicine. Screening for nonviral sexually transmitted infections in adolescents and young adults. *Pediatrics.* 2014;134(1):e302-e311

EVIDENCE AND RATIONALE

Tobacco, Alcohol, or Drug Use

Tobacco Use

The USPSTF recommends "primary care clinicians provide interventions, including education or brief counseling, to prevent initiation of tobacco use among adolescents" (Grade B). The USPSTF made the same recommendation for pregnant women (Grade A) and for adults (≥18 years) who are not pregnant (Grade A).

The AAP has developed comprehensive reports regarding tobacco use prevention and cessation and recommends asking about tobacco use and secondhand smoke exposure, using office systems that require documentation of tobacco use and secondhand smoke exposure and providing anticipatory guidance by age 5 years.

The AAP recommends that pediatric health care professionals increase their capacity in substance use detection, assessment, and intervention and suggests that research-informed Screening, Brief Intervention, and Referral to Treatment practices can be applied across the variety of practice settings and health care professionals who provide health care to adolescents.

Alcohol Use

The USPSTF has concluded that current evidence is insufficient to recommend for or against screening and behavioral interventions for adolescents for alcohol misuse in primary care settings (I Statement).[20] However, the USPSTF recommends screening adults 18 years and older for alcohol misuse and recommends brief behavioral counseling interventions to reduce alcohol misuse for "persons engaged in risky of hazardous drinking" (Grade B).

Drug Use

The USPSTF has concluded that current evidence is insufficient to recommend for or against screening adolescents, adults, and pregnant women for illicit drug use (I Statement). The USPSTF further concluded that current evidence is insufficient to recommend for or against primary care behavioral interventions to prevent or reduce illicit drug use in children and adolescents who do not have a substance use disorder (I Statement).[21]

Tobacco, Alcohol, or Drug Use: Universal	
Bright Futures Visits	**Adolescents (11 Through 21 Year)**
US Preventive Services Task Force	Moyer VA; US Preventive Services Task Force. Screening and behavioral counseling interventions in primary care to reduce alcohol misuse: US Preventive Services Task Force recommendation statement. *Ann Intern Med.* 2013;159(3):210-218
Citation	American Academy of Pediatrics Committee on Substance Abuse. Substance use Screening, Brief Intervention, and Referral to Treatment. *Pediatrics.* 2016;138(1):e20161210

EVIDENCE AND RATIONALE

Tuberculosis

The USPSTF is reviewing the topic of screening for latent tuberculosis infection in populations that are at increased risk. The USPSTF draft recommendation is for screening adults who are at increased risk for tuberculosis (Grade B).

There is no evidence of benefit or harm from screening asymptomatic children and adolescents for tuberculosis (TB). Questionnaires that address contact with a person who has TB, birth in or travel to endemic areas, regular contact with high-risk adults, and HIV infection in the child have been shown to have adequate sensitivity and specificity when compared with a positive tuberculin skin test.

Tuberculosis: Selective	
Bright Futures Visits	**1, 6, 12 Month; Annually Beginning at 2 Year Through 17 Year**
Risk assessment	Children who should have annual tuberculin skin test • Children infected with human immunodeficiency virus (HIV) Validated questions for determining risk of latent tuberculosis (TB) infection in children in the United States • Has a family member or contact had tuberculosis disease? • Has a family member had a positive tuberculin skin test? • Was your child born in a high-risk country (countries other than the United States, Canada, Australia, New Zealand, or Western European countries)? • Has your child traveled (had contact with resident populations) to a high-risk country for more than 1 week?
Citation	American Academy of Pediatrics. Tuberculosis. In: Kimberlin DW, Brady MT, Jackson MA, Long SS. *Red Book: 2015 Report of the Committee on Infectious Diseases.* 30th ed. Elk Grove Village, IL: American Academy of Pediatrics; 2015:814-831
Bright Futures Visits	**Annually Beginning at 18 Year**
US Preventive Services Task Force	Young adults at increased risk, including those • Born in, or former residents of, countries with increased TB prevalence • Living in, or who have lived in, high-risk congregate settings (eg, homeless shelters, correctional facilities) • Immunocompromised or living with HIV
Citation	US Preventive Services Task Force. Screening for latent tuberculosis infection in adults: US Preventive Services Task Force recommendation statement. *JAMA.* 2016;316(9):962-969

EVIDENCE AND RATIONALE

Vision

Children should have an assessment for eye problems in the newborn period and at all subsequent routine health supervision visits.

Infants and children at high risk of eye problems or with a concerning finding at physical examination should be referred for specialized eye examination by an ophthalmologist experienced in treating children. This includes children who are very premature; those with family histories of congenital cataracts, retinoblastoma, and metabolic or genetic diseases; those who have significant developmental delay or neurologic difficulties; and those with systematic diseases associated with eye abnormalities.

The USPSTF has concluded that current evidence is insufficient to recommend for or against vision screening for children younger than 3 years (I Statement).[22] Although instrument-based screening devices can be used to screen young children, not enough evidence is available for *Bright Futures Guidelines* to recommend for or against their use in children younger than age 3 years.

Strong evidence shows that identifying amblyopia risk factors can lead to therapeutic measures that prevent persistent vision loss. There is no evidence that instrument-based screeners (eg, auto-refractors, photo-screeners) are superior to repeated traditional vision screening tests at health supervision visits over time. However, instrument-based screeners require less cooperation on the part of the child. Examination of the eyes, including assessment for ocular motility and the cover-uncover test, is included in Bright Futures Visits.

The USPSTF recommends vision screening "for all children at least once between the ages of 3 and 5 years, to detect the presence of amblyopia or its risk factors" (Grade B). Traditional vision testing requires a cooperative, verbal child and cannot be performed reliably until ages 3 to 4 years. Strong evidence shows that vision screening tests have reasonable accuracy in identifying strabismus, amblyopia, and refractive error in children with these conditions and that treatment of strabismus and amblyopia for children aged 3 through 5 can improve visual acuity and reduce long-term amblyopia.

Bright Futures supports the screening recommendations for ages 6 to 21 years that are found in the guidelines developed by the AAP, American Association of Certified Orthoptists, American Association for Pediatric Ophthalmology and Strabismus, and American Academy of Ophthalmology.

Vision: Universal	
Bright Futures Visits	**3, 4, 5 Year**
US Preventive Services Task Force	US Preventive Services Task Force. Vision screening for children 1 to 5 years of age: US Preventive Services Task Force recommendation statement. *Pediatrics.* 2011;127(2):340-346
	Donahue SP, Ruben JB; American Academy of Ophthalmology, American Academy of Pediatrics Ophthalmology Section, American Association for Pediatric Ophthalmology and Strabismus, Children's Eye Foundation, American Association of Certified Orthoptists. US Preventive Services Task Force vision screening recommendations. *Pediatrics.* 2011;127(3):569-570

continued

Vision: Universal *(continued)*

Bright Futures Visits	6, 8, 10, 12, 15 Year
Citation	American Academy of Pediatrics Committee on Practice and Ambulatory Medicine, Section on Ophthalmology; American Association of Certified Orthoptists; American Association for Pediatric Ophthalmology and Strabismus; American Academy of Ophthalmology. Visual system assessment in infants, children, and young adults by pediatricians. *Pediatrics.* 2016;137(1):e20153596

Vision: Selective

Bright Futures Visits	Newborn, First Week; 1, 2, 4, 6, 9, 12, 15, 18 Month; 2, 2½, 7, 9, 11, 13, 14, 16, 17, 18 Through 21 Year
Risk assessment	**Birth to Age 3 Years**
	Eye evaluation should include • Ocular history • Vision assessment • External inspection of the eyes and lids • Ocular motility assessment • Pupil examination • Red reflex examination **Ocular history.** Parents' observations are valuable. Questions that can be asked include • Do your child's eyes appear unusual? • Does your child seem to see well? • Does your child exhibit difficulty with near or distance vision? • Do your child's eyes appear straight, or do they seem to cross? • Do your child's eyelids droop, or does one eyelid tend to close? • Has your child ever had an eye injury? Relevant family histories regarding eye disorders or preschool or early childhood use of glasses in parents or siblings should be explored.
	≥3 Years
	Above criteria plus • Age-appropriate visual acuity measurement • Attempt at ophthalmoscopy
Citation	Donahue SP, Baker CN; American Academy of Pediatrics Committee on Practice and Ambulatory Medicine, Section on Ophthalmology; American Association of Certified Orthoptists; American Association for Pediatric Ophthalmology and Strabismus; American Academy of Ophthalmology. Procedures for the evaluation of the visual system by pediatricians. *Pediatrics.* 2016;137(1)

EVIDENCE AND RATIONALE

References

1. Grossman DC, Kemper AR. Confronting the need for evidence regarding prevention. *Pediatrics.* 2016;137(2):1-3

2. Siu AL; US Preventive Services Task Force. Screening for iron deficiency anemia in young children: US Preventive Services Task Force recommendation statement. *Pediatrics.* 2015;136(4):746-752

3. Siu AL; US Preventive Services Task Force. Screening for autism spectrum disorder in young children: US Preventive Services Task Force recommendation statement. *JAMA.* 2016;315(7):691-696

4. Siu AL; US Preventive Services Task Force. Screening for high blood pressure in adults: US Preventive Services Task Force recommendation statement. *Ann Intern Med.* 2015;163(10):778-786

5. Moyer VA; US Preventive Services Task Force. Screening for primary hypertension in children and adolescents: US Preventive Services Task Force recommendation statement. *Pediatrics.* 2013;132(5):907-914

6. Moyer VA; US Preventive Services Task Force. Screening for cervical cancer: US Preventive Services Task Force recommendation statement. *Ann Intern Med.* 2012;156(12):880-891

7. Siu AL; US Preventive Services Task Force. Screening for depression in children and adolescents: US Preventive Services Task Force recommendation statement. *Pediatrics.* 2016;137(3):1-8

8. LeFevre ML; US Preventive Services Task Force. Screening for suicide risk in adolescents, adults, and older adults in primary care: US Preventive Services Task Force recommendation statement. *Ann Intern Med.* 2014;160(10):719-726

9. Siu AL; US Preventive Services Task Force. Screening for depression in adults: US Preventive Services Task Force recommendation statement. *JAMA.* 2016;315(4):380-387

10. Siu AL; US Preventive Services Task Force. Screening for speech and language delay and disorders in children aged 5 years or younger: US Preventive Services Task Force recommendation statement. *Pediatrics.* 2015;136(2):e474-e481

11. Noritz GH, Murphy NA; Neuromotor Screening Expert Panel. Motor delays: early identification and evaluation. *Pediatrics.* 2013;131(6):e2016-e2027

12. US Preventive Services Task Force. Screening for lipid disorders in children and adolescents: US Preventive Services Task Force recommendation statement. *JAMA.* 2016;316(6):625-633

13. American Academy of Pediatrics Task Force on Newborn and Infant Hearing. Newborn and infant hearing loss: detection and intervention. *Pediatrics.* 1999;103(2):527-530

14. US Preventive Services Task Force. Screening for elevated blood lead levels in children and pregnant women. *Pediatrics.* 2006;118(6):2514-2518

15. Marinho VC, Worthington HV, Walsh T, Clarkson JE. Fluoride varnishes for preventing dental caries in children and adolescents. *Cochrane Database Syst Rev.* 2013;(7):CD002279

16. Screening for idiopathic scoliosis in adolescents. *Pediatrics.* 2016;137(4):e20160065

17. Hresko MT, Talwalkar VR, Schwend RM. Screening for the Early Detection for Idiopathic Scoliosis in Adolescents. Scoliosis Research Society Web site. https://www.srs.org/about-srs/quality-and-safety/position-statements/screening-for-the-early-detection-for-idiopathic-scoliosis-in-adolescents. Accessed August 11, 2016

18. US Preventive Services Task Force. *Final Summary: Idiopathic Scoliosis in Adolescents: Screening.* US Preventive Services Task Force. Web site. http://www.uspreventiveservicestaskforce.org/Page/Document/UpdateSummaryFinal/idiopathic-scoliosis-in-adolescents-screening?ds=1&s=scoliosis. Updated July 2015. Accessed August 24, 2016

19. LeFevre ML; US Preventive Services Task Force. Screening for chlamydia and gonorrhea: US Preventive Services Task Force recommendation statement. *Ann Intern Med.* 2014;161(12):902-910

20. Moyer VA; US Preventive Services Task Force. Screening and behavioral counseling interventions in primary care to reduce alcohol misuse: US Preventive Services Task Force recommendation statement. *Ann Intern Med.* 2013;159(3):210-218

21. Moyer VA; US Preventive Services Task Force. Primary care behavioral interventions to reduce illicit drug and nonmedical pharmaceutical use in children and adolescents: US Preventive Services Task Force recommendation statement. *Ann Intern Med.* 2014;160(9):634-639

22. US Preventive Services Task Force. Vision screening for children 1 to 5 years of age: US Preventive Services Task Force recommendation statement. *Pediatrics.* 2011;127(2):340-346

EVIDENCE AND RATIONALE

Infancy Visits

Prenatal Through 11 Months

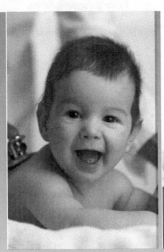
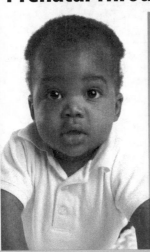
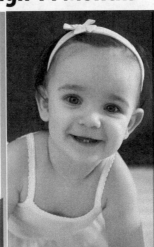
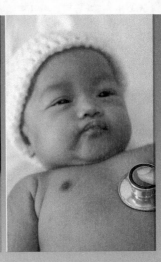

Infancy
Prenatal Visit

Context

A Prenatal Visit is recommended for all expectant families as an important first step in establishing a child's medical home. Some parents use this opportunity to select a health care professional, and this first visit is about establishing a relationship. It provides an opportunity to introduce parents to the practice, gather basic information, provide guidance, identify high-risk situations, and promote parenting skills.[1] The Prenatal Visit is especially valuable for first-time parents; single parents; families with high-risk pregnancies, pregnancy complications, or multiple pregnancies; parents who anticipate health problems for the newborn; parents who have experienced a perinatal or infant death; and parents who are planning to adopt a child. Health evaluation for newly adopted children has been reviewed, with recommendations provided.[2]

Optimally, the Prenatal Visit entails a full office visit during which the expectant parents have the opportunity to meet with the health care professional. Among issues for discussion are the importance of early skin-to-skin contact and routine newborn screening, including blood, bilirubin, hearing, and critical congenital heart disease tests. Other issues for discussion are the anticipated timing of the newborn's discharge from the nursery, common health care concerns for a newborn during the first week of life, and normal early newborn behaviors. This visit also provides an opportunity to provide an overview of health supervision during the first year and to discuss the practice's routines for handling telephone or electronic communication for questions, the procedure for scheduling appointments, and after-hours care.

During the Prenatal Visit, the health care professional can review the importance of a healthy maternal diet for fetal development as well as identify any unique dietary concerns for the family, including any food allergies or intolerances, cultural feeding practices, and the use of herbal or complementary products. The Prenatal Visit also presents an opportunity to inquire about, and document, important aspects of pregnancy history, including potential exposures to toxins (eg, lead, alcohol, drugs) as well as to reiterate messages about healthy behaviors. Breastfeeding promotion is a key aspect of this visit, in particular for expectant mothers who have not yet decided on a feeding method or who are unsure about the benefits or their ability to successfully breastfeed. The benefits of breastfeeding for the mother and baby can be emphasized and parental questions or concerns about breastfeeding and human milk can be addressed.

The health care professional also can inquire about the family constellation; the family's genetic history and health beliefs; the mother's health and wellness, including her mental health, life stressors, status of health insurance coverage for the mother and other family members, and support systems; and the couple's developmental adaptation to becoming parents. The family's preparations for the newborn's birth and homecoming can be assessed during this discussion, as can potential safety concerns and resource needs. This will help

INFANCY
PRENATAL VISIT

the health care professional determine the availability of support for the family at home and within the community.

The health care professional should reach out to the prospective parents, emphasizing the importance of each parent's role in the health, development, and nurturing of the child, and encouraging the parents and other important caregivers to attend subsequent health supervision visits, if possible.

Before a baby's birth, many parents do not have the opportunity to meet their baby's health care professional during a full prenatal office visit. However, a practice may use alternative strategies to obtain information once the parents have decided to use the practice for their primary care and medical home. These strategies can include group prenatal visits, a prenatal/family history completed by the parents, or telephone contact.

Priorities for the Prenatal Visit

The first priority is to attend to the concerns of the parents.

In addition, the Bright Futures Infancy Expert Panel has given priority to the following topics for discussion in this visit:

▶ Social determinants of health[a] (risks [living situation and food security, environmental risks, pregnancy adjustment, intimate partner violence, maternal drug and alcohol use, maternal tobacco use], strengths and protective factors [becoming well informed, family constellation and cultural traditions])

▶ Parent and family health and well-being (mental health [perinatal or chronic depression], diet and physical activity, prenatal care, complementary and alternative medicine)

▶ Newborn care (introduction to the practice as a medical home, circumcision, newborn health risks [handwashing, outings])

▶ Nutrition and feeding (breastfeeding guidance, prescription or nonprescription medications or drugs, family support of breastfeeding, formula-feeding guidance, financial resources for infant feeding)

▶ Safety (car safety seats, heatstroke prevention, safe sleep, pets, firearm safety, safe home environment)

---

[a] Social determinants of health is a new priority in the fourth edition of the *Bright Futures Guidelines*. For more information, see the *Promoting Lifelong Health for Families and Communities* theme.

Health Supervision

The *Bright Futures Tool and Resource Kit* contains Previsit Questionnaires to assist the health care professional in taking a history, conducting developmental surveillance, and performing medical screening.

History

The prenatal history may be obtained according to the concerns of the family and the health care professional's preference or style of practice.

General Questions

- How has your pregnancy gone so far? What are similarities and differences from what you expected? From previous pregnancies? Have you had any prenatal testing done?
- What questions do you or other family members have about your baby after you deliver? Are there any concerns about the health of your baby?
- What have you heard about the purpose of routine child health care? What have you heard about immunizations?
- What do you think might be the most delightful aspect of being a parent? What do you think might be the most challenging aspect of being a parent?
- Where do you get information when you have questions about health issues or caring for your baby? How do you prefer to receive information?

Family History

- Obtain a comprehensive family health history. A family history questionnaire can be found in the *Bright Futures Tool and Resource Kit.*

Social History

- See the Social Determinants of Health priority in Anticipatory Guidance for social history questions.

Surveillance of Development

What have you heard about what newborns can do at birth?

- Newborns are able to smell (especially their mother's breast milk), hear their parents' voices, see up to a distance of under 1 foot (eg, they can see their parent's face when being held), and respond to different types of touch (soothing touch and alerting touch).
- Newborns communicate through crying and through behaviors such as facial expressions, body movements, and movement of their arms and legs. Initially, these behaviors may seem random, but, gradually, it will be possible to understand this early nonverbal language.
- Newborns learn to anticipate and trust their world through their parents' consistent and predictable caregiving (eg, through feeding and how parents respond to their cries).
- For the first months of life, newborns learn to live in a world that is very different from the womb. In the womb, the baby is in a dark environment, is in a curled-up position with arms and legs close to the body, and feels swaying movements when you walk. The baby is used to a small space with limited movements. Your baby hears constant swishing sounds of the placenta and your heartbeat.
- During the first month after birth, babies have a lot to learn—how to feed well and how to coordinate sucking, swallowing, and breathing while breastfeeding or feeding from a bottle. They also must learn how to handle the world around them—the sights, sounds, tactile stimulation (touch)—while learning to control their movements. All these are important steps in a young infant's development.

Review of Systems

Not applicable.

Observation of the Family Dynamic

During the visit, the health care professional acknowledges and reinforces positive parent interactions and discusses any concerns. Observation focuses on

- Who asks questions and who provides responses to questions? (Observe mother's relationship with her partner, other children, or support people present during the visit.)
- Verbal and nonverbal behaviors and communication between family members indicating support and understanding, or differences and conflicts.

Physical Examination

Not applicable.

Screening

Discuss the purpose and importance of the routine newborn screening tests, including newborn blood screening (metabolic, endocrine, hemoglobinopathy), jaundice, congenital heart disease, and hearing, that will be performed in the hospital before the baby is discharged. Explain that the hospital, state health department, and the health care professional work together to ensure that family gets these test results and the appropriate follow-up if any test results are not normal or are not able to be completed before the baby goes home.

Inquire about any maternal prenatal testing (eg, alpha fetoprotein, diabetes [GTT/GCT, HgA1$_c$], hepatitis B, syphilis, human immunodeficiency virus [HIV], cytomegalovirus, group B *Streptococcus*), any abnormal findings seen on ultrasound, and any maternal conditions that may affect the developing fetus or newborn.

Immunizations

Discuss the importance of routine initiation of immunizations, including routine newborn hepatitis B immunization and any state-specific recommendations for immunization before discharge.

Infants younger than 6 months are at risk of complications from influenza, but are too young to be vaccinated for seasonal influenza. Encourage **influenza vaccine** for caregivers of infants younger than 6 months and recommend **pertussis immunization (Tdap)** for adults who will be caring for the infant. *The Centers for Disease Control and Prevention (CDC) Advisory Committee on Immunization Practices (ACIP) recommends that every pregnant woman receive Tdap with each pregnancy.* The Tdap is safe after 20 weeks' gestation and immediately postpartum for women who have not received Tdap in the previous year.

The health care professional also can use this opportunity to assess vaccination status for other children in the family. Their vaccination status not only affects their health but also that of the newborn.

Consult the CDC/ACIP or American Academy of Pediatrics (AAP) Web sites for the current immunization schedule.

CDC National Immunization Program **www.cdc.gov/vaccines**

AAP *Red Book:* **http://redbook.solutions.aap.org**

Anticipatory Guidance

The following sample questions, which address the Bright Futures Infancy Expert Panel's Anticipatory Guidance Priorities, are intended to be used selectively to invite discussion, gather information, address the needs and concerns of the family, and build partnerships. Use of the questions may vary from visit to visit and from family to family. Questions can be modified to match the health care professional's communication style. The accompanying anticipatory guidance for the family should be geared to questions, issues, or concerns for that particular infant and family. Tools and handouts to support anticipatory guidance can be found in the *Bright Futures Tool and Resource Kit*.

Priority

Social Determinants of Health

Risks: Living situation and food security, environmental risks (dampness and mold, lead, pica), pregnancy adjustment, intimate partner violence, maternal drug and alcohol use, maternal tobacco use

Strengths and protective factors: Becoming well informed, family constellation and cultural traditions

Risks: Living Situation and Food Security

Parents in difficult living situations or with limited means may have concerns about their ability to care for their newborn. Suggest community resources that help with finding quality child care, accessing transportation, or getting an infant car safety seat and crib, or addressing issues such as financial concerns, inadequate resources to cover health care expenses, parental inexperience, or lack of social support. Other community groups or agencies can address inadequate or unsafe housing and limited food resources (eg, food or nutrition assistance programs, such as the Commodity Supplemental Food Program, Supplemental Nutrition Assistance Program [SNAP], or Special Supplemental Nutrition Program for Women, Infants, and Children [WIC]).

Sample Questions

Tell me about your living situation. Do you live in an apartment or a house? Is permanent housing a worry for you?

Do you have the things you need to take care of the baby, such as a crib, a car safety seat, and diapers? Does your home have enough heat, hot water, electricity, and working appliances? Do you have health insurance for yourself? How about for the baby?

Within the past 12 months, were you ever worried whether your food would run out before you got money to buy more? Within the past 12 months, did the food you bought not last and you did not have money to get more?

Anticipatory Guidance

- Community agencies are available to help you with concerns about your living situation.
- Programs and resources are available to help you and your baby. You may be eligible for the WIC or housing or transportation assistance programs. Several food programs, such as the Commodity Supplemental Food Program and SNAP, the program formerly known as Food Stamps, can help you. If you are breastfeeding and eligible for WIC, you can get nutritious food for yourself and support from peer counselors.

Risks: Environmental Risks—Dampness and Mold

Explain the risks of dampness and mold and discuss strategies for minimizing these risks.

Sample Questions

Are you aware of any health concerns in your family related to dampness or mold in your home? Have you had problems with bugs, rodents, or peeling paint or plaster in your home?

Anticipatory Guidance

- Some homes may have health risks that may affect your baby. Exposure to damp and moldy environments can cause a variety of health effects in people sensitive to mold. Mold exposure can cause nasal stuffiness, throat irritation, coughing or wheezing, eye irritation, or, in more severe cases, breathing difficulties.
- Mold will grow in places with a lot of moisture, such as around leaks in roofs, windows, or pipes, or where there has been flooding. Mold grows easily on paper products, cardboard, ceiling tiles, and wood products.
- To control mold, prevent water leaks, ventilate well, clean gutters, and drain water away from your house's foundation.
- Mold can be removed from hard surfaces with commercial cleaners, soap and water, or a bleach solution of 1 part bleach in 4 parts of water.

Risks: Environmental Risks—Lead

Exposure to lead, whether during pregnancy or after the baby's birth, can have harmful effects on the health and developmental of the baby. Prenatal lead exposure affects children's neurodevelopment, placing them at increased risk for developmental delay, reduced IQ, and behavioral problems. Risk factors for lead exposure above normal day-to-day environmental levels differ in pregnant women from those described in young children.

Women and children with iron deficiency anemia are at particularly high risk for lead poisoning. Other risk factors for lead exposure in pregnant women include recent immigration; pica practices; occupational exposure (eg, working at a battery manufacturing plant); culturally specific practices, such as the use of traditional remedies or imported cosmetics; and the use of traditional lead-glazed pottery for cooking and storing food. Lead-based paint is less likely to be an important exposure source for pregnant women than it is for children, except during renovation or remodeling in older homes.

Some states have lead screening guidelines and follow-up requirements for pregnant women by physicians or other health care professionals. The CDC encourages mothers with blood lead levels less than 40 µg/dL to breastfeed. However, mothers with higher blood lead levels are encouraged to pump and discard their breast milk until their blood lead levels drop below 40 µg/dL.

Sample Questions

Do you have concerns about lead exposure in your home or neighborhood? How old is your home or apartment building? Was it built before 1978? Do you know if there have been any recent renovations on your house, or have you done any? Is your house near a freeway or busy roadway? Does anyone in your house work in a job that exposes him or her to lead?

Anticipatory Guidance

- If your home was built before 1978, it will likely have lead-based paint. You can obtain information about testing your home for lead by contacting the **National Lead Information Center** at **800-424-LEAD** or calling your local state or city health department.
- You can protect your baby and other young children from lead exposure. Avoid using traditional home remedies and cosmetics that may contain lead. When you store or cook foods or liquids, avoid using containers, cookware, or tableware that is not shown to be lead-free. Use only cold water from the tap for drinking, cooking, and making baby formula because hot water is more likely to contain higher levels of lead.
- Avoid exposing children and women who are pregnant or breastfeeding to areas where old paint is being sanded or chipped. Wait until the work is completed and area completely wiped down.
- Lead dust can come into your home on your clothes or body of people who work with lead. After people who live with a woman who is pregnant or breastfeeding finish a task that involves working with lead-based products, such as renovating older housing, stained glass work, bullet making, or using a firing range, they should change their clothes before they enter the home and shower as soon as they return home. Women who are pregnant or breastfeeding should avoid activities that involve working with lead.

Risks: Environmental Risks—Pica

The most common source of lead exposure in pregnant women is pica, or a craving to eat nonfood items. In addition to dirt, clay, and plaster, pregnant women with pica may consume burnt matches, stones, charcoal, mothballs, cornstarch, toothpaste, soap, sand, coffee grounds, baking soda, and cigarette ashes. Pica can interfere with the body's ability to absorb nutrients from healthy foods and actually cause a nutrient deficiency. Pica cravings are a concern because nonfood items may contain toxic elements, like lead or parasitic organisms. In some instances, pica cravings may indicate an underlying physical or mental disorder.

Sample Question

Do you ever have the urge to eat dirt, clay, plaster, or other nonfood items? Tell me about them.

Anticipatory Guidance

- Eating nonfood substances can harm both you and your baby. Please let me know if you have these cravings. I can help you understand why it can be risky.
- If you do have these cravings, talk with your own health care professional. He or she will check your iron status and review your vitamin and mineral intake.
- When a pica craving occurs, try chewing sugarless gum instead. Tell family members or friends about your cravings so they can help you avoid nonfood items.

Risks: Pregnancy Adjustment

Discuss the parents' feelings about the pregnancy and gauge whether disagreements or conflicts in the parents' relationship are likely to be a problem. Suggest community sources of help, if appropriate.

Sample Questions

How do you feel about your pregnancy? What has been the most exciting aspect? What has been the hardest part? Pregnancy can be a stressful time for expectant families; do you have any specific worries? How have you been feeling physically and emotionally? Is this a good time for you to be pregnant? How does your family feel about it? Is it a wanted pregnancy? How does your partner feel about it? Is your pregnancy a source of discord between you and your partner? What works in your family for communicating with each other, making decisions, managing stress, and handling emotions?

Anticipatory Guidance

- It's great that you are happy about having your baby. Working on open communication with your partner and making decisions together will help you both get through the stresses of introducing a new baby into your home and family.
- Taking advantage of support from family and friends and community groups can be a big help in the first few days after you get home with your new baby.
- Pregnancy is a time of personal growth and learning about yourself and your partner. If you and your partner disagree a lot or have many conflicts, consider contacting community resources that can help you work out these difficulties. It is important to work on resolving differences or conflicts because of the stress they may cause. Resolving these problems also can help you be emotionally ready for the baby's birth.

Risks: Intimate Partner Violence

According to the CDC, 1.5 million women are battered by their intimate partner every year, and 324,000 of those women are pregnant. Homicide is the leading cause of death for pregnant and recently pregnant women.[3] When inquiring, avoid asking about abuse or domestic violence. Instead, use descriptive terms, such as *hit, kicked, shoved, choked,* and *threatened.* Provide information on the effect of intimate partner violence on the fetus and children and the community resources that provide assistance. Recommend resources and support groups.

To avoid causing upset to families by questioning about sensitive and private topics, such as family violence, alcohol and drug use, and similar risks, it is recommended to begin screening about these topics with an introductory statement, such as, "I ask all patients standard health questions to understand factors that may affect health of their child as well as their own health."

Sample Questions

Because violence is so common in so many people's lives, I've begun to ask about it. I don't know if this is a problem for you, but many children I see have parents who have been hurt by someone else. Some are too afraid or uncomfortable to bring it up, so I've started asking all my patients about it routinely. Do you always feel safe with your partner? Has your partner, or another significant person in your life, ever hit, kicked, or shoved you, or physically hurt you in any way? Has he or she ever threatened to hurt you or someone close to you? Do you have any questions about your safety at home? What will you do if you feel afraid? Do you have a plan? Would you like information on where to go or who to contact if you ever need help? Can we help you develop a safety plan for you and your other children?

Anticipatory Guidance

- If your partner, or another significant person in your life, is hitting or threatening you, one way that I and other health care professionals can help you is to support you and provide information about local resources that can help you.
- You can also call the toll-free **National Domestic Violence Hotline** at **800-799-SAFE (7233)**.

Risks: Maternal Drug and Alcohol Use

Any substance taken during pregnancy should be evaluated for its risk to the developing fetus, including prescription drugs, over-the-counter preparations, pain relievers, herbal substances, marijuana, and other illegal substances.

Alcohol is a particular risk in pregnancy. During medical screening at this visit, if the pregnant woman acknowledges alcohol use, discuss the concerns about both neurobehavioral disorder associated with prenatal alcohol exposure (ND-PAE) and fetal alcohol spectrum disorder (FASD) to the developing fetus. Both ND-PAE and FASD have lifelong effects on the baby that can include physical problems and problems with behavior and learning. Fetal alcohol exposure, including the timing during the pregnancy, quantity, and duration, is important to document for later diagnosis of FASD. The pregnant woman should be advised to stop drinking and a brief intervention and referral for drug and alcohol counseling is recommended. Referrals to community social service agencies and drug and alcohol treatment programs can be provided if the mother is not already linked to these services.

If the mother acknowledges illicit drug or alcohol use, also discuss state- and hospital-specific policies related to child protection referrals and practices related to child custody.

The newborn will need referral to the state Early Intervention Program, often referred to as IDEA Part C, based on the newborn's clinical findings at birth and state-specific policy.

Sample Questions

How often do you drink beer, wine, or liquor in your household?

For any response other than "Never," ask the following questions: *In the 3 months before you knew you were pregnant, how many times did you have 4 or more drinks in a day? After you knew you were pregnant, how many times did you have 4 or more drinks in a day?*

Depending on the responses to any of the above questions, the health care professional can, if desired, follow up to determine frequency and extent of consumption by asking the following questions: *During your pregnancy on average, how many days per week have you had a drink? During your pregnancy on a typical day when you've had an alcoholic beverage, how many drinks did you have?*

Are you using marijuana, cocaine, pain pills, narcotics, or other controlled substances? What have you heard about the drug's effects on the baby during pregnancy or after the baby is born? Are you getting any help to cut down/stop your drug use?

If any maternal at-risk drinking is identified, a brief intervention and referral is recommended.

Are you taking any medicines or vitamins now? Are you using any prescription or over-the-counter medications or pain relievers? Have you used any health remedies or special herbs or teas to improve your health since you have been pregnant? Is there anything that you used to take, but stopped using when you learned that you were pregnant?

Anticipatory Guidance

- The reason we are concerned about a pregnant woman's use of alcohol or drugs is because of the effects on the baby's mental, physical, and social development. We know that a mother's alcohol or drug use affects her unborn baby and we have no way to know whether any alcohol is safe. Therefore, our recommendation is that women not drink alcohol while they are pregnant. If you are drinking alcohol, we encourage you to stop.
- Alcohol and drug cessation programs are available in our community and we would like to help you connect to these services.
- Community agencies are available to help women during their pregnancy as well as after their baby arrives so that they can safely care for their baby and themselves. Your obstetrics provider also can refer you to programs that help pregnant women stop using drugs and alcohol.
- To understand how over-the-counter medications or herbal products may affect your baby, it is important to know what, if any, of these products you are taking.
- It is important that you have accurate information about the safety in pregnancy of any over-the-counter drugs or remedies that you are using.

Risks: Maternal Tobacco Use

Address how smoking affects the baby, including increasing the risk of low birth weight, preterm delivery, premature rupture of the membranes, placental abruption, sudden infant death syndrome (SIDS), asthma, cleft lip and palate, acute otitis media and middle ear effusion, and respiratory infections. Provide smoking cessation strategies and make specific referrals. Consider the safety of various treatments during pregnancy for patients who are committed to smoking cessation.

800-QUIT-NOW (800-784-8669); TTY 800-332-8615 is a national telephone triage and support service that is routed to local resources. Additional resources are available at www.cdc.gov. Specific information for women is available at http://women.smokefree.gov. Health care professionals also may investigate what is available in their own communities, through their hospitals and health departments and through Internet-based resources such as the American Cancer Society (www.cancer.org) or the American Lung Association (www.lungusa.org).

Sample Questions

Have you smoked during this pregnancy? Do you use any other forms of nicotine delivery, such as e-cigarettes? Does anyone else in your home smoke or use e-cigarettes? Have you thought about cutting down or quitting now that you are pregnant? Have you been able to cut down the daily number of cigarettes or even quit? Do you know where to get help with stopping smoking?

Anticipatory Guidance

- It is important to keep your car, home, and other places where your baby spends time free of tobacco smoke and e-cigarette vapor. Smoking affects the baby by increasing the risk of sudden infant death, asthma, ear infections, and respiratory infections.

Strengths and Protective Factors: Becoming Well Informed

Discuss the parents' support system at home and access to health information.

Be ready to provide parents with trusted sources of maternal and child health information, and provide these links on your own Web site.

Parents of hospitalized babies or whose babies have special health care needs may be more likely to seek out virtual networks for support and information. Trusted Web sites with accurate information can be recommended.

Sample Questions

Tell me about whom you ask for information and where else you go for answers about health questions. How do you decide if the information you get is something you can trust? Are going to believe? To try? Do you enjoy connecting with other parents using social media? What sites, including blogs and birth groups, do you use for networking and finding information about pregnancy, birth, parenting, and caring for a new baby?

Anticipatory Guidance

- Social media tools can be useful in building social networks, but they should not be relied on for maternal and child health advice.
- The AAP HealthyChildren.org is one resource that you may find helpful. Its Web site is **www.HealthyChildren.org,** and its Twitter address is @healthychildren.

Strengths and Protective Factors: Family Constellation and Cultural Traditions

New parents look to family and friends for support and answers to their questions about their children's health and development.

Inquire about other children, older family members and others living in the home, family routines, and relationships. Anticipatory guidance regarding the infant's health and safety will vary, based on the specific cultural traditions of the family.

Sample Questions

Tell me about yourself and your family. Are there other children in your home? How old are they? How have they responded to your pregnancy and the thought of becoming a big brother or sister? Do you have any children or family members living with you who have special health care needs?

Who will be helping you take care of the baby and yourself when you go home from the hospital? How will you handle your other children's needs? Are you working outside the home or attending school now? Who do you go to for help when you need a hand? Do you have friends or relatives that you can call on for help? Do they live near you? How are decisions made in your family? Is there anyone that you rely on to help you with decisions? Is there anyone that you want me to include in our discussions about the baby? If you are returning to school or work, do you have child care arrangements?

Anticipatory Guidance

- It can be a challenge to provide care to several children at once, especially knowing and understanding the unique needs of each family member.
- Older children in the home at any age may express a variety of feelings—from happiness and excitement to anger, sadness, or guilt—about the new baby or your need to devote extra time and attention to the baby. Make the most of your other children's positive feelings and support their emotional needs as they adapt to a new sibling. Helping your other children feel that they have a role in the care and emotional support of the baby is a good way to strengthen family bonds.
- It is important to take the time to get to know your new baby and her personality. This will help you and the rest of your family learn how to help her grow and develop.
- Take advantage of your support network, whether it's friends, family members, or community contacts. This network can be an important strength for you as you prepare to welcome a new baby into your life.
- The information you share with me about your family traditions and your sources of support and assistance will help me learn about your family, its strengths, and how we can best partner in your baby's health care decisions.

Priority

Parent and Family Health and Well-being

Mental health (perinatal or chronic depression), diet and physical activity, prenatal care, complementary and alternative medicine

Mental Health (Perinatal or Chronic Depression)

An estimated 10% to 20% of women struggle with major depression before, during, and after delivery of a baby. Perinatal depression has substantial personal consequences and interferes with quality of child-rearing, adversely affecting parent-child interactions, maternal responsiveness to infant vocalizations and gestures, and other stimulation essential for optimal child development. Fathers also can experience depression.

New mothers may wonder why they are being asked about signs of depression. Because pregnancy and childbirth are supposed to be a joyous occasion, women may feel that they are going to be bad mothers if they are depressed. It is important for apprehensive patients to understand what perinatal depression is, to know that many women experience similar feelings, and to realize that untreated perinatal depression may have adverse effects on women's health and their children's health and development.

Sample Questions

Over the past 2 weeks, have you ever felt down, depressed, or hopeless? Over the past 2 weeks, have you felt little interest or pleasure in doing things?

Anticipatory Guidance

- Although a birth of a baby is considered a wonderful experience, it is important not to ignore the stress that often occurs during parenting a newborn, and the life changes that come with this responsibility. In addition to taking care of your baby and family, you need to make sure to take care of yourself. This stress can take a toll on any parents' mental health and their interactions with the child. It can affect your partner as well.
- It is common for women during and after pregnancy to feel down or depressed. Fathers can also be affected in similar ways. It is very important to address these feelings to ensure your health and your baby's health.
- Emphasizing healthy life behaviors, like getting enough sleep, eating healthy foods, and finding time for walking or other light physical activity, can help you feel better.
- If you are sad or down for more than 2 days in a row, please speak with me about options for treatment. Talk therapy or counseling generally helps very quickly.

Diet and Physical Activity

Pregnant women need a balanced diet and should also take a prenatal vitamin containing folic acid, vitamin D, choline, and iron in amounts that will help protect the mother's and baby's health.

A pregnant woman's diet should include an average daily intake of 200 to 300 mg of the omega-3 long-chain polyunsaturated fatty acid (PUFA) docosahexaenoic acid (DHA) to guarantee a sufficient concentration of preformed DHA in the milk. Consumption of one to two 3-oz portions of seafood weekly will supply sufficient DHA. Women who are pregnant and breastfeeding should avoid the 4 types of fish that are high in mercury. These are tilefish, shark, swordfish, and king mackerel.

Additionally, a pregnant woman's diet should include 550 mg/day of choline because human milk is rich in choline and depletes the mother's tissue stores. Eggs, milk, chicken, beef, and pork are the biggest contributors of choline in the diet. For vegan mothers, who consume no animal products in the diet, a daily multi-vitamin including iron, zinc, vitamin B_{12}, omega-3 fatty acids, and 550 mg/day of choline is recommended.

Pregnant women also should be encouraged to engage in moderate-intensity physical activity for at least 30 minutes at least 5 days of the week to help ensure appropriate prenatal weight gain and to improve blood glucose levels. Pregnant women who habitually engage in vigorous-intensity aerobic activity or who are highly active can continue physical activity during pregnancy and the postpartum period, provided that they remain healthy and discuss with their health care professional how and when activity should be adjusted over time.

Sample Questions

Are you able to eat a healthy diet? Has your obstetrician or nurse midwife prescribed a vitamin for you to take every day? Do you eat fish at least 1 to 2 times per week? Do you have protein-containing foods every day, such as eggs, chicken, beef or pork, or dairy? Are you able to exercise most days?

Anticipatory Guidance

- Eating a small serving of fish 1 to 2 times a week provides important nutrients to your baby. Canned light tuna, salmon, trout, and herring are the best choices to give your baby the neurobehavioral benefits of an adequate intake of an important fat called DHA.
- It is best to avoid 4 kinds of fish that are high in mercury. These fish are tilefish, shark, swordfish, and king mackerel.
- Consuming small amounts of milk, eggs, or meat every day is recommended.
- Talk with your own health care professional about how physically active you should be now and how to adjust your activity after the baby is born.

Prenatal Care

Reinforce adherence to recommended prenatal care and encourage the mother to share her concerns with her obstetrician or other health care professional. If she has not already been tested for HIV during this pregnancy or if she does not know her HIV status, encourage her to seek HIV testing and counseling.

Sample Question

What have you been doing to keep yourself and your baby healthy during your pregnancy?

Anticipatory Guidance

- It is important to maintain your own health by getting prenatal care and going to all your prenatal care appointments, getting enough sleep, and regular physical activity, as well as eating a healthy diet with an appropriate weight gain.
- It also is important to maintain good oral health care and to make sure that you get regular dental checkups.
- All mothers should know their HIV status because early treatment for themselves, and particularly for their baby, is so important. If you do not know your status already, we recommend that you get tested, because proper treatment before, during, and after delivery can protect your baby from getting the virus.

Complementary and Alternative Medicine

A family's health beliefs and use of any complementary and alternative health practices need to be examined and, if safe, considered for incorporation into the child's health care plan.

Sample Questions

Are there any special family health concerns that I should know about to better care for your baby and family? What health practices do you follow to keep your family healthy?

Anticipatory Guidance

- Recognizing your family values, health beliefs, health practices, and learning styles will allow me to better answer your questions about the care of your baby.

Priority

Newborn Care

Introduction to the practice as a medical home, circumcision, newborn health risks (handwashing, outings)

Introduction to the Practice as a Medical Home

Families new to the practice will want to learn information about the practice. This information includes the need for follow-up visits within 48 to 72 hours of nursery discharge and 24-hour access phone numbers to call in case of any particular concerns (eg, jaundice, breastfeeding problems or questions, concerns about infant's intake or feeding skills, fever or suspected illness). Information about the practice policies for after-hours and weekend routines and when parents should contact the health care professional should be included as well.

First-time parents may need detailed information about typical early infant care and supply needs for their newborn. Mothers who have had a cesarean delivery may have additional information and referral needs. Special considerations may also be necessary depending on the number of other children in the home or if any individuals in the home have special health care needs to which the new mother must attend. If the mother is ill herself, it may limit or constrain her ability to fully care for her infant. These should be assessed and plans developed to support the needs of the infant and mother. Home health care or public health nursing referrals for post-discharge assessment and supportive care may be appropriate.

Sample Questions

Most new parents worry that they may not be ready to care for a baby. Do you have any concerns about being ready to take care of your baby? What are you looking forward to? What challenges do you think you will face as new parents?

Anticipatory Guidance

- Because your family is new to the practice, we will give you information about the practice, such as names and background of the health care professionals, staff, appointment scheduling, and urgent and emergency access information.
- Preparing to become a parent can seem daunting, but the best way to be a terrific parent to your baby is to learn as much about your baby as possible. You will learn to read your baby's personality and understand how to help her adjust to her new environment.
- If you have other children in the home, you will also figure out how best to help them adapt to having another family member who needs a lot of your time and attention.

INFANCY
PRENATAL VISIT

Circumcision

Discussion about the parents' views on circumcision would be appropriate at this time, but must be handled in a culturally sensitive manner. The parents' decision may be based on family beliefs and cultural or religious practices. If parents are interested in having their baby circumcised, provide information about methods for performing circumcisions, pain relief during the procedure, and early care of the circumcised penis. If parents choose not to circumcise their son, provide information about early care of the uncircumcised penis.

Sample Questions

If you have a son, have you decided about circumcision? If you are planning on circumcision, who will be performing the procedure?

Anticipatory Guidance

- Circumcision has potential medical benefits and advantages, as well as risks. A recent analysis by the AAP concluded that the medical benefits of circumcision outweigh the risks.[4]
- The AAP recommends that the decision to circumcise is one best made by parents in consultation with their pediatrician, taking into account what is in the best interests of the child, including medical, religious, cultural, and ethnic traditions and personal beliefs.

Newborn Health Risks (Handwashing, Outings)

Remind all family members or guests to wash their hands before handling the baby. Remind the family to protect the baby from anyone with colds or illnesses, especially for the first couple of months.

Sample Questions

What other suggestions have you heard about that will keep your baby healthy? How do you plan to protect your baby from getting infections?

Anticipatory Guidance

- Wash your hands frequently with soap and water or a non-water antiseptic, and always after diaper changes and before feeding the baby.
- For the first few weeks, it is important to limit the baby's exposure to people with colds or to large groups where people may have illnesses.
- Breastfeeding provides important protection for the baby and reduces the frequency of illnesses in babies.

Priority

Nutrition and Feeding

Breastfeeding guidance, prescription or nonprescription medications or drugs, family support of breastfeeding, formula-feeding guidance, financial resources for infant feeding

Breastfeeding Guidance

Feeding guidance will be based on the mother's plan for feeding her baby (ie, breastfeeding, formula feeding, or a combination of both) and any perceived barriers or contraindications to breastfeeding. The Prenatal Visit is a perfect opportunity to address any concerns parents have about breastfeeding their newborn, provide information, and dispel any myths the parents may have heard. A woman's knowledge about newborn feeding is significantly linked with a decision to breastfeed. Potential barriers to successfully meeting the mother's breastfeeding goals, such as pain, worry about how much the baby is getting, returning to work, embarrassment, and family influences, should be discussed along with strategies to overcome them. Relevant information and appropriate resources should be given. Maternal history of breast surgery or implants or past breastfeeding concerns may need in-depth discussions, and a lactation consultant may be a resource to provide support and answer these questions. In addition, pregnant women may benefit from attending local community breastfeeding support group meetings, such as through the health department or La Leche League (**www.llli.org**). These meetings provide role models and peer support for breastfeeding.

Mothers with a strong family history of allergies need to understand that their babies may benefit from breastfeeding through the first year of life.

Mothers who are considering combining breastfeeding and formula feeding should be counseled to wait until lactation is well established (usually 2–4 weeks) before introducing formula. Discuss the benefits of exclusive breastfeeding and breastfeeding duration. Ultimately, the decision is up to the mother (parents), and the health care professional should respect the decision and understand that the mother may change her mind by the time the baby arrives.

Sample Questions

What are your plans for feeding your baby? What have you heard about breastfeeding? Do you have questions about breastfeeding that I can answer for you? What kinds of experiences have you had feeding babies? Did you breastfeed your other children? How did that go? Do you have concerns about these experiences that we should talk about if they will affect the new baby? Do you have any concerns about having support for breastfeeding, privacy, having enough breast milk, or changes in your body? Have you had any breast surgery? Do you or does anyone in your family have a history of food allergy or intolerance?

Have you attended any classes that taught you how to breastfeed your baby? Do you know anyone who breastfeeds her baby? Did any of your family or friends breastfeed? Would you be able to get help from them as you are learning to breastfeed? Will they support your decision? Do you have a breast pump? If you plan to return to work, do you have time, space, and enough privacy to use a breast pump?

Anticipatory Guidance

- Successful breastfeeding begins with knowledge and information. Prenatal classes through local hospitals can be very helpful for new parents. In addition, many communities have lactation consultants and nurses who are available to assist with breastfeeding. Having these resources available helps you be comfortable with breastfeeding and can help you get off to a good start.

- Put your baby to the breast as soon as possible after the baby is born. Start in the delivery room if you can.

- Breastfeeding exclusively for about the first 6 months of life, and then combining it with solid foods from 6 to 12 months of age, provides the best nutrition and supports the best possible growth and development. You can continue to breastfeed for as long as you and your baby want.

Prescription or Nonprescription Medications or Drugs

Share information about the known effects for an expectant mother of any drugs, medications, or herbal or traditional health remedies that she may be taking. If the mother is planning on breastfeeding, provide information about the safety of continued medication or herbal use while breastfeeding. (Many herbal teas contain ephedra and other substances that may be harmful to the baby.)

A general vitamin-mineral supplement that contains 100% of the daily recommended intake for iron, vitamin D, folic acid, and vitamin B_{12} is recommended for all women who are breastfeeding. Women should also be encouraged to drink plenty of fluids and to eat a healthy diet while breastfeeding. Docosahexaenoic acid supplements are generally safe to consume during pregnancy and lactation.

Sample Questions

Are you taking any prescribed or over-the-counter medications now or have you taken any in the past? Have you used any special or traditional health remedies to improve your health since you have been pregnant? Do you drink alcohol, drink any special teas, or take any herbs? Is there anything that you were taking, but stopped using when you learned that you were pregnant?

Anticipatory Guidance

- Because some medications, herbs, or, especially, alcohol can be passed into human milk, it is important to know what these might be so that you can be advised appropriately when you are breastfeeding.

INFANCY
PRENATAL VISIT

Family Support of Breastfeeding

Most mothers are able to successfully breastfeed their babies. Babies with medical conditions that make breastfeeding challenging may still breastfeed. Their mothers benefit greatly from appropriate breastfeeding consultation and close monitoring. Babies who have a very low birth weight or have special health care needs particularly benefit from expressed human milk if they are unable to breastfeed from their mother.

Describe actions that the other parent or caregiver can take to support breastfeeding, including cuddling, bathing, and diapering the baby. Family members, significant others, or friends should be included in breastfeeding education. Share options for engaging family members in the care of both the mother and baby. Provide information about community resources if the mother does not have an adequate, positive family and friend support network.

Emphasize the need for a follow-up visit within 48 to 72 hours of discharge at the health care professional's office, to check on the baby's feeding, weight, and how the mother is doing and whether she has any questions or concerns. Other options for breastfeeding follow-up may include a visit by a home health nurse, if this is covered by insurance, or by a public health nurse, if available. Provide parents with specific information about who they may contact with questions. Encourage parents with phrases such as, "From our discussion, it seems you are going to do very well with breastfeeding."

Sample Question
Do you know how to contact support groups or lactation consultants?

Anticipatory Guidance
- Resources for help with breastfeeding are available through the hospital, lactation consultants, and some public health programs.
- We will be able to answer your breastfeeding questions and help you get the support that you need to be successful.

Formula-Feeding Guidance

For babies who are unable to breastfeed or tolerate expressed human milk (classic galactosemia), or parents who choose not to breastfeed, iron-fortified formula is the recommended alternative for feeding the baby during the first year of life.

An explanation of the rationale for iron fortification, that iron-fortified formulas are well tolerated, and that studies show that iron-fortified formulas do not cause constipation, can help ensure that parents choose iron-fortified formula.

Encourage parents to discuss choice of formula and any proposed changes in formula with the health care professional. Review steps for preparing formula and reinforce the need to carefully read the directions on the cans. Mixing directions differ among powdered formulas. Provide written information about the importance of food safety with formula, including heating and cleaning bottles and nipples.

Sample Questions

What have you read or heard about the different infant formulas, such as iron-fortified, soy, lactose-free, and others? Would you like some guidance about choosing an appropriate formula for your baby? How do you plan to prepare the formula? What have you heard about formula safety? Do you have any other questions about formula feeding?

Anticipatory Guidance

- If you are unable to breastfeed or choose not to breastfeed your baby, iron-fortified formula is the recommended substitute for breast milk for feeding your full-term baby during the first year of life.

Financial Resources for Infant Feeding

Parents may need referrals about resources for community food or nutrition assistance programs for which they are eligible (eg, Commodity Supplemental Food Program, SNAP, or WIC), and housing or transportation, if needed. The WIC provides nutritious foods for infants and children, foods for mothers who breastfeed, nutrition education, peer support for breastfeeding, and referrals to health and other social services. Mothers who choose to breastfeed can receive enhanced food packages, breast pumps, breastfeeding supplies, and support through peer counselors.

Sample Questions

Are you concerned about having enough money to buy food or infant formula? Would you be interested in resources that may help you afford to care for you and your baby?

Anticipatory Guidance

- Programs and resources are available to help you and your baby. You may be eligible for food, nutrition, or housing or transportation assistance programs. Several food programs, such as the Commodity Supplemental Food Program and SNAP, can help you. The SNAP used to be called Food Stamps. If you are breastfeeding and eligible for WIC, you can get nutritious food for yourself and support from peer counselors.

Priority

Safety

Car safety seats, heatstroke prevention, safe sleep, pets, firearm safety, safe home environment

Car Safety Seats

Although the rate of motor vehicle crash injury deaths has declined over time, it is still the leading cause of death in childhood. Car safety seats significantly reduce the risk of death and injury and are essential for every trip in any vehicle, starting with the first ride home from the hospital. The type of transportation the family uses will determine counseling about car safety seats. Many families rely on other family members or friends for transportation and may not be familiar with car safety seat information. It is important to explore the parents' beliefs about seat belt use and their understanding of car safety seat use for infants. The family must obtain a car safety seat and learn how to install it properly before the birth, so this visit is a good opportunity to review this information.

The parents' own safe driving behaviors (including using seat belts at all times, not driving under the influence of alcohol or drugs, and not using a cell phone or other handheld device) are important to the health of their children. The use of seat belts during pregnancy is especially critical. Lap belts should be worn below the belly and shoulder belts across the mid-chest.

Sample Questions

Do all members in the family use a seat belt every time they ride in the car? What type of car safety seat do you have for the baby? Have you tried installing it?

Anticipatory Guidance

- Using a seat belt during pregnancy is the best way to protect you and your unborn baby, even if your vehicle has an air bag and even when you ride in the back seat. Wear the lap belt across your hips/pelvis and below your belly; place the shoulder belt across your chest between your breasts and away from your neck; and move your seat as far away from the steering wheel as you can while still allowing you to drive easily.
- All babies and children younger than 2 years should always ride in a rear-facing car safety seat in the back seat of the car. There are different types of rear-facing car safety seats. Rear-facing–only seats have a carry handle and typically attach to a base that stays installed in the vehicle. Convertible and 3-in-1 car safety seats are used in the rear-facing position and later convert in the forward-facing position. They typically have higher height and weight limits for the rear-facing position, allowing you to keep your child rear facing for a longer period of time. However, they may not fit small newborns as well as rear-facing–only seats. Do not use any extra products, like cold-weather buntings or inserts, that did not come in the box with the car safety seat. If the weather is cold, tuck a blanket around the baby over the straps.

- Bring your newborn home from the hospital in a rear-facing car safety seat, as this provides the best protection for infants and toddlers. You can choose either a rear-facing–only seat or a convertible car safety seat. The car safety seat should be installed in the back seat of the vehicle at the angle recommended by the manufacturer. If you use a convertible seat, choose one with a lower weight limit for rear facing that is no more than the weight of your baby.
- Even if you do not own a vehicle, you should still have a car safety seat for your child and know how to install it when you are riding in a taxi or in someone else's vehicle.
- Learn how the car safety seat straps are adjusted and how to install the seat in your vehicle. You can get help from a local certified Child Passenger Safety Technician. The National Highway Traffic Safety Administration (NHTSA) also has information for parents on its Web site that includes videos on how to install and use a child's car safety seat.
- Your own safe driving habits are important to the health of your children. Always use a seat belt and never drive under the influence of alcohol or drugs. Don't text or use cell phones or other handheld devices while you are driving.
- Never put a rear-facing car safety seat in the front seat of a vehicle.

For information about car safety seats and actions to keep your baby safe in and around cars, visit the NHTSA Web site at www.safercar.gov/parents.

Find a Child Passenger Safety Technician: http://cert.safekids.org. Click on "Find a Tech."

Toll-free Auto Safety Hotline: 888-327-4236

Heatstroke Prevention

Each year, children die of heatstroke after being left in a car that becomes too hot. More than half of the deaths are infants and children younger than 2 years. In most cases, the parent or caregiver forgot the child was in the car, often because there was a change in the usual routine or schedule. Even very loving and attentive parents can forget a child in the car. Additionally, some children have died while playing in the vehicle or after getting in the vehicle without the caregiver's knowledge.

The temperature inside a car can rise to a dangerous level quickly, even when the temperature outside is as low as 60 degrees. Leaving the windows open will not prevent heatstroke. Because children have proportionally less surface area than adults and less ability to regulate internal temperature, their bodies overheat up to 5 times more quickly than adults' bodies.

Parents should establish habits early to help prevent their baby from being forgotten in a vehicle.

Sample Question
Every year, babies die of heatstroke after being left in a hot car. Would you like to talk about creating a plan so this doesn't happen to you?

Anticipatory Guidance

- Never leave your child alone in a car for any reason, even briefly.
- Start developing habits that will help prevent you from ever forgetting your baby in the car. Consider putting your purse, cell phone, or employee identification in the back seat to help form the habit of checking the back seat before you walk away.
- Check the back seat before walking away, every time you park your vehicle.

Safe Sleep

The incidence of sleep-related infant death has been dramatically reduced by safe sleep policies promoted in the past 15 years.[5,6] Sudden unexpected infant death (SUID) describes sudden infant death that is explained or unexplained. After autopsy, case review, and death scene investigation, a SUID may be determined to be caused by asphyxiation, suffocation, parental overlie, infection, or other medical causes. The diagnosis of SIDS is reserved for infant deaths that are unexpected and unexplained. Culturally sensitive information should be provided about what is known about safe sleep environments for babies.

A supine position ("back to sleep") is best for babies, including premature babies, because of the reduction of SIDS. However, parents should avoid using wedges or other positioning devices, as they are a suffocation hazard. Room sharing is recommended, with the baby in a separate, but nearby, sleep space. Bed sharing (sleeping in the same bed as the parents, another adult, or a child) is not recommended. Bed sharing increases the risk of SUID. Likewise, sleeping together on a non-bed surface, such as a sofa or chair, places a baby at risk for entrapment, suffocation, and death. It is important to explore the parents' intended infant sleep practices at home and to offer guidance to ensure the safest sleep environment for the newborn.

Common beliefs and concerns expressed by families as justification for not placing their babies to sleep in the supine position include the fear of infant choking/aspiration, perceived uncomfortable/less peaceful sleep, concern about a flat occiput and hair loss, and family beliefs about appropriate infant sleep patterns, position, and sleep location. Different cultures may view infant sleep differently than current safe sleep recommendations. These concerns should be sought and discussed with the parents.

Swaddling can be a useful calming technique with an *awake* infant and is appropriately used for positioning in early breastfeeding. However, swaddling is no longer generally recommended and it is *not for sleep*. Swaddled infants have been associated with a 3-fold increase in SUID when compared to infants in a footed blanket sleeper or a sleepsack. Before 2 months of age, if parents swaddle their awake infant, they should be encouraged to remove the wrap before putting their baby down for sleep because this can establish a habit that can be hard to change and the risk of harm appears to increase with age. After 2 months of age, swaddling should *never* be used for sleep. Deaths have been reported among babies 2 to 2½ months of age who are swaddled and end up on their stomachs. Tight swaddling for a prolonged period of time is a risk factor for worsening of developmental hip dysplasia. Recommendations for what is now referred to as "modern swaddling" for *awake* infants in their parent's arms are based on the principle that infants have startle reflexes they are not able to control. If the blanket is snug around the chest, but loose around the legs, infants have the benefits of swaddling without the risk to the hips. The blanket should be loose enough at the chest that a hand can fit between the blanket and the baby's chest, but not so loose that it unravels. There is currently no evidence supporting a safe swaddling technique for sleep.

Parents need strategies that will assist them in engaging relatives, friends, and child care providers to follow safe sleep practices for the baby. A consistent message about back to sleep provides family members with the best information.

Sample Questions

What have you heard about safe sleep for infants? Where will your baby sleep? How about at naptime?

Anticipatory Guidance

- It is best to always have your baby sleep on her back because it reduces the risk of sudden infant death. We recommend this sleep position for babies even if they are born premature or have problems with reflux, which is frequent vomiting after feeding. Do not use a wedge or other product to keep your baby on her back, as the baby can wiggle down and suffocate against the wedge.

- For at least the first 6 months, your baby should sleep in your room in her own crib, but not in your bed. Think about some strategies you might use to soothe your baby without bringing her into your bed, where the risks of suffocation, entrapment, and death are increased.

- If possible, use a crib purchased after June 28, 2011, as cribs sold in the United States after that date are required to meet a new, stronger safety standard. If you use an older crib, choose one with slats that are no more than 2⅜ inches (60 mm) apart and with a mattress that fits snugly, with no gaps between the mattress and the crib slats. Drop-side cribs are no longer recommended.

- If you choose a mesh play yard or portable crib, consider choosing one that was manufactured after a new, stronger safety standard was implemented on February 28, 2013. If you use an older product, the weave should have openings less than ¼ inch (6 mm) and the sides should always stay fully raised.

- The baby's sleep space should be kept empty, with no toys or soft bedding, such as pillows, bumpers, or blankets.

- The safest cover for the baby is a sleepsack or footed pajamas that can keep the baby warm without concern about suffocating under a blanket. This also allows the baby to move her legs as opposed to swaddling, which has the potential to cause poor development of her hips and increases your baby's risk of suffocation and death.

- Some babies with very sensitive startle reflexes appear more comfortable having their arms close to their body. Swaddling can help with this sensitivity. If you swaddle your baby, be sure to keep it loose around her legs, but snug—not tight—around her chest. To make sure your baby can breathe, leave enough space so that you can fit your hand between the blanket and her chest. Also, be sure that there are no loose ends of blanket around her neck, as these can increase your baby's risk of suffocating.

- Swaddling should only be used with babies younger than 2 months and is recommended only when your baby is awake. Older babies can roll over and risk suffocation if they are swaddled.

Pets

Pet guidance is based on the specific animals in the home (eg, domestic and exotic birds, cats, dogs, ferrets, or reptiles). Discussion points may include the need for maintaining physical separation of the pet from the child, introducing the pet to the new baby, avoiding contact with animal waste, the importance of handwashing, and limiting indoor air contamination with animal dander or waste products.

Sample Questions

Do you have any pets at home or do you handle any animals? If you have handled cats, have you ever been tested for antibodies to a parasitic infection called toxoplasmosis that some cats are infected with?

Anticipatory Guidance

- Pets may be dangerous for babies and young children. Cats and dogs can become jealous just like humans. Learn about the risks that may occur with your pets and determine the best method of protecting your baby.
- If you work with or handle cats, we suggest that you talk to your own health care professional about getting tested for toxoplasmosis.

Firearm Safety

Discuss firearm safety in the home and the danger to family members and children. Homicide and suicide are more common in homes in which firearms are kept. The AAP recommends that firearms be removed from the places children live and play, and that, if it is necessary to keep a firearm, it should be stored unloaded and locked, with the ammunition locked separately from the firearm.

Sample Questions

Do you keep firearms at home? Are they unloaded and locked? Is the ammunition locked and stored separately? Are there firearms in the homes where you visit, such as the homes of grandparents, other relatives, or friends?

Anticipatory Guidance

- Homicide and suicide and unintentional firearm injuries are more common in homes that have firearms. The best way to keep your child safe from injury or death from firearms is to never have a firearm in the home.
- If it is necessary to keep a firearm in your home or if the homes of people you visit have firearms, they should be stored unloaded and locked, with the ammunition locked separately from the firearm. Make sure the firearm is stored safely before your baby starts crawling and exploring your home.

Safe Home Environment

Discuss other home safety precautions with parents, including appropriate water heater setting and smoke and carbon monoxide detector/alarms.

Sample Question

What home safety precautions have you taken for your unborn baby or any children in your home?

Anticipatory Guidance

- **To protect your child from tap water scalds, the hottest temperature at the faucet should be no higher than 120°F.** In many cases, you can adjust your water heater.

- Milk and formula should never be heated in the microwave because they can heat unevenly, causing pockets of liquid that are hot enough to scald your baby's mouth.

- Make sure you have a working smoke alarm on every level of your home, especially in the furnace and sleeping areas. Test the alarms every month. It's best to use smoke alarms that use long-life batteries, but, if you don't, change the batteries at least once a year. Plan several escape routes from the house and conduct home fire drills.

- Install a carbon monoxide detector/alarm, certified by Underwriters Laboratories (UL), in the hallway near every separate sleeping area of the home.

Infancy
Newborn Visit

Context

Tremendous excitement accompanies the birth of a baby, but new parents also often feel overwhelmed and fatigued. During the typically short postpartum hospital stay, mothers are recovering from the birth, working to establish exclusive breastfeeding, and getting to know their newborns. At the same time, they are navigating visits from elated family and friends and dealing with frequent interruptions from hospital personnel. During this time, the mother needs to be able to focus on establishing breastfeeding and attaching to and caring for her newborn and herself while she recovers from the delivery.

The number of visits in the immediate newborn period will depend on the mode of delivery and the presence of maternal or neonatal complications. The duration of each visit also will vary, based on the specific needs of the baby and family. Prior parental experience with newborns, the newborn's health status, the new mother's own physical and emotional health needs, and the presence of social support influence the parents' responses and guide the health care professional's interactions with the family. New parents always ask one question first: "Is the baby OK?" Once they hear that the baby is healthy, the parents want to learn how to feed and care for her, establish a good schedule, recover physically and emotionally from the birth, and go home to begin their new adventure.

Examining the newborn in the mother's room within the first 24 hours following delivery gives the health care professional an important opportunity to learn more about the family and to demonstrate the newborn's abilities, observe the parents' interactions with the baby, and model behaviors that engage and support the newborn during this transition time. The health care professional can assess the newborn's response to voices and other forms of stimulation, such as noises in the room, touch, light, movement, being undressed, and being comforted. If this visit also is the first meeting between the health care professional and the mother, questions from the Prenatal Visit may need to be incorporated into this visit to gain a more comprehensive understanding of the family's values and beliefs, strengths, resources, and needs.

This interaction with the family gives the health care professional the chance to build a medical home partnership with the family. Answering questions and addressing concerns during this visit will reassure parents and lessen the anxiety they may be feeling about taking their baby home. Knowing that the health care professional will be available after they leave the hospital will add to the parents' comfort and confidence as they embark on this new phase of their lives.

Priorities for the Newborn Visit

The first priority is to attend to the concerns of the parents.

In addition, the Bright Futures Infancy Expert Panel has given priority to the following topics for discussion in this visit:

▶ Social determinants of health[a] (risks [living situation and food security, environmental tobacco exposure, intimate partner violence, maternal alcohol and substance use], strengths and protective factors [family support, parent-newborn relationship])

▶ Parent and family health and well-being (maternal health and nutrition, transition home [assistance after discharge], sibling relationships)

▶ Newborn behavior and care (infant capabilities, baby care [infant supplies, skin and cord care], illness prevention, calming your baby)

▶ Nutrition and feeding (general guidance on feeding, breastfeeding guidance, formula-feeding guidance)

▶ Safety (car safety seats, heatstroke prevention, safe sleep, pets, safe home environment)

---

[a] Social determinants of health is a new priority in the fourth edition of the *Bright Futures Guidelines*. For more information, see the *Promoting Lifelong Health for Families and Communities* theme.

Health Supervision

The *Bright Futures Tool and Resource Kit* contains Previsit Questionnaires to assist the health care professional in taking a history, conducting developmental surveillance, and performing medical screening.

History

The prenatal and birth history may be obtained according to the concerns of the family and the health care professional's preference or style of practice.

General Questions

- How did you and your partner feel about becoming a parent when you first found out you were pregnant? How was the delivery? How are you feeling now?
- Have you named the baby yet? *(Families may delay naming because of cultural beliefs.)*
- Has the baby been able to stay with you since your delivery? Were you able to spend time with the baby skin-to-skin and breastfeed after the baby was born?
- How have things been going with the baby? *(Use the baby's name if it is given.)*
- What questions do you have about your baby? Do you have any concerns about taking care of your baby?

Prenatal, Labor, and Delivery History

- Prenatal history
  - Pregnancy history, including maternal conditions potentially affecting the baby's health—preexisting maternal health conditions (asthma, diabetes, obesity, poor oral health, thyroid disease, chronic cardiac or kidney disease), pregnancy complications (gestational diabetes, hypertensive disorders of pregnancy), special dietary restrictions, infections (group B *Streptococcus*, chorioamnionitis, urinary tract infection, HIV, hepatitis B, sexually transmitted infections, toxoplasmosis, cytomegalovirus)
- Prenatal diagnoses and maternal or fetal interventions
  - Maternal medications, including mental health prescriptions; vitamin, mineral, and other nutrition-related supplements; complementary medicine; environmental exposures
- Maternal or family use of tobacco, alcohol, or other drugs
- Prior adverse pregnancy outcome

Delivery

- Mother's hepatitis B, HIV, group B *Streptoccocus,* and blood group and Rh status
- Preterm labor, premature rupture of the membranes
- Mode of delivery—vaginal or cesarean; indication for cesarean; instrumentation—forceps, vacuum
- Medications used—tocolytics, magnesium sulfate, pitocin, analgesics, antenatal steroids, antibiotics
- Anesthesia used—epidural, spinal, general
- Use of episiotomy (degree) or lacerations
- Duration of labor, length of delivery, indications for delivery/induction
- Complications of labor and delivery—fever, infection, bleeding, preeclampsia including HELLP syndrome (hemolysis, elevated liver enzymes, and low platelet count) and toxemia

Newborn at Delivery

- Delivery history
  - Fetal distress—heart rate tracing abnormalities, decreased fetal movement, meconium-stained amniotic fluid, oligohydramnios or polyhydramnios, mode of delivery
  - Complications—intrauterine growth restriction, macrosomia, maternal hypertensive disease, diabetes, infection, intrapartum anesthesia/analgesia or other medical conditions affecting the fetus or newborn (eg, antenatal diagnosis of hydronephrosis), birth trauma
  - Gestational age, birth weight, and Apgar score; appropriateness of growth
  - Newborn transition problems—respiratory distress, cyanosis, hypoglycemia, poor feeding, temperature instability, jitteriness, lethargy
- Risk of withdrawal from maternal substance use
- Administration of vitamin K and eye prophylaxis

Neonatal Course

Information obtained about the postnatal course of the mother and newborn will influence further interactions, assessments, and recommendations for the care of the newborn and mother. This information includes underlying maternal health, including the level of maternal discomfort and pain medication use, effect on and interaction with baby, perspectives on breastfeeding, attempts at breastfeeding, and perceived success with breastfeeding.

Neonatal History and Initial Assessments

- Newborn blood type and direct Coombs test.
- Vital signs (temperature, respirations, heart rate).
- If at risk, newborn's blood sugar.
- Weight loss/gain.
- Feeding history—breastfeeding LATCH scores,[7] frequency, duration.
- Type of infant formula used, if not breastfeeding.
- State regulation and sleep pattern—ease of awakening, pattern of sleep-wake, and duration of sleep cycles.
- Elimination pattern—meconium passage, number of wet diapers.
- Risk assessment for severe neonatal jaundice—blood group incompatibility, prematurity, racial background, exclusive breastfeeding and not feeding well; recommendations for follow-up after discharge.
- Presence of 1 major anomaly or 3 or more minor anomalies, a combination of major and minor anomalies, or a recognized pattern or distribution of anomalies suggesting a need for genetic evaluation.
- The family's cultural beliefs relating to illness and disability, and their reaction to screening, particularly if the screening is mandated. Screening requirements may violate some cultural and religious beliefs. If the family's religious or cultural beliefs include acceptance of disabilities or illness, pursuit of some types of interventions may not fit family values.

Family History

- A comprehensive family health history is recommended to be obtained at the 1 Month Visit. Health care professionals wishing to record a family history at this visit can find a questionnaire in the *Bright Futures Tool and Resource Kit*.

Social History

- See the Social Determinants of Health priority in Anticipatory Guidance for social history questions.

Surveillance of Development

What have you heard about what newborns can do at birth?

Clinicians using the *Bright Futures Tool and Resource Kit* Previsit Questionnaires or another tool that includes a developmental milestones checklist, or those who use a structured developmental screening tool, need not ask about these developmental surveillance milestones. *(For more information, see the Promoting Healthy Development theme.)*

Social Language and Self-help

Does your child

- Have periods of wakefulness?
- Look at and study you when awake?
- Look in your eyes when being held?
- Calm when picked up?
- Respond differently to soothing touch and alerting touch?

Verbal Language (Expressive and Receptive)

Does he

- Communicate discomfort through crying and through behaviors such as facial expressions, body movements, and movement of arms and legs?
- Move or calm to your voice?

Gross Motor

Does she

- Move in response to visual or auditory stimuli?
- Move her arms and legs symmetrically and reflexively when startled?

Fine Motor

Does he

- Keep his hands in a fist?
- Automatically grasp others' fingers or objects?

Review of Systems

The Bright Futures Infancy Expert Panel recommends a complete review of systems as a part of every health supervision visit. This review can be done by asking the following questions:

Do you have concerns about your newborn's

- Head
  - Shape
- Eyes
  - Discharge
- Ears, nose, and throat
- Breathing
- Stomach or abdomen
  - Vomiting or spitting
  - Bowel movements
  - Umbilical stump
- Genitals or rectum
- Skin
- Development
  - Muscle strength, movement of arms or legs, any developmental concerns

Observation of Parent-Newborn Interaction

During the visit, the health care professional acknowledges and reinforces positive parent-newborn interactions and discusses any concerns. Observation focuses on

- Who asks questions and who provides responses to questions?
- Do the verbal and nonverbal behaviors/communication between family members indicate support, understanding, or differences of opinion/conflicts?
- Do the parents recognize and respond to the baby's needs?
- Are they comfortable when feeding, holding, or caring for the baby?
- Do they have visitors or any other signs of a support network?

Physical Examination

A complete physical examination is included as part of every health supervision visit.

When performing a physical examination, the health care professional's attention is directed to the following components of the examination that are important for a newborn this age:

- **Measure and plot on appropriate World Health Organization (WHO) Growth Chart**
  - Recumbent length
  - Weight
  - Head circumference
  - Weight-for-length

- **General observations**
  - Assess alertness and if in any apparent distress.
  - Observe for congenital anomalies.

- **Skin**
  - Note skin lesions or jaundice.

- **Head**
  - Observe shape (sutures, molding), size, and fontanels.
  - Note evidence of birth trauma.

- **Eyes**
  - Inspect eyes and eyelids.
  - Examine pupils for opacification and red reflexes.
  - Assess visual acuity using fixate and follow response.

- **Ears**
  - Observe shape and position of pinnae, patency of auditory canals, and presence of pits or tags.

- **Nose**
  - Observe for patency, septal deviation.

- **Oral**
  - Note clefts of lip or palate.
  - Note presence of natal teeth, Epstein pearls.

- **Heart**
  - Auscult rate, rhythm, heart sounds, murmurs.
  - Palpate femoral pulses.

- **Abdomen**
  - Examine umbilical cord and cord vessels.

- **Genitalia/rectum**
  - Determine that testes are descended; observe for penile anomalies or labial or vaginal anomalies.
  - Assess position and patency of anus.

- **Musculoskeletal**
  - Note any deformities of the back and spine.
  - Note any foot or arm/hand abnormalities.
  - Palpate clavicles for crepitus.

- **Developmental hip dysplasia**
  - Perform Ortolani and Barlow maneuvers.
- **Neurologic**
  - Demonstrate primitive reflexes.
  - Observe symmetry of limb posture and extremity movement.
  - Observe muscle tone.

Screening

Universal Screening	Action
Hearing	All newborns should receive an initial hearing screening before being discharged from the hospital.[a]
Newborn: Bilirubin	All newborns should be screened for hyperbilirubinemia before nursery discharge or at the first newborn visit if the baby is born at home or at a birth facility.
Newborn: Blood	Conduct screening as required by state-specific newborn screening requirements. Know the conditions that are screened for in your state.
Newborn: Critical Congenital Heart Disease	All newborns should be screened for critical congenital heart disease using pulse oximetry before nursery discharge or at the first newborn visit if the baby is born at home or at a birth facility.

Selective Screening	Risk Assessment[b]	Action if Risk Assessment Positive (+)
Blood Pressure	Children with specific risk conditions	Blood pressure measurement
Vision	+ on risk screening questions	Ophthalmology referral

[a] Any newborn who does not pass the initial screen must be rescreened. Any failure at rescreening should be referred for a diagnostic audiologic assessment, and any newborn with a definitive diagnosis should be referred to the state Early Intervention Program.

[b] See the *Evidence and Rationale chapter* for the criteria on which risk screening questions are based.

Immunizations

Discuss the importance of routine newborn hepatitis B immunization before discharge. Verify that the mother is hepatitis surface antigen negative.

Babies younger than 6 months are at risk of complications from influenza, but are too young to be vaccinated for seasonal influenza. Encourage **influenza vaccine** for caregivers of babies younger than 6 months and recommend **pertussis immunization (Tdap)** for adults who will be caring for the baby.

Consult the CDC/ACIP or AAP Web sites for the current immunization schedule.

CDC National Immunization Program: **www.cdc.gov/vaccines**

AAP *Red Book:* **http://redbook.solutions.aap.org**

Anticipatory Guidance

The following sample questions, which address the Bright Futures Infancy Expert Panel's Anticipatory Guidance Priorities, are intended to be used selectively to invite discussion, gather information, address the needs and concerns of the family, and build partnerships. Use of the questions may vary from visit to visit and from family to family. Questions can be modified to match the health care professional's communication style. The accompanying anticipatory guidance for the family should be geared to questions, issues, or concerns for that particular baby and family. Tools and handouts to support anticipatory guidance can be found in the *Bright Futures Tool and Resource Kit*.

Priority

Social Determinants of Health

Risks: Living situation and food security, environmental tobacco exposure, intimate partner violence, maternal alcohol and substance use

Strengths and protective factors: Family support, parent-newborn relationship

Risks: Living Situation and Food Security

Parents in difficult living situations or with limited means may have concerns about their ability to care for their newborn. Provide information and referrals, as needed, for community resources that help with finding quality child care, accessing transportation or getting a car safety seat or an infant crib so that the baby can sleep safely, or addressing issues such as financial concerns, inadequate or unsafe housing, or limited food resources. Public health agencies can be excellent sources of help because they work with all types of community agencies and family needs. Facilitate referrals.

Sample Questions

Tell me about your living situation. Do you live in an apartment or a house? Is permanent housing a worry for you?

Do you have the things you need to take care of the baby, such as a crib, a car safety seat, and diapers? Does your home have enough heat, hot water, electricity, and working appliances? Do you have health insurance for yourself? How about for the baby?

Within the past 12 months, were you ever worried whether your food would run out before you got money to buy more? Within the past 12 months, did the food you bought not last and you did not have money to get more?

Anticipatory Guidance

- Community agencies are available to help you with concerns about your living situation.
- Programs and resources are available to help you and your baby. You may be eligible for the WIC food and nutrition program, or housing or transportation assistance programs. Several food programs, such as the Commodity Supplemental Food Program and SNAP, the program formerly known as Food Stamps, can help you. If you are breastfeeding and eligible for WIC, you can get nutritious food for yourself and support from peer counselors.

Risks: Environmental Tobacco Exposure

Address how smoking affects a baby's health and increases the baby's chance for respiratory infections, SIDS, ear infections, and asthma. Provide smoking cessation strategies and make specific referrals. If one or both of the parents quit during the pregnancy, congratulate them and encourage them to continue to remain abstinent from tobacco.

Sample Questions

Did you smoke or use e-cigarettes before or during this pregnancy? Does anyone in your home smoke or use e-cigarettes? Have you been able to cut down the daily number of cigarettes? Do you know where to get help with stopping smoking?

Anticipatory Guidance

- It's important to keep your car, home, and other places where your baby spends time free of tobacco smoke and e-cigarette vapor. Smoking affects the baby by increasing the risk of asthma, ear infections, respiratory infections, and sudden infant death.
- **800-QUIT-NOW (800-784-8669);** TTY **800-332-8615** is a national telephone helpline that is routed to local resources. Additional resources are available at **www.cdc.gov.** Specific information for women is available at **http://women.smokefree.gov.**

Risks: Intimate Partner Violence

According to the CDC, 1.5 million women are battered each year by their intimate partner and 324,000 of these women are pregnant. Homicide is the leading cause of death for pregnant and recently pregnant women. When inquiring, avoid asking about abuse or domestic violence. Instead, use descriptive terms, such as *hit*, *kicked*, *shoved*, *choked*, and *threatened*. Be mindful about who is with the mother at the time you conduct the visit. If you suspect intimate partner violence, you may not want to ask the question directly, but provide a paper and pencil screening form. Place flyers or information about abuse and intimate partner violence in women's restrooms so that mothers can obtain the information in a safe and confidential manner without threat that the perpetrator may bear witness to it.

To avoid causing upset to families by questioning about sensitive and private topics, such as family violence, alcohol and drug use, and similar risks, it is recommended to begin screening about these topics with an introductory statement, such as, "I ask all patients standard health questions to understand factors that may affect health of their child as well as their own health."

Sample Questions

Because violence is so common in so many people's lives, I've begun to ask about it. I don't know if this is a problem for you, but many children I see have parents who have been hurt by someone else. Some are too afraid or uncomfortable to bring it up, so I've started asking all my patients about it routinely. Do you always feel safe with your partner? Has your partner, or another significant person in your life, ever hit, kicked, or shoved you, or physically hurt you in any way? Has he or she ever threatened to hurt you or someone close to you? Do you have any questions about your safety at home? What will you do if you feel afraid? Do you have a plan? Would you like information on where to go or who to contact if you ever need help? Can we help you develop a safety plan for you and your children?

Anticipatory Guidance

- If your partner, or another significant person in your life, is hitting or threatening you, one way that I and other health care professionals can help you is to support you and provide information about local resources that can help you.
- You can also call the toll-free **National Domestic Violence Hotline** at **800-799-SAFE (7233).**

Risks: Maternal Alcohol and Substance Use

Any substance taken during or after pregnancy should be evaluated for its overall risk to the newborn, including prescription drugs, over-the-counter preparations, pain relievers, herbal substances, and illegal substances.

Any alcohol is a particular risk in pregnancy. If the mother acknowledges alcohol use during pregnancy and this was not previously discussed as part of the prenatal history, discuss the concerns for the developing fetus of both ND-PAE and other FASD. Both ND-PAE and FASD have lifelong effects on the baby that can include physical problems and problems with behavior and learning. Fetal alcohol exposure, including the timing during the pregnancy, quantity, and duration, is important to document for later diagnosis of FASD.

Marijuana should be discontinued during pregnancy and breastfeeding. In utero exposure is associated with impaired cognition and increased sensitivity to drugs of abuse.[8] Data regarding the effects of marijuana on infants are insufficient, but its use should be avoided.

Referrals to community social service agencies and drug treatment programs can be provided if the mother is not already linked to these services. Newborns determined to be at risk can be referred to support programs, such as a local Early Intervention Program agency, often referred to as IDEA Part C.

Sample Questions

How often do you drink beer, wine, or liquor in your household? **For any response other than "Never," ask the following questions:** *In the 3 months before you knew you were pregnant, how many times did you have 4 or more drinks in a day? After you knew you were pregnant, how many times did you have 4 or more drinks in a day?*

Depending on the responses to any of the above questions, the health care professional can, if desired, follow up to determine frequency and extent of consumption by asking the following questions:

During the pregnancy on average, how many days per week did you have a drink? During the pregnancy on a typical day when you had an alcoholic beverage, how many drinks did you have? Do you, or does anyone you ride with, ever drive after having a drink? Does your partner use alcohol? What kind and for how long?

If any maternal at-risk drinking is identified, a brief intervention and referral is recommended.

Are you using marijuana, cocaine, pain pills, narcotics, or other controlled substances? What have you heard about the drug's effects on the baby during pregnancy or after the baby is born? Are you getting any help to cut down/stop your drug use?

Are you taking any medicines or vitamins at the present time? Are you using any prescription or over-the-counter medications or pain relievers? Have you used any health remedies or special herbs or teas to improve your health since you have been pregnant? Is there anything that you used to take, but stopped using when you learned that you were pregnant?

Anticipatory Guidance

- Because alcohol is passed into the breast milk, it is important for mothers to avoid alcohol for 2 to 3 hours before breastfeeding or during breastfeeding. This also means that, because newborns breastfeed so frequently (every 2 to 3 hours), it may be prudent for you to avoid alcohol during the first several months of your baby's life.
- Most medications are compatible with breastfeeding, but should be checked on an individual basis. To understand how any over-the-counter medications or herbal product may affect your baby, it is important to know what you are taking.
- The reason we are concerned about a parent's use of alcohol or drugs is because of the effects on the baby's mental, physical, and social development. Alcohol misuse can harm a parent's interaction with the baby and lead to poor decisions about the baby's care.
- Drug and alcohol cessation programs are available in our community and we would like to help you connect to these services.
- Community agencies are available to help women during their pregnancy as well as after their baby arrives so that they can safely care for their baby and themselves.

Strengths and Protective Factors: Family Support

The newborn period is a time of great adjustment and change for parents. Discuss and provide suggestions about making life easier during the first week at home. Parents need support and help from their family, friends, and community. Many parents feel overwhelmed by a new baby. Knowing appropriate coping strategies can prevent parents from harming their baby when they feel tired, overwhelmed, or frustrated.

Sample Questions

Do you have family and friends you can call who are willing and able to help you and your baby when you have a question or need help, or in case of an emergency? How easily can you get help from others? Is there someone who can help you care for the baby? Can someone help with transportation? Is there someone you can leave the baby with?

Anticipatory Guidance

- It's important to have people you can turn to when you need help with the baby. Consider talking with family members or friends and making arrangements with them so that they can be prepared to help if needed. These people usually are willing to help, but may need specific information about ways in which they can be most helpful.

Strengths and Protective Factors: Parent-Newborn Relationship

Skin-to-skin contact and stimulation is a special way of enhancing the attachment experience for parents and baby, just as breastfeeding does for mother and baby. First-time parents and young parents gain self-confidence and become more proficient in their nurturing abilities through this exchange and it helps to promote child and family development and parental well-being.

Sample Question

What do you do to help the baby feel safe and comfortable?

Anticipatory Guidance

- Make touching your baby (caressing, massaging, holding in your arms or skin-to-skin, carrying, and rocking) an important part of all the everyday care activities of feeding, diapering, bathing, and bedtime. This physical contact helps your baby feel secure and understand that he is loved and cared for. It is a special way for you and your partner to develop a strong bond with your baby and it will help you grow together as a family.
- Physical contact also offers important health and developmental benefits if your baby was premature or has special health care needs. It can improve his sleep, help him regulate his sleep and wake times, and promote the parent-baby attachment that may have been delayed or disrupted because of prolonged or repeated hospitalizations.

Priority

Parent and Family Health and Well-being

Maternal health and nutrition, transition home (assistance after discharge), sibling relationships

Maternal Health and Nutrition

New mothers need to take care of their baby and themselves. This includes getting enough rest and making sure they have adequate resources to feed themselves and their baby. The WIC provides nutritious foods for children, foods for mothers who exclusively breastfeed their babies, nutrition education, and referrals to health and other social services. All breastfeeding mothers should continue to take a prenatal vitamin containing iron. Iron and zinc may be deficient in the diets of certain mothers who have restrictive diets and they may need additional supplementation. Mothers who breastfeed should ingest 500 μg of folate or folic acid daily by taking a daily prenatal vitamin or a multivitamin in addition to eating a nutritious diet.

Sample Questions

Have you been able to get enough rest? What vitamin or mineral supplements do you take or plan to take?

Anticipatory Guidance

- Getting rest is important to your recovery after delivery. It can be difficult while you are in the hospital; you can ask the staff to put a sign on your door saying that you are resting.
- Getting rest or having quiet time to spend with your baby can be a challenge, especially as babies sleep in short stretches at a time, wake easily and often to feed, and are often most awake at night. Don't be afraid to ask visitors to come at times that are convenient for you, or to ask staff members to try to cluster their care, so that you and the baby can have time to get to know each other and establish feeding patterns and recognize feeding cues, and so that you can rest when possible.
- If you are in pain, be sure to let your nurse and obstetric health care professional know so they can make sure you are getting the right pain medicines or treat any problems that are causing you pain.
- You may continue to take your prenatal vitamin with iron every day to ensure adequate intake of vitamins and minerals. If you do not consume any animal products in your diet and follow a vegan diet, your supplement should include vitamins D and B_{12}.

Transition Home (Assistance After Discharge)

It is important to not only assess the newborn's status but also listen and observe for concerns the parents may have in obtaining adequate support during the transition period right after the birth that may indicate the need for a referral to home care services. It also is important to provide contact information for lactation consultants, parenting classes, support groups, community resources, or social services to help parents care for their baby and reduce feelings of isolation.

Sample Questions

When you go home, what are your plans to help you get the rest you need and get back into your usual routines? How do you think your baby will change your lives? Will you be able to take time for yourself, individually and as a couple?

Anticipatory Guidance

- You'll probably want to spend most of your time and attention on the new baby. Taking care of yourself, too, will help you stay healthy and happy for your baby.
- Here are a few suggestions about making life easier the first week at home.
  - Tell family and friends about needing family time with just your baby, and partner, as well as what they can do to really help.
  - Identify the activities that are more difficult for you to do, such as grocery shopping, laundry, and vacuuming, now that you are a new mom so that you can ask others to help.
- Many mothers feel tired or overwhelmed in the first weeks at home. These feelings usually don't last more than 1 to 2 weeks. However, for some mothers, these feelings do last for a long time or seem to get worse as time goes by. If you find that you are continuing to feel very tired, overwhelmed, or depressed, you need to let your partner, your own health care professional, and me know so that we can help you get better.

Sibling Relationships

Parent concerns about sibling reactions to the baby are best guided according to the siblings' developmental ages and responses. Behavior regression and jealousy sometimes occur with older siblings.

Sample Questions

Are there other children in your home? How old are they? How did they respond to your pregnancy and the thought of becoming a big brother/sister? What do they think about the new baby?

Anticipatory Guidance

- Older children in the home may exhibit feelings of insecurity, behavioral regression, or, in some instances, anger or embarrassment with the birth of a sibling. It is important to support the emotional needs of your other children as they adapt to a new sibling and to help them to find a role in the care and emotional support of the baby.
- To help your older children adjust to the new baby and still feel wanted and loved, ask for their help in caring for the baby. Make sure not to ask them to do anything beyond their capability. Do not leave the baby unsupervised with young or inexperienced brothers or sisters.
- Spend individual time every day with your other children doing things they like to do. Provide each of your children with love and reassurance that they are important and loved, and that their place in the family is secure.

Priority

Newborn Behavior and Care

Infant capabilities, baby care (infant supplies, skin and cord care), illness prevention, calming your baby

Infant Capabilities

Encourage parents to learn about their baby's temperament and how it affects the way he relates to the world. Demonstrate the newborn's skills and his competence and readiness to respond to his parents and handle his environment. Acknowledge the parents' abilities as they respond to and care for their newborn to reinforce their sense of competence. By effectively managing stress, parents feel better and can provide more nurturing attention, which enables their child to form a secure attachment. Because families from some cultures may be uncomfortable with publicly praising the newborn because of concerns about this bringing on harm, it may be best to note these skills in a neutral way until ascertaining the parents' feelings about this issue.

Sample Question

How do you think your baby sees, hears, and reacts to you?

Anticipatory Guidance

- Your baby is already beginning to know you. See how he brightens when he hears your voice? He shows you that he likes it when you hold him, feed him, and talk to him. You will soon learn what your baby is trying to tell you when he cries, looks at you, turns away, or smiles.
- From an early age, your baby learns when he hears words spoken. Hearing words spoken by you and other caregivers will help his brain develop.
- Your baby is adjusting to the world around him while learning to let you know what he needs through his cries and movements. Newborns also have to learn how to respond to all the new sights, sounds, and physical contacts, such as touch, they are exposed to after birth. Some babies will have an easy time of this; others will need your help to learn to calm down or soothe themselves.

Baby Care (Infant Supplies, Skin and Cord Care)

Discuss newborn supplies and safety precautions. Most babies use 8 to 12 diapers a day, or a diaper before or after each feeding. Often, this is not a supply or expense that parents anticipate. Thus, this information may be helpful in their decision to use disposable versus cloth diapers.

Parents are often counseled by family members on cultural and family beliefs about skin care. Listening to parents' plans for skin care provides information about how to approach skin-care counseling. Because parents are fearful of touching the "soft spot," they hesitate to wash the baby's scalp, although washing is a safe and necessary practice.

Parents and caregivers need to know about the possibility of some vaginal bleeding in female newborns as a result of maternal hormones.

Sample Questions

What questions do you have about your baby's skin care? Is there any special care or treatment you or your family provides to the umbilical cord?

Anticipatory Guidance

- A newborn's skin is sensitive. Using fragrance-free soaps and lotions for bathing and fragrance-free detergents for washing clothing will reduce the likelihood of rashes. In addition, oils and heavy lotions tend to clog pores and increase the likelihood of rashes. The baby has natural skin oils that are protective and do not need to be removed or altered. Powders are not recommended because of the possibility of inhalation and possible respiratory problems.

- Also, because your baby's skin is sensitive, do not expose him to direct sunlight. As much as possible, keep your baby out of the sun. If he has to be in the sun, use a sunscreen made for children. For babies younger than 6 months, sunscreen may be used on small areas of the body, such as the face and backs of the hands, if adequate clothing and shade are not available.

- Your baby's skin does not need to be washed daily with soap.

- To prevent diaper rash, clean your baby after wet diapers or stools and change his diaper frequently. Good cleaning and air drying before replacing the diaper are best for your baby's skin.

- Current cord care recommendations include air-drying, by keeping the diaper below the cord until the cord falls off, which will happen by about 10 to 14 days. There may be some slight bleeding for a day or two after the cord falls off. Belly bands and alcohol on the cord are not recommended. Call our office if there is a bad smell, redness, or fluid from the cord area.

Illness Prevention

Parents may welcome guidance about issues such as knowing how to keep their baby healthy and strategies for how to prevent illness.

Sample Questions

What suggestions have you heard about things you can do to keep your baby healthy? How do you plan to protect your baby from getting infections?

Anticipatory Guidance

- One of the most important steps in keeping your baby healthy is to wash your hands frequently with soap and water or a non-water antiseptic and always after diaper changes and before feeding your baby. You also should ask all family members and guests to wash their hands before handling the baby.

- Newborns are susceptible to illnesses in the first few months of life and need to be protected from anyone with colds or other illnesses. Outings to gatherings with a lot of people, including restaurants, and movies, should be considered carefully and avoided during cold and flu season.

- As long as you wash your hands before breastfeeding, you can continue to breastfeed through most illnesses that you or your baby have.

- Make sure that you and all adults who will have contact with the newborn have had pertussis and influenza immunizations.

Calming Your Baby

The first weeks with a new baby are a stressful time of transitions in which parents and other family members must learn how to care for the baby and adjust to new roles. New mothers also must focus on their physical recovery from the birth. If there are other children at home, this is a time of adjustment to a new schedule and responsibilities.

Sample Questions

Has your baby been with you since he was born? How has it been having the baby with you? Have you been able to rest or get sleep? What do you do to calm your baby? What do you do if that doesn't work?

Anticipatory Guidance

- The first days and weeks caring for a newborn are exhausting. You and your baby have to get to know each other while, at the same time, you are recovering from giving birth.
- A baby does not cry or fuss to intentionally bother us. When babies cry, it's because they need us. He may be hungry or wet, or too cold or too warm. He is adjusting to his new environment and needs your help to become comfortable.
- As you try to soothe your baby, you will begin to recognize that he may not always be consolable. Actions such as stroking your baby's head or gentle, repetitive rocking may help you calm him.
- Your baby may be calmed if swaddled in your arms while you rock and softly say, "Shush." To ensure safe sleep, remove the swaddling before putting your baby down for sleep.
- Your baby's head is fragile. It is very important to never shake your baby because of the damage this can cause to his head and brain.
- It is normal for parents to feel upset or frustrated sometimes when there's a new baby at home. All parents get upset sometimes. When you have these feelings, put the baby down in a safe place, like a crib or cradle. It helps if you have somebody to call or ask for help when you feel upset.

Priority

Nutrition and Feeding
General guidance on feeding, breastfeeding guidance, formula-feeding guidance

General Guidance on Feeding

Parents find great enjoyment and satisfaction when their newborn feeds. It is a time the newborn is awake and alert, looking intently at her parent. Most parents gauge their early parenting ability with their success in feeding their baby. Therefore, providing guidance, assurance, and early assistance with any feeding concerns is a critical element of the Newborn Visit.

Many parents find early feeding a challenge because of difficulties in waking the newborn and the newborn's immature ability to organize sucking, swallowing, and breathing. Mothers of newborns with special health care needs may benefit from specialized assistance with feeding and nutrition. Consider including a lactation consultant in your medical home to support early and continued attempts at breastfeeding so that mothers can gain confidence.

Observing a feeding episode, whether at the breast or when bottle-feeding, often provides insight into the newborn's neuromotor abilities and the parent-newborn interaction. This examination is of value for all babies, but especially for babies who are at risk of feeding difficulties, or if there is concern about the parent-newborn interaction. The mother's comfort in feeding the newborn, eye contact between the mother and newborn, the mother's interaction with the newborn, the mother's and newborn's responses to distractions in the environment, and the newborn's ability to suck can be assessed with observation. Burping frequency varies for breastfed and formula-fed babies and is affected by technique.

Newborns typically lose 7% to 10% of their birth weight during the first 3 to 4 days of life. Birth weight is typically regained by 14 days of age. A newborn who is growing appropriately will gain on average 20 to 30 g per day after birth weight is regained. Newborns who have not passed urine by 24 hours of age or stool by 48 hours of age will require evaluation.

Sample Question
How many wet diapers and stools has your baby had so far?

Anticipatory Guidance
- The baby's first stools are called meconium. The stools look greenish black and tarry. All babies should have their first stool by 2 days of age. You may notice that your baby is passing frequent meconium stools, especially each time she feeds. Most babies will pass urine by the time they are 1 day old.
- Your baby should have about 6 to 8 wet diapers in 24 hours when she reaches 3 to 4 days of age. She may have stools as frequently as every time she feeds. If you are breastfeeding, your baby's stools will be loose and yellowish. This is normal and is not diarrhea.

Sample Question

How easy is it to burp your baby during or after a feeding?

Anticipatory Guidance

▪ Burp your baby at natural breaks (eg, midway through or after a feeding) by gently rubbing or patting her back while holding her against your shoulder and chest or supporting her in a sitting position on your lap.

Breastfeeding Guidance

Cultural beliefs and family beliefs have an important effect on infant feeding practices. For example, in some cultures, people may believe that colostrum is harmful to the baby and that breastfeeding should not begin until the full milk has come in, or that the addition of formula offers health benefits. Explore what the family thinks about infant feeding and breastfeeding, and provide education that is tailored to their needs or concerns so that the parents can then make an informed decision that is best for them. It is important to get the breastfeeding mother off to a good start by assessing her plans, making sure she is eating healthy foods and taking vitamin and mineral supplements, and that there are no contraindications to breastfeeding. Very few contraindications to breastfeeding exist, and most need to be considered on a case-by-case basis. Breastfeeding is contraindicated for a baby with classic galactosemia. Additional contraindications include HIV-positive status (see the CDC Web site at **www.cdc.gov** for most current recommendations), substance use, tuberculosis (only until treatment is initiated and the mother is no longer infectious), herpetic lesions localized to the breast, and chemotherapy or other contraindicated drugs.

Before talking with the mother about how feedings are going, it is advisable to determine the weight difference from birth (percentage weight loss); the type, frequency, and duration of feedings; and number of wet diapers and stools. These details will give the mother specific information about the adequacy of feeding and to identify any possible concerns.

Mothers who breastfeed should ingest 500 µg of folate or folic acid daily by taking a daily prenatal vitamin or a multivitamin in addition to eating a nutritious diet. The mother's diet should include an average daily intake of 200 mg to 300 mg of the omega-3 long-chain PUFA DHA to guarantee a sufficient concentration of preformed DHA in the milk. This is obtained either through supplementation or consumption of 1 to 2 portions (3 oz each) of fish (eg, herring, canned light tuna, salmon) per week. The concern regarding the possible risk from intake of excessive mercury or other contaminants is offset by the neurobehavioral benefits of an adequate DHA intake and can be minimized by avoiding the intake of 4 types of fish that are high in mercury. These are tilefish, shark, swordfish, and king mackerel. Additionally, the mother's diet should include 550 mg/day of choline because human milk is rich in choline and depletes the mother's tissue stores. In the diets of women, eggs, milk, chicken, beef, and pork are the biggest contributors of choline.

For vegan mothers, who consume no animal products in their diet, a daily multivitamin including iron, zinc, vitamin B₁₂, omega-3 fatty acids, and 550 mg of choline is recommended.

Sample Questions

How is breastfeeding going for you and your baby? What questions or concerns do you have about feeding? Are you having pain with breastfeeding? Are your nipples cracked or sore?

How often does your baby feed? How long does it generally take for a feeding? How does the baby behave during a feeding? Pulls away, arches back, is irritable, or is calm? Has your baby received any other fluids from a bottle?

How does the baby behave after feedings? Is she still rooting? Or does your baby look satisfied?

How do you know whether your baby is hungry? How do you know if she has had enough to eat?

Anticipatory Guidance

- Breastfeeding should not hurt, and pain is a warning sign that something is not right. You may experience nipple tenderness at first, but this should be mild. Anything other than mild tenderness should be checked. Speak with your nurse or lactation professional to make sure your baby is positioned and latching on correctly. She can also help you with treating your sore or cracked nipples.

- Breastfeeding exclusively for about the first 6 months of life provides ideal nutrition and supports the best possible growth and development. For mothers who have difficulties with breastfeeding their baby or who choose not to breastfeed, iron-fortified infant formula is the recommended substitute for breast milk for feeding the full-term infant during the first year of life.

- You should feed your baby when she is hungry. A baby's usual signs of hunger include putting her hand to her mouth, sucking, rooting, pre-cry facial grimaces, and fussing. Crying is a late sign of hunger. You can avoid crying by responding to the baby's subtler cues. Once a baby is crying, feeding may become more difficult, especially with breastfeeding, as crying interferes with latching on.

- In the first days after your delivery, encourage your baby to breastfeed between 8 to 12 times per day. This will ensure that she receives small, but frequent feedings of colostrum, the early milk that helps your baby's immune system and stimulates increased milk production.

- Around day 2 to 4 after delivery, your milk supply increases and you will notice that your breasts feel full and warm. You may notice milk leaking from your breasts. If you have not experienced this increase by day 5, let me know.

- At about 3 to 4 days after birth, babies will often increase the frequency and length of their feedings. They often want to breastfeed very frequently. This is when babies begin to gain weight. They should be back to their birth weight by about 2 weeks of age. As your baby breastfeeds more, you will see your milk supply increase to meet your baby's needs.

- At about 1 week of age, your baby should feed every 1 to 3 hours in the daytime, and every 3 hours at night with one longer 4- to 5-hour stretch between feedings. For the first few weeks, your baby should breastfeed between 8 to 12 times in 24 hours.

- Feed your baby until she seems full. Signs of fullness are gently releasing the nipple, closing the mouth, and relaxing the hands. If she is sleeping more than 4 hours at a time during the first 2 weeks, she should be awakened for feeding. Keeping her close by rooming-in while in the hospital and at home will make it easier for you to recognize her early feeding cues.

- A newborn is usually very alert for the first 3 to 4 hours after delivery, and then is typically sleepy for the rest of the first day. She may need gentle stimulation (such as rocking, patting, or stroking or undressing) and time to come to an alert state for feeding. These movements also are helpful for consoling your baby.

INFANCY NEWBORN VISIT

- Healthy babies do not require anything other than mother's milk. It is not necessary to give your baby anything other than your breast milk unless there is a medical reason.

Formula-Feeding Guidance

If a woman is unable or chooses not to breastfeed, a cow's milk–based, iron-fortified infant formula is the recommended substitute for feeding the full-term infant for the first year of life. Information regarding formula preparation and storage, formula safety, infant holding, and burping should be provided by the birthing hospital staff as part of the routine infant care to ensure safe and appropriate formula preparation and feeding.

Sample Questions

What formula are you planning to use? What do you know about preparing formula and keeping formula safe? How often does your baby feed? How much does your baby take at a feeding? How long does it take to complete a feeding? How does your baby like to be held when you feed her? Are you able to get the baby to burp during or at the end of a feeding? Is the baby falling asleep while you feed her?

Anticipatory Guidance

- Carefully read the instructions on the formula can. It will give you important information about how to prepare the formula and store it safely. The nurses will review how to safely prepare the baby's milk before you go home from the hospital. Talk with me or another health care professional if you have any questions about how to prepare formula or before switching to a different brand or kind of formula.
- Choose plastic bottles made from new, safer plastics or tempered glass baby bottles.
- Never heat a bottle in a microwave. If you wish to warm a bottle, a hot water bath is recommended.
- Formula-fed babies should be fed on cue, usually at least 8 times in 24 hours. The baby's stomach size increases after birth over the first few days. Newborns will typically take ½ to 1 oz per feeding in the first day or 2, and then gradually increase to 1 to 1½ oz by day 2 to 4. Take care not to overfeed your baby.
- Because formula is expensive, you may be hesitant to throw away any that is left in the bottle. For food safety reasons, if your baby has not taken all of the formula at one feeding, you may use it for the next feeding, but be sure to put it back in the refrigerator. Do not mix this formula with new formula. If the formula has been heated and has been out of the refrigerator for 1 hour or more, discard it.
- Do not cut bottle nipples or make the holes larger to increase the amount of formula the baby receives or to speed up feeding times.
- As your baby's appetite increases over time, you will need to prepare and offer larger quantities of formula.
- It is important for you to always hold your baby close when feeding, in a semi-upright position, so that you are able to sense her behavioral cues of hunger, being full, comfort, and distress. Hold your baby so you can look into her eyes during feeding.
- When you feed your baby with a bottle, do not prop the bottle in her mouth. Propping increases the risk that she may choke, get an ear infection, and develop early tooth decay. Holding your baby in your arms and holding the bottle for her gives you a wonderful opportunity for warm and loving interaction with her.

Priority

Safety

Car safety seats, heatstroke prevention, safe sleep, pets, safe home environment

Car Safety Seats

Although the rate of motor vehicle crash injury deaths has declined over time, it is still the leading cause of death in childhood. Car safety seats significantly reduce the risk of death and injury and are essential for every trip in any vehicle, starting with the first ride home from the hospital. The type of transportation the family uses will determine counseling about car safety seats. Many families rely on other family members or friends for transportation and may not be familiar with car safety seat information. It is important to explore the parents' beliefs about seat belt use and their understanding of car safety seat use for infants. The family should have obtained a car safety seat and learned how to install it properly before the birth, so this visit is a good opportunity to check that the family is prepared and knows how to transport the baby safely.

If the baby is born preterm, less than 37' weeks gestation, or is at risk of cardiorespiratory compromise (neurologic impairment, craniofacial anomalies affecting breathing, severe cardiac or pulmonary disease), it is important to ensure that a car safety seat tolerance screening will be performed before the baby is discharged from the hospital. The screening will determine if the baby needs any special precautions during travel or while positioned in the infant seat. For all babies, car safety seats should be used only for travel, not for sleep or positioning outside the vehicle.

The parents' own safe driving behaviors (including using seat belts at all times, not driving under the influence of alcohol or drugs, and not using a cell phone or other handheld device) are important to the health of their children.

Sample Questions

Do all members in the family use a seat belt every time they ride in the car? What type of car safety seat do you have for the baby? Have you tried installing it?

Anticipatory Guidance

- All babies and children younger than 2 years should always ride in a rear-facing car safety seat in the back seat of the car. There are different types of rear-facing car safety seats: rear-facing–only seats have a carry handle and typically attach to a base that stays installed in the vehicle. Convertible and 3-in-1 car safety seats are used rear facing and later convert to forward facing; they typically have higher height and weight limits for the rear-facing position, allowing you to keep your child rear facing for a longer period of time. However, they may not fit small newborns as well as rear-facing–only seats. Do not use any extra products, like cold-weather buntings or inserts, that did not come in the box with the car safety seat. If the weather is cold, tuck a blanket around the baby over the straps.

INFANCY
NEWBORN VISIT

- Bring your newborn home from the hospital in a rear-facing car safety seat, as this provides the best protection for babies. You can choose either a rear-facing–only seat or a convertible car safety seat. The car safety seat should be installed in the back seat of the vehicle at the angle recommended by the manufacturer. If you use a convertible seat, choose one with a lower weight limit for rear facing that is no more than the weight of your baby. Even if you do not own a vehicle, you should still have a car safety seat for your child and know how to install it when you are riding in a taxi or in someone else's vehicle.
- Learn how the car safety seat straps are adjusted and how to install the seat in your vehicle. You can get help from a local certified Child Passenger Safety Technician. The NHTSA also has information for parents on its Web site that includes videos on how to install and properly use a child's car safety seat.
- Your own safe driving habits are important to the health of your children. Always use a seat belt and do not drive under the influence of alcohol or drugs. Don't text or use a cell phone or other handheld device while you are driving.

For information about car safety seats and actions to keep your baby safe in and around cars, visit the NHTSA Web site at www.safercar.gov/parents.

Find a Child Passenger Safety Technician: http://cert.safekids.org. Click on "Find a Tech."

Toll-free Auto Safety Hotline: 888-327-4236

Heatstroke Prevention

Each year, an average of 37 children die of heatstroke after being left in a car that becomes too hot. More than half of the deaths are children younger than 2 years. In most cases, the parent or caregiver forgot the child was in the car, often because there was a change in the usual routine or schedule. Even very loving and attentive parents can forget a child in the car. Additionally, some children have died while playing in the vehicle or after getting in the vehicle without the caregiver's knowledge.

The temperature inside a car can rise to a dangerous level quickly, even when the temperature outside is as low as 60 degrees. Leaving the windows open will not prevent heatstroke. Because children have proportionally less surface area than adults and less ability to regulate internal temperature, their bodies overheat up to 5 times more quickly than adults' bodies.

Parents should establish habits early to help prevent their child from being forgotten in a vehicle.

Sample Question
Every year, children die of heatstroke after being left in a hot car. Would you like to talk about creating a plan so this doesn't happen to you?

Anticipatory Guidance
- Never leave your child alone in a car for any reason, even briefly.
- Start developing habits that will help prevent you from ever forgetting your baby in the car. Consider putting an item that you need, like your purse, cell phone, or employee ID, in the back seat of the vehicle, so you will see the child when you retrieve the item before leaving the car.
- Check the back seat before walking away, every time you park your vehicle.

Safe Sleep

Culturally sensitive information should be provided about what is known about safe-sleep environments for babies. A supine position is best for babies, including premature babies, because it reduces the risk of SIDS. However, parents should avoid using wedges or other positioning devices, as they are a suffocation hazard. Room sharing is recommended, with the baby in a separate, but nearby, sleep space. Bed sharing (sleeping in the same bed as the parents, another adult, or a child) increases the risk of SUID. Parents should never bed share or sleep with their baby in a chair or on a couch. Bed sharing is not required for successful breastfeeding and the clinician can share other approaches for soothing the baby other than putting the baby in their bed. It is important to explore the parents' intended infant sleep practices at home and to offer guidance to ensure the safest sleep environment for the newborn.

Common beliefs and concerns expressed by families as justification for not placing their babies to sleep in the supine position include the fear of infant choking or aspiration, perceived uncomfortable or less peaceful sleep, concern about a flat occiput and hair loss, and family beliefs about appropriate infant sleep patterns, position, and sleep location. Different cultures may view infant sleep differently than current safe sleep recommendations. These concerns should be sought and discussed with the parents.

Swaddling can be a useful calming technique with an *awake* infant and is appropriately used for positioning in early breastfeeding. However, swaddling is no longer generally recommended and it is *not for sleep*. Swaddled infants have been associated with a 3-fold increase in SUID when compared to infants in a footed blanket sleeper or a sleepsack. Before 2 months of age, if parents swaddle their awake infant, they should be encouraged to remove the wrap before putting their baby down because this can establish a habit that can be hard to change and the risk of harm appears to increase with age. After 2 months of age, swaddling should *never* be used for sleep. Deaths have been reported among babies 2 to 2½ months of age who are swaddled and end up on their stomachs. Tight swaddling for a prolonged period of time is a risk factor for worsening of developmental hip dysplasia. Recommendations for what is now referred to as "modern swaddling" for *awake* babies in their parent's arms are based on the principle that babies have startle reflexes they are not able to control. If the blanket is snug around the chest, but loose around the legs, babies have the benefits of swaddling without the risk to the hips. The blanket should be loose enough at the chest that a hand can fit between the blanket and the baby's chest, but not so loose that it unravels. There is currently no evidence supporting a safe swaddling technique for sleep.

Parents need strategies that will assist them in engaging relatives, friends, and child care providers to follow safe sleep practices for the baby. A consistent message about "back to sleep" provides family members with the best information.

Sample Questions

What have you heard about how babies should sleep? Where will your baby sleep? How about at naptime?

Anticipatory Guidance

- It is best to always have your baby sleep on his back because it reduces the risk of sudden death. We recommend this sleep position for babies even if they are born premature or have problems with reflux, which is frequent vomiting after feeding. Do not use a wedge or other product to keep your baby on his back, as he can wiggle down and suffocate against the wedge.
- Your baby should sleep in your room in his own crib, but not in your bed. Think about some strategies you might use to soothe your baby without bringing him into your bed, where the risks of suffocation, entrapment, and death are increased.
- If possible, use a crib purchased after June 28, 2011, as cribs sold in the United States after that date are required to meet a new, stronger safety standard. If you use an older crib, choose one with slats that are no more than 2⅜ inches (60 mm) apart and with a mattress that fits snugly, with no gaps between the mattress and the crib slats. Drop-side cribs are no longer recommended.
- If you choose a mesh play yard or portable crib, consider choosing one that was manufactured after a new, stronger safety standard was implemented on February 28, 2013. If you use an older product, the weave should have openings less than ¼ inch (6 mm) and the sides should always stay fully raised.
- The baby's sleep space should be kept empty, with no toys or soft bedding, such as pillows, bumpers, or blankets.
- The safest cover for the baby is a sleepsack or footed pajamas that can keep him warm without concern about suffocating under a blanket. This also allows the baby to move his legs, as opposed to swaddling, which has the potential to cause poor development of his hips and increases his risk of suffocation and death.
- Newborn sleeping patterns may be different from one baby to another. Usually, in the first few weeks, the baby's pattern may vary from day to day, but most babies will sleep 16 to 20 hours out of 24. They may wake and need to be fed as often as every 1 to 2 hours and often have one period when they sleep for 3 to 4 hours.

Pets

Pet guidance is based on the specific animals in the home (eg, domestic and exotic birds, cats, dogs, ferrets, or reptiles). Discussion points may include the need for maintaining physical separation of the pet from the baby, introducing the pet to the new baby, avoiding contact with animal waste, the importance of handwashing, and limiting indoor air contamination with animal dander or waste products.

Sample Question

Do you have any pets at home or do you handle any animals?

Anticipatory Guidance

- Pets may be dangerous for infants and young children. Cats and dogs can become jealous just like humans. Learn about the risks that may occur with your pets and determine the best method of protecting your baby.

Safe Home Environment

Discuss other home safety precautions with parents.

Sample Question

What home safety precautions have you taken for your baby and any other children in your home?

Anticipatory Guidance

- **To protect your child from tap water scalds, the hottest temperature at the faucet should be no higher than 120°F.** In many cases, you can adjust your water heater.
- If you bathe your baby in the kitchen sink, do not run the dishwasher at the same time. Hot water from the dishwasher can come up the sink drain and scald the baby.
- Milk and formula should not be heated in the microwave because they can heat unevenly, causing pockets of liquid that are hot enough to scald your baby's mouth.
- Make sure you have a working smoke alarm on every level of your home, especially in the furnace and sleeping areas. Test the alarms every month. It's best to use smoke alarms that use long-life batteries, but, if you don't, change the batteries at least once a year. Plan several escape routes from the house and conduct home fire drills.
- Install a UL-certified carbon monoxide detector/alarm in the hallway near every separate sleeping area of the home.

Infancy
First Week Visit (3 to 5 Days)

Context

Families need a clear plan, tailored to their individual needs, for continuing care of their newborn. Current recommendations for timing the initial post-nursery continuing care visit are based on the known health risks for a newborn during the first week of life—jaundice, feeding difficulties, hydration problems that cause excessive weight loss, suspected sepsis, and detection of serious congenital malformations that were not apparent on the initial examinations, but became symptomatic during the first weeks of life. A follow-up visit should, therefore, occur within 3 to 5 days after birth and within 48 to 72 hours after discharge.

Early discharge at 48 hours or less after delivery may be appropriate following the normal vaginal birth of a healthy, full-term newborn (39–40%⁷ weeks' gestation). Late preterm newborns, defined as 34%⁷ to 36%⁷ weeks' gestation, typically require a longer hospitalization. These younger newborns have higher rates of neonatal complications and adverse outcomes when compared with the full-term newborn. In this younger group, the likelihood is greater within the first 2 weeks of life for neonatal morbidities. These include respiratory distress, difficulties with feeding, problems with glucose homeostasis and temperature regulation, suspected sepsis, and severe hyperbilirubinemia requiring specialized newborn care or rehospitalization.

Despite recommendations and evidence supporting the utility of follow-up care within the first week of life for newborns discharged within 48 hours of birth, most of these newborns are not receiving timely post-discharge follow-up care. Early follow-up care may not be feasible in some rural communities and adherence may be poor among families who do not have a previously established medical home. Health care professionals may use a variety of approaches (both office-based and home visits conducted by a hospital home health program, public health nurse, or community outreach worker) to ensure follow-up care within the first week of life.

The recommendation for babies delivered by cesarean delivery and whose hospital stay is 96 hours or longer is for a first office visit up to a week after discharge. The exact timing of this visit depends on the specific issues, health concerns, and needs of the baby and mother. Potential risks to consider at the First Week Visit (3 to 5 Days) include prematurity, risk factors for severe hyperbilirubinemia (blood group incompatibility or other causes of neonatal hemolytic anemia), bruising, cephalohematoma, maternal conditions that may affect the newborn (maternal diabetes, thyroid disease, substance/psychotropic medication use), as well as breastfeeding difficulties or problems with feeding or state regulation (alertness, orientation, and regulatory capacity). Assessment for perinatal depression and observation of parent-newborn interactions are additional aspects of importance to this visit.

The completion of routine newborn screening, including blood, bilirubin, hearing, and critical congenital heart disease tests, needs to be confirmed, available results reviewed, and plans made for communication with the family for pending results.

If these tests were not performed during the newborn's hospital stay, the pediatric primary care professional will need to assess the newborn and ensure that screening is completed in the office, or that the newborn has follow-up appointments for the necessary screening.

Appropriate specialty referral or consultation must be arranged promptly for babies with special health care needs. Mothers and families who have experienced a perinatal complication or the need for specialized newborn care require extra attention, as they may experience depression, anxiety, guilt, a sense of loss of control, reduced satisfaction with the birth experience, and even loss of self-esteem. Family members may need extra support to resolve their feelings and additional time to understand their newborn's condition and appreciate their newborn's unique characteristics and strengths rather than only the newborn's special needs.

Priorities for the First Week Visit (3 to 5 Days)

The first priority is to attend to the concerns of the parents.

In addition, the Bright Futures Infancy Expert Panel has given priority to the following topics for discussion in this visit:

▶ Social determinants of health[a] (risks [living situation and food security, environmental tobacco exposure], strengths and protective factors [family support])

▶ Parent and family health and well-being (transition home, sibling adjustment)

▶ Newborn behavior and care (early brain development, adjustment to home, calming, when to call [temperature taking] and emergency readiness, CPR, illness prevention [handwashing, outings] and sun exposure)

▶ Nutrition and feeding (general guidance on feeding [weight gain, feeding strategies, holding, burping, hunger and satiation cues], breastfeeding guidance, formula-feeding guidance)

▶ Safety (car safety seats, heatstroke prevention, safe sleep, safe home environment: burns)

---

[a] Social determinants of health is a new priority in the fourth edition of the *Bright Futures Guidelines*. For more information, see the *Promoting Lifelong Health for Families and Communities* theme.

Health Supervision

The *Bright Futures Tool and Resource Kit* contains Previsit Questionnaires to assist the health care professional in taking a history, conducting developmental surveillance, and performing medical screening.

History

The interval history may be obtained according to the concerns of the family and the health care professional's preference or style of practice.

General Questions

- Tell me how things are going for you and your baby.
- What questions or concerns do you have at this time?
- How are you feeling?
- How have things been going since you got home from the hospital?
- What has been easier or harder than you expected?
- How are things going for you and your family?

Family History

- A comprehensive family health history is to be obtained at the 1 Month Visit. If this is the first visit to the health care professional or practice, then a detailed family, pregnancy, delivery, and initial newborn care history is needed. A family history questionnaire can be found in the *Bright Futures Tool and Resource Kit*.

Social History

- See the Social Determinants of Health priority in Anticipatory Guidance for social history questions.

Surveillance of Development

Do you or any of your baby's caregivers have any specific concerns about your baby's learning, development, or behavior?

Clinicians using the *Bright Futures Tool and Resource Kit* Previsit Prescreening Questionnaires or another tool that includes a developmental milestones checklist, or those who use a structured developmental screening tool, need not ask about these developmental surveillance milestones. *(For more information, see the Promoting Healthy Development theme.)*

Social Language and Self-help

Does your child

- Sustain periods of wakefulness for feeding?
- Make brief eye contact with adult when held?

Verbal Language (Expressive and Receptive)

Does she

- Cry with discomfort?
- Calm to adult's voice?

Gross Motor

Does he

- Lift his head briefly when on his stomach and turn it to the side?
- Move his arms and legs symmetrically and reflexively when startled?

Fine Motor

Does she

- Keep her hands in a fist?

Review of Systems

The Bright Futures Infancy Expert Panel recommends a complete review of systems as a part of every health supervision visit. This review can be done by asking the following questions:

Do you have concerns about your baby's

- Head
  - Shape
- Eyes
  - Discharge
- Ears, nose, and throat
- Breathing
- Stomach or abdomen
  - Vomiting or spitting
  - Bowel movements
  - Umbilical stump
- Genitals or rectum
- Skin
- Development
  - Muscle strength, movement of arms or legs, any developmental concerns

Observation of Parent-Newborn Interaction

During the visit, the health care professional acknowledges and reinforces positive parent-newborn interactions and discusses any concerns. Observation focuses on

- Do the parents and newborn respond to each other (gazing, talking, smiling, holding, cuddling, comforting, showing affection)?
- Do the parents appear content, happy, at ease, depressed, tearful, angry, anxious, fatigued, overwhelmed, or uncomfortable?
- Are the parents aware of, responsive to, and effective in responding to the newborn's distress?
- Do the parents appear confident in holding, comforting, feeding, and understanding the newborn's cues or behaviors?
- What are the parents' and newborn's interactions around comforting, dressing, changing diapers, and feeding?
- Are both parents present and do they support each other or show signs of disagreement?

Physical Examination

A complete physical examination is included as part of every health supervision visit.

When performing a physical examination, the health care professional's attention is directed to the following components of the examination that are important for a baby this age:

- **General observations**
  - Assess alertness.
  - Assess for congenital anomalies and note any dysmorphic features.

- **Measure and plot on appropriate WHO Growth Chart**
  - Recumbent length
  - Weight
  - Head circumference
  - Weight-for-length

- **Skin**
  - Inspect for rashes or jaundice.
  - Assess hydration.

- **Head**
  - Observe shape (sutures, molding), size, and fontanels.
  - Note evidence of birth trauma.

- **Eyes**
  - Inspect eyes and eyelids.
  - Examine pupils for opacification and red reflexes.
  - Assess visual acuity using fixate and follow response.

- **Heart**
  - Auscult for murmurs.
  - Palpate femoral pulses and compare against upper extremity pulses.

- **Abdomen**
  - Inspect umbilical cord and umbilicus.
  - Palpate for masses.

- **Genitourinary**
  - Palpate testes in male newborn.
  - Inspect external female genitalia.

- **Musculoskeletal**
  - Perform Ortolani and Barlow maneuvers.
  - Examine the spine and back for deformities, sinus tracts, dimples, hair tufts.

- **Neurologic**
  - Note posture, tone, activity level, symmetry of movement, neonatal reflexes and state regulation (alertness, orientation, and regulatory capacity).

Screening

Universal Screening	Action
Hearing	If not yet done, hearing screening test should be completed.[a]
Newborn: Blood	Verify screening was obtained and review results of the state newborn metabolic screening test. Unavailable or pending results must be obtained immediately. If there are any abnormal results, ensure that appropriate retesting has been performed and all necessary referrals are made to subspecialists. State newborn screening programs are available for assistance with referrals to appropriate resources.

Selective Screening	Risk Assessment[b]	Action if Risk Assessment Positive (+)
Blood Pressure	Children with specific risk conditions	Blood pressure measurement
Vision	+ on risk screening questions	Ophthalmology referral

[a] Any newborn who does not pass the initial screen must be rescreened. Any failure at rescreening should be referred for a diagnostic audiologic assessment, and any newborn with a definitive diagnosis should be referred to the state Early Intervention Program.

[b] See the *Evidence and Rationale chapter* for the criteria on which risk screening questions are based.

Immunizations

Provide hepatitis B vaccine, if not administered during the newborn stay. Verify that the mother is hepatitis surface antigen negative.

Babies younger than 6 months are at risk of complications from influenza, but are too young to be vaccinated for seasonal influenza. Encourage **influenza vaccine** for caregivers of babies younger than 6 months and recommend **pertussis immunization (Tdap)** for adults who will be caring for the baby.

Review the immunization status of siblings in the home.

Consult the CDC/ACIP or AAP Web sites for the current immunization schedule.

CDC National Immunization Program: **www.cdc.gov/vaccines**

AAP *Red Book:* **http://redbook.solutions.aap.org**

Anticipatory Guidance

The following sample questions, which address the Bright Futures Infancy Expert Panel's Anticipatory Guidance Priorities, are intended to be used selectively to invite discussion, gather information, address the needs and concerns of the family, and build partnerships. Use of the questions may vary from visit to visit and from family to family. Questions can be modified to match the health care professional's communication style. The accompanying anticipatory guidance for the family should be geared to questions, issues, or concerns for that particular infant and family. Tools and handouts to support anticipatory guidance can be found in the *Bright Futures Tool and Resource Kit*.

Priority

Social Determinants of Health

Risks: Living situation and food security, environmental tobacco exposure

Strengths and protective factors: Family support

Risks: Living Situation and Food Security

Probe for stressors, such as return to work or school or the inability to return to work or school, competing family needs, or loss of social or financial support. Provide guidance, referrals, and help in connecting with community resources as needed.

Suggest community resources that help with finding quality child care, accessing transportation or getting an infant car safety seat and crib, or addressing issues such as financial concerns, inadequate means to cover health care expenses, inadequate or unsafe housing, parental inexperience, or lack of social support. If the family is having difficulty obtaining sufficient formula or nutritious food, provide information about WIC, SNAP, local food shelves, and local community food programs.

Sample Questions

Tell me about your living situation. Do you live in an apartment or a house? Is permanent housing a worry for you?

Do you have the things you need to take care of the baby, such as a crib, a car safety seat, and diapers? Does your home have enough heat, hot water, electricity, and working appliances? Do you have health insurance for yourself? How about for the baby?

Within the past 12 months, were you ever worried whether your food would run out before you got money to buy more? Within the past 12 months, did the food you bought not last and you did not have money to get more?

Have you ever tried to get help for these issues? What happened? What barriers did you face?

How do you deal with family members who criticize you or offer suggestions that are not helpful?

Anticipatory Guidance

- Programs and resources are available to help you and your baby. You may be eligible for the WIC food and nutrition program. Several food programs, such as the Commodity Supplemental Food Program and SNAP, the program formerly known as Food Stamps, also can help you. If you are breastfeeding and eligible for WIC, you can get nutritious food for yourself and support from peer counselors. Would you like their numbers? Would you like someone from our office to help you get in touch with them?

- It's good that these things are not a concern for you right now. If things change, please consider us a place where you can get ideas about whom to contact for help. We know how important these things are to helping you keep your baby and your family healthy and safe.

- One way to deal with unwanted advice from family and friends is to acknowledge their concerns and desire to help and then change the subject to something you do agree on. Trying to justify your desire to follow the recommendations of your health care professional may only lead to a long and futile conversation.

Risks: Environmental Tobacco Exposure

Address how smoking affects a young baby's health and increases the baby's chance for respiratory infections, SIDS, ear infections, and asthma. Provide smoking cessation strategies and make specific referrals as needed. If either parent quit smoking during the pregnancy, congratulate the parent and encourage him or her to continue remaining abstinent from tobacco.

Sample Questions

Did you smoke or use e-cigarettes before or during this pregnancy? Does anyone else in your home smoke? Do you or anyone you live with use e-cigarettes? Have you been able to cut down the daily number of cigarettes? Do you know where to get help with stopping smoking?

Anticipatory Guidance

- It's important to keep your car, home, and other places where your baby spends time free of tobacco smoke and vapor from e-cigarettes. Smoking affects the baby by increasing the risk of asthma, ear infections, respiratory infections, and sudden infant death.

- **800-QUIT-NOW (800-784-8669);** TTY **800-332-8615** is a national telephone triage and support service that is routed to local resources. Additional resources are available at **www.cdc.gov.** Specific information for women is available at **http://women.smokefree.gov.**

Strengths and Protective Factors: Family Support

Parents look to many people and information sources for answers to their questions about their children's health and development. They need a support network, whether with friends or family members or through community programs.

Social media can allow parents to share parenting tips and resources, and create a virtual support network. Ask the parents what sites (including blogs and birth groups) they are using for networking and finding information regarding parenting and their new baby. Explore how they sort through all the varied online information and decide what they believe is valuable. Be ready to provide parents with trusted sources of maternal and child health information, and provide these links on your own Web site. The AAP's HealthyChildren.org is one resource that health care professionals can provide to parents (Web site: **www.HealthyChildren.org,** Twitter: @healthychildren). Parents of hospitalized babies or whose babies have special health care needs may be more likely to seek out virtual networks for support and information. Trusted Web sites with accurate information can be recommended.

Sample Questions
Where do you go for answers about health questions? How do you decide if the information you are given is something you are going to try or believe?

Anticipatory Guidance
- Social media tools can be useful in building social networks, but do not rely on them for maternal and child health advice. I can answer your questions and give you useful and reliable information.
- It is important that parents have people they can turn to when they need help with the baby. Talking with family members or friends and making arrangements with them so that they can be prepared to help if needed is one way to address this issue. These people usually are willing to help, but may need specific information about ways in which they can be most helpful.

Priority

Parent and Family Health and Well-being
Transition home, sibling adjustment

Transition Home

The first weeks with a new baby are a stressful time of transitions in which parents and other family members must learn how to care for the baby and adjust to new roles. New mothers also must focus on their physical recovery from the birth. Counsel the new parents on this transitional time and provide strategies for settling into a routine.

Review expectations, perspectives, and satisfaction with parenthood, as well as how well any siblings and the extended family are functioning.

Sample Questions

How is the adjustment to the new baby going? How are your partner or other family members helping with the baby?

Anticipatory Guidance

- The first week home is a time of transitions. It is normal for you to feel uncertain, overwhelmed, and very tired at times. As you and your baby get to know each other, it gets much better!
- Making sure to rest and sleep when the baby sleeps is one way to help you maintain your sense of well-being. Another is to let your partner and other family members do things for you and participate in the care of the baby by holding, bathing, changing, dressing, and calming him.

Sibling Adjustment

Parent concerns about sibling reactions to meeting the baby are best guided according to the siblings' developmental ages and responses. Behavior regression and jealousy sometimes occur with an older sibling. Inquire about other children, older family members and others living in the home, family routines, and relationships. Anticipatory guidance regarding the newborn's health and safety will vary, based on the specific cultural traditions of the family.

Sample Questions

Are there other children in your home? How old are they? How did they respond to your pregnancy and the thought of becoming a big brother/sister? How are your other children coping with the new baby? Is that difficult for you? Do you have any children or family members living with you who have special health or developmental care needs?

Anticipatory Guidance

- Older children in the home, no matter what their age, may show feelings of insecurity, behavioral regression, or, in some instances, anger or embarrassment with the birth of a sibling. Older children may express anger, sadness, guilt, or a mix of these feelings about the baby or your need to devote extra time and attention to the new baby.
- Your other children need special time with you and your partner. Try to spend individual time every day with your other children doing things they like to do.
- Acknowledge your older children's possible negative feelings and regression.
- To help your older children adjust to the new baby and still feel wanted and loved, ask for their help in caring for the baby, if they have reached a level of development and maturity where they can do so without harming the baby.
- Maintaining routines as much as possible can help reduce stress.
- Provide each of your children with love and reassurance that they are important and loved, and that their place in the family is secure.

Priority

Newborn Behavior and Care

Early brain development, adjustment to home, calming, when to call (temperature taking) and emergency readiness (CPR), illness prevention (handwashing, outings) and sun exposure

Early Brain Development

Singing, talking, and reading to even young babies enhance early brain development and have been shown to improve early language skills and lifelong literacy. Television (TV) and other media distract a parent's attentiveness and reduce the language to which the baby is exposed. As more families and children have access to and exposure to digital media, it is important to assess for the use of such devices and offer guidance about consequences of media use for a child this age.

Sample Questions

Do you have books to read with your baby? Have you found good times to talk and read together? Is there a TV or other digital media device on in the background while your baby is in the room?

Anticipatory Guidance

- Whenever you can, sing and talk to your baby. Begin to communicate interactively and see how your baby responds more and more each week.
- Set a time each day to sit together and read. Your baby won't understand the story, but she will love hearing the sound of your voice, and the physical closeness of sitting together will enhance your bonding. Be sure to turn off TVs, radios, smartphones, and other digital media. Babies cannot learn language from TV.
- Having a TV on in the background can distract you from reading your baby's cues. Reading her cues is important to learning about her patterns of behavior and developing sensitive interactions with her. These interactions between you and your baby are crucial for language, cognitive, and emotional development.

Adjustment to Home

Healthy newborns breastfeed at least 8 to 12 times in 24 hours and often much more frequently. Breastfeedings may occur in clusters and without obvious patterns. Newborns tend to waken about equally, day and night.

Newborns with rapid state changes from sleep or drowsiness to crying, or newborns whose parents are concerned with excessive crying, may need additional counseling.

Sample Questions

How has the baby been adjusting since you got home? About how often does your baby feed each day? Where does she sleep? Is she able to come to an alert state for feeding? What have you found works to wake up your baby for feedings or to calm her for sleep?

Anticipatory Guidance

- At this age, newborns usually lack a day and night schedule. They may or may not sleep for a longer stretch during the day.
- The room temperature should be comfortable and the baby should be kept from getting too warm or too cold while sleeping.
- Newborn sleeping patterns may be different from one baby to another. Usually, in the first few weeks, the baby's pattern may vary from day to day, but most babies will sleep 16 to 20 hours out of 24. They need to be fed on cue about every 1 to 2 hours, and have one period where they may sleep for up to 3 hours.
- A newborn is often tired after delivery, just like her parents. Medications you received can prolong this sleepy period. For your baby to feed consistently through the day and night, she may need help waking up for feedings. Use a variety of stimulating actions, such as rocking, patting, stroking, diaper changes, and undressing, to help her come to an alert state for feeding.
- Other types of actions, such as stroking your baby's head or gentle repetitive rocking, help put your baby to sleep and are useful for consoling her.

Calming

The newborn period is a time of great adjustment and change for parents. Encourage parents to learn about their baby's temperament and how it affects the way she relates to the world. Some spirited babies will need help from their parents to learn to calm down. Acknowledge the parents' abilities as they respond to and care for their newborn to reinforce their sense of competence. By effectively managing stress, parents feel better and can provide more nurturing attention, which provides a protective environment for their newborn. Parents can learn effective ways to calm their baby and reach out to friends and family for support, when needed. Evidence of ambivalence or stress caused by the home situation or the care of the newborn may require referrals to community support systems, such as public health nursing, home care, or other community agencies.

Sample Questions

How do you feel when you have the baby with you? Have you been able to rest or get sleep? What is it like for you when your baby cries? What do you do for her when she cries?

Anticipatory Guidance

- Even though taking care of a newborn can be tiring, it can also be great fun as you watch the baby adjust to her new surroundings and begin to recognize you.
- Your baby has to adjust to the world around her while learning to let you know what she needs through her cries and movements. Newborns also have to learn how to respond to all the new sights, sounds, and physical contacts, like touch, that they are exposed to after birth. Some babies will have an easy time of this; others will need your help to learn to calm down or soothe themselves.

- A baby does not cry or fuss to intentionally bother us. When babies cry, it's because they need us. She may miss the warmth and gentle swaying of your body and the sounds of your heartbeat and voice that she felt and heard while she was still inside you. She may be hungry or wet, or too cold or too warm. She is adjusting to her new environment and needs your help to become comfortable.

- It is normal for parents to feel upset or frustrated sometimes when there's a new baby at home. All parents get upset sometimes.

- Never shake your baby to try to get her to calm down or stop crying. If you feel you may lose control, put the baby in a safe place, like a crib or a cradle. Your crying baby will be OK while you regain your calm.

When to Call (Temperature Taking) and Emergency Readiness (CPR)

It may take some time for parents of newborns to develop confidence in their ability to care for their baby. They may welcome guidance about issues such as knowing when to call the practice, knowing how to determine and prevent illness in their baby, and knowing how to handle emergencies.

Sample Questions

What type of thermometer do you have? Do you know how to use it? Do you know what to do in an emergency or if you have concerns or questions about your baby? Do you know how to call our office so we can work with you to ensure your baby's health and well-being? Do you know how we handle your after office–hours care?

Anticipatory Guidance

- In the first year of life, taking your baby's temperature rectally is the only accurate method. A rectal temperature of 100.4°F/38.0°C or higher is considered a fever. Home ear or skin temperatures are not accurate enough.

- You can call our office any time with questions.

- Here are some emergency preparedness strategies.
  - Complete an American Heart Association or American Red Cross first aid or infant CPR program.
  - Have a family first aid kit.
  - Make a list of the local emergency telephone numbers, including our office and after-hours number and the national **Poison Help line (800-222-1222).** Post these numbers at every telephone and store them in your cell phone.

- Have a family emergency preparedness plan and become familiar with your community's emergency plan.

Illness Prevention (Handwashing, Outings) and Sun Exposure

In spite of protective maternal antibodies, infants are at risk for communicable illness.

Sun exposure risk in babies is best prevented by avoiding the sun.

Sample Questions

What questions do you have about going out with your baby? Going to public places, such as parks or faith-based activities? What to tell visitors about handling your baby?

Anticipatory Guidance

- To protect your baby in the first month of life, do not let her be handled by many people. Avoid crowded places, overdressing, and exposure to very hot or cold temperatures.
- Make sure to wash your hands often, especially after diaper changes and before feeding the baby.
- Make sure that you and all adults who will have contact with your baby have had pertussis and influenza immunizations.
- As much as possible, keep your baby out of the sun. If she has to be in the sun, use a sunscreen made for children. For babies younger than 6 months, sunscreen may be used on small areas of the body, such as the face and backs of the hands, if adequate clothing and shade are not available.

Priority

Nutrition and Feeding

General guidance on feeding (weight gain, feeding strategies, holding, burping, hunger and satiation cues), breastfeeding guidance, formula-feeding guidance

General Guidance on Feeding (Weight Gain, Feeding Strategies, Holding, Burping, Hunger and Satiation Cues)

One of the first tasks for parents during their newborn's first week is learning when and how much their baby needs either for breastfeeding or formula. The First Week Visit usually provides parents with reassurance that their baby has started to gain weight after the initial weight loss and is thus getting the appropriate feedings. Close supervision and counseling are needed to assist parents in ensuring that their newborn awakens for feedings to ensure adequate hydration.

Providing parents with guidance to recognize their baby's signals for both hunger and satiety will help them provide an appropriate feeding amount and frequency, as well as avoid overfeeding.

Counseling may be needed to discuss the best ways of holding the baby during feedings. It also may be advisable to actually observe the newborn feeding. For example, some newborns with reflux will arch their back and pull away from the parent, leaving the parent with the impression that the newborn does not like the human milk, formula, or being held. This is an important cue that the family needs additional counseling and assistance. If the family is having difficulty obtaining sufficient formula or nutritious food, provide information about WIC, SNAP, local food shelves, and local community food programs.

Sample Questions

How is feeding going? How are you feeding your baby? How does your baby like to be held when you feed him? How easy is it to burp your baby during or after feedings?

Are you comfortable that your baby is getting enough to eat? How many wet diapers and stools does your baby have each day?

How do you know if your baby is hungry? How do you know if he has had enough to eat?

Anticipatory Guidance

- If you are bottle-feeding, do not prop the bottle, as this puts your baby at risk of choking, ear infections, and early childhood caries or tooth decay. Holding your baby close while you feed him gives you the opportunity for warm and loving interaction with him.
- Babies usually burp at natural breaks (eg, midway through or after a feeding). Help him burp by gently rubbing or patting his back while holding him against your shoulder and chest or supporting him in a sitting position on your lap.
- Your baby is getting enough milk if he has 6 to 8 wet cloth diapers (5 or 6 disposable diapers) and 3 or 4 stools per day and is gaining weight appropriately.
- Breastfed newborns usually have loose, frequent stools. After several weeks, the number of bowel movements may decrease. Breastfed babies who are 4 weeks and older may have stools as infrequently as every 3 days or more.
- Healthy babies do not require extra water, as breast milk and formula, when properly prepared, are adequate to meet the newborn's fluid needs.
- A baby's usual signs of hunger include putting his hand to his mouth, sucking, rooting, facial grimaces, and fussing. Crying is a late sign of hunger.
- You can tell he's full because he will gently release the nipple, close his mouth, or relax his arms and hands.

Breastfeeding Guidance

Mothers

Mothers who breastfeed should ingest 500 µg of folate or folic acid daily by taking a daily prenatal vitamin or a multivitamin in addition to eating a nutritious diet. The mother's diet should include an average daily intake of 200 mg to 300 mg of the omega-3 long-chain PUFA DHA to guarantee a sufficient concentration of preformed DHA in the milk. This is obtained either through supplementation or consumption of 1 to 2 portions (3 oz each) of fish (eg, herring, canned light tuna, salmon) per week. The concern regarding the possible risk from intake of excessive mercury or other contaminants is offset by the neurobehavioral benefits of an adequate DHA intake and can be minimized by avoiding the intake of 4 types of fish that are high in mercury. These are tilefish, shark, swordfish, and king mackerel. Additionally, the mother's diet should include 550 mg/day of choline because human milk is rich in choline and depletes the mother's tissue stores. In the diets of women, eggs, milk, chicken, beef, and pork are the biggest contributors of choline.

For vegan mothers, who consume no animal products in their diet, a daily multivitamin including iron, zinc, vitamin B$_{12}$, omega-3 fatty acids, and 550 mg of choline is recommended.

Infants

Vitamin D supplementation (400 IU per day) is recommended for breastfed babies beginning at hospital discharge.

Sample Questions

How is breastfeeding going for you and your baby? How often does your baby breastfeed? How long do feedings last? Does it seem like your baby is breastfeeding more often or for longer periods of time, compared with the first couple of days? How can you tell whether your baby is satisfied at the breast?

What concerns do you have about breastfeeding? Is breastfeeding uncomfortable or do you have sore nipples?

Are you continuing to take prenatal vitamins? What over-the-counter or prescription medications are you taking? Are you taking any vitamin-mineral or herbal supplements? What questions do you have about any condition that might prevent you from breastfeeding?

Are you offering the baby breast milk in a bottle? Are you using a pacifier? Will you be able to breastfeed your baby if you return to work or school?

Do you eat fish at least 1 to 2 times per week? Do you have protein-containing foods every day, such as eggs, chicken, beef or pork, or dairy?

Anticipatory Guidance

- Exclusive breastfeeding continues to be the ideal source of nutrition for about the first 6 months of life.
- At about 1 week of age, your baby should feed every 1 to 3 hours in the daytime, and every 3 hours at night, with one longer 4- to 5-hour stretch between feedings. For the first few weeks, your baby should breastfeed between 8 to 12 times in 24 hours.
- You can help your baby by paying attention to his sleep cycles in the day. When he comes to a drowsy state, change his diaper and wake him for a feeding about every 2 to 3 hours.
- Breastfeeding may be challenging for mothers, whether or not they have breastfed before. Every baby is different and catches on a little differently. That is why lactation consultants and breastfeeding support groups are valuable for consultation, education, and support as you and your baby are beginning to breastfeed. I can give you contact information for community groups and a lactation consultant.
- If you are breastfeeding your baby, be sure that you are giving him vitamin D drops.
- You may continue to take your prenatal vitamin with iron every day to ensure adequate intake of vitamins and minerals. If you do not consume any animal products in your diet and follow a vegan diet, your supplement should include vitamins D and B_{12}.
- Eating a small serving of fish 2 times a week provides important nutrients to your baby. Canned light tuna, salmon, trout, and herring are the best choices to give your baby the neurobehavioral benefits of an adequate intake of an important fat called DHA.
- It is best to avoid 4 kinds of fish that are high in mercury. These fish are tilefish, shark, swordfish, and king mackerel.
- Consuming small amounts of protein-containing foods, such as lean meat, poultry, dairy products, beans and peas, eggs, processed soy products, and nuts and seeds, every day is recommended.
- Because newborns feed so frequently, you should avoid alcohol in the first several months of your baby's life. Alcohol easily passes into breast milk and can remain in breast milk for 2 to 3 hours.

Formula-Feeding Guidance

A newborn who is growing appropriately will average 20 oz of formula per day, with a range of 16 to 24 oz per day. Formula preparation and formula safety information is needed for parents, especially the length of time over which formula from one feeding can be offered to the newborn. Parents also need to know why it is important to seek professional guidance before changing to a different formula.

Sample Questions

Do you have any concerns about formula? What concerns do you have about cost, nutrient content, and differences across brands? Are you able to get your baby's formula from WIC? What questions do you have about preparing formula and storing it safely?

Anticipatory Guidance

- Make sure to always use iron-fortified formula. At first, give your baby 2 oz of prepared formula every 2 to 3 hours. Give him more if he still seems hungry. As he grows and his appetite increases, you will need to prepare larger amounts.
- Because formula is expensive, you may be hesitant to throw away any that is left in the bottle. For food safety reasons, if your baby has not taken all of the formula at one feeding, you may use it for the next feeding, but be sure to put it back in the refrigerator. Do not mix this formula with new formula. If the formula has been heated and has been out of the refrigerator for 1 hour or more, discard it.
- Never heat a bottle in a microwave. If you wish to warm a bottle, a hot water bath is recommended.
- If you are thinking about switching brands of formula, talk to me first.

Priority

Safety
Car safety seats, heatstroke prevention, safe sleep, safe home environment: burns

Car Safety Seats

Parents should not place their baby's car safety seat in the front seat of a vehicle with a passenger air bag because the air bags deploy with great force against a car safety seat and cause serious injury or death.

Counsel parents that their own safe driving behaviors (including using seat belts at all times and not driving under the influence of alcohol or drugs) are important to the health of their children.

Babies with special health care needs require special consideration for safe transportation. Refer parents to a local, specially trained Child Passenger Safety Technician for assistance with special positioning and restraint devices (**http://cert.safekids.org**).

Sample Questions

Is your baby fastened securely in a rear-facing car safety seat in the back seat every time she rides in a vehicle? Do you have any problems using your baby's car safety seat?

Anticipatory Guidance

- A rear-facing car safety seat should always be used to transport your baby in all vehicles, including taxis and cars owned by friends or other family members.
- The back seat is the safest place for children to ride. The harnesses should be snug and the car safety seat should be positioned at the recommended angle so that the baby's head does not fall forward. (Check the instructions to find the right angle and how to adjust it.) Babies with special needs, such as premature babies or babies in casts, need special consideration for safe transportation.
- Your baby needs to stay in her car safety seat at all times during travel. If she becomes fussy or needs to breastfeed, stop the vehicle and take her out of the car safety seat to attend to her needs. Strap her safely back into her seat before traveling again.
- Car safety seats should be used only for travel, not for positioning outside the vehicle. Keep the harnesses snug whenever your baby is in the car safety seat. This will help prevent falls out of the seat and strangulation on the harnesses.
- Your own safe driving habits are important to the health of your children. Always use a seat belt and do not drive under the influence of alcohol or drugs. Never text or use a cell phone or other handheld device while driving.

For information about car safety seats and actions to keep your baby safe in and around cars, visit www.safercar.gov/parents.

Find a Child Passenger Safety Technician: http://cert.safekids.org. Click on "Find a Tech."

Toll-free Auto Safety Hotline: 888-327-4236

Heatstroke Prevention

Each year, an average of 37 children die of heatstroke after being left in a car that can become too hot. More than half of the deaths are infants and children younger than 2 years. In most cases, the parent or caregiver forgot the child was in the car, often because there was a change in the usual routine or schedule. Even very loving and attentive parents can forget a child in the car. Additionally, some children have died while playing in the vehicle or after getting in the vehicle without the caregiver's knowledge.

The temperature inside a car can rise to a dangerous level quickly, even when the temperature outside is as low as 60 degrees. Leaving the windows open will not prevent heatstroke. Because children have proportionally less surface area than adults and less ability to regulate internal temperature, their bodies overheat up to 5 times more quickly than adults' bodies.

Sample Question

Every year, children die of heatstroke after being left in a hot car. Would you like to talk about creating a plan so this doesn't happen to you?

Anticipatory Guidance

- Never leave your child alone in a car for any reason, even briefly.
- Start developing habits that will help prevent you from ever forgetting your baby in the car. Consider putting an item that you need, like your purse, cell phone, or employee ID, in the back seat of the vehicle, so you will see your baby when you retrieve the item before leaving the car.
- Check the back seat before walking away, every time you park your vehicle.

Safe Sleep

A family's beliefs and cultural traditions will have a significant effect on where and how the baby sleeps, and whether the family or other caregivers follow the safe to sleep message. Counsel parents about appropriate sleep positioning and sleep location for the baby. In many cultures, family sleep arrangements are viewed as a part of the parent's commitment to their children's well-being.

Culturally sensitive information should be provided about what is known about safe-sleep environments for babies. A supine position ("back to sleep") is best for babies, including premature babies, because of the reduction of SIDS. However, parents should avoid using wedges or other positioning devices, as they are a suffocation hazard. Room sharing is recommended for at least the first 6 months of life, with the baby in a separate, but nearby, sleep space. Bed sharing (sleeping in the same bed as the parents, another adult, or a child), and sleeping on couches or recliners, increases the risk of SUID by entrapment or parental overlie and suffocation. Swaddling is *not for sleep*. It is important to explore the parents' intended infant sleep practices at home and to offer guidance to ensure the safest sleep environment for the newborn.

Common beliefs and concerns expressed by families as justification for not placing their babies to sleep in the supine position include the fear of choking or aspiration, perceived uncomfortable or less peaceful sleep, concern about a flat occiput and hair loss, and family beliefs about appropriate sleep patterns, position, and sleep location. Sleeping in a semi-reclined position, such as in a swing or car seat, increases the risk of decreasing oxygen levels when an infant assumes an improper head and neck position. A semi-reclined position may also worsen gastroesophageal reflux. Different cultures may view infant sleep differently than current safe sleep recommendations. These viewpoints should be sought and discussed with the parents.

Parents need strategies that will assist them in engaging relatives, friends, and child care providers to follow safe sleep practices for the newborn. A consistent message about back to sleep provides family members with the best information when they ask about side sleeping.

Sample Questions

What have you heard about how babies should sleep? Where will your baby sleep? How about at naptime?

Anticipatory Guidance

- It is best to always have your baby sleep on her back because it reduces the risk of sudden death. We recommend this sleep position for babies even if they are born premature or have problems with reflux, which is frequent vomiting after feeding. Do not use a wedge or other product to keep your baby on her back, as the baby can wiggle down and suffocate against the wedge.

- Your baby should sleep in your room in her own crib, but not in your bed. Think about some strategies you might use to soothe your baby without bringing her into your bed, where the risks of suffocation, entrapment, and death are increased.

- If possible, use a crib purchased after June 28, 2011, as cribs sold in the United States after that date are required to meet a new, stronger safety standard. If you use an older crib, choose one with slats that are no more than 2⅜ inches (60 mm) apart and with a mattress that fits snugly, with no gaps between the mattress and the crib slats. Drop-side cribs are no longer recommended.

- If you choose a mesh play yard or portable crib, consider choosing one that was manufactured after a new, stronger safety standard was implemented on February 28, 2013. If you use an older product, the weave should have openings less than ¼ inch (6 mm) and the sides should always stay fully raised. The baby's sleep space should be kept empty, with no toys or soft bedding, such as pillows, bumpers, or blankets.

- The safest cover for the baby is a sleepsack or footed pajamas that can keep the baby warm without concern about suffocating under a blanket. This also allows the baby to move her legs as opposed to swaddling, which has the potential to cause poor development of her hips and increases your baby's risk of suffocation and death.

- Some babies with very sensitive startle reflexes appear more comfortable having their arms close to their body. Swaddling can help with this sensitivity. If you swaddle your baby, be sure to keep it loose around her legs, but snug—not tight—around her chest. To make sure your baby can breathe, leave enough space so that you can fit your hand between the blanket and her chest. Also, be sure that there are no loose ends of blanket around her neck, as these can increase her risk of suffocating.

- Swaddling should only be used with babies younger than 2 months and is recommended only when your baby is awake. Older babies can roll over and risk suffocation if they are swaddled.

- Your baby should sleep in a crib or bassinet, not in a swing, bouncer, or car safety seat. Sleeping in a semi-reclined position can contribute to decreased oxygen levels in a newborn. If your baby falls asleep in one of these places, move him to a crib or bassinet as soon as possible.

Safe Home Environment: Burns

Sample Question
Have you made any changes in your home to keep your baby safe?

Anticipatory Guidance
- Do not drink hot liquids while holding the baby.
- **To protect your child from tap water scalds, the hottest temperature at the faucet should be no higher than 120°F.** In many cases, you can adjust your water heater. Before bathing the baby, always test the water temperature with your wrist to make sure it is not too hot.

Infancy
1 Month Visit

Context

Within the first month, parents become increasingly attuned to their baby as they learn to interpret the meanings of their baby's cues and how their caregiving responses to the baby's behaviors may influence her behaviors. Through their growing understanding of their newborn, parents learn strategies to support the baby's emerging personality and self-regulation. The primary focus of parents' caregiving relates to feedings, sleep and wake patterns, elimination, and assimilation into the family.

The frequency of visits during the first 2 months of life will depend on the baby's health status and the family's needs. Babies who were premature or sick at birth, those entering foster care or adoptive families, those with special health or developmental needs, and first-time or anxious parents likely will need more frequent visits. In addition to offering counseling and reassurance to the parents, the health care professional may need to arrange referrals for comprehensive evaluation and management of the infant's problems and for community-based family support services. As coordinator of the infant's medical home, the health care professional will ascertain and assist the family in ensuring that appropriate linkages are in place for any needed subspecialty medical or surgical care and early intervention services.

The 1 Month Visit encompasses routine health surveillance, response to parental concerns, and encouragement, support, and practical guidance about the infant's growth and nutrition, development, and normal sleep patterns. For the infant born preterm or with a health condition that makes feeding a challenge, additional attention will need to be directed toward feeding skills, the adequacy of nutrient and caloric intake, and infant growth. The results of newborn screening, including blood, hearing, and critical congenital heart disease, and hearing screening tests should be reviewed, and repeat testing, as required, should be arranged or completed. Risk factors requiring future testing should be documented. If the parents will be returning to work or school in the near future, guidance regarding the selection of safe child care may be provided. The mother's plans regarding infant feeding also should be explored. Discussion points may include human milk pumping and storage and the introduction of bottle-feeding (expressed human milk or infant formula) in the exclusively breastfeeding infant.

Families experiencing adjustment difficulties, and mothers manifesting postpartum psychological symptoms, will require close involvement and interaction with the health care professional and may need referral to resources to support their material or emotional needs.

Priorities for the 1 Month Visit

The first priority is to attend to the concerns of the parents.

In addition, the Bright Futures Infancy Expert Panel has given priority to the following topics for discussion in this visit:

▶ Social determinants of health[a] (risks [living situation and food security, environmental tobacco exposure, dampness and mold, radon, pesticides, intimate partner violence, maternal alcohol and substance use], strengths and protective factors [family support])

▶ Parent and family health and well-being (postpartum checkup, maternal depression, family relationships)

▶ Infant behavior and development (sleeping and waking, fussiness and attachment, media, playtime, medical home after-hours support)

▶ Nutrition and feeding (feeding plans and choices, general guidance on feeding, breastfeeding guidance, formula-feeding guidance)

▶ Safety (car safety seats, safe sleep, preventing falls, emergency care)

[a] Social determinants of health is a new priority in the fourth edition of the *Bright Futures Guidelines*. For more information, see the *Promoting Lifelong Health for Families and Communities* theme.

Health Supervision

The *Bright Futures Tool and Resource Kit* contains Previsit Questionnaires to assist the health care professional in taking a history, conducting developmental surveillance, and performing medical screening.

History

The interval history may be obtained according to the concerns of the family and the health care professional's preference or style of practice.

General Questions

- Do you have any concerns, questions, or problems that you would like to discuss today?
- How are how things going for you and your family? If there are other children in the home, how are your children adjusting to having a new baby at home?
- What are some of the best times of day with your baby? What are some of the most difficult times of day with your baby?
- Have you been feeling tired or blue?
- How are feedings going?
- Have you and your partner had some time for yourselves?
- Who helps you with the baby? Do you have any conflicts with those who help you about what is safe and healthy for your baby?
- How often does your baby have wet diapers? Stool? Any concerns?
- Tell me some things that you are doing to keep your baby safe and healthy. Have any relatives developed medical problems since your last visit?

Family History

- Obtain a comprehensive family health history. A family history questionnaire can be found in the *Bright Futures Tool and Resource Kit*.

Social History

- See the Social Determinants of Health priority in Anticipatory Guidance for social history questions.

Surveillance of Development

Do you or any of your baby's caregivers have any specific concerns about your baby's learning, development, or behavior?

Clinicians using the *Bright Futures Tool and Resource Kit* Previsit Questionnaires or another tool that includes a developmental milestones checklist, or those who use a structured developmental screening tool, need not ask about these developmental surveillance milestones. *(For more information, see the Promoting Healthy Development theme.)*

Social Language and Self-help

Does your child

- Look at you?
- Follow you with her eyes?
- Have self-comforting behaviors, such as bringing hands to mouth?
- Start to become fussy when bored?
- Calm when picked up or spoken to?
- Look briefly at objects?

Verbal Language (Expressive and Receptive)

Does he

- Make brief short vowel sounds?
- Alert to unexpected sound?
- Quiet or turn to your voice?
- Show signs of sensitivity to his environment (such as excessive crying, tremors, or excessive startles) or a need for extra support to handle activities of daily living?
- Have different types of cries for hunger and tiredness?

Gross Motor

Does she

- Move both arms and both legs together?
- Hold her chin up when on her stomach?

Fine Motor

Does he

- Open his fingers slightly when at rest?

Review of Systems

The Bright Futures Infancy Expert Panel recommends a complete review of systems as a part of every health supervision visit. This review can be done by asking the following questions:

Do you have concerns about your infant's

- Head
  - Shape
- Eyes
  - Discharge
- Ears, nose, and throat
- Breathing
- Stomach or abdomen
  - Vomiting or spitting
  - Bowel movements
  - Umbilical stump
- Genitals or rectum
- Skin
- Development
  - Muscle strength, movement of arms or legs, any developmental concerns

Observation of Parent-Infant Interaction

During the visit, the health care professional acknowledges and reinforces positive parent-infant interactions and discusses any concerns. Observation focuses on

- Do the parents respond to their baby, such as by holding or comforting, and to each other?
- Does the mother engage with her infant while breastfeeding or bottle-feeding?
- Do parents attend to and support the baby during the visit, especially during the examination or immunizations?
- How do the parents respond to the infant's hunger and satiation cues, tiredness, need for comforting?
- Do any parent behaviors or expressions indicate stress (eg, fatigue, tears, anger, anxiety, seeming to be overwhelmed, discomfort, uncertainty, parental tension)?

Physical Examination

A complete physical examination is included as part of every health supervision visit.

When performing a physical examination, the health care professional's attention is directed to the following components of the examination that are important for an infant this age:

- **Measure and plot on appropriate WHO Growth Chart**
  - Recumbent length
  - Weight
  - Head circumference
  - Weight-for-length

- **Skin**
  - Inspect for skin lesions, birthmarks, and bruising.

- **Head**
  - Note positional skull deformities.
  - Palpate fontanels.

- **Eyes**
  - Inspect eyes and eyelids.
  - Examine pupils for opacification and red reflexes.
  - Assess visual acuity using fixate and follow response.

- **Heart**
  - Auscult for murmurs.
  - Palpate femoral pulses.

- **Abdomen**
  - Search for masses.
  - Note healing of the umbilicus.

- **Musculoskeletal**
  - Perform Ortolani and Barlow maneuvers.

- **Neurologic**
  - Observe and examine for asymmetries, movement quality, tone, and posture.
  - Assess tone and neurodevelopmental status, including attentiveness to visual and auditory stimuli.

- **Genitourinary**

  MALE
  - Assess testicular position.

Screening

Universal Screening	Action
Depression: Maternal	Maternal depression screen
Hearing	If not yet done, hearing screening test should be completed.[a]
Newborn: Blood	Verify documentation of newborn blood screening results, and that any positive results have been acted upon with appropriate rescreening, needed follow-up, and referral.

Selective Screening	Risk Assessment[b]	Action if Risk Assessment Positive (+)
Blood Pressure	Children with specific risk conditions or change in risk	Blood pressure measurement
Tuberculosis	+ on risk screening questions	Tuberculin skin test
Vision	+ on risk screening questions	Ophthalmology referral

[a] Positive screenings should be referred for a diagnostic audiologic assessment, and an infant with a definitive diagnosis should be referred to the state Early Intervention Program.

[b] See the *Evidence and Rationale chapter* for the criteria on which risk screening questions are based.

Immunizations

Newborns and infants younger than 6 months are at risk of complications from influenza, but are too young to be vaccinated for seasonal influenza. Encourage **influenza vaccine** for caregivers of infants younger than 6 months and recommend **pertussis immunization (Tdap)** for adults who will be caring for the infant.

Discuss the importance of the immunization schedule and what to expect at the 2 Month Visit.

Review the immunization status of siblings in the home.

Consult the CDC/ACIP or AAP Web sites for the current immunization schedule.

CDC National Immunization Program: **www.cdc.gov/vaccines**

AAP *Red Book:* **http://redbook.solutions.aap.org**

Anticipatory Guidance

The following sample questions, which address the Bright Futures Infancy Expert Panel's Anticipatory Guidance Priorities, are intended to be used selectively to invite discussion, gather information, address the needs and concerns of the family, and build partnerships. Use of the questions may vary from visit to visit and from family to family. Questions can be modified to match the health care professional's communication style. The accompanying anticipatory guidance for the family should be geared to questions, issues, or concerns for that particular infant and family. Tools and handouts to support anticipatory guidance can be found in the *Bright Futures Tool and Resource Kit*.

Priority

Social Determinants of Health

Risks: Living situation and food security, environmental tobacco exposure, dampness and mold, radon, pesticides, intimate partner violence, maternal alcohol and substance use

Strengths and protective factors: Family support

Risks: Living Situation and Food Security

Probe for stressors, such as return to work or school or the inability to return to work or school, competing family needs, or loss of social or financial support. Suggest community resources that help with finding quality child care, accessing transportation, getting a car safety seat and crib, or addressing issues such as financial concerns, inadequate resources to cover health care expenses, inadequate or unsafe housing, parental inexperience, or lack of social support. If the family is having difficulty obtaining sufficient formula or nutritious food, provide information about WIC, SNAP, local food shelves, and local community food programs.

For mothers or caregivers who have a limited support network, community services and resources may be able to help the family.

Support family connection to the community through social, faith-based, cultural, volunteer, and recreational organizations or programs.

Sample Questions

Tell me about your living situation. Do you have enough heat, hot water, and electricity? Do you have appliances that work? Do you have problems with bugs, rodents, or peeling paint or plaster?

How are your resources for caring for your baby? Do you have enough knowledge to feel comfortable in caring for your baby? Do you have health insurance? Do you have enough money for food, clothing, diapers, and child care?

Within the past 12 months, were you ever worried whether your food would run out before you got money to buy more? Within the past 12 months, did the food you bought not last and you did not have money to get more?

Have you ever tried to get help for these issues? What happened? What barriers did you face?

Anticipatory Guidance

- If you have problems with your living situation or with getting enough food, let me know. I can tell you about community services, such as WIC and SNAP, the program formerly known as Food Stamps, that can help you.

Risks: Environmental Tobacco Exposure

Discuss the risks to the infant of environmental tobacco smoke exposure. Encourage parents who are quitting, and provide information about smoking cessation strategies and resources for those who are considering quitting.

Sample Question

Does anyone who lives in or visits the home smoke or use e-cigarettes?

Anticipatory Guidance

- It is important to keep your car, home, and other places the baby stays free of tobacco smoke and vapor from e-cigarettes. Exposure to tobacco smoke can increase your baby's risk of sudden infant death, as well as asthma, ear infections, and respiratory infections.
- **800-QUIT-NOW (800-784-8669);** TTY **800-332-8615** is a national telephone helpline that is routed to local resources. Additional resources are available at **www.cdc.gov.** Specific information for women is available at **http://women.smokefree.gov.**

Risks: Dampness and Mold

Explain the risks of dampness and mold, and discuss strategies for minimizing these risks.

Sample Questions

Are you aware of any health concerns in your family related to your home caused by dampness or mold? Do you have water leaks in your home? Have you had problems with mold or dampness?

Anticipatory Guidance

- Some homes may have health risks that may affect your baby. Exposure to damp and moldy environments can cause a variety of health effects in people sensitive to mold. Mold exposure can cause nasal stuffiness, throat irritation, coughing or wheezing, eye irritation, or, in more severe cases, breathing difficulties.
- Mold will grow in places with a lot of moisture, such as around leaks in roofs, windows, or pipes, or where there has been flooding. Mold grows easily on paper products, cardboard, ceiling tiles, and wood products.

- To control mold, prevent water leaks, ventilate well, clean gutters, and drain water away from your house's foundation.
- Mold can be removed from hard surfaces with commercial cleaners, soap and water, or a bleach solution of 1 part bleach in 4 parts of water.

Risks: Radon

Radon is a gas that is a product of the breakdown of uranium in soil and rock. It also may be in water, natural gas, and building materials. High levels of radon enter homes in many regions of the United States through cracks or openings in the walls, foundation, and floors, or occasionally in well water. It does not cause health problems immediately upon inhalation. Over time, however, it can increase the risk of lung cancer. In fact, next to cigarette smoking, radon is thought to be the most common cause of lung cancer in the United States.

Sample Question

If your home has a basement, has it been checked for radon?

Anticipatory Guidance

- Test your house for radon. If the level is unknown or high (above 4 pCi/L), avoid using your basement for sleeping and playing.
- If your radon level is high, consider taking action to reduce it to an acceptable level. Call **800-SOS-RADON.**

Risks: Pesticides

Pesticides are often used in a variety of products for the control of pests both in the indoor and outdoor environments. They may affect children's health in a variety of ways. Thousands of cases of pesticide poisonings are reported to poison control centers every year.

Sample Question

Do you use pesticides inside or outside the home?

Anticipatory Guidance

- Avoid using pesticides. Instead, choose the least toxic methods for pest control, commonly referred to as integrated pest management. These include repairing all cracks in your house to prevent pests from getting in and making sure that your food is securely sealed.
- If needed, use baits, traps, or gels instead of fogging, bombing, or spraying. Store and dispose of these items safely.

Risks: Intimate Partner Violence

Discuss intimate partner relationships. When inquiring, avoid asking about abuse or domestic violence. Instead, use descriptive terms, such as *hit, kicked, shoved, choked,* and *threatened.* Provide information about the effect of family violence on children and about community resources that provide assistance. Recommend resources for parent education and parent support groups.

To avoid causing upset to families by questioning about sensitive and private topics such as family violence, alcohol and drug use, and similar risks, it is recommended to begin screening about these topics with an introductory statement, such as, "I ask all patients standard health questions to understand factors that may affect health of their child as well as their own health."

Sample Questions

Because violence is so common in so many people's lives, I've begun to ask about it. I don't know if this is a problem for you, but many children I see have parents who have been hurt by someone else. Some are too afraid or uncomfortable to bring it up, so I've started asking all my patients about it routinely. Do you always feel safe in your home? Has your partner, or another significant person in your life, ever hit, kicked, or shoved you, or physically hurt you or the baby? Are you scared that you or other caregivers may hurt the baby? Do you have any questions about your safety at home? What will you do if you feel afraid? Do you have a plan? Would you like information on where to go or who to contact if you ever need help?

Anticipatory Guidance

- One way that I and other health care professionals can help you if your partner, or another significant person in your life, is hitting or threatening you is to support you and provide information about local resources that can help you.
- You can also call the toll-free **National Domestic Violence Hotline** at **800-799-SAFE (7233).**

Risks: Maternal Alcohol and Substance Use

Any substance taken during pregnancy should be evaluated for its overall risk to the newborn, including prescription drugs, over-the-counter preparations, pain relievers, herbal substances, and illegal substances.

Alcohol use during pregnancy is a particular risk for an infant. If the mother acknowledges alcohol use during pregnancy and this was not previously discussed as part of the prenatal history, discuss the concerns to the developing fetus about both ND-PAE and other FASD. Both ND-PAE and FASD have lifelong effects on the infant that can include physical problems and problems with behavior and learning. Fetal alcohol exposure, including the timing during the pregnancy, quantity, and duration, is important to document for later diagnosis of FASD.

Referrals to community social service agencies and drug treatment programs can be provided if the mother is not already linked to these services. Newborns determined to be at risk can be referred to support programs, such as a local Early Intervention Program agency, often referred to as IDEA Part C.

Sample Questions

How often do you drink beer, wine, or liquor in your household? **For any response other than "Never," continue by asking the following questions:** *In the 3 months before you knew you were pregnant, how many times did you have 4 or more drinks in a day? After you knew you were pregnant, how many times did you have 4 or more drinks in a day?*

Depending on the responses to any of the above questions, the health care professional can, if desired, follow up to determine frequency and extent of consumption by asking the following questions: *During the pregnancy, on average, how many days per week did you have a drink? During the pregnancy on a typical day when you had an alcoholic beverage, how many drinks did you have?*

Do you, or does anyone you ride with, ever drive after having a drink? Does your partner use alcohol? What kind and for how long?

If any maternal at-risk drinking is identified, a brief intervention and referral is recommended.

Are you using marijuana, cocaine, pain pills, narcotics, or other controlled substances? What have you heard about the drug's effects on the baby during pregnancy or after the baby is born? Are you getting any help to cut down or stop your drug use?

Are you taking any medicines or vitamins at the present time? Are you using any prescription or over-the-counter medications or pain relievers? Have you used any health remedies or special herbs or teas to improve your health since you have been pregnant? Is there anything that you used to take, but stopped using when you learned that you were pregnant?

Anticipatory Guidance

- Because alcohol is passed into the breast milk, it is important for mothers to avoid alcohol for 2 to 3 hours before breastfeeding or during breastfeeding. This also means that, because newborns breast-feed so frequently (every 2–3 hours), you most likely will have to avoid alcohol during the first several months of your baby's life.
- Most medications are compatible with breastfeeding, but should be checked on an individual basis. To understand how they may affect your baby, it is important to know what over-the-counter medications or herbal products you are taking.
- The reason we are concerned about a parent's use of alcohol or drugs is because of the effects on the baby's mental, physical, and social development. Alcohol misuse can harm a parent's interaction with the baby and lead to poor decisions about the baby's care.
- Drug and alcohol cessation programs are available in our community and we would like to help you connect to these services so that you can safely care for your baby and yourself.

Strengths and Protective Factors: Family Support

By the time an infant is 1 month of age, parents are beginning to think about options for caring for their child if they are considering returning to work or school. Parents need strategies to help juggle multiple responsibilities and garner support from each other and other family members. Help parents understand the importance of asking for help when they need it. Recognize that fathers also will need support, as they may feel conflicted about their desire to be with and support the mother and baby, while needing to return to work. In many cultures, the grandmother or other female relative provides for, or supervises the care of, the young infant. However, many of today's families, including immigrant families, may not have this resource available to them. Parents need to be aware of the many different kinds of child care arrangements that are available in the community.

Parents who are planning on returning to work have many feelings about leaving their baby and need assistance in finding high-quality child care and, for the mother, in determining how to continue breastfeeding. It is important at this time to assess for connections to community and parents' ability to get information about child care options that match their needs.

Sample Questions

How do you feel about returning to work or school? Do you wonder about how returning to work or school may affect your relationship with your baby? **For mothers:** *How it may affect breastfeeding? Have you spoken with your employer about continuing to breastfeed when you return to work?*

Who will take care of the baby while you are at work/school? Have you made arrangements for child care? What factors did you or are you taking into account when deciding on a child care provider for your baby— factors such as affordability, quality, comfort, and access? Would you like any information about things to consider when selecting an affordable, safe child care provider?

Anticipatory Guidance

- Returning to work is often a hard thing to do, but many people are willing to help new parents find a situation they feel comfortable with. Finding a good child care arrangement that you trust will help you feel better about this decision. There are helpful resources and written guides as well as community resources available to assist you in selecting the right child care for you and your child.
- I also can give you advice and information about resources that can help you identify child care and help you continue breastfeeding after you go back to work/school.

Priority

Parent and Family Health and Well-being
Postpartum checkup, maternal depression, family relationships

Postpartum Checkup

Discuss the mother's postpartum physical and emotional health and provide information about her needs during this period. Any suggestion of depression should trigger screening questions for increased drug and alcohol use. Explore issues of substance abuse (with legal and illegal drugs) as self-medication of mood. As needed, refer the mother to her obstetrician or other health care professional and appropriate community-based mental health services. Ask the mother what other medical visits that she has had in the interim for herself or the infant and whether she has health insurance.

Sample Questions
What have you heard from your obstetrician or other health care professional about resuming your normal daily activities after delivery? When is your postpartum checkup? How are you managing any pain or discomfort from delivery? How is breastfeeding going?

Anticipatory Guidance
- Typically, a 6-week postpartum checkup should be scheduled to discuss how you are feeling and make any arrangement you wish about birth control. Sometimes, moms are so tired or busy they forget or just don't make their postpartum appointment.
- If you are still feeling discomfort from the delivery, you should talk with your obstetrician or health care professional.

Maternal Depression

An estimated 10% to 20% of women struggle with major depression before, during, and after delivery of a baby. Perinatal depression has substantial personal consequences and interferes with quality of child-rearing, adversely affecting parent and infant interactions, maternal responsiveness to infant vocalizations and gestures, and other stimulation essential for optimal child development.

Because pregnancy and childbirth are supposed to be a joyous occasion, women may feel that they are going to be bad mothers if they are depressed. It is important for apprehensive patients to understand what postpartum depression is, to know that many women experience similar feelings, and to realize that untreated postpartum depression may have adverse effects on women's health and their children's health and development.

Sample Questions

What are some of your best, and most difficult, times of day with the baby? How are you feeling emotionally? Have you been feeling sad, blue, or hopeless since the delivery? Are you still interested in activities you used to enjoy? Do you find that you are drinking, using herbs, or taking drugs to help make you feel less depressed, less anxious, less frustrated, and calmer? Who has been available to assist you at home? Who has been the most help to you?

Over the past 2 weeks, have you ever felt down, depressed, or hopeless? Over the past 2 weeks, have you felt little interest or pleasure in doing things? Do you have any physical symptoms, like headache, chest pain, or palpitations?

Anticipatory Guidance

- Many mothers feel tired or overwhelmed in the first weeks at home. These feelings should not continue, however. If you find that you are still feeling very tired or overwhelmed, or you are using over-the-counter or prescription medication, drugs, or alcohol to feel better, let your partner, your own health care professional, or me know so that you can get the help you need.
- It is common for women during and after pregnancy to feel down or depressed. It is very important to address these feelings to ensure your health and your baby's health.
- Emphasizing healthy life behaviors, like getting enough sleep, eating healthy foods, and finding time for walking or other light physical activity, can help you feel better.
- If you are sad or down for more than 2 days, please speak with me about options for treatment. Talk therapy or counseling is generally rapidly helpful.

Family Relationships

Families who are living with others (eg, their elders, those who are helping them from being homeless, or teen parents living with their parents) may have little control over their environment and caregiver roles and responsibilities. For some families, gender roles may preclude women from asking men for help. In a culturally sensitive way, health care professionals need to develop strategies with parents and the family about how to support the mother's needs.

If parents are feeling stressed or if they are having difficulty getting along together, they need referral to an appropriate mental health care professional.

Sample Questions

How are you finding taking care of yourself and the baby? Are you able to find time for your other children? Who helps you with the baby? Are your partner or other family members able to help care for the baby or with things around the house? How are your other children reacting to the baby? Have you observed any behavior changes, jealousy, or anything that concerns you? How are you handling this?

Anticipatory Guidance

- Finding time for yourself can be a challenge. Talking with your partner and problem-solving together will help your partner feel involved and identify ways to help you. It also may be important to have someone to talk with if you feel isolated and alone.
- Please let us know if you are feeling isolated or alone so that we can provide you with community contacts that can help you.

Priority

Infant Behavior and Development

Sleeping and waking, fussiness and attachment, media, playtime, medical home after-hours support

Sleeping and Waking

Discuss the infant's sleep patterns and the ways in which the parents respond. Parents may need reassurance that infants' sleep patterns are highly variable, and that their need for frequent night feedings is normal. An infant's inability to sleep may result from illness or allergy, but not from a failure to learn how to sleep.

Sample Questions

How is your baby sleeping? Does he use a pacifier? When do you use the pacifier?

Anticipatory Guidance

- Putting the baby in his crib either awake or drowsy, not in a deep sleep, will help him make the transition from being awake to asleep in the crib. This will avoid problems with night waking later on because, when he wakes up, he will be in a familiar place.
- The room temperature should be comfortable and the baby should be kept from getting too warm or too cold while sleeping.
- Using a pacifier during sleep is strongly associated with a reduced risk of sudden infant death. After your baby is about 1 month old, consider offering a pacifier when he lies down for sleep. If your baby drops the pacifier, rinse it with water before reinserting it. It is important not to lick the pacifier to clean it, as you can transfer bacteria from your mouth to the baby's. Do not coat the pacifier with formula or a sweet solution.

Fussiness and Attachment

Offer strategies to support the infant's state regulation (alertness, orientation, and regulatory capacity) and behavioral maturation, including ways to engage the infant and console and calm him. This is particularly important if the infant was preterm or exhibits signs of easily being overstimulated or overwhelmed or if the baby is difficult to engage. Encourage parents to learn about their baby's temperament and how it affects the way he relates to the world.

If the intensity, frequency, duration, and constancy of the infant's crying are worrisome or stressful for parents, it should be evaluated. Discuss with parents strategies to support their infant and her responses.

The safest cover for the baby is a sleepsack or footed sleeper that can keep the baby warm without concern about suffocating under a blanket. This also allows the baby to move his legs, as opposed to swaddling, which has the potential to cause hip dysplasia.

If swaddling is used, it should *not* be used for sleep. The swaddle wrap should be snug, but not too tight, around the chest and loose around the baby's legs. When done correctly, swaddling can be an effective tool in helping to calm the infant.

Concerns about infant attachment or parent-infant interaction should prompt the health care professional to refer the family to community parenting and support programs. If concerns about infant development are evident, consider referral to the local Early Intervention Program agency, often referred to as IDEA Part C.

Counsel parents about how fragile an infant's brain is and how it is important to protect an infant from shaking and other forms of abuse. Parents can help their baby's other caregivers appreciate the infant's vulnerabilities and understand how to handle their frustrations with the infant's behavior. For babies who cannot be easily consoled, parents may need guidance on how to first check for the baby's safety, and then put the baby down in order to take a break. Parents can learn effective ways to calm their baby and reach out to friends and family for support, when needed.

Parents can be encouraged to seek support from their natural support network for respite. Not all families will have this resource accessible to them. Health care professionals can give parents the telephone numbers for community resources that can help.

Sample Questions

Tell me how you know what your baby wants. What is his cry like? Are the cries different at different times? What do you think they mean?

How much is your baby crying? How often? What seems to help? Do you swaddle your baby?

What do you do when you are feeling overwhelmed as a parent or frustrated with your baby? What are some of the ways you have found to calm your baby when he is crying? What do you do if they don't work? Who is helping you at home? What helps you keep calm and centered when you are stressed?

Anticipatory Guidance

- A young infant cannot be "spoiled" by holding, cuddling, and rocking him, or by talking and singing to him. Responding quickly to your baby's cry will not spoil him, but it will teach him that he will be cared for.
- Many babies have fussy periods in the late afternoon or evening. Babies can't always calm themselves. Strategies to calm a fussy infant include feeding him again; being there with him; talking to, patting, or stroking him; bundling or containing him; holding and rocking him; and letting him suck. Sometimes it is hard to console a fussy or crying baby, no matter what you do.
- It will be a while before your baby is developmentally ready for self-consoling and will need your attention in the meantime. If you feel you're at the end of your rope and in danger of physically harming your crying baby, call for help right away.
- An infant's developmental progress toward self-consoling includes putting his hands to his mouth or sucking on his fingers, thumb, and pacifier.
- Holding a baby in a front carrier or sling may decrease crying, but these may not be safe for infants who are premature or who have neuromuscular, respiratory, or neurologic problems.

- If you swaddle your baby, be sure to keep the blanket loose around his legs, but snug—not tight—around his chest. To make sure your baby can breathe, leave enough space so that you can fit your hand between the blanket and his chest. Also, be sure that there are no loose ends of blanket around his neck, as these can increase his risk of suffocating.
- Swaddling should only be used with babies younger than 2 months and is recommended only when your baby is awake. Older babies can roll over and risk suffocation if they are swaddled.
- All new parents feel overwhelmed, frustrated, exhausted, or angry occasionally. Remember that your baby is not trying to make you angry. He is just having a rough time and still needs someone to be there. You could ask a family member, neighbor, or trusted friend to stay with your crying baby for a few minutes to allow you to take a break. If you are alone, you can try putting the baby in his crib, closing the door, and checking on him every few minutes.
- Never, ever, shake your baby or otherwise harm your baby, because it could cause permanent injury, including brain damage. If you ever feel that you need help because your baby is crying so much, contact me or other community resources that can help you.

Media

As more families and children have access to and exposure to digital media, it is important to assess for the use of such devices and offer guidance regarding media in the home.

Sample Question

Is there a TV or other digital media device on in the background while your baby is in the room?

Anticipatory Guidance

- Babies this young should not watch TV or videos. Some parents try to calm their fussy babies by sitting them in front of a TV show or video, but this may make them fussier in the long run, and doesn't help them learn ways to soothe themselves. Try other ways to soothe your baby when he is fussy, such as taking a walk, holding him in a carrier, decreasing the amount of stimulation and noise in the home, or using infant massage. You can also ask someone else to hold the baby so you can take a break.
- Having a TV on in the background can distract you from reading your baby's cues. Reading infant cues is important to learning about your baby's patterns of behavior and developing sensitive interactions with the baby. These interactions between you and your baby are crucial for language, cognitive, and emotional development.

Playtime

Spending time playing and talking during quiet, alert states helps strengthen the parent-infant bond by building a trusting relationship.

Sample Question

Tell me what happens with you and the baby when he is alert and awake.

Anticipatory Guidance

- Playing is fun for you, but essential for your baby's brain development.
- Babies need "tummy time" to develop head control and to get used to being on their stomach. This time is important because it stimulates muscle development and can help prevent the development of a flat area on the back of the head. During these times, place your baby in a position where he can see around the room and you can talk and interact with him even if you are doing other chores.

Medical Home After-hours Support

The health care professional should clearly explain the office practice plan for telephone triage, secure e-mail communication, after-hours calls, and same-day illness appointments. Parents are welcome to call about any change in the infant's activity, appearance, or behavior that makes them uncomfortable.

Sample Questions

Do you know when to call the health care professional? What type of thermometer do you have? Are you comfortable using it and knowing when to call the office if your child has a fever?

Anticipatory Guidance

- Wash your hands with soap and water often, or use a non-water antiseptic, and always after diaper changes and before feeding your baby.
- You can call our office anytime with questions.
- A rectal temperature of 100.4°F/38°C is considered a fever. Use of a rectal digital thermometer is preferred. Do not take the baby's temperature by mouth until he is 4 years old.

Priority

Nutrition and Feeding

Feeding plans and choices, general guidance on feeding, breastfeeding guidance, formula-feeding guidance

---

Feeding Plans and Choices

Helping parents develop a confident and pleasurable feeding relationship during the first 6 months not only establishes adequate nutrition and growth for their baby but also supports a positive parent-infant relationship. Encouraging parents to hold their baby and meet her needs will help the baby trust that she will be cared for.

An infant who cries inconsolably for several hours a day and passes a lot of gas may have colic or reflux. Exploring the consistency and predictability of the baby's day, especially for feeding and sleeping, will help to identify strategies that parents can implement that can significantly resolve infant fussiness. This information also can shed light on other issues that may need medical intervention.

Feeding strategies and information depends on whether the mother is breastfeeding or formula feeding her baby, or both. Solid foods, including cereals, are not indicated until about 6 months of age.

If a parent gives the infant over-the-counter medications (eg, teas, digestive aids, or sleep or discomfort remedies), discuss the possible adverse effects. Discussion about use of these products should be conducted within the family's cultural context, recognizing that, for many families, these are important practices believed to protect the child's health and well-being.

Sample Questions

How is feeding going? What are you feeding her at this time? How often are you feeding your baby during the day? During the night? Tell me about all foods and fluids you are offering the baby. Has anyone given her cereal or other food?

As you are beginning to look for a child care provider, have you thought about talking with the child care provider about your baby's daily routines for feeding and sleep or how he or she might support you in continuing to breastfeed?

How many wet diapers and stools does your baby have each day?

Are you giving your baby any supplements, herbs, special tea, or vitamins?

What vitamin or mineral supplements do you take or plan to take? Are you taking any herbs or drinking any special teas? What medications do you use, such as prescription, over-the-counter, homeopathic, or street drugs?

Anticipatory Guidance

- Mothers who exclusively breastfeed provide ideal nutrition for their babies for about the first 6 months of life. For infants who are not breastfeeding, iron-fortified formula is the recommended substitute.
- Feed your baby when she shows signs of hunger, usually every 1 to 3 hours in the daytime, and every 3 hours at night, with one longer 4- to 5-hour stretch between feedings, for a total of 8 to 12 times in 24 hours. Babies should not be overfed.
- Do not offer your baby food other than breast milk or formula until she is developmentally ready, which is at about 6 months old.
- Healthy babies do not require extra water. Breast milk and formula (when properly prepared) are adequate to meet your baby's fluid needs. Juice is not recommended.
- Infants often go through growth spurts between 6 and 8 weeks of age and significantly increase their milk intake during that time.
- Your baby is getting enough milk if she has 6 to 8 wet cloth diapers (5 or 6 disposable diapers) and a variable number of stools per day and is gaining weight appropriately.
- Most medications are compatible with breastfeeding, but check them out individually with me or your other health care professionals.
- If your baby is a full-term, formula-fed infant, you do not need to give her vitamin supplements if the formula is iron fortified and your baby is consuming an adequate volume of formula for appropriate growth.

General Guidance on Feeding

Sample Questions

How do you know if your baby is hungry? How do you know if she has had enough to eat?

For formula feeding: *How do you hold your baby when you feed her? Do you ever prop the bottle to feed or put your baby to bed with the bottle?*

How easily does your baby burp during or after a feeding?

Anticipatory Guidance

- Signs of fullness are turning the head away from the nipple, closing the mouth, and showing interest in things other than eating.
- Exclusive breastfeeding or formula meets all the nutritional needs of your baby for about 6 months. At that time, breastfed infants will need zinc- and iron-rich supplementary foods to meet their zinc and iron needs.
- Wait to introduce solid foods or liquids until about 6 months. Introducing solid foods earlier will not help your baby sleep through the night.
- If you are bottle-feeding your baby, always hold her in your arms in a partly upright position. This will allow you to look into her eyes during feedings and watch her cues for when she has had enough or needs to take break from feeding. Feeding is a wonderful opportunity for warm and loving interaction with your baby.

- It is very important to not prop a bottle in your baby's mouth or put her to bed with a bottle containing juice, milk, or other sugary liquids. Propping and putting her to bed with a bottle increases the risk of choking and developing early tooth decay.
- Burp your baby at natural breaks, such as midway through or after a feeding. Gently rub or pat her back while holding her against your shoulder and chest or supporting her in a sitting position on your lap.

Breastfeeding Guidance

Mothers

Mothers who breastfeed should ingest 500 μg of folate or folic acid daily by taking a daily prenatal vitamin or a multivitamin in addition to eating a nutritious diet. The mother's diet should include an average daily intake of 200 to 300 mg of the omega-3 long-chain PUFA DHA to guarantee a sufficient concentration of preformed DHA in the milk. This is obtained either through supplementation or consumption of 1 to 2 portions (3 oz each) of fish (eg, herring, canned light tuna, salmon) per week. The concern regarding the possible risk from intake of excessive mercury or other contaminants is offset by the neurobehavioral benefits of an adequate DHA intake and can be minimized by avoiding the intake of 4 types of fish that are high in mercury. These are tilefish, shark, swordfish, and king mackerel. Additionally, the mother's diet should include 550 mg/day of choline because human milk is rich in choline and depletes the mother's tissue stores. In the diets of women, eggs, milk, chicken, beef, and pork are the biggest contributors of choline.

For vegan mothers, who consume no animal products in their diet, a daily multivitamin including iron, zinc, vitamin B_{12}, omega-3 fatty acids, and 550 mg of choline is recommended.

Infants

Breastfed preterm or low birth weight infants will need multivitamin drops and iron supplementation by 2 to 6 weeks of age (2 weeks in very low birth weight infants) before solid foods are introduced.

Vitamin D supplementation (400 IU per day) is recommended for breastfed infants beginning at hospital discharge.

Sample Questions

How is breastfeeding going for you and your baby? Are you breastfeeding exclusively? If not, what else is the baby getting? Do you need any help with breastfeeding? In what ways is breastfeeding different now from when you were last here? How can you tell if your baby is satisfied at the breast?

What vitamin or mineral supplements are you giving your infant? What vitamin or mineral supplements do you take or plan to take?

Has your baby received breast milk or other fluids from a bottle?

Anticipatory Guidance

- Exclusive breastfeeding continues to be the baby's best source of nutrition for about the first 6 months of life.
- You can be reassured about your baby's weight gain by reviewing the growth chart.
- If you are breastfeeding your baby, be sure that you are giving her vitamin D drops.
- Continue to take a daily prenatal vitamin or a multivitamin, in addition to eating a nutritious diet. If you do not consume any animal products in your diet and follow a vegan diet, your supplement should include vitamins D and B_{12} as well as iron and zinc.
- Avoid using any bottles and supplements, unless medically indicated, until breastfeeding is well established. For most infants, this occurs around 4 to 6 weeks of age.
- If you wish to introduce a bottle to your breastfeeding baby, pick a time when she is not overly hungry or full. Have someone other than you offer the bottle. Allow the baby to explore the bottle's nipple and take it in her mouth. Experiment with different bottle nipples and flow rates. Once you find a nipple that works well for your baby, it is important to stay with that type so that she can get used to a consistent flow of milk. Over time, as her suck becomes stronger, she may need a nipple with a slower flow rate.

Formula-Feeding Guidance

Proper preparation, heating, and storage of infant formula should be reinforced. If there is evidence of inadequate formula availability to meet the infant's needs, appropriate referrals to WIC and other community resources should be provided.

Infants will take an average of 24 to 27 oz of formula daily, with a range from 20 to 31 oz per day.

Sample Questions

How is formula feeding going for you and your baby? What formula do you use and how do you prepare it? Do you have enough formula for your baby? Is the formula iron fortified? How often does your baby feed? How much does your baby take at a feeding? Have you offered your baby anything other than formula? What concerns do you have about the formula, such as cost, preparation, and nutrient content?

Anticipatory Guidance

- You will need to prepare and offer more infant formula as your baby's appetite increases and she goes through growth spurts.
- Never heat a bottle in a microwave. If you wish to warm a bottle, a hot water bath is recommended.

Priority

Safety

Car safety seats, safe sleep, preventing falls, emergency care

Car Safety Seats

Parents should not place their baby's car safety seat in the front seat of a vehicle with a passenger air bag because the air bags deploy with great force against a car safety seat and cause serious injury or death.

Counsel parents that their own safe driving behaviors (including using seat belts at all times and not driving under the influence of alcohol or drugs) are important to the health of their children.

Infants with special needs require special consideration for safe transportation. Refer parents to a local, specially trained Child Passenger Safety Technician for assistance with special positioning and restraint devices (**www.preventinjury.org**).

Sample Question

Are you having any problems using the baby's car safety seat?

Anticipatory Guidance

- A rear-facing car safety seat should always be used to transport your baby in all vehicles, including taxis and cars owned by friends or other family members.
- The back seat is the safest place for children to ride. Babies are best protected in the event of a crash when they are in the back seat and in a rear-facing car safety seat.
- Never place your baby's car safety seat in the front seat of a vehicle with a passenger air bag because air bags deploy with great force. When it hits the car safety seat, it causes serious injury or death.
- Your baby needs to remain in the car safety seat at all times during travel. If he becomes fussy or needs to breastfeed, stop the car and remove him from the car safety seat to attend to his needs. Strap him safely back into his seat before traveling again.
- Your own safe driving behaviors are important to the health of your children. Use a seat belt at all times, do not drive after using alcohol or drugs, and do not text or use mobile devices while you are driving.

For information about car safety seats and actions to keep your baby safe in and around cars, visit www.safercar.gov/parents.

Find a Child Passenger Safety Technician: http://cert.safekids.org. Click on "Find a Tech."

Toll-free Auto Safety Hotline: 888-327-4236

Safe Sleep

Counsel parents about the very real risks of bed sharing with a caregiver or with other children, and appropriate cautions regarding bed and bedding type, avoiding infant overheating, and the effects of parental exhaustion, obesity, tobacco, alcohol, medication, or substance use by the caregiver. Health care professionals should be sensitive to parents' cultural traditions and beliefs about infant sleep and sleep location.

The health care professional can provide suggestions about how to keep the infant from getting too warm or too cold while sleeping.

Discuss with parents who are anticipating using child care whether it will be a family member or a child care center, and whether they have discussed safety issues, especially safe sleep and using a similar sleep/wake routine for their baby.

Sample Questions

Where does your baby sleep now? What have you heard about "back to sleep" and tummy to play? Have you talked with your child care provider about safe sleep practices for your baby?

Anticipatory Guidance

- Always put your baby down to sleep on his back, not his tummy or side. Ask your relatives and caregivers to also put your baby back to sleep.
- Experts recommend that your baby sleep in your room in his own crib and not in your bed. If you breastfeed or bottle-feed your baby in your bed, return him to his own crib or bassinet when you both are ready to go back to sleep.
- Do not use loose, soft bedding, such as blankets, comforters, sheepskins, quilts, pillows, pillow-like bumper pads, or soft toys, in the baby's crib because they can suffocate the baby.
- If possible, use a crib purchased after June 28, 2011, as cribs sold in the United States after that date are required to meet a new, stronger safety standard. If you use an older crib, choose one with slats that are no more than 2⅜ inches, or 60 mm, apart and with a mattress that fits snugly, with no gaps between the mattress and the crib slats. Drop-side cribs are no longer recommended.
- If you choose a mesh play yard or portable crib, consider choosing one that was manufactured after a new, stronger safety standard was implemented on February 28, 2013. If you use an older product, the weave should have openings less than ¼ inch (6 mm) and the sides should always stay fully raised.
- If you use a mesh play yard or portable crib, the weave should have small openings less than ¼ inch (6 mm).

Preventing Falls

Discuss strategies that parents can use to keep their baby safe from falls.

Sample Question

What actions are you taking to keep your baby safe from falls?

Anticipatory Guidance

- Always keep one hand on your baby when changing diapers or clothing on a changing table, couch, or bed, especially as he begins to roll over. Falls are the most frequent reason for emergency department visits for injury.
- Bracelets, toys with loops, or string cords should be kept away from your baby, and string or necklaces should never be around his neck. Dangling electrical, telephone, window blind, or drapery cords should be far from his reach.

Emergency Care

Parents will appreciate discussion of what sort of problems can be handled at the medical home and what will require emergency care. CPR and emergency and disaster preparedness may be discussed.

Culturally based practices to prevent illness, such as tying amulets or strings, and any other related safety issues, are important to discuss.

Sample Questions

Do you know what to do in an emergency? Do you have a list of emergency numbers? Do you know when and where to go to an emergency department? Do you have access to a telephone for emergencies?

Anticipatory Guidance

- I encourage you to complete an American Heart Association or American Red Cross first aid or infant CPR program.
- You also should learn what to do if your baby begins to choke.
- Make sure you have a first aid kit, know the local emergency telephone numbers, and are aware of concerns that might require a 911 call. Post emergency phone numbers next to every phone and store them in your cell phone.
- Think about the steps you can take to prepare for disasters or other unexpected events. Making a plan for how to deal with a storm or power outage is a great start.

Infancy
2 Month Visit

Context

By 2 months after birth, parents and their baby are communicating with each other. The parent and baby can gain each other's attention and respond to each other's cues. The baby looks into his parents' eyes, smiles, coos, and vocalizes reciprocally. He is attentive to his parents' voices, and reacts with enjoyment when his senses are stimulated with pleasant sights, sounds, and touch. The infant's responses to his parents when they cuddle him or talk and sing to him provide important feedback that helps the parents feel pleasure and competence. Likewise, the parents' prompt responses to his cries and other subtler cues help teach him cause and effect and, most important, trust.

Typically, parents have settled into their new roles, learning how to divide the tasks of caring for their baby, themselves, and the needs of the family. They may still feel tired and express a desire for rest. Other relatives and members of the support network feel a connection to the baby, and the parents are comfortable with them holding or caring for the baby.

The baby can now hold his head upright for brief periods of time while he is being held. His weight, length, and head circumference should increase along his predicted growth curve. Parents appreciate the health care professional's review of early milestone development because it helps them understand and anticipate the resolution of newborn reflexes. The Moro reflex, reflex grasp, and tonic neck reflexes disappear before purposeful motor skills emerge. Opportunities for motor activity when the baby is awake, such as "tummy time," should be encouraged because they promote head control.

Frequent feedings are still normal for the breastfed baby. The formula-fed baby may need to be fed less frequently. As the baby is able to consolidate longer sleep cycles, night feedings may occur less frequently. However, many babies have not yet begun to consolidate sleep, and many of those who have begun are likely to regress at times. Parents need to be counseled on delaying the introduction of solid foods until the middle of the first year of the baby's life and when the baby shows definite signs of readiness. These signs include increasing volume of human milk or formula consumed, and continuing physical development. Although it is a common belief, adding cereal to the diet will not increase the hours of sleep at night. Rather, the frequency and duration of feedings, regular naptimes, and active playtimes are more likely to encourage a consolidation of nighttime sleep cycles and longer sleep duration.

As the infant and family settle into a routine, parents begin to resume more of their previous activities, reengage with other family members and friends, and return to school or work. Siblings and other members of the family can be encouraged to participate in the baby's care, fostering their involvement and connection to the baby. Ideally, parents make plans to spend adult time together. Single parents may choose to spend time on outside interests and relationships. It also is important that other children in the family have some time alone with their parents for activities they enjoy.

Parents can encourage responsible siblings to participate in the care of the baby to help them feel a valued connection with their little sibling. Arranging for quality, affordable child care is an important priority.

The mother's health (both physical and emotional) will determine her emotional and physical availability to care for her infant. Thus, she should consider talking with her partner and health care professional about completing her postpartum checkup and making family-planning arrangements.

At this visit, it is important for the health care professional to review infant safety measures, including appropriate sleep position and sleep practices, because families and other caregivers may have modified the recommended safe-sleeping measures because of perceived infant or caregiver needs. For example, the parents or other caregivers may feel that the infant's sleep is less comfortable or that spitting up poses a choking threat if the infant is on his back. It is important to ask the parents about their caregiving practices or preferences to determine whether they differ from recommended practices. In addition, consideration should be given to the family's environment and living circumstances, as some aspects of the child's caregiving may not be under the control of the parent or primary caregiver. Health care professionals should be sensitive to cultural practices, gender roles, parental age, functional abilities, and financial independence of the parents.

Priorities for the 2 Month Visit

The first priority is to attend to the concerns of the parents.

In addition, the Bright Futures Infancy Expert Panel has given priority to the following topics for discussion in this visit:

- Social determinants of health[a] (risks [living situation and food security], strengths and protective factors [family support, child care])
- Parent and family health and well-being (postpartum checkup, depression, sibling relationships)
- Infant behavior and development (parent-infant relationship, parent-infant communication, sleeping, media, playtime, fussiness)
- Nutrition and feeding (general guidance on feeding and delaying solid foods, hunger and satiety cues, breastfeeding guidance, formula-feeding guidance)
- Safety (car safety seats, safe sleep, safe home environment: burns, drowning, and falls)

[a] Social determinants of health is a new priority in the fourth edition of the *Bright Futures Guidelines*. For more information, see the *Promoting Lifelong Health for Families and Communities* theme.

Health Supervision

The *Bright Futures Tool and Resource Kit* contains Previsit Questionnaires to assist the health care professional in taking a history, conducting developmental surveillance, and performing medical screening.

History

The interval history may be obtained according to the concerns of the family and the health care professional's preference or style of practice.

General Questions

- How are you feeling?
- How are things going for your family?
- How are things going for your baby? Tell me about your baby's day. What are some of the best times of day with your baby? Some of the most difficult?
- What are some of the things you are doing to keep your baby healthy and safe? Does your child live with or spend time with anyone who smokes or uses e-cigarettes? Other than your baby's birth, have there been any major changes in your family?

Past Medical History

- Has your baby received any specialty or emergency care since the last visit?

Family History

- Has your child or anyone in the family, such as parents, brothers, sisters, grandparents, aunts, uncles, or cousins, developed a new health condition or died? **If the answer is Yes:** Ascertain who in the family has or had the condition, and ask about the age of onset and diagnosis. If the person is no longer living, ask about the age at the time of death.

Social History

- See the Social Determinants of Health priority in Anticipatory Guidance for social history questions.

Surveillance of Development

Do you or any of your baby's caregivers have any specific concerns about your infant's learning, development, or behavior?

Clinicians using the *Bright Futures Tool and Resource Kit* Previsit Questionnaires or another tool that includes a developmental milestones checklist, or those who use a structured developmental screening tool, need not ask about these developmental surveillance milestones. *(For more information, see the Promoting Healthy Development theme.)*

Social Language and Self-help

Does your child

- Smile responsively?
- Make sounds that let you know he is happy or upset?

Verbal Language (Expressive and Receptive)

Does she

- Make short cooing sounds?

Gross Motor

Does he

- Lift head and chest when on stomach?
- Keep head steady when held in a sitting position?

Fine Motor

Does she

- Open and shut hands?
- Briefly bring hands together?

Review of Systems

The Bright Futures Infancy Expert Panel recommends a complete review of systems as a part of every health supervision visit. This review can be done by asking the following questions:

Do you have concerns about your infant's

- Head
  - Shape
- Eyes
  - Discharge
- Ears, nose, and throat
- Breathing
- Stomach or abdomen
  - Vomiting or spitting
  - Bowel movements
  - Belly button
- Genitals or rectum
- Skin
- Development
  - Muscle strength, movement of arms or legs, any developmental concerns

Observation of Parent-Infant Interaction

During the visit, the health care professional acknowledges and reinforces positive parent-infant interactions and discusses any concerns. Observation focuses on

- Are the parents responsive to the baby, to hunger or satiation cues, distress, or need for attention?
- How do the parents interact with their baby, such as through gazing, talking, smiling, holding, cuddling, comforting, and showing affection?
- What are the parents' appearance and emotional state? Do they support each other, and demonstrate confidence with the baby's care and contentment? Are they depressed, tearful, angry, anxious, fatigued, overwhelmed, or uncomfortable?

Physical Examination

A complete physical examination is included as part of every health supervision visit.

When performing a physical examination, the health care professional's attention is directed to the following components of the examination that are important for an infant this age:

- **Measure and plot on appropriate WHO Growth Chart**
  - Recumbent length
  - Weight
  - Head circumference
  - Weight-for-length
- **Skin**
  - Inspect for skin lesions, birthmarks, and bruising.
- **Head**
  - Palpate fontanelles occipital shape (flatness).
- **Eyes**
  - Examine pupils for opacification and red reflexes.
  - Assess visual acuity using fixate and follow response.
- **Heart**
  - Auscult for murmurs.
  - Palpate femoral pulses.
- **Musculoskeletal**
  - Perform Ortolani and Barlow maneuvers.
  - Inspect for torticollis.
- **Neurologic**
  - Evaluate tone, strength, and symmetry of movements.

Screening

Universal Screening	Action	
Depression: Maternal	Maternal depression screen	
Hearing	If not done previously, verify documentation of newborn hearing screening results and appropriate rescreening.[a]	
Newborn: Blood Screening	Verify documentation of newborn blood screening results, and that any positive results have been acted upon with appropriate rescreening, needed follow-up, and referral.	
Selective Screening	**Risk Assessment[b]**	**Action if Risk Assessment Positive (+)**
Blood Pressure	Children with specific risk conditions or change in risk	Blood pressure measurement
Vision	+ on risk screening questions	Ophthalmology referral

[a] Positive screenings should be referred for a diagnostic audiologic assessment, and an infant with a definitive diagnosis should be referred to the state Early Intervention Program.

[b] See the *Evidence and Rationale chapter* for the criteria on which risk screening questions are based.

Immunizations

Newborns and infants younger than 6 months are at risk of complications from influenza, but are too young to be vaccinated for seasonal influenza. Encourage **influenza vaccine** for caregivers of infants younger than 6 months and recommend **pertussis immunization (Tdap)** for adults who will be caring for the infant.

Consult the CDC/ACIP or AAP Web sites for the current immunization schedule.

CDC National Immunization Program: **www.cdc.gov/vaccines**

AAP *Red Book:* **http://redbook.solutions.aap.org**

Anticipatory Guidance

The following sample questions, which address the Bright Futures Infancy Expert Panel's Anticipatory Guidance Priorities, are intended to be used selectively to invite discussion, gather information, address the needs and concerns of the family, and build partnerships. Use of the questions may vary from visit to visit and from family to family. Questions can be modified to match the health care professional's communication style. The accompanying anticipatory guidance for the family should be geared to questions, issues, or concerns for that particular infant and family. Tools and handouts to support anticipatory guidance can be found in the *Bright Futures Tool and Resource Kit.*

Priority

Social Determinants of Health

Risks: Living situation and food security

Strengths and protective factors: Family support, child care

Risks: Living Situation and Food Security

Probe for stressors, such as return to work or school or the inability to return to work or school, competing family needs, or loss of social or financial support. Provide guidance, referrals, and help in connecting with community resources as needed.

Suggest community resources that help with finding quality child care, accessing transportation or getting an infant car safety seat and crib, or addressing issues such as financial concerns, inadequate means to cover health care expenses, inadequate or unsafe housing, limited food resources, parental inexperience, or lack of social support.

Sample Questions

Tell me about your living situation. Do you live in an apartment or a house? Is permanent housing a worry for you?

Do you have the things you need to take care of the baby, such as a crib, a car safety seat, and diapers? Does your home have enough heat, hot water, electricity, and working appliances? Do you have health insurance for yourself? How about for the baby?

Within the past 12 months, were you ever worried whether your food would run out before you got money to buy more? Within the past 12 months, did the food you bought not last and you did not have money to get more?

Have you ever tried to get help for these issues? What happened? What barriers did you face?

How do you deal with family members who criticize you or offer suggestions that are not helpful?

Anticipatory Guidance

- Programs and resources are available to help you and your baby. You may be eligible for the WIC food and nutrition program. Several food programs, such as the Commodity Supplemental Food Program and SNAP, the program formerly known as Food Stamps, also can help you. Would you like their numbers? Would you like someone from our office to help you get in touch with them?
- It's good that these things are not a concern for you right now. If things change, please consider us a place where you can get ideas about whom to contact for help. We know how important these things are to helping you keep your baby and your family healthy and safe.
- One way to deal with unwanted advice from family and friends is to acknowledge their concerns and desire to help and then change the subject to something you do agree on. Trying to justify your desire to follow the recommendations of your health care professional may only lead to a long and futile conversation.

Strengths and Protective Factors: Family Support

Parents reach out to families and friends for support and information for strategies in caring for their child. Making friends with adults who have a child the same age can help parents establish a support network that is useful in planning same-age playgroups and visiting neighborhood playgrounds. Families who are living with others (eg, their elders, those who are helping them from being homeless, or teen parents living with their parents) may have little control over their environment and caregiver roles and responsibilities. For some families, gender roles may preclude women from asking men for help. In a culturally sensitive way, health care professionals can develop strategies with parents and the family about how to support the mother's needs.

Sample Questions

What help do you have with the baby? Are you getting enough rest? Have you been out of the house without the baby? Who takes care of the baby when you go out? How does your baby handle this separation? Do you know parents of babies your baby's age? Do you feel you can reach out to them for help and advice? What are your plans for returning to school or work? Would you like any help in locating affordable, safe, quality child care?

Anticipatory Guidance

- It is important to take time for yourself as well as time with your partner. Your baby has a strong need to be with you. This need is stronger for some babies than for others. Let me know if you would like some suggestions for how to arrange time away from the baby or ideas for creative ways to spend time with your partner that do not compromise your baby's needs, such as activities when she is sleeping.
- It is important for you to identify ways to keep in contact with your friends and family members so that you do not become socially isolated.

Strengths and Protective Factors: Child Care

At this time, parents may need to return to work or school and should make plans for quality, affordable child care. Parents may benefit from guidance in finding child care and ensuring that caregivers are providing developmental stimulation as well as physical care. Reassure parents about how their baby can thrive in child care. It is important for them to find a person or place they can trust, that will keep their baby safe and consider her developmental needs, while engaging the parents in their infant's progress through sharing of daily activities.

Parents may need reassurance during this time of transition to someone else sharing the care of their baby. Separation usually is hard, and the parent may feel guilty and will need to be able to trust or receive support from family members and the child care provider. Changes in routine and separation also may be hard on the infant, and parents may find it helpful to spend extra time comforting the infant during the transition.

Sample Questions

What have you done about locating someone for child care when you return to work or school, need to run errands, or go out with family? Are you comfortable with these arrangements?

How do you feel now about leaving your baby with someone else? Have you talked with your child care provider about your baby's routines and how to let you know how your baby did during the day?

Anticipatory Guidance

- We can give you suggestions about how to find good child care, if you wish. Standards for child care exist. You should look for licensed child care centers and family child care centers that meet specific criteria. It is important to visit and spend time in any setting where you will be leaving your baby to make sure you know how it operates.
- You can expect a good child care provider to have good infection control practices in place and to give you a daily activity report about your baby's feedings, sleep, play, and elimination.
- It is not uncommon for mothers to have strong feelings about leaving their baby. Knowing that your baby is with someone you trust and who will take good care of her is a very important first step.
- Regular and predictable routines build your child's social and emotional competence.

Priority

Parent and Family Health and Well-being
Postpartum checkup, depression, sibling relationships

Postpartum Checkup

Discuss the mother's perspective of her own health and steps she is taking to care for herself. Mothers at this stage may feel sad, exhausted, frustrated, discouraged, or disappointed in their ability to care for their infant. Health care professionals should take into account economic pressures on the family, the need for the mother to return to work quickly, the need to care for other children, and neighborhood issues, such as safety and lack of sidewalks and recreational space. Provide phone numbers and contact information if the mother expresses any concerns about taking care of herself, and provide follow-up to ensure that she is able to access these resources.

Sample Questions
To both parents: *How are you feeling?*

To the mother: *Have you had a postpartum checkup? Did you discuss family-planning arrangements at this checkup? With your partner? What have you heard from your obstetrician about resuming your normal daily activities after delivery? What do you do to take care of yourself?*

Anticipatory Guidance
- Because your role as parents requires both physical and emotional energy, you must take care of yourselves so you can care for your baby.

Depression

An estimated 10% to 20% of women struggle with major depression before, during, and after delivery of a baby. Perinatal depression has substantial personal consequences and interferes with quality of childrearing, adversely affecting parent-infant interactions, maternal responsiveness to infant vocalizations and gestures, and other stimulation essential for optimal child development.

Because pregnancy and childbirth are supposed to be a joyous occasion, women may feel that they are going to be bad mothers if they are depressed. It is important for apprehensive patients to understand what postpartum depression is, know that many women experience similar feelings, and realize that untreated postpartum depression may have adverse effects on women's health and their baby's health and development.

Sample Questions

What are some of your best, and most difficult, times of day with your baby? How are you feeling emotionally? Have you been feeling sad, blue, or hopeless since the delivery? Are you still interested in activities you used to enjoy? Do you find that you are drinking, using herbs, or taking drugs to help make you feel less depressed, less anxious, less frustrated, and calmer? Who has been available to assist you at home? Who has been the most help to you?

Anticipatory Guidance

- Many mothers feel tired or overwhelmed in the first weeks at home. These feelings should not continue, however. If you find that you are still feeling very tired or overwhelmed, or you are using over-the-counter or prescription medication, drugs, or alcohol to feel better, let your partner, your own health care professional, or me know so that you can get the help you need.

Sibling Relationships

Sibling adjustment is a process over time and not yet complete at only 2 months of age. Behavior regression and jealousy sometimes occur and are normal.

Parents can help older siblings by including them in the care of the new baby in developmentally appropriate ways. Reading, talking, and singing together assures older siblings of their importance to parents and their value in the family.

Sample Questions

How are your other children? Are you able to spend time with each of them individually?

Anticipatory Guidance

- One of the ways that you can meet the needs of your other children is by appropriately engaging them in the care of the baby. Having them bring supplies and hold the baby's hand are 2 ways they can help. Giving them a "baby doll" of their own to hold, feed, and diaper is important; so is setting aside regular one-on-one time with your other children to read, talk, and do things together.

Priority

Infant Behavior and Development
Parent-infant relationship, parent-infant communication, sleeping, media, playtime, fussiness

Parent-Infant Relationship

The parents are beginning to experience some of the joys of their baby's behavior, such as an emerging smile, longer periods of alertness, and responsiveness. Parent uncertainty or nervousness, an uninvolved partner, or a statement that caring for the baby is "work," without relaxed or pleasant moments, requires further exploration and counseling. Additionally, a lack of parental involvement, as shown by a lack of questions about the baby and her development, or a demeanor of sadness, withdrawal, or anger, should trigger further exploration and counseling.

Sample Questions
What do you and your partner enjoy most about your baby? What are some of your best times of day with her? What are you enjoying about caring for your baby? What is challenging about caring for your baby?

Has your child care provider expressed any concerns about your baby's development?

Anticipatory Guidance
- At 2 months of age, your baby is beginning be alert and awake for longer stretches of time. She also will begin to respond more actively to you now by smiling and babbling. Make the most of this new development by cuddling, talking, and playing with your baby.
- It is important to know that a young infant cannot be "spoiled" by holding, cuddling, and rocking her, or by talking and singing to her. Spending time playing and talking during quiet, alert states helps strengthen your relationship with your baby by building trust between both of you.

Parent-Infant Communication

Assist the parents in becoming attuned to their infant's ability to handle stimulation and movement, and how best to incorporate activity into their infant's daily routine. Resources for parents to learn infant massage can be provided if parents are interested.

Sample Questions

What sounds does your baby make? Does the baby startle or respond to sounds and voices? Does she look at you and watch you as you move your face when you talk? What do you think your baby is feeling and trying to tell you? How does it make you feel? How do you know what your baby wants? Have you noticed any differences in her cries?

How would you describe your baby's personality? How does she respond to you? Is it easy or hard to know what she wants? What does your baby do with her hands?

Anticipatory Guidance

- Responding to your baby's sounds by making sounds, too, and by showing your face as you talk, encourages her to "talk back," especially during dressing, bathing, feeding, playing, and walking. This kind of "turn taking" is a foundation of language and conversation. Singing and talking during these typical daily routines also encourages language, as does reading aloud, looking at books, and talking about the pictures. Gradually, your baby will increase the variety and frequency of the sounds she makes as well as how she responds to sounds, especially her parents' voices.

- It is important to understand and recognize your infant's early temperament and personality so that you know how to adjust to meet her needs. As you learn about her temperament and the way she processes sensory stimulation, such as whether she is active, quiet, sensitive, demanding, or easily distracted, you will be better able to understand how it affects the way your baby relates to the world.

- Getting in tune with your baby's likes and dislikes also can help you feel comfortable and confident in your abilities as a parent. Infant massage is a helpful way for you to understand what your baby likes or dislikes. It can help you calm and relax her, and it enhances your baby's ability to go to sleep easily. Infant massage also offers important health and developmental benefits for premature infants and babies with special health care needs. It helps them sleep, regulate, and organize their waking and sleeping patterns, and promotes muscle tone and infant movement.

Sleeping

Parents with atypical and inconsistent sleeping patterns of their own, and parents of infants with difficulty developing consistent sleep patterns, irritability, difficulty consoling, or difficulty with feeding, may also need additional counseling because all these problems may be related to poor sleep patterns.

Sample Questions

How is your baby sleeping? What are some of your favorite routines with your baby?

Anticipatory Guidance

- Your baby is still developing regular sleep patterns. Help her by paying attention to her cues for sleep and by sticking to a regular schedule for naps and nighttime sleep. Infant irritability usually is caused by lack of sleep.
- By this point, you may be waiting for your baby to sleep through the night. It's normal for babies this age to continue to wake frequently at night. Placing your baby in her crib in a drowsy state encourages her to learn to sleep on her own.

Media

As more families and children have access to and exposure to digital media, it is important to assess for the use of such devices and offer guidance regarding media in the home.

Sample Question

Is there a TV or other digital media device on in the background while your baby is in the room?

Anticipatory Guidance

- Babies this young should not watch TV or other digital media. Some parents try to calm their fussy babies by sitting them in front of a TV show or video, but this may make them fussier in the long run, and doesn't help them learn ways to soothe themselves. Try other ways to soothe your baby when she is fussy, such as taking a walk, holding her in a carrier, decreasing the amount of stimulation and noise in the home, or using infant massage; or, ask someone else to hold the baby and take a break.
- Having a TV on in the background can distract you from reading your baby's cues. Reading infant cues is important to learning about your baby's patterns of behavior and developing sensitive interactions with the baby. These interactions between you and your baby are crucial for language, cognitive, and emotional development.

Playtime

While observing the infant in prone position, discuss the importance of tummy time in the baby's daily activities. During the physical examination, demonstrate how the infant will try to grasp objects held close to her hand and learn to put her hands in her mouth, which aids in self-consoling.

Sample Question

Physical activity is important for all of us, even young children. How is your baby moving about now?

Anticipatory Guidance

- When babies are awake, they enjoy looking around their environment and moving their bodies. One of the first skills babies must learn is holding their head up. One of the ways babies learn to do this is through tummy time. Although babies need to sleep on their backs, we want to encourage them to play on their tummies. Tummy time also can help prevent the development of a flat area on the back of the head.

Fussiness

Counsel parents that the infant's crying may increase at this age, but the crying spells will decrease over time. Parents may need strategies that will help them find ways to console their baby, and they need to be counseled about the fragility of an infant's head. Help parents understand that they are teaching the infant to trust that she will be cared for when they quickly respond to their infant's crying. This responsiveness will not spoil the infant, as many parents believe.

The safest cover for the infant is a sleepsack or footed sleeper, which can keep the baby warm without the concern of suffocation from a blanket. Swaddling is discouraged after 2 months of age.

Putting their hands to their mouth and sucking is an important self-comforting strategy used by infants, and it is an important step in self-regulation. Explain that this strategy helps infants with the earliest feelings of competence and mastery.

If the infant is very irritable, parents need to find a way to avoid frustration. They need to be cautioned to never shake their infant or leave her with someone who may harm her, because it causes severe, permanent brain damage. Provide telephone numbers for local community resources that can help parents.

Sample Questions

How much is your baby crying? How often? What are some of the ways you have found to calm your baby when she is crying? What do you do if that does not work? Do you still swaddle your baby?

Do you ever feel that you or other caregivers may hurt the baby? What makes you feel that way? How do you handle the feeling?

Anticipatory Guidance

- Spending time playing and talking to your baby during the quiet, alert times during the day supports her continuing brain development. Many babies have fussy periods in the late afternoon or evening. These are normal. There are many possible strategies for calming your baby, including just being there with her, talking, patting or stroking, bundling or containing, holding, wearing in a sling or carrier, and rocking. Other calming strategies include caressing or dancing with your infant, walking with her in a carriage or stroller, and going on car rides. Remember that your baby is not trying to make you angry—she is just having a rough time and still needs someone to be there. Ask a family member, neighbor, or trusted friend to stay with your crying baby for a few minutes to allow you to take a break. If you are alone, you can try putting the baby in her crib, closing the door, and checking on her every few minutes.

- It is no longer safe to swaddle your baby unless you are holding her in your arms. If your baby rolls to her tummy while swaddled tightly, she may not be able to move her head and keep her airway open. This can increase her risk of suffocation.

- At this age, your baby is developing the ability to put her hands to her mouth, suck on her fingers or her thumb, or use a pacifier. This is one of the ways your baby will learn to calm herself, and it is normal, age-appropriate behavior. She will use these methods until she is able to use other self-calming strategies.

- Never, ever, shake your baby or otherwise harm your baby, because it could cause permanent injury, including brain damage. If you ever feel that you need help because your baby is crying so much, contact me or other community resources that can help you.

Priority

Nutrition and Feeding

General guidance on feeding and delaying solid foods, hunger and satiety cues, breastfeeding guidance, formula-feeding guidance

General Guidance on Feeding and Delaying Solid Foods

By the second month of life, infant growth and the parent's comfort in feeding their infant should be well established. Infants who are struggling with maintaining a good growth pattern or parents who are struggling with feeding routines, extremely long feedings, or infrequent feedings should have additional support, guidance, and counseling to determine potential underlying infant developmental concerns or parenting knowledge issues.

Sample Questions

How is your baby's feeding going? Tell me about all the foods and fluids you are offering your baby. What questions or concerns do you have about feeding?

Anticipatory Guidance

- Exclusive breastfeeding for about the first 6 months of life provides ideal nutrition and supports the best possible growth and development. If you are still breastfeeding, congratulations!
- If your baby is not breastfed, iron-fortified formula is the recommended substitute during the first year of life.
- Do not give your baby food other than breast milk or formula until he is developmentally ready, which is at about 6 months of age.
- Usually, healthy babies do not require extra water. On very hot days with no air conditioning, babies will benefit from some extra water. Breast milk and formula, when properly prepared, are adequate to meet the baby's fluid needs. Juice is not recommended.

Hunger and Satiety Cues

Parents begin to learn their infant's cues for hunger and satiety.

Sample Questions

How do you know if your baby is hungry? How do you know if he has had enough to eat? How easily does your baby burp during or after a feeding?

Anticipatory Guidance

- Breastfed and formula-fed infants have different needs for the frequency of feeding, although both breast milk and formula provide all the nutrition that infants need until about 6 months of age.
- To prevent overfeeding, which often leads to more frequent spit-ups, recognize your baby's individual signs of hunger and fullness. An infant's stomach is still small. Therefore, your baby still needs to eat every 2 to 4 hours, even during the night. Hopefully, your baby will have one longer stretch at night of 4 to 5 hours without feeding.
- Burp your baby at natural breaks, such as midway through or after a feeding, by gently rubbing or patting his back while holding him against your shoulder and chest or supporting him in a sitting position on your lap.

Breastfeeding Guidance

Explain that as infants grow, they are more easily distracted during feeding and may need gentle repetitive stimulation, such as rocking, patting, or stroking. The infant may need a quiet environment, perhaps with low lighting and without other people present. Feeding times offer a wonderful opportunity for social interaction between the infant and the mother.

Counsel mothers on safe storage of human milk.

Vitamin D supplementation (400 IU per day) is recommended for all full-term breastfed infants beginning at hospital discharge. Breastfed preterm or low birth weight infants will need multivitamin drops and iron supplementation at 2 mg/kg/day by 2 to 6 weeks of age until solid food introduction.

Sample Questions

How is breastfeeding going for you and your baby? Is your baby breastfeeding exclusively? If not, what else is the baby getting? Do you need any help with breastfeeding? Does it seem like your baby is breastfeeding more often or for longer periods of time? In what ways is breastfeeding different now from when you were last here? How can you tell if your baby is satisfied at the breast? Is your child care provider supporting your breastfeeding efforts?

Are you planning to return to work or school? If so, will you express your breast milk? Does your school or workplace have a place where you can pump your milk in privacy? How will you store your milk? How long will you keep it?

Do you eat fish at least 1 to 2 times per week? Do you have protein-containing foods every day, such as eggs, chicken, beef or pork, or dairy? Are you able to be physically active most days?

Anticipatory Guidance

- Breastfed infants continue to need about 8 to 12 feedings in 24 hours. They may feed more frequently when they go through growth spurts. By 3 months of age, breastfed infants generally will be feeding every 2 to 3 hours. If your baby is receiving frequent feedings during the day and continuing to receive between 8 and 12 feedings in 24 hours, he may have one longer stretch of 4 to 5 hours at night between feedings.

- Consider how to plan your activities and schedules to make things easier when you are home or out with your baby. Storing breast milk properly is very important. If you are interested, I can give you written guidelines to help you make sure your stored breast milk remains safe for your baby.

- I can help you with strategies to support breast milk production if you will be away from the baby for extended periods.

- If you are breastfeeding your baby, be sure that you are giving him vitamin D drops.

- You may continue to take your prenatal vitamin with iron every day to ensure adequate intake of vitamins or minerals. Discuss with your obstetric team how long you should continue to take it. If you do not consume any animal products in your diet and follow a vegan diet, your supplement should include vitamins D and B_{12} as well as iron and zinc.

- Eating a small serving of fish 2 times a week provides important nutrients for your baby. Canned light tuna, salmon, trout, and herring are the best choices to give your baby the neurobehavioral benefits of an adequate intake of an important fat called DHA.

- It is best to avoid 4 kinds of fish that are high in mercury. These fish are tilefish, shark, swordfish, and king mackerel.

- Consuming small amounts of protein-containing foods, like lean meat, poultry, dairy products, beans and peas, eggs, processed soy products, and nuts and seeds, every day is recommended.

Formula-Feeding Guidance

If parents feel that they do not have time to hold the bottle, review the importance of the feeding relationship and the benefits of holding the infant during feeding, as well as the risks of propping the bottle. Parents also may need to be reminded not to put the baby to bed with a bottle.

The usual amount of formula for a 2-month-old in 24 hours is about 26 to 28 oz, with a range of 21 to 32 oz.

Sample Questions

How is formula feeding going for you and your baby?

What formula do you use? Is the formula fortified with iron? How often does your baby feed? How much does he drink at a feeding? Have you offered your baby anything other than formula? What questions or concerns do you have about the formula, such as cost, preparation, and nutrient content?

How do you hold your baby when you feed him? Do you ever prop the bottle to feed or put your baby to bed with the bottle?

Anticipatory Guidance

- Babies who receive formula usually will feed every 3 to 4 hours, with one longer stretch at night of up to 5 or 6 hours at night between feedings. Overall, a 2-month-old still needs about 6 to 8 feedings in 24 hours.
- When feeding your baby, always hold him in your arms in a partly upright position. This will prevent him from choking and will allow you to look into his eyes during feedings. Feeding is a wonderful opportunity for warm and loving interaction with your baby.
- Do not prop a bottle in your baby's mouth or put him to bed with a bottle containing juice, milk, or other sugary liquid. Propping and putting him to bed with a bottle increases the risk of choking and of developing early tooth decay.
- Never heat a bottle in a microwave. If you wish to warm a bottle, a hot water bath is recommended.

Priority

Safety
Car safety seats, safe sleep, safe home environment: burns, drowning, and falls

Car Safety Seats

Review car safety seat guidelines with the parents.

Counsel parents that their own safe driving behaviors, including using seat belts at all times and not driving under the influence of alcohol or drugs, are important to the health of their infant.

Sample Question
Do you have any questions about using your car safety seat?

Anticipatory Guidance
- A rear-facing car safety seat that is properly secured in the back seat should always be used to transport your baby in all vehicles, including taxis and cars owned by friends or other family members.
- Never place your baby's car safety seat in the front seat of a vehicle with a passenger air bag because air bags deploy with great force. When it hits a car safety seat, it causes serious injury or death.
- Car safety seats should be used only for travel, not for positioning outside the vehicle. Keep the harnesses snug whenever your baby is in the car safety seat. This will help prevent falls out of the seat and strangulation on the harnesses.
- Your own safe driving behaviors are important to the health of your children. Use a seat belt at all times, do not drive after using alcohol or drugs, and do not text or use mobile devices while driving.

For information about car safety seats and actions to keep your baby safe in and around cars, visit www.safercar.gov/parents.

Find a Child Passenger Safety Technician: http://cert.safekids.org. Click on "Find a Tech."

Toll-free Auto Safety Hotline: 888-327-4236

Safe Sleep

It is recommended that the infant sleep in a separate, but proximate, sleep environment. The infant should sleep in a crib, bassinet, or cradle in the same room as the parents. Infants should not share a bed with parents or any other caregivers or children. A pacifier should be offered when the baby is falling asleep. At the same time, health care professionals should be aware of parents' cultural traditions and beliefs about infant sleep and sleep location.

Sample Questions

Where does your baby sleep? What position does your baby sleep in? Is your baby having any difficulty sleeping on her back? Do you provide your child with a pacifier when she falls asleep? Where does your baby sleep when in child care?

Anticipatory Guidance

- Don't forget to reduce the risk of sudden infant death, by following "back to sleep" and "tummy to play." Make sure that any others who put your baby down to sleep also follow back to sleep.
- Your baby should sleep in your room in her own crib, but not in your bed.
- Offer your baby a pacifier when she is falling asleep.
- The room temperature should be kept comfortable. Make sure your baby doesn't get too warm or cold while sleeping.
- If possible, use a crib purchased after June 28, 2011, as cribs sold in the United States after that date are required to meet a new, stronger safety standard. If you use an older crib, choose one with slats that are no more than 2⅜ inches (60 mm) apart and with a mattress that fits snugly, with no gaps between the mattress and the crib slats. Drop-side cribs should never be used.
- If you choose a mesh play yard or portable crib, consider choosing one that was manufactured after a new, stronger safety standard was implemented on February 28, 2013. If you use an older product, the weave should have openings less than ¼ inch (6 mm) and the sides should always stay fully raised.
- If your baby is cared for by others, such as in a child care setting or with a relative, be sure to emphasize the importance of safe sleep practices with that caregiver.

INFANCY
2 MONTH VISIT

Safe Home Environment: Burns, Drowning, and Falls

As the baby develops more fine and gross motor skills, it is important to review with the parents how to keep the home environment safe. Discuss the importance of not leaving the baby alone in a tub of water—even for a second—even when using a bath seat. Also, the baby should never be left unattended in high places, such as changing tables, beds, sofas, or chairs.

Safety issues apply to all homes where the baby spends time, including child care and at grandparents' and friends' homes.

Sample Question
Have you made any changes in your home to keep your baby safe?

Anticipatory Guidance
- Do not drink hot liquids while holding the baby.
- **To protect your child from tap water scalds, the hottest temperature at the faucet should be no higher than 120°F.** In many cases, you can adjust your water heater. Before bathing the baby, always test the water temperature with your wrist to make sure it is not too hot.
- Never leave your baby alone in a tub of water, even for a moment. A bath seat or bath ring is not a safety device and is not a substitute for adult supervision. Your baby can drown in even a few inches of water, including in the bathtub, play pools, buckets, or toilets. A supervising adult should be within an arm's reach, providing "touch supervision," whenever babies are in or around water.
- Leaving the baby on a changing table, couch, infant seat, or bed is never safe because of your baby's ability to roll or push off. At this age, your baby's legs are getting stronger now and her newborn reflexes that prevent rolling over are gradually fading away. Because your baby is now bigger and stronger, it is important to always keep one hand on the baby when changing diapers or clothing on a changing table, couch, or bed, especially as she begins to roll over.
- Do not put your baby in a bouncy seat, recliner, or positioning seat on an elevated surface like a countertop or coffee table. Keep these devices on the floor when they are in use.

Infancy
4 Month Visit

Context

The relationship between parents and their 4-month-old is pleasurable and rewarding. The baby's ability to smile, coo, and laugh encourages her parents to talk and play with her. Clear and predictable cues from the infant are met with appropriate and predictable responses from her parents, promoting mutual trust. During this period, the infant masters early motor, language, and social skills by interacting with those who care for her.

The infant's fussiness should begin to decrease as she develops self-consoling skills and improved self-regulation. If crying is still a concern, parents need additional specific strategies for calming their baby. An irritable child who cries frequently or does not sleep through the night may clash temperamentally with a family that values regularity and tranquility. Evaluation of the infant's temperament and parent temperament may be needed to help the parents understand the importance of these strategies.

Responding to the sights and sounds around her, the 4-month-old raises her body from a prone position with her arms and holds her head steady. She may be so interested in her world that she sometimes refuses to settle down to eat. She may stop feeding from the breast or bottle after just a minute or so to check out what else is happening in the room. Parents may need to feed her in a quiet, darkened room for the next few weeks.

Milk is still sufficient nutrition, but parents may begin to ask about introducing solid foods. Infants become developmentally ready to start eating solid foods by about 6 months of age. Keep in mind that every baby is different and if a baby was born premature, her adjusted age should be used for any recommendations. Parents may have been told to start giving their babies cereal and other solid foods much earlier in life, often in an attempt to help their babies sleep longer at night, despite evidence to the contrary. Some families may wish to begin introducing solid foods before 6 months of age because the baby's ability to become an active participant in eating solid foods is growing, as is her physiological ability to handle these foods.

As key social and motor abilities become apparent at 4 months of age, the infant who appears to have a delay in achieving these skills may benefit from a formal developmental assessment. If developmental delays are found, exploring their origin and making referrals for early intervention will be important.

Most employed mothers will have returned to work by the time their infant is 4 months old, and it is important that the child care arrangements be of high quality and work well for both the infant and the family. Family problems, such as inadequate finances, few social supports, or low parental self-esteem, may impair the parents' ability to nurture. It is important that parents seek help when they feel sad, discouraged, depressed, overwhelmed, or inadequate. Parents who have the support they need can be warmly rewarded by their interactions with their 4-month-old.

Priorities for the 4 Month Visit

The first priority is to attend to the concerns of the parents.

In addition, the Bright Futures Infancy Expert Panel has given priority to the following topics for discussion in this visit:

- ▶ Social determinants of health[a] (risks [environmental risk: lead] strengths and protective factors [family relationships and support, child care])

- ▶ Infant behavior and development (infant self-calming, parent-infant communication, consistent daily routines, media, playtime)

- ▶ Oral health (maternal oral health, teething and drooling, good oral hygiene [no bottle in bed])

- ▶ Nutrition and feeding (general guidance on feeding, feeding choices [avoid grazing], delaying solid foods, breastfeeding guidance, supplements and over-the-counter medications, formula-feeding guidance)

- ▶ Safety (car safety seats, safe sleep, safe home environment)

---

[a] Social determinants of health is a new priority in the fourth edition of the *Bright Futures Guidelines*. For more information, see the *Promoting Lifelong Health for Families and Communities* theme.

Health Supervision

The *Bright Futures Tool and Resource Kit* contains Previsit Questionnaires to assist the health care professional in taking a history, conducting developmental surveillance, and performing medical screening.

History

The interval history may be obtained according to the concerns of the family and the health care professional's preference or style of practice.

General Questions

- Do you have any concerns, questions, or problems you would like to discuss today?
- How are you feeling today?
- How is your family doing? Siblings?
- What changes have you noticed in your baby?
- How are feeding and sleep going?
- What are you doing to keep your baby safe and healthy?
- What are some of the most enjoyable times of day now with your baby? What are some of the most challenging times of day?

Past Medical History

- Has your infant received any specialty or emergency care since the last visit?

Family History

- Has your child or anyone in the family, such as parents, brothers, sisters, grandparents, aunts, uncles, or cousins, developed a new health condition or died? **If the answer is Yes:** Ascertain who in the family has or had the condition, and ask about the age of onset and diagnosis. If the person is no longer living, ask about the age at the time of death.

Social History

- See the Social Determinants of Health priority in Anticipatory Guidance for social history questions.

Surveillance of Development

Do you or any of your baby's caregivers have any specific concerns about your baby's learning, development, or behavior?

Clinicians using the *Bright Futures Tool and Resource Kit* Previsit Questionnaires or another tool that includes a developmental milestones checklist, or those who use a structured developmental screening tool, need not ask about these developmental surveillance milestones. *(For more information, see the Promoting Healthy Development theme.)*

Social Language and Self-help

Does your child

- Laugh aloud?
- Look for you or another caregiver when upset?

Verbal Language (Expressive and Receptive)

Does he

- Turn to voices?
- Make extended cooing sounds?

Gross Motor

Does she

- Support herself on elbows and wrists when on stomach?
- Roll over from stomach to back?

Fine Motor

Does he

- Keep his hands unfisted?
- Play with fingers in midline?
- Grasp objects?

Review of Systems

The Bright Futures Infancy Expert Panel recommends a complete review of systems as a part of every health supervision visit. This review can be done by asking the following questions:

Do you have concerns about your infant's

- Head
  - Shape
- Eyes
  - Discharge
- Ears, nose, and throat
- Breathing
- Stomach or abdomen
  - Vomiting or spitting
  - Bowel movements
  - Belly button
- Genitals or rectum
- Skin
- Development
  - Muscle strength, movement of arms or legs, any developmental concerns

Observation of Parent-Infant Interaction

During the visit, the health care professional acknowledges and reinforces positive parent-infant interactions and discusses any concerns. Observation focuses on

- Do the parents respond to their baby through mutual gaze, talking, smiling, holding, cuddling?
- How do the parents respond to their infant's cues and what is the infant's response to the parents?
- How do the parents attempt to comfort their baby when crying? Are they successful?
- Do the parents attend to and support their infant during the examination?
- How do the parents interact with each other?

Physical Examination

A complete physical examination is included as part of every health supervision visit.

When performing a physical examination, the health care professional's attention is directed to the following components of the examination that are important for an infant this age:

- **Measure and plot on appropriate WHO Growth Chart**
  - Recumbent length
  - Weight
  - Head circumference
  - Weight-for-length

- **Skin**
  - Inspect for skin lesions, birthmarks, and bruising.

- **Head**
  - Palpate for positional skull deformities.

- **Eyes**
  - Examine pupils for opacification and red reflexes.
  - Assess visual acuity using fixate and follow response.

- **Heart**
  - Auscult for heart murmurs.
  - Palpate femoral pulses.

- **Musculoskeletal**
  - Assess for developmental hip dysplasia by examining for leg length discrepancy, thigh-fold asymmetry, and appropriate abduction.

- **Neurologic**
  - Evaluate tone, strength, and symmetry of movements.
  - Diminishing primitive reflexes.

Screening

Universal Screening	Action	
Depression: Maternal	Maternal depression screen	
Selective Screening	**Risk Assessment[a]**	**Action if Risk Assessment Positive (+)**
Anemia	Preterm and low birth weight infants and formula-fed infants not on iron-fortified formula	Hematocrit or hemoglobin
Blood Pressure	Children with specific risk conditions or change in risk	Blood pressure measurement
Hearing	+ on risk screening questions	Referral for diagnostic audiologic assessment
Vision	+ on risk screening questions	Ophthalmology referral

[a] See the *Evidence and Rationale chapter* for the criteria on which risk screening questions are based.

Immunizations

Infants younger than 6 months are at risk of complications from influenza, but are too young to be vaccinated for seasonal influenza. Encourage **influenza vaccine** for caregivers of infants younger than 6 months and recommend **pertussis immunization (Tdap)** for adults who will be caring for the infant.

Consult the CDC/ACIP or AAP Web sites for the current immunization schedule.

CDC National Immunization Program: **www.cdc.gov/vaccines**

AAP *Red Book:* **http://redbook.solutions.aap.org**

Anticipatory Guidance

The following sample questions, which address the Bright Futures Infancy Expert Panel's Anticipatory Guidance Priorities, are intended to be used selectively to invite discussion, gather information, address the needs and concerns of the family, and build partnerships. Use of the questions may vary from visit to visit and from family to family. Questions can be modified to match the health care professional's communication style. The accompanying anticipatory guidance for the family should be geared to questions, issues, or concerns for that particular infant and family. Tools and handouts to support anticipatory guidance can be found in the *Bright Futures Tool and Resource Kit.*

Priority

Social Determinants of Health

Risks: Environmental risk (lead)

Strengths and protective factors: Family relationships and support, child care

Risks: Environmental Risk (Lead)

Explain the risks of lead and discuss strategies for minimizing this risk. It is important to plan for creating a safe environment for the infant as mobility increases and he spends more time on the floor.

Work-related exposures, such as working in a battery plant, or home-related exposures, such as renovating an old home that has lead-based paint, can bring lead into the home through the clothing or body of the person doing the work.

Sample Questions

Do you know how to assess the risk of lead poisoning in your home?

Do you or anyone else in your household work outside the home in an environment where there might be concerns about exposure to harmful substances, such as lead?

Anticipatory Guidance

- Lead can be found in the paint of older homes (built before 1978), pottery and pewter, folk medicines, insecticides, industry, and hobbies, as well as other sources. Lead is toxic, and it is important to be aware of any sources of lead in your home to prevent lead exposure for your family.
- Lead dust can come into your home on your clothes or body of people who work with lead. After someone finishes a task that involves working with lead-based products, such as renovating older housing, stained glass work, bullet making, or using a firing range, they should change their clothes before they enter the home and shower as soon as they return home. Women who are breastfeeding should avoid activities that involve working with lead.

Strengths and Protective Factors: Family Relationships and Support

Usually by the time their infant is 4 months old, parents are truly enjoying their role as parents and beginning to gain confidence in their ability to care for their infant. Parents who are juggling work or school and child care and parenting may be less likely to find this time as enjoyable and may begin to feel the stress of their many responsibilities. Staying in touch with family and friends helps to avoid social isolation. Inquire about who helps them with their child. If fewer than 3 sources of help are offered, ask parents what family lives nearby, and about neighbors with children and friends from work, faith-based groups, or child care.

Sample Questions

What do you do when problems really get to you? Who do you turn to at times like that? How are you and your partner getting along together? Have you and your partner been able to find time alone? Who helps you care for your infant? How are your other children doing? Do you spend time with each of them individually? Who helps you take care of your baby?

Anticipatory Guidance

- Stay in touch with friends and family members. It will help you avoid social isolation.
- Talk to me or another health care professional if you and your partner are in conflict.
- Take some time for yourself and spend some individual time with your partner.
- Make sure you meet the needs of your other children by spending time with them each day doing things they like to do. Help them enjoy the baby by appropriately engaging them in the care of the baby, such as by bringing you supplies or holding the baby's hand.
- If you have few people in your family or at home who can help you care for your child, consider asking neighbors with children, friends from work, faith-based groups, or child care providers.

Strengths and Protective Factors: Child Care

Parents need help in identifying and evaluating their child care options. Provide written material or contact information for community resources that are available to assist parents in identifying family home care or child care centers that meet their requirements.

Parents of children with special needs often will have significant difficulty locating child care resources and, therefore, may particularly benefit from being connected to local public health resources as well as contacts through the local Early Intervention Program agency, often referred to as IDEA Part C. These contacts can help with developmental concerns and also for links to other community resources.

Sample Questions

Have you returned to work or school, or do you plan to do so? What are your child care arrangements? Who takes care of the baby when you go out?

How are your child care arrangements working out for you? Do you feel they are supporting your efforts to breastfeed your baby? Do they give you a daily report on your baby's activities, including feeding, elimination, sleep, and playtime?

Anticipatory Guidance

- If you are returning to work, talk with me or another health care professional about child care arrangements and your feelings about leaving your baby. Choose babysitters and caregivers who are mature, trained, responsible, and recommended by someone you trust.

- Getting a report from your child care provider helps you to stay connected to your child during his day. This also helps you to continue with the same routine and schedule. When it works for you, observe your baby and spend time at the child care setting. This may reassure you about the care he is getting.

Priority

Infant Behavior and Development

Infant self-calming, parent-infant communication, consistent daily routines, media, playtime

---

Infant Self-calming

Four-month-olds still will have fussy times, and parents need to have a variety of strategies to calm their infant. Setting up a variety of play activities so that the infant can be moved easily from one to the other is often helpful in adjusting for the infant's increasing awake time and short attention span. As they try to console their baby, sometimes unsuccessfully, parents begin to recognize that their baby may not always be consolable. Discuss additional strategies for calming the infant when this occurs. Swaddling is no longer recommended at this age, with evidence that it increases the risk of suffocating, leading to SUID.

Sample Questions

What do you do to calm your baby? What do you do if that does not work? Do you ever feel that you or other caregivers may hurt the baby? What will you do if you feel this way? Do you have a plan? How do you handle the feeling?

Anticipatory Guidance

- If your baby is being very fussy and you have checked that she is fed, clean, and safe and you are beginning to get upset and frustrated, put the baby in her crib and give yourself a break—make a cup of tea or call a friend. Babies cry a lot at this age; it gets better as they get older. Crying won't hurt your baby. If this happens consistently, though, call me for advice.

Parent-Infant Communication

As parents learn about their infant through observing her behaviors, they are able to respond appropriately to her ever-changing needs. Helping parents have "watchful wonder" about their baby's behaviors allows them to discover the uniqueness of their baby's own temperament and sensory processing, and how it affects the way she relates to the world. To demonstrate this watchful wonder, during the physical examination, describe the infant's behaviors and responses to being handled and engaged in play. This can lead to a discussion about what is developmentally appropriate and, if needed, when and how it is appropriate to redirect the infant's behavior.

Sample Questions

Tell me about your baby. What do you like best about her? What does your partner enjoy most about her? What do you think your baby is trying to tell you when she cries, looks at you, turns away, or smiles?

Bright Futures Guidelines for Health Supervision of Infants, Children, and Adolescents

Anticipatory Guidance

- Babies use their behaviors to communicate their likes and dislikes. Each baby has a unique way of communicating. By watching your baby closely, and how she responds to you and the world around her, you become the expert on your baby and the best way to meet her needs.
- As you begin to understand and recognize your infant's temperament and personality, you also will begin to feel more comfortable in knowing how to adjust your responses to meet her needs. This also will help your baby better understand how she relates to the world.
- It is important to know that an infant cannot be "spoiled" by holding, cuddling, and rocking her, or by talking and singing to her. Spending time playing and talking with your baby helps to strengthen the parent-child relationship by building trust between you and your baby.

Consistent Daily Routines

To receive adequate calories, most 4-month-olds continue to wake at night for feeding. Parents often see the infant not sleeping through the night as a problem, and they want solutions. This visit is a good time to explore the importance of a consistent daily routine and its effect on sleep, typical sleep patterns, ways to establish a good sleep routine, and the overall relationship among feeding, sleep, and play activities. Also, it may be important to clarify sleeping through the night. Some parents may expect an infant to sleep 12 hours at night, although actually having a longer stretch of sleep for 5 to 6 hours is more typical.

Parents who describe infants with inconsistent and unpredictable behaviors, or parents who are unable to describe their baby's schedule, may need additional monitoring and intervention.

Discuss difficulties integrating the routines of the infant with that of scheduling demands of older siblings and family members.

Sample Questions
What type of daily routine do you have for your baby? How long is your baby sleeping at night? Do you have a bedtime routine for your baby?

Anticipatory Guidance
- Creating a daily routine for feedings and naps and a bedtime routine is a good idea because they will help establish eventual longer sleeping stretches at night.
- It also is important to help your baby learn to put herself to sleep by placing her in her crib when she is drowsy, talking gently to her, and even patting her to sleep.
- Continuing to provide regular structure and routines for the baby will increase her sense of security.

INFANCY
4 MONTH VISIT

444

Media

As more families and children have access to, and exposure to, digital media, it is important to assess for the use of such devices and offer guidance regarding media in the home. Discuss alternatives to infants watching TV. Discourage any TV, computer, tablet, smartphone, or viewing or play for children at this age.

Sample Question

Is there a TV or other digital media device on in the background while your baby is in the room?

Anticipatory Guidance

- Babies this young should not watch TV or videos. Some parents try to calm their fussy babies by sitting them in front of a TV show or video, but this may make them fussier in the long run, and doesn't help them learn ways to soothe themselves. Try other ways to soothe your baby when she is fussy, such as taking a walk, holding her in a carrier, decreasing the amount of stimulation and noise in the home, or using infant massage; or, ask someone else to hold the baby and take a break.
- Having a TV on in the background can distract you from reading your baby's cues. Reading infant cues is important to learning about your baby's patterns of behavior and developing sensitive interactions with the baby. These interactions between you and your baby are crucial for language, cognitive, and emotional development.

Playtime

Counsel parents on the steps in development that are likely to occur during the next 2 months, based on the baby's current development and how the daily physical activities of the baby encourage normal development. Encourage parents to use both active and quiet playtime.

Babies who are described as excessively active or extremely quiet should be monitored. Management assistance is extremely important for parents who are sad or unhappy, or who rarely sleep. Consider referring parents for mental health evaluation and treatment.

Health care professionals can use the physical examination to demonstrate the integration of the newborn reflexes and emergence of the protective reflexes, and discuss what these reflexes, plus the infant's head control and sitting with support, mean in terms of the infant's ability to roll over and sit. As the infant improves her ability to move on her own, parents must begin to use extra caution about protecting her from rolling off the bed or couch or changing table. During the physical examination, demonstrate the protective reflexes, if emerging.

Sample Questions

What are some of your baby's new achievements? What are some of your baby's favorite activities? Favorite toys? How is she getting around now? How is "tummy time" working for your baby? How have you been able to fit together your physical activities with the baby? How would you describe your baby's personality? How does she act around other people? Is she responsive or withdrawn with family members?

Anticipatory Guidance

- Use both quiet and active playtime with your baby. Quiet playtime activities include reading or singing to your baby or sitting together outside in the park. For active playtime activities, give your baby age-appropriate toys to play with, such as a floor play gym so that, when she is placed on her back, she can reach for the toys or kick them with her feet. Another choice is a colorful blanket, a mirror, or toys for her to look at when she is on her tummy. Make sure your baby has safe opportunities to explore her environment.

- Babies at 4 months of age find that interacting with their parents is their favorite activity. Their emerging social play and interaction can be a delight, but also frustrating for parents who are balancing other responsibilities. Understanding ways to engage your baby in activities, even for a short time, will help provide some time to accomplish your other responsibilities.

Priority

Oral Health

Maternal oral health, teething and drooling, good oral hygiene (no bottle in bed)

Maternal Oral Health

Most parents are not aware that their own oral health has an effect on their baby's eventual dental health. Therefore, it is important to discuss this with parents.

Sample Questions

When was your last dental checkup? What is your daily dental care routine?

Anticipatory Guidance

- Sharing spoons and cleaning a dropped pacifier in your mouth may increase the growth of bacteria in your baby's mouth and increase the risk that he will develop tooth decay, also called dental caries, when his teeth come in.
- To protect your child's eventual dental health, it is important for you to maintain good dental health. Because you may be the source of caries-promoting bacteria for your baby, it is important you visit the dentist, reduce the amount of sugary drinks in your diet, take careful care of your teeth through brushing and flossing, and use a fluoridated toothpaste or rinse.

Teething and Drooling

Teething typically begins between 4 and 7 months of age. This is an appropriate time to address the family's concerns. Describe the teething syndrome and its management.

Sample Question

Is your baby beginning to drool?

Anticipatory Guidance

- If your baby is teething, he may drool, become fussy, or put things in his mouth. A cold, not frozen, teething ring may help ease his discomfort. Talk with me if his symptoms persist.

Good Oral Hygiene (No Bottle in Bed)

Discuss with parents the care of the infant's mouth and gums to prevent dental caries in their baby's primary teeth.

Sample Questions

Your baby will be getting his first tooth soon, if he has not already. Do you know how to keep his teeth clean? What are you doing now to care for your baby's mouth and gums?

Anticipatory Guidance

- To avoid developing a habit that will harm your baby's teeth, do not put him to bed with a bottle containing juice, milk, or other sugary liquid. Always hold your baby for a bottle-feeding and do not prop the bottle in his mouth or allow him to graze, meaning drinking from a bottle at will during the day. When you begin feeding your baby, at around 6 months of age, avoid baby foods or juices that are sucked out of a bag or pouch. A baby's teeth and gums will be in contact with the pureed food longer than necessary, which can lead to tooth decay. It's always best to use a spoon.

- Use a soft cloth or soft toothbrush with tap water and a small smear of fluoridated toothpaste, no more than a grain of rice, to gently clean your baby's gums and any teeth that develop. This should be done twice a day—after the baby's last feeding before nighttime sleep, and then again in the morning.

Priority

Nutrition and Feeding

General guidance on feeding, feeding choices (avoid grazing), delaying solid foods, breastfeeding guidance, supplements and over-the-counter medications, formula-feeding guidance

General Guidance on Feeding

At age 4 months, feeding can be one of the most enjoyable experiences for parents, and both parents often share in this responsibility. Babies continue to gain about ½ pound a week, or 2 pounds a month. Their feedings may become less frequent, with 6 to 10 feedings in 24 hours. Only one parent might be present at this visit and a complete feeding history may not be available. This is particularly true if the infant is in child care. If there are concerns with feeding, irritability, or weight gain, it may be advisable to have the parents work together with the child care provider to complete a 24-hour or 3-day diet history that can be reviewed for nutritional adequacy. A referral can be made to a dietitian, if needed.

Sample Questions

How is feeding going? What questions or concerns do you have about feeding? Tell me about what you are feeding your baby. How often are you feeding your baby? How much does she take at a feeding? About how long does a feeding last? Are you feeding your baby any foods besides breast milk or formula?

Anticipatory Guidance

- Exclusive breastfeeding provides the ideal source of nutrition for all infants for about the first 6 months of life. For those infants who are not breastfed, iron-fortified formula is the recommended substitute.
- Formula-fed infants do not need vitamin supplements if the formula is fortified with iron and the baby is consuming an adequate volume of formula for appropriate growth.

Feeding Choices (Avoid Grazing)

Parents continue to need reassurance that their infant is getting enough to eat when feeding patterns change because of a temporary increase in the frequency of feedings caused by growth spurts. Discuss the meaning of the growth chart and the relationship between the infant's birth weight and current weight and length.

As babies learn that they can put their hands in their mouth for chewing and sucking, they use this technique to calm themselves. Some parents think this means their baby is still hungry and they use it as a rationale for starting solid foods. Solid foods are not recommended until about 6 months of age.

Vitamin D (400 IU) supplements are recommended for all breastfed infants, but are not needed for formula-fed infants because vitamin D is present in the formula. Some preterm infants will require supplementation of additional vitamins.

Oral iron supplementation (1 mg/kg/day) should be provided to exclusively breastfed infants beginning at 4 months of age and should continue until iron- and zinc-rich complementary foods (baby meats and iron-fortified cereals) are introduced. It may take 1 to 2 months following introduction of these foods for infants to consume sufficient iron from complementary foods alone. Red meat is a better source of iron than iron-fortified cereals for older infants because a higher percentage of the iron in red meat is absorbed.

At 4 months, babies become very interested in their environment and it is not uncommon for them to vigorously begin a feeding and then become distracted by siblings or other activities in the environment and not complete a feeding. However, in an hour or so they begin to fuss because they are hungry again.

Sample Questions

How long does a typical feeding last now? How long between feedings? Do you feel that your baby finishes a feeding in one sitting or eats small amounts and then is hungry again in about an hour? Are you continuing to provide vitamin D?

Anticipatory Guidance

- It is important for you to help your baby avoid getting into the habit of grazing or snacking and then crying to be fed again soon. For breastfed babies, this may not be uncommon, however, when they are going through a growth spurt. The difference is that a growth spurt does not usually last more than a week.
- Be sure to continue your baby's vitamin D supplement. An iron supplement is now also necessary and we will begin it today.
- To help your baby finish a feeding, it may help to find a quiet and less distractible environment.
- In addition, because your baby loves to see your face, watch your expressions, and hear your voice, you can be the most interesting thing to watch while feeding. Position your baby so that she can see your face, and talk with her about her feeding, what is going on around her, and what will happen during the day. You can use touch, changes in your voice, and even slight changes in her position to help her refocus on feeding.

Delaying Solid Foods

At 4 months of age, human milk or formula remains the best food for babies. Solid feeding is discouraged until about 6 months of age.

Sample Question

Have you thought about when you will know that your baby is ready to begin solid foods?

Anticipatory Guidance

- Exclusive breastfeeding for about the first 6 months of life provides ideal nutrition and supports the best possible growth and development.
- If your baby is not breastfed, iron-fortified formula is the recommended substitute during the first year of life.
- Do not give your baby food other than breast milk or formula until she is developmentally ready, which is at about 6 months of age.
- Usually, healthy babies do not require extra water. On very hot days with no air conditioning, she will benefit from some extra water. Breast milk and formula, when properly prepared, are adequate to meet your baby's fluid needs. Juice is not recommended.

Breastfeeding Guidance

Commend mothers who are still breastfeeding. Reinforce that exclusive breastfeeding is the ideal source of nutrition for about the first 6 months of age, followed, as solid foods are introduced, by continued breastfeeding for 1 year or longer as mutually desired by the mother and child.

Discuss how demand for more frequent breastfeeding is usually related to an infant's growth spurt and is nature's way of increasing human milk supply. If an increased demand continues for a few days, is not affected by increased breastfeeding, and is unrelated to illness, teething, or changes in routine, it may be a sign that the breastfed infant is ready for solid foods.

Counsel mothers on safe storage of human milk.

Sample Questions

How is breastfeeding going for you and your baby? In what ways is breastfeeding different now from when you were last here? How often does your baby breastfeed? Does it seem as though she is breastfeeding more often or for longer periods of time? How can you tell whether your baby is satisfied at the breast? Has she received breast milk or other fluids from a bottle? How are you storing pumped breast milk?

Anticipatory Guidance

- Congratulations for continuing to breastfeed your baby! It is not unusual for babies to go through growth spurts during the first year of life and, whenever this occurs, your baby will begin to breastfeed more frequently, and often at night. This is nature's way of increasing your milk supply. This is a temporary situation and it does not indicate that your baby is not getting enough to eat.
- Storing breast milk properly is very important. If you are interested, I can give you written guidelines to help you make sure your stored breast milk remains safe for your baby.
- As your baby gets closer to 6 months of age, you may begin to see signs that she is ready for solid foods.

Supplements and Over-the-counter Medications

Medications and supplements often pass through the human milk to the baby. It is important to know what supplements and over-the-counter medications mothers are taking. Assess their safety for the infant.

Sample Question

Do you take any supplements, herbs, vitamins, or medications?

Anticipatory Guidance

- It is important to tell me about any medications, supplements, herbs, or vitamins you may be taking. This information will help me give you the best care and advice since you are breastfeeding. However, some medications may decrease your milk supply. Knowing what you are taking helps me determine whether they are safe with medications or treatments your baby might receive.
- Most medications are compatible with breastfeeding, but should be checked on an individual basis.

INFANCY
4 MONTH VISIT

Formula-Feeding Guidance

Discuss with parents that as the infant's appetite increases and she grows, they will need to continue to prepare and offer a little more infant formula. Instruct parents to feed the infant when she is hungry (usually 8–12 times in 24 hours).

Discuss with parents that iron-fortified formula is the most important nutrition for the infant at this time. Other foods or drinks are not advised unless recommended by the health care professional.

The usual amount of formula for a 4-month-old in 24 hours is about 30 to 32 oz of formula per day, with a range of 26 to 36 oz.

Sample Questions

How is feeding going? What formula are you using now? Is the formula fortified with iron? Have you tried other formulas? How often does your baby feed? How much at a feeding? How much in 24 hours? How does your baby show she is hungry or full? Has your baby begun to put her hands around the bottle? Are you still holding your baby for feedings? What questions or concerns do you have about the formula, such as cost, preparation, and nutrient content? Have you offered your baby anything other than formula?

Anticipatory Guidance

- Your baby is now able to clearly show when she is hungry or full. It also is not unusual for her to want different amounts of formula at different times of the day. She may take more at a morning feeding than at a noon feeding. It is important to respond to your baby's behaviors for feeding to avoid underfeeding or overfeeding. Overfeeding can lead to spitting up. Holding your baby during feeding also helps you understand the meaning of her behaviors. This will help you meet her needs and reduce fussiness. It will even help with her learning as she watches you and listens to your voice.

- It is important to hold your baby for all bottle-feedings to reduce the risks of choking and to ensure that your baby gets enough of the formula. To reduce the risk of your baby developing tooth decay, do not prop the bottle.

- If you have concerns about the cost of formula now that your baby is drinking larger amounts, you may want to contact community resources, like WIC, that can provide formula for your baby.

- Never heat a bottle in a microwave. If you wish to warm a bottle, a hot water bath is recommended.

Priority

Safety
Car safety seats, safe sleep, safe home environment

Car Safety Seats

Remind parents about proper car safety seat use and the importance of putting the infant in the rear seat of the vehicle.

Remind parents that their own safe driving behaviors (including using seat belts at all times and not driving under the influence of alcohol or drugs) are important to the health of their children.

Sample Questions
Do you use a rear-facing car safety seat in the back seat every time the baby rides in a vehicle? Do you know when to change from an infant-only car safety seat to a convertible car safety seat?

Anticipatory Guidance
- The back seat is the safest place for babies and children to ride. Babies are best protected in the event of a crash when they are in the back seat and in a rear-facing car safety seat.
- Never place your baby's car safety seat in the front seat of a vehicle with a passenger air bag because air bags deploy with great force. When it hits a car safety seat, it causes serious injury or death. Keep your baby's car safety seat rear facing in the back seat of the vehicle until your baby is 2 years of age or until he reaches the highest weight or height allowed by his car safety seat's manufacturer.
- When your baby outgrows the weight or height limit of a rear-facing–only seat, switch to a convertible seat used rear facing. Convertible seats can be used rear facing to higher weights and heights.
- Do not start the engine until everyone is buckled in.
- Your own safe driving behaviors are important to the health of your children. Use a seat belt at all times, do not drive after using alcohol or drugs, and do not text or use mobile devices while driving.

For information about car safety seats and actions to keep your baby safe in and around cars, visit www.safercar.gov/parents.

Find a Child Passenger Safety Technician: http://cert.safekids.org. Click on "Find a Tech."

Toll-free Auto Safety Hotline: 888-327-4236

Safe Sleep

Remind parents of the continuing importance of "back to sleep, tummy to play."

Sample Questions

Do you have any difficulty getting your baby to sleep on his back? Have you discussed with your child care provider the importance of safe sleep and back to sleep and tummy time to play?

Anticipatory Guidance

- Continue to put your baby to sleep on his back to reduce the risk of sudden infant death, but, if he rolls in his sleep, it is not necessary to return him to his back. Relatives and child care providers should be reminded to follow the same practice.
- To reduce the risk of suffocation, do not put loose, soft bedding, such as blankets, quilts, sheepskins, comforters, pillows, and bumpers or soft toys, in the crib.
- Be sure your baby's crib is safe both at home and at the babysitter's home. It is best to use a crib made after June 28, 2011, that meets the newest safety standard. If you must use an older crib, the slats should be no more than 2⅜ inches (60 mm) apart. The mattress should be firm and fit snugly into the crib. Drop-side cribs should not be used.
- Lower the crib mattress before the baby can sit up by himself.
- If you choose a mesh play yard or portable crib, consider choosing one that was manufactured after a new, stronger safety standard was implemented on February 28, 2013. If you use an older product, the weave should have openings less than ¼ inch (6 mm) and the sides should always stay fully raised.

Safe Home Environment

As the baby develops more fine and gross motor skills and becomes more active, it is important to review with parents how to keep the home environment safe. This applies to all homes where the baby spends time, including child care and grandparents' and friends' homes.

Sample Questions

Where does your baby spend awake time during the day? Have you made any changes in your home to help keep your baby safe?

Anticipatory Guidance

- **To protect your child from tap water scalds, the hottest temperature at the faucet should be no more than 120°F.** In many cases, you can adjust your water heater.
- Drinking hot liquids, cooking, ironing, smoking cigarettes, or using e-cigarettes while holding your baby puts him at risk of burns.
- To prevent choking, keep small objects, sibling's toys, pieces of plastic, and latex balloons out of the baby's reach as he develops skills with reaching.
- Always keep one hand on your baby when changing diapers or clothing on a changing table, couch, or bed, especially as he begins to roll over. Falls are the most common reason for emergency department visits for injury.

- A baby should not be left alone for even a second in a tub of water, even if using a bath seat, or on high places such as changing tables, beds, sofas, or chairs.
- Infant walkers should not be used by young children at any age. They are frequently associated with falls and can slow development of motor skills in children.
- The kitchen is the most dangerous room for children. A safer place for your child while you are cooking, eating, or unable to provide your full attention is the play yard, crib, or stationary activity center, or buckled into a high chair.

Infancy
6 Month Visit

Context

Parents cherish their interactions with their social 6-month-old, who smiles and vocalizes back at them, but has not yet mastered the ability to move from one place to another. The feelings of attachment between the parents and their child create a secure emotional attachment that will help provide stability to the changing family. The major developmental markers of a 6-month-old are social and emotional. A 6-month-old likes and needs to interact with people. He increasingly engages in reciprocal and face-to-face play and often initiates these games. From these reciprocal interactions, he develops a sense of trust and self-efficacy. His distress is less frequent than in previous weeks.

The infant also is starting to distinguish between strangers and those with whom he wants to be sociable. He usually prefers interacting with familiar adults. At 6 to 8 months, he may appear to be afraid of new people.

The 6-month-old can sit with support, and he smiles or babbles with a loving adult. He may have a block, toy, or book in his hand. As he watches his hands, he can reach for objects, such as cubes, and grasp them with his fingers and thumbs. He can transfer objects between his hands and may attempt to obtain small objects by raking with all his fingers. He also may mouth, shake, bang, and drop toys or other objects. The infant's language has moved beyond making razzing noises to single-consonant vocalizing. The 6-month-old produces long strings of vocalizations in play, usually during interactions with adults. He also can stand with help and enjoys bouncing up and down in the standing position. He may rock back and forth on his hands and knees, in preparation for crawling forward or backward.

An infant who lies on his back, shows little interest in social interaction, avoids eye contact, and smiles and vocalizes infrequently is indicating either developmental problems or a lack of attention from his parents and other caregivers. He needs formal developmental assessment and referral to early intervention, as well as increased health supervision, and he may need more nurturance.

Over the next few months, as the infant develops an increasing repertoire of motor skills for mobility, such as crawling and pulling to a stand, parents must be vigilant about falls. The expanding world of the infant must be looked at through his eyes to make exploration as safe as possible. The infant will do more than most parents anticipate, and sooner. Toys must be sturdy and have no small parts that could be swallowed or inhaled. Baby walkers should never be used at any age. To avoid possible injury, it is never too early to secure safety gates at the top and bottom of stairs and install window guards.

Parents need to understand developmentally appropriate strategies to redirect their child's behavior when safety is threatened or inappropriate behaviors occur.

Priorities for the 6 Month Visit

The first priority is to attend to the concerns of the parents.

In addition, the Bright Futures Infancy Expert Panel has given priority to the following topics for discussion in this visit:

▶ Social determinants of health[a] (risks [living situation and food security; tobacco, alcohol, and drugs; parental depression], strengths and protective factors [family relationships and support, child care])

▶ Infant behavior and development (parents as teachers, communication and early literacy, media, emerging infant independence, putting self to sleep, self-calming)

▶ Oral health (fluoride, oral hygiene/soft toothbrush, avoidance of bottle in bed)

▶ Nutrition and feeding (general guidance on feeding, solid foods, pesticides in vegetables and fruits, fluids and juice, breastfeeding guidance, formula-feeding guidance)

▶ Safety (car safety seats, safe sleep, safe home environment: burns, sun exposure, choking, poisoning, drowning, falls)

[a] Social determinants of health is a new priority in the fourth edition of the *Bright Futures Guidelines*. For more information, see the *Promoting Lifelong Health for Families and Communities* theme.

Health Supervision

The *Bright Futures Tool and Resource Kit* contains Previsit Questionnaires to assist the health care professional in taking a history, conducting developmental surveillance, and performing medical screening.

History

The interval history may be obtained according to the concerns of the family and the health care professional's preference or style of practice.

General Questions

- How are things going for you and your family?
- What questions or concerns do you have about your baby?
- What is working best for you in caring for your baby?
- What is most challenging?
- Are there differences in your views about the baby and those of your partner?

Past Medical History

- Has your infant received any specialty or emergency care since the last visit?

Family History

- Has your child or anyone in the family, such as parents, brothers, sisters, grandparents, aunts, uncles, or cousins, developed a new health condition or died? **If the answer is Yes:** Ascertain who in the family has or had the condition, and ask about the age of onset and diagnosis. If the person is no longer living, ask about the age at the time of death.

Social History

- See the Social Determinants of Health priority in Anticipatory Guidance for social history questions.

Surveillance of Development

Do you or any of your baby's caregivers have any specific concerns about your baby's learning, development, or behavior?

Clinicians using the *Bright Futures Tool and Resource Kit* Previsit Questionnaires or another tool that includes a developmental milestones checklist, or those who use a structured developmental screening tool, need not ask about these developmental surveillance milestones. *(For more information, see the Promoting Healthy Development theme.)*

Social Language and Self-help

Does your child

- Pat or smile at his reflection?
- Look when you call his name?

Verbal Language (Expressive and Receptive)

Does she

- Babble?
- Make sounds like "ga," "ma," or "ba"?

Gross Motor

Does he

- Roll over from back to stomach?
- Sit briefly without support?

Fine Motor

Does she

- Pass a toy from one hand to another?
- Rake small objects with 4 fingers?
- Bang small objects on surface?

Review of Systems

The Bright Futures Infancy Expert Panel recommends a complete review of systems as a part of every health supervision visit. This review can be done by asking the following questions:

Do you have concerns about your infant's

- Head
  - Shape
- Eyes
  - Discharge
  - Cross-eyed
- Ears, nose, and throat
- Breathing
- Stomach or abdomen
  - Vomiting or spitting
  - Bowel movements
  - Belly button
- Genitals or rectum
- Skin
- Development
  - Muscle strength, movement of arms or legs, any developmental concerns

Observation of Parent-Infant Interaction

During the visit, the health care professional acknowledges and reinforces positive parent-infant interactions and discusses any concerns. Observation focuses on

- Are the parents and infant responsive to one another (eg, holding, talking, smiling, providing toys for play and distraction, especially during the examination)?
- Are the parents aware of, responsive to, and effective in responding to the infant?
- Do the parents express and show comfort and confidence with their infant?
- Does the parent-infant relationship demonstrate comfort, adequate feeding/eating, and response to the infant's cues?
- If the infant is given a book, what is the parents' response (eg, react with pleasure, show puzzlement, put book away)?
- Do parents appear to be happy, content, at ease, depressed, tearful, angry, anxious, fatigued, overwhelmed, or uncomfortable?
- Do the parents/partners support each other or show signs of disagreement?

Physical Examination

A complete physical examination is included as part of every health supervision visit.

When performing a physical examination, the health care professional's attention is directed to the following components of the examination that are important for an infant this age:

- **Measure and plot on appropriate WHO Growth Chart**
  - Recumbent length
  - Weight
  - Head circumference
  - Weight-for-length

- **Skin**
  - Inspect for skin lesions, birthmarks, and bruising.

- **Eyes**
  - Assess ocular mobility.
  - Examine pupils for opacification and red reflexes.
  - Assess visual acuity using fixate and follow response.

- **Heart**
  - Auscult for murmurs.
  - Palpate for femoral pulses.

- **Musculoskeletal**
  - Assess for developmental hip dysplasia by examining for leg length discrepancy, thigh-fold asymmetry, and appropriate abduction.

- **Neurologic**
  - Evaluate tone, strength, and symmetry of movements.

Screening

Universal Screening	Action	
Depression: Maternal	Maternal depression screen	
Oral Health	Administer the oral health risk assessment. Apply fluoride varnish after first tooth eruption.	

Selective Screening	Risk Assessment[a]	Action if Risk Assessment Positive (+)
Blood Pressure	Children with specific risk conditions or change in risk	Blood pressure measurement
Hearing	+ on risk screening questions	Referral for diagnostic audiologic assessment
Lead	+ on risk screening questions	Lead blood test
Oral Health	Primary water source is deficient in fluoride.	Oral fluoride supplementation
Tuberculosis	+ on risk screening questions	Tuberculin skin test
Vision	+ on risk screening questions	Ophthalmology referral

[a] See the *Evidence and Rationale chapter* for the criteria on which risk screening questions are based.

Immunizations

Consult the CDC/ACIP or AAP Web sites for the current immunization schedule.

CDC National Immunization Program: **www.cdc.gov/vaccines**

AAP *Red Book:* **http://redbook.solutions.aap.org**

Anticipatory Guidance

The following sample questions, which address the Bright Futures Infancy Expert Panel's Anticipatory Guidance Priorities, are intended to be used selectively to invite discussion, gather information, address the needs and concerns of the family, and build partnerships. Use of the questions may vary from visit to visit and from family to family. Questions can be modified to match the health care professional's communication style. The accompanying anticipatory guidance for the family should be geared to questions, issues, or concerns for that particular infant and family. Tools and handouts to support anticipatory guidance can be found in the *Bright Futures Tool and Resource Kit.*

Priority

Social Determinants of Health

Risks: Living situation and food security; tobacco, alcohol, and drugs; parental depression

Strengths and protective factors: Family relationships and support, child care

Risks: Living Situation and Food Security

Parents in difficult living situations or with limited means may have concerns about their ability to obtain affordable housing, food, or other resources. Provide information and referrals, as needed, for community resources that help with finding quality child care, accessing transportation, getting a car safety seat or an infant crib so that the baby can sleep safely, or addressing issues such as financial concerns, inadequate or unsafe housing, or limited food resources. Public health agencies can be excellent sources of help because they work with all types of community agencies and family needs.

Sample Questions

Tell me about your living situation. Do you live in an apartment or a house? Is permanent housing a worry for you?

Do you have the things you need to take care of the baby, such as a crib, a car safety seat, and diapers? Does your home have enough heat, hot water, electricity, and working appliances? Do you have health insurance for yourself? How about for the baby?

Within the past 12 months, were you ever worried whether your food would run out before you got money to buy more? Within the past 12 months, did the food you bought not last and you did not have money to get more?

Have you ever tried to get help for these issues? What happened? What barriers did you face?

Anticipatory Guidance

- Community agencies are available to help you with concerns about your living situation.
- Programs and resources are available to help you and your baby. You may be eligible for the WIC food and nutrition program, or housing or transportation assistance programs. Several food programs, such as the Commodity Supplemental Food Program and SNAP, the program formerly known as Food Stamps, can help you. If you are breastfeeding and eligible for WIC, you can get nutritious food for yourself and support from peer counselors.

Risks: Tobacco, Alcohol, and Drugs

The use of tobacco, alcohol, and other drugs has adverse health effects on the entire family. Focusing on the effect on health is often the most helpful approach and may help some family members with quitting or cutting back on substance use.

Sample Questions

Does anyone in your home smoke or use e-cigarettes? Are you worried about any family members and how much they smoke, drink, or use drugs?

How often do you drink beer, wine, or liquor in your household? Do you, or does anyone you ride with, ever drive after having a drink? Does your partner use alcohol? What kind and for how long?

Are you using marijuana, cocaine, pain pills, narcotics, or other controlled substances? Are you getting any help to cut down or stop your drug use?

Anticipatory Guidance

- It's important to keep your car, home, and other places where your child spends time free of tobacco smoke and vapor from e-cigarettes. Smoking affects your child by increasing the risk of asthma, ear infections, and respiratory infections.
- **800-QUIT-NOW (800-784-8669); TTY 800-332-8615** is a national telephone helpline that is routed to local resources. Additional resources are available at **www.cdc.gov.**
- Drug and alcohol cessation programs are available in our community and we would like to help you connect to these services.

Risks: Parental Depression

An estimated 10% to 20% of women struggle with major depression before, during, and after delivery of a baby. Fathers also may experience major depression in this period. A prior history of depression increases risk for both mothers and fathers. Parental depression has substantial personal consequences and interferes with quality of child-rearing, adversely affecting parent-infant interactions, maternal responsiveness to infant vocalizations and gestures, and other stimulation essential for optimal child development.

Sample Questions

What are some of your best, and most difficult, times of day with the baby? How are you feeling emotionally? Have you been feeling sad, blue, or hopeless since the delivery? Are you still interested in activities you used to enjoy? Do you find that you are drinking alcohol, using herbs, or taking drugs to help make you feel less depressed, less anxious, less frustrated, and calmer? Who has been available to assist you at home? Who has been the most help to you?

Anticipatory Guidance

- Many mothers feel tired or overwhelmed with a new baby. These feelings should not continue, however. If you find that you are still feeling very tired or overwhelmed, or you are using over-the-counter or prescription medication, drugs, or alcohol to feel better, let your partner, your own health care professional, or me know so that you can get the help you need.

Strengths and Protective Factors: Family Relationships and Support

As the infant becomes increasingly awake and alert and demands attention, parents may find new challenges in balancing responsibilities with wanting to interact with a responsive and engaging infant. Mothers may find that family support systems that were available earlier are less available now. It is important to periodically review the family's living circumstances and familial relationships, and who is currently responsible for decision-making and caregiving to the child and family. Remind parents it is OK to ask for help and to be specific in expressing their needs to family and close friends.

Sample Questions

Who are you able to rely on to help you with the baby or when you are tired? How are you balancing your roles of partner and parent? How do you feel you are managing in meeting the needs of your family? Who are you able to go to when you need help with your family?

Anticipatory Guidance

- When you are feeling stressed or overwhelmed, you need to be able to use the support network that is available to help you. If you are having difficulty doing this or are hesitant to do so, we may be able to give you additional counseling and support.
- If your family is living with others, such as elders or those who are helping you from being homeless, or if you are a teen parent living with your parents, you may have little control over your environment and caregiver roles and responsibilities. If you are in this situation, you can talk to me about things you can do to reduce the stress and make the most of your circumstances.

Strengths and Protective Factors: Child Care

Review parents' selection of child care providers, including what they may expect from a child care provider, safeguards in place, and the importance of their infant having a consistent child care provider with regular and predictable daily routines.

Sample Questions

What are your child care arrangements? Do you have a reliable person to care for your baby when you need or want to go out? Are you satisfied with the arrangements? How many hours is your child in child care each day?

Anticipatory Guidance

- It is important that you have a child care provider whom you like and trust and who gives your baby a healthy and predictable daily routine that is similar to what you provide.
- If you are at home with your infant and you are not getting out, you may want to join a playgroup or invite other mothers and babies over for a playdate.

Priority

Infant Behavior and Development

Parents as teachers, communication and early literacy, media, emerging infant independence, putting self to sleep, self-calming

---

Parents as Teachers

Parents' expectations about their infant's development should evolve as the parent-infant attachment evolves, particularly of their infant's desire for independence. Parents need to understand the developmental next steps that are likely to occur after each visit as well as their role as teachers and the importance of using appropriate behavioral management strategies appropriate for the child's developmental age. Infants learn about their environment through visual exploration, mouthing toys, and, eventually, imitation. Show parents examples of age-appropriate books such as "touch and feel" and other soft plastic or board books that cannot be damaged by the infant's ripping or chewing.

Sample Questions

How do you think your baby is learning? Does he watch you as you walk around the room?

Anticipatory Guidance

- Your baby's vision gradually improves during the first year of life. By 6 months of age, he should be able to follow you around the room with his eyes. Putting your baby in a high chair or an upright seat during awake time (as opposed to a crib), will allow him to visually explore and verbally interact with you and his brothers and sisters.

Communication and Early Literacy

As the baby matures, parents will need to expand their strategies to support their child's neurobehavioral maturation, self-regulation, and ability to tolerate specific sensory stimuli. Encourage parents to engage in interactive, reciprocal play with their infants, as this promotes emotional security as well as language development. This playtime should not be a teaching session, but rather a time to follow the infant's interests and expand the play with simple words.

Sample Questions

What have you noticed about changes in your baby's development and behaviors around you and other people? How does your baby adapt to new situations, such as people or places? Is he sensitive to any particular stimulation? Does he seem to get anxious or easily upset? **If yes:** *What things seem to trigger these reactions?*

How does your baby communicate or tell you what he wants and needs? With gestures? Does he point? What sounds is your baby making, such as "ga," "ma," "ba"?

How does your baby respond when you look at books together?

Anticipatory Guidance

- Your baby's temperament and sensory processing and how they affect the way he relates to the world will become more evident at 6 months of age. Understanding your baby's temperament will help you respond to his needs and fussy behaviors appropriately.
- Babies learn to communicate during typical daily routines, such as bedtime, naptime, baths, diaper changes, and dressing. Here are some things you can do to help your baby develop these communication skills.
  - Talk with your baby during routine activities.
  - Play music and sing.
  - Imitate vocalizations.
  - Play games such as pat-a-cake, peekaboo, and "so big."
- Place your baby in your lap and look at picture books together. Point to and name things in the book. Respond if he pats a picture or turns a page.
- Anticipate short attention spans.

Media

As more families and children have access to and exposure to digital media, it is important to assess for the use of such devices and offer guidance regarding media in the home.

Sample Questions

How much time each day does your baby spend watching TV or playing on a tablet, smartphone, or other digital device? Is there a TV or other digital media device on in the background while your baby is in the room?

Anticipatory Guidance

- Babies may start to seem interested in mobile devices and TV at this age, but it is mostly because they are attracted to the lights and sounds, and because they are naturally interested in whatever their caregivers are paying attention to.
- Research shows that babies this age cannot learn information from screens, even though many toys and videos claim to teach babies skills. Babies learn by interacting with caregivers; being read, talked, and sung to; and exploring their environment by grabbing, mouthing, crawling, and cruising. Make special time for this tech-free type of play every day.
- Most babies are starting to eat sitting in high chairs now. Make this an opportunity for face-to-face learning interactions. Don't have the TV or other digital media on during meals, which distracts babies from learning.
- Starting healthy media habits now is important, because they are much harder to change when children are older.

Emerging Infant Independence

Consistent and predictable daily routines help infants develop their own self-regulation in the first year of life, which leads to better self-regulation later. Parents who cannot provide this type of environment for their infant may need additional counseling, monitoring, and intervention.

Monitor infants who are excessively active or extremely quiet. Additional counseling and assistance for parents who are sad or unhappy, or who rarely sleep or sleep more than expected, is extremely important. Infants, especially those with special health care needs, such as premature infants or babies with chronic health or developmental conditions, who exhibit any stereotypical behaviors or sensory issues may need additional assistance. Parents who are excessively anxious, or, conversely, parents who are unaware of potential dangers, also need additional assistance.

Sample Questions

What is your baby's typical day like? When does he wake up, eat, play, nap, and go to sleep for the night?

Anticipatory Guidance

- As much as possible, maintain a consistent and predictable daily routine for your baby. This will help him learn how to manage his own behavior appropriately now and as he gets older.

Putting Self to Sleep

By 6 months of age, some, but not all, babies are sleeping for longer stretches at night (6–8 hours), which parents consider "through the night." Parents need to support their infant's increasing ability to put himself to sleep initially and put himself back to sleep after awakening at night.

Suggestions about establishing a bedtime routine, putting the infant to bed when he is awake, and other habits to discourage night waking help parents help their baby learn to console himself. In many cultures, family sleep arrangements are viewed as a part of the parent's commitment to their children's well-being. Infant sleep patterns are often among the last traditions to change among immigrant families.

Sample Question

How is your baby learning to go to sleep by himself?

Anticipatory Guidance

- Placing your baby in the crib when he is drowsy, but not asleep, will help your baby learn that he can go to sleep on his own. Then, when he awakens at night, he will be more likely to be able to go back to sleep without your help. This approach will help both you and your baby get a good night's sleep.

Self-calming

At 6 months of age, infants may still have periods of fussiness and irritability. Remind parents that the baby is not trying to make them angry—he is just having a rough time and still needs someone to be there. Parents can ask a family member, neighbor, or trusted friend to stay with the crying baby for a few minutes to allow the parent to take a break.

Review the importance of protecting an infant's head even though the baby has head control. Never shake or hit an infant, as even unintentional shaking or hitting may cause brain damage.

Sample Questions

How does your baby calm himself? How much does your baby cry? What helps to calm your baby? What do you do if that does not work? Do you ever feel that you or other caregivers may hurt the baby because of the crying? What will you do if you feel this way? Do you have a plan? How do you handle the feeling?

Anticipatory Guidance

- At 6 months of age, your baby may still have fussy periods. If he is clean, dry, and not hungry, his fussiness may be telling you that he is tired or bored. Regular daily naps and giving him a variety of short play activities are 2 good strategies for dealing with overtiredness and boredom.
- You can ask a family member, neighbor, or trusted friend to stay with your crying baby for a few minutes to allow you to take a break. If you are alone, you can try putting the baby in his crib, closing the door, and checking on him every few minutes.
- By 6 months of age, your baby will have different strategies that will allow him to begin calming himself, such as grasping safe and appropriate toys, oral exploration, and visual exploration.

Priority

Oral Health

Fluoride, oral hygiene/soft toothbrush, avoidance of bottle in bed

Fluoride, Oral Hygiene/Soft Toothbrush, Avoidance of Bottle in Bed

To promote preventive dental care, counseling for parents about their infant's oral health needs to begin early. This includes parental awareness of the importance of their own dental health and modeling of brushing their teeth. The oral health risk assessment recommended by the American Academy of Pediatric Dentistry is recommended to begin at 6 months of age.

Sample Questions

What have you thought about doing to protect your infant's teeth during this first year? What are your plans for protecting your baby's teeth? Where does your baby take her bottle? Do you continue to hold it for her?

Anticipatory Guidance

- All infants need a source of fluoride at 6 months. If your water does not contain fluoride, it is time to begin fluoride supplementation. Our local health department may be a resource for information about local community fluoride levels.
- Early dental care, with the eruption of the first tooth, means using a soft toothbrush or cloth to clean your baby's teeth with a small smear of fluoridated toothpaste, no more than a grain of rice, twice a day—after the baby's first feeding in the morning and then after the last feeding before nighttime sleep.
- Continue to hold your baby for bottle-feeding. Do not prop the bottle or let your baby graze, which means drinking from a bottle at will during the day.
- Putting your baby to bed with a bottle or grazing with a bottle containing juice, milk, or other sugary liquid will lead to tooth decay.
- Avoid baby foods or juices that babies suck out of a bag or pouch. A baby's teeth or gums will be in contact with pureed food longer than necessary, leading to tooth decay. It's always best to use a spoon.
- Avoid sharing a spoon or putting the pacifier in your mouth because this introduces your own bacteria into your baby's mouth, which can contribute to tooth decay.

Priority

Nutrition and Feeding

General guidance on feeding, solid foods, pesticides in vegetables and fruits, fluids and juice, breast-feeding guidance, formula-feeding guidance

General Guidance on Feeding

By reviewing the growth chart with parents at each visit, parents become aware of the importance of growth and nutrition and become partners in providing appropriate nutrition for their child. This review also will determine the need for more in-depth assessment of nutritional adequacy and anticipatory guidance about the use of nutritional supplements (eg, vitamins, herbs, alternative formulas, and foods). Infants who take longer than 35 to 45 minutes to feed should be evaluated carefully for developmental and nutritional concerns.

Significant transitions in feeding occur during the next 3 months, and parents need clear guidance about what to expect. Managing this transition includes a discussion about cultural or extended family beliefs about introduction of solid foods and types and textures of foods. The concept of the division of responsibility between parent and infant with feeding is especially helpful. In this division, the parent is responsible for providing appropriate foods and the infant is responsible for how much to eat.

Sample Questions

What questions or concerns do you have about your baby's growth and feeding? What are you feeding your baby at this time? How often are you feeding your baby? How much does he eat or drink? When you begin feeding him solid foods, where will he sit when you feed him? Are you feeding your baby any drinks or foods besides breast milk or formula? About how long do feedings last?

Anticipatory Guidance

- In the next 6 months, it is typical for your baby's growth to slow down a little, as you can see on the growth chart.
- Breastfeeding exclusively for about 6 months of life and then combining breast milk with solid foods from about 6 to 12 months of age provides the best nutrition and supports the best possible growth and development. You can continue breastfeeding for as long as you and your baby want.
- For infants who are not breastfed, iron-fortified infant formula, with the addition of solid foods after 6 months of age, is the recommended alternative through the first year of life.
- As you begin solid foods, it is important to feed your baby in a bouncy seat or high chair that is adjusted to support your baby's head, trunk, and feet, so you can look at each other. Your baby's arms also should be free, as this is his way of communicating with you. Of course, when offering the bottle, it is still very important to continue to hold your baby so that you can see each other and communicate with each other. Your baby then will be able to let you know when he is still hungry and when he is full.

- Responding appropriately to your baby's behaviors during feedings lets him know that you understand his needs so you can provide the appropriate amount of food at a feeding. Remember, you are responsible for providing a variety of nutritious foods, but he is responsible for deciding how much to eat.

Solid Foods

Parents need specific verbal or written guidance on the introduction of solid foods. The order in which they are introduced is not critical as long as essential nutrients are provided. For the breastfed infant, emphasize the need to include a good dietary source of iron to prevent iron deficiency and an oral vitamin D supplement (400 IU/day). Some breastfed infants may need an iron supplement.

Parents can offer store-bought and home-prepared baby food as well as soft table foods. As the infant progresses from purees to foods with more consistency, encourage parents to offer finger foods, such as soft bananas and cereal. Advise parents that infants do not need salt or sugar added to their food.

After the introduction of solid foods, the next few months are a sensitive period for learning to chew. A gradual exposure to solid textures during this time may decrease the risk of feeding problems, such as rejecting certain textures, refusing to chew, or vomiting.

The WIC can provide information and guidance on introducing solid foods.

Sample Questions

How are you planning to introduce solid foods, such as cereal, meats, fruits, vegetables, and other foods? How much does your baby eat at a time? How does your baby let you know when he likes a certain food? Does your baby have any favorite foods?

Anticipatory Guidance

- Adding solid foods to your baby's diet is very individualized. Transitioning from breast milk or formula at about 6 months of age to table foods at 12 months of age involves a number of steps.
- A key step is to determine when your baby is ready for solid foods.
  - One of the signs that a baby is ready to eat solid foods is the fading of the baby's tongue-thrust reflex. This is when the baby pushes food out of his mouth.
  - Another sign is that the baby can elevate his tongue to move pureed food to the back of his mouth and, as he sees a spoon approach, he opens his mouth in anticipation of the next bite. At this stage, your baby sits with arm support and has good head and neck control, so he can indicate a desire for food by opening his mouth and leaning forward.
  - He can tell you he's full or doesn't want food by leaning back and turning away.
- Introduce single-ingredient new foods, one at a time, and watch for adverse reactions over several days.
- Good sources of zinc- and iron-rich foods include zinc- and iron-fortified infant cereal and pureed meats, especially red meats. One ounce (30 g) of infant cereal provides the daily iron requirement, particularly if you give it to him along with vitamin C–rich foods, such as fruit, which enhance iron absorption from the cereal. Some breastfed infants may need to continue oral iron drops.

- Gradually introduce other pureed or soft fruits and vegetables after your baby has accepted zinc- and iron-fortified, single-grain infant cereal and/or pureed or soft meats. Offer solid food 2 to 3 times per day and let him decide how much to eat.
- As with all feeding interactions, watch your baby's verbal and nonverbal cues and respond appropriately. If a food is rejected, move on and try it again later. Don't force him to eat or finish foods.
- Give your baby an initial taste of one of these foods *at home* rather than at day care or a restaurant. Most reactions occur in response to what is believed to be the initial try.
- Repeated exposure to foods enhances acceptance of new foods by both breastfed and formula-fed infants. It may take up to 10 to 15 experiences before a new food is accepted, because of the transition to textures as well as tastes.
- The only foods to be avoided are raw honey or large chunks of food that could cause choking. Newer data suggest that the early introduction of all foods may actually *prevent* individual food allergies.
- If your baby has no apparent reaction, introduce the food in gradually increasing amounts. Continue introducing other new foods in the same manner if no adverse reactions occur.
- Giving your baby foods of varying textures, such as pureed, blended, mashed, finely chopped, and soft lumps, will help him successfully go through the change from gumming to chewing foods. Slowly introducing solid textures during this time may decrease the risk of feeding problems, refusing to chew, or vomiting. Gradually increase table foods. Avoid mixed textures, like broth with vegetables, because they are the most difficult for infants to eat.

Pesticides in Vegetables and Fruits

Many families wonder whether they should choose organic fruits and vegetables over conventional to reduce pesticides exposure in their child's diet. The key message is to encourage vegetable and fruit consumption—eating a diet rich in a variety of fruits and vegetables, either conventional or organic, has well-established health benefits. Choosing organic fruits and vegetables can reduce exposures to pesticides in the diet.

Sample Question
What fruits and vegetables does your child eat?

Anticipatory Guidance
- The most important thing is to encourage your baby to eat a variety of vegetables and fruits.
- Wash vegetables and fruits before serving.
- Consider buying organic, if possible.

INFANCY
6 MONTH VISIT

Fluids and Juice

Parents can begin offering sips of human milk, formula, or water from a small cup held by the feeder, but an infant this age is unlikely or unable to take adequate amounts of fluids and energy needs in a cup. Caution parents to limit juice to 2 to 4 oz of 100% juice in any one day and to avoid the use of sweetened drinks, such as sodas and artificially flavored "fruit" drinks that provide calories without other nutrients.

Sample Question

What types of fluids is your baby getting in the bottle or cup?

Anticipatory Guidance

- Give your baby only 2 to 4 oz of 100% juice in any one day, as it is not considered a snack or food. Avoid the use of sweetened drinks, such as sodas and artificially flavored fruit drinks that provide calories without other nutrients.

Breastfeeding Guidance

Congratulate the mother for continuing to breastfeed.

Weaning ages vary considerably from child to child. Although breastfeeding is recommended for at least 12 months, or longer as mutually desired by the mother and infant, some infants are ready to wean earlier. Refer mothers to breastfeeding support groups or a lactation consultant as needed for questions or concerns.

Vitamin D supplementation (400 IU per day) is recommended for all breastfed infants, but is not needed for formula-fed infants, as vitamin D is present in the formula. Some preterm infants will require supplementation of additional vitamins.

Oral iron supplementation (1 mg/kg/day) for exclusively breastfed infants should continue until iron- and zinc-rich complementary foods (baby meats and iron-fortified cereals) are introduced. It may take a month or two following the introduction of these foods for infants to consume sufficient iron from complementary foods alone. Red meat is a better source of iron than iron-fortified cereals for older infants because a higher percentage of the iron in red meat is absorbed.

Sample Questions

How is breastfeeding going? In what ways is breastfeeding different now from when you were last here? How often are you breastfeeding your baby? For how long on each breast? Are you continuing to provide vitamin D drops and iron drops? Does it seem like your baby is breastfeeding more often or for longer periods of time? How can you tell if he is satisfied at the breast? What are your plans for continuing to breastfeed?

Anticipatory Guidance

- At 6 months of age, breast milk with solid foods continue to be your baby's best source of nutrition. You should try to continue to breastfeed for the first year of your baby's life and for as long thereafter as you and your baby want to continue.
- Be sure to continue your baby's vitamin D until your baby is taking at least 16 oz of vitamin D–fortified milk each day.
- Continue your baby's iron supplement until he is eating red meat or iron-fortified cereal every day.

Formula-Feeding Guidance

Older infants generally consume 24 to 32 oz of formula per day with solid food, but larger infants (6 months old, 90th percentile for weight) may take as much as 42 oz of formula per day without solid foods. Often, at this age, parents may consider using a less expensive formula and may need guidance based on the individual needs of the infant.

Sample Questions

How is formula feeding going? What formula are you using now? Have you tried other formulas or are you thinking of using other formulas? How often does your baby feed in 24 hours and how much does he take at a feeding? Day feeding versus night feedings? Do you have any concerns about the formula, such as cost, preparation, or nutrient content?

Anticipatory Guidance

- Continue to feed your baby when he shows hunger cues, usually 5 to 6 times in 24 hours.
- Supplements are not needed if the formula is iron fortified and your baby is consuming an adequate volume of formula for appropriate growth.
- During the first year of life, babies continue to need iron-fortified formula. If the cost of the formula is a concern, programs such as WIC or other community services may be able to help you.
- Never heat a bottle in a microwave. If you wish to warm a bottle, a hot water bath is recommended.

Priority

Safety

Car safety seats, safe sleep, safe home environment: burns, sun exposure, choking, poisoning, drowning, falls

Car Safety Seats

If parents are concerned that their baby has outgrown her infant car safety seat or the infant has reached the maximum weight or height allowed for use of her rear-facing–only car safety seat, counsel them to switch to a rear-facing convertible or 3-in-1 car safety seat. These seats typically allow more room for the infant's legs and are designed to be used rear facing to higher weights and heights. Advise parents that their child should ride rear facing as long as possible, or at least to age 2 years. The rear-facing position offers the best possible protection to the infant's head, neck, and spine. Convertible and 3-in-1 car safety seats have weight and height limits that will accommodate even large toddlers up to 24 months rear facing.

Remind parents that their own safe driving behaviors (including using seat belts at all times, not driving under the influence of alcohol or drugs, and avoiding use of electronic devices while driving) are important to the health of their children.

Sample Question

How well does your baby fit in her rear-facing car safety seat?

Anticipatory Guidance

- The back seat is the safest place for all babies and children to ride.
- Keep your baby's car safety seat rear facing in the back seat of your vehicle until your baby is at least 2 years old.
- Never place your baby's car safety seat in the front seat of a vehicle with a passenger air bag because air bags deploy with great force. When it hits a car safety seat, it causes serious injury or death.
- Babies are best protected in the event of a crash when they are in the back seat and in a rear-facing car safety seat. They should be in a 5-point harness at all times.
- Infants who reach the maximum height or weight allowed by their rear-facing–only car safety seat should use a convertible or 3-in-1 seat that is approved for use rear facing to higher weights and heights (up to 50 pounds and 49 inches, depending on the seat). Your baby will be safest if she rides rear facing to the highest weight or height allowed by the manufacturer.
- Do not start the engine until everyone is buckled in.
- Your own safe driving behaviors are important to the health of your children. Use a seat belt at all times, do not drive after using alcohol or drugs, and do not text or use mobile devices when driving.

For information about car safety seats and actions to keep your baby safe in and around cars, visit **www.safercar.gov/parents.**

Find a Child Passenger Safety Technician: **http://cert.safekids.org.** Click on "Find a Tech."

Toll-free Auto Safety Hotline: **888-327-4236**

Safe Sleep

Parents also may have questions about their ability to keep their infant on her back now that she has learned to roll over. Information on continuing to keep the crib safe is important in providing reassurance.

Sample Questions

Do you continue to place your baby on her back for sleep? Where does she sleep?

Anticipatory Guidance

- Continue to put your baby to sleep on her back to reduce the risk of sudden infant death, but, if she rolls in her sleep, it is no longer necessary to return her to her back. Relatives and child care providers should be reminded to follow the same practice. Bed sharing increases the risk of sudden infant death. Your baby should continue to sleep in her own crib, not in your bed. If you breastfeed or bottle-feed your baby in your bed, return her to her own crib before you go back to sleep.
- Be sure your baby's crib is safe. It is best to use a crib made after June 28, 2011, that meets the newest safety standard. If you must use an older crib, the slats should be no more than 2⅜ inches (60 mm) apart. The mattress should be firm and fit snugly into the crib, and drop sides should not be used.
- The crib mattress should be at its lowest point before the baby begins to stand. Keep bumpers, pillows, and other items out of the crib to prevent suffocation and so they cannot be used as steps over the crib railing to a fall.
- If you choose a mesh play yard or portable crib, consider choosing one that was manufactured after a new, stronger safety standard was implemented on February 28, 2013. If you use an older product, the weave should have openings less than ¼ inch (6 mm) and the sides should always stay fully raised.

Safe Home Environment: Burns, Sun Exposure, Choking, Poisoning, Drowning, Falls

As their baby develops more fine and gross motor skills, it is important to review with the parents how to keep the home environment safe. No home is ever childproof, but parents can initiate changes to make the environment safer. This applies to all homes where the baby spends time, including child care and grand-parents' and friends' homes.

Sample Questions

What other things are you doing to keep your baby safe and healthy? Do you spend time outside with your baby? Do you use a front or back carrier to carry her?

Anticipatory Guidance

- As your baby begins to crawl, it is a good idea to do a safety check of your home and the home of family or friends.
- Before bathing your baby, test the water temperature on your wrist to make sure it is not too hot. **To protect your child from tap water scalds, the hottest temperature at the faucet should be no more than 120°F.** In many cases, you can adjust your water heater. Never set a cup of coffee or any hot liquid on a table that is within your child's reach.
- Don't leave your baby alone, even for a second, in a tub of water, even if you use a bath seat. Never leave your baby alone on high places such as changing tables, beds, sofas, or chairs.
- Use appropriate barriers around space heaters, wood stoves, and kerosene heaters.
- Babies this age explore their environment by putting anything and everything into their mouths. NEVER leave small objects, electrical cords, or latex balloons within your baby's reach.
- To prevent choking, limit finger foods to soft bits not much larger than a Cheerio. Infants and children younger than 4 years should not eat hard food like nuts or popcorn, compressible foods like hot dogs or marshmallows, or sticky foods like spoonfuls of peanut butter.
- Be sure to keep household products, such as cleaners, chemicals, and medicines, locked up and out of your child's sight and reach. If your child does eat something that could be poisonous, call the **Poison Help line** at **800-222-1222** immediately. Post the number next to every phone and store it in your cell phone. Do not make your child vomit.
- The kitchen is the most dangerous room for children. A safer place for your child while you are cooking, eating, or unable to provide your full attention is the play yard, crib, or stationary activity center, or buckled into a high chair.
- Your baby may be able to crawl as early as 6 months of age. Use gates on stairways and close doors to keep her out of rooms where she might get hurt.
- Do not use a baby walker. Your baby may tip the walker over, fall out of it, or fall down the stairs and seriously injure her head. Baby walkers let children get to places where they can pull heavy objects or hot food on themselves.
- Babies this age are not ready for formal swimming lessons. Although some programs claim to teach infants how to save themselves from drowning, there is no evidence that lessons for babies younger than 1 year reduce the risk of drowning. Such lessons may influence parents to be less vigilant around water, thinking that their baby can save herself from drowning, and are not recommended.
- The best sun protection is to avoid the sun. Your baby's head and face are exposed in a front or back carrier. Always have her wear a hat. Apply sunscreen with an SPF greater than 15 to any exposed skin.

Infancy
9 Month Visit

Context

The 9-month-old has made some striking developmental gains and displays growing independence. She is increasingly mobile and will express explicit opinions about everything, from the foods she eats to her bedtime. These opinions often will take the form of protests. She will say, "No," in her own way, from closing her mouth and shaking her head when a parent wants to feed her, to screaming when she finds herself alone. The baby also has gained a sense of object permanence (ie, she understands that an object or person, such as a parent, exists in spite of not being visible at the moment).

The 9-month-old's behaviors are an adaptation to her uncertainties about how the world works. Though certain that an unseen object exists, she is not yet fully confident that the out-of-sight object or the absent person will reappear. Her protests when a parent leaves show her attachment and her ability to fear loss. Her insecurity about the whereabouts of her parents may lead to night waking. Until this age, she was waking during her normal sleep cycle, but usually fell back to sleep. Many babies who were sleeping through the night revert to night waking. Knowing that this is a normal developmental stage may help parents accept the temporary return to earlier patterns.

As a result of these developments, the parents' tasks have changed dramatically. The infant's increasing activity and protests necessitate setting limits. The parents must decide when it is important for them to say, "No." This requires self-esteem, confidence in their role as responsible parents, and a great deal of energy. Parents also view their infant's growing independence with a sense of loss. No longer content to be held, cuddled, and coddled, the baby will now wiggle, want to be put down, and may even crawl away. This physical independence requires a heightened vigilance about safety around the house.

Recognizing and responding appropriately to infant cues associated with basic care, such as nurturing and feeding, now require complex skills. As the baby's first birthday approaches, the parents' attitudes and expectations, based in part on their own early childhood experiences, will become a significant factor. At the 9 Month Visit, it is important for the health care professional to assess the parents' attitudes and abilities to cope with their infant's growing independence of body and mind. The health care professional also should provide the parents with basic skills and resources for making decisions about methods of managing their infant's behavior.

At 9 months of age, infants are at the height of stranger awareness. The intensity of their responses to strangers is highly variable. Although they may have been friendly and cooperative at the previous visit, they are far more likely to become upset with the physical examination at this age. The health care professional can minimize this reaction by approaching the infant very slowly, by examining the infant in a parent's arms, by first touching the infant's shoe or leg and gradually moving to the chest, and by distracting the infant with a toy or stethoscope during the examination.

481

This is an appropriate age to start guidance for the parents about discipline. Discuss the difference between discipline (which involves the parent teaching appropriate behaviors) and punishment (which places emphasis only on negative behaviors). Assist parents in making their baby's environment safe rather than trying to teach their baby how to be safe. Emphasize that yelling, spanking, and hitting are ineffective punishment in changing behaviors. Also point out that, at this age, an infant is NOT capable of learning or remembering rules.

Priorities for the 9 Month Visit

The first priority is to attend to the concerns of the parents.

In addition, the Bright Futures Infancy Expert Panel has given priority to the following topics for discussion in this visit:

▶ Social determinants of health[a] (risks [intimate partner violence], strengths and protective factors [family relationships and support])

▶ Infant behavior and development (changing sleep pattern [sleep schedule], developmental mobility and cognitive development, interactive learning and communication, media)

▶ Discipline (parent expectations of child's behavior)

▶ Nutrition and feeding (self-feeding, mealtime routines, transition to solid foods [table food introduction], cup drinking, plans for weaning)

▶ Safety (car safety seats, heatstroke prevention, firearm safety, safe home environment: burns, poisoning, drowning, falls)

[a] Social determinants of health is a new priority in the fourth edition of the *Bright Futures Guidelines*. For more information, see the *Promoting Lifelong Health for Families and Communities* theme.

Health Supervision

The *Bright Futures Tool and Resource Kit* contains Previsit Questionnaires to assist the health care professional in taking a history, conducting developmental surveillance, and performing medical screening.

History

The interval history may be obtained according to the concerns of the family and the health care professional's preference or style of practice.

General Questions

- How are you? How are things going in your family?
- What questions or concerns do you have today? What questions do you have about your baby's care?
- Tell me about your baby.
  - What do you like best about your baby?
  - What is most challenging about caring for your baby?
  - What works best for you to deal with these challenges?

Past Medical History

- Has your child received any specialty or emergency care since the last visit?

Family History

- Has your child or anyone in the family, such as parents, brothers, sisters, grandparents, aunts, uncles, or cousins, developed a new health condition or died? **If the answer is Yes:** Ascertain who in the family has or had the condition, and ask about the age of onset and diagnosis. If the person is no longer living, ask about the age at the time of death.

Social History

- See the Social Determinants of Health priority in Anticipatory Guidance for social history questions.

Surveillance of Development

Do you or any of your baby's caregivers have any specific concerns about your baby's learning, development, or behavior?

Clinicians using the *Bright Futures Tool and Resource Kit* Previsit Questionnaires or another tool that includes a developmental milestones checklist, or those who use a structured developmental screening tool, need not ask about these developmental surveillance milestones. *(For more information, see the Promoting Healthy Development theme.)*

Social Language and Self-help

Does your child

- Use basic gestures, such as holding arms out to be picked up or waving bye-bye?
- Look for dropped objects?
- Play games like peekaboo and pat-a-cake?
- Turn consistently when name is called?

Verbal Language (Expressive and Receptive)

Does he

- Say *Dada* or *Mama* nonspecifically?
- Look around when you say things like "Where's your bottle?" or "Where's your blanket?"
- Copy sounds that you make?

Gross Motor

Does she

- Sit well without support?
- Pull to stand?
- Transition well between sitting and lying?
- Crawl on hands and knees?

Fine Motor

Does he

- Pick up food and eat it?
- Pick up small objects with 3 fingers and thumb?
- Let go of objects intentionally?
- Bang objects together?

Review of Systems

The Bright Futures Infancy Expert Panel recommends a complete review of systems as a part of every health supervision visit. This review can be done by asking the following questions:

Do you have concerns about your infant's

- Head
  - Shape
- Eyes
  - Discharge
  - Cross-eyed
- Ears, nose, and throat
- Breathing
- Stomach or abdomen
  - Vomiting or spitting
  - Bowel movements
  - Belly button
- Genitals or rectum
- Skin
- Development
  - Muscle strength, movement of arms or legs, any developmental concerns

Observation of Parent-Infant Interaction

During the visit, the health care professional acknowledges and reinforces positive parent-infant interactions and discusses any concerns. Observation focuses on

- Do the parents respond to the infant's cues?
- Do the parents stimulate the infant with language and play?
- Do the parents and infant demonstrate a reciprocal engagement while playing and around feeding and eating?
- Is the infant free to move away from the parent to explore and check back with the parent visually and physically?
- Are the parents' developmental expectations appropriate?
- How do the parents respond to their infant's autonomy or independent behavior within a safe environment?

Physical Examination

A complete physical examination is included as part of every health supervision visit.

When performing a physical examination, the health care professional's attention is directed to the following components of the examination that are important for an infant this age:

- **Measure and plot on appropriate WHO Growth Chart**
  - Recumbent length
  - Weight
  - Head circumference
  - Weight-for-length

- **Head**
  - Palpate for positional skull deformities.

- **Eyes**
  - Assess ocular motility.
  - Examine pupils for opacification and red reflexes.
  - Assess visual acuity using fixate and follow responses.

- **Heart**
  - Auscult for murmurs.
  - Palpate femoral pulses.

- **Musculoskeletal**
  - Assess for developmental hip dysplasia by examining for abduction.

- **Neurologic**
  - Evaluate tone, strength, and symmetry of movements.
  - Elicit parachute reflex.

Screening

Universal Screening	Action	
Development	Developmental screen	
Oral Health	Oral health risk assessment. Apply fluoride varnish after first tooth eruption.	
Selective Screening	Risk Assessment[a]	Action if Risk Assessment Positive (+)
Blood Pressure	Children with specific risk conditions or change in risk	Blood pressure measurement
Hearing	+ on risk screening questions	Referral for diagnostic audiologic assessment
Lead	+ on risk screening questions	Lead blood test
Oral Health	Primary water source is deficient in fluoride.	Oral fluoride supplementation
Vision	+ on risk screening questions	Ophthalmology referral

[a] See the *Evidence and Rationale chapter* for the criteria on which risk screening questions are based.

Immunizations

Consult the CDC/ACIP or AAP Web sites for the current immunization schedule.

CDC National Immunization Program: **www.cdc.gov/vaccines**

AAP *Red Book:* **http://redbook.solutions.aap.org**

Anticipatory Guidance

The following sample questions, which address the Bright Futures Infancy Expert Panel's Anticipatory Guidance Priorities, are intended to be used selectively to invite discussion, gather information, address the needs and concerns of the family, and build partnerships. Use of the questions may vary from visit to visit and from family to family. Questions can be modified to match the health care professional's communication style. The accompanying anticipatory guidance for the family should be geared to questions, issues, or concerns for that particular infant and family. Tools and handouts to support anticipatory guidance can be found in the *Bright Futures Tool and Resource Kit*.

Priority

Social Determinants of Health
Risks: Intimate partner violence
Strengths and protective factors: Family relationships and support

Risks: Intimate Partner Violence

Children who are exposed to intimate partner violence are at increased risk of adverse mental and physical health outcomes. Intimate partner violence cannot be determined through observation, but is best identified through direct inquiry. Avoid asking about abuse or domestic violence, but use descriptive terms, such as *hit, kick, shove, choke,* or *threaten.* Provide information about the effect of violence on children and about community resources that provide assistance. Recommend resources for parent education and/or parent support groups.

To avoid causing upset to families by questioning about sensitive and private topics, such as family violence, alcohol and drug use, and similar risks, it is recommended to begin screening about these topics with an introductory statement, such as, "I ask all patients standard health questions to understand factors that may affect health of their child as well as their own health."

Sample Questions

Because violence is so common in so many people's lives, I've begun to ask about it. I don't know if this is a problem for you, but many children I see have parents who have been hurt by someone else. Some are too afraid or uncomfortable to bring it up, so I've started asking all my patients about it routinely. Do you always feel safe in your home? Has your partner, or another significant person in your life, ever hit, kicked, or shoved you, or physically hurt you or the baby? Are you scared that you or other caregivers may hurt the baby?

How do you stay calm and centered when things are getting overwhelming? Do you have any questions about your safety at home? What will you do if you feel afraid? Do you have a plan? Would you like information on where to go or who to contact if you ever need help?

Anticipatory Guidance

- One way that I and other health care professionals can help you if your partner, or another significant person in your life, is hitting or threatening you is to support you and provide information about local resources that can help you.
- You can also call the toll-free **National Domestic Violence Hotline** at **800-799-SAFE (7233).**

Strengths and Protective Factors: Family Relationships and Support

The increasingly mobile infant brings joy to his parents with his new abilities to move around the home. Keeping him safe and entertained often leaves parents very little time for themselves. Discuss whether the parents have time to themselves, with each other, and with other family and friends. Social contacts and activities apart from the baby can help maintain parental well-being. Ideally, both partners are involved in health supervision visits and infant care.

Sample Questions

Do you have regular time for yourself? How often do you see friends and get out of the house to do other activities? What do you do to take care of yourself?

Anticipatory Guidance

- All parents need time alone and individual time with their partner.
- Staying in touch with friends and family members and participating in activities without the baby helps avoid social isolation.

Priority

Infant Behavior and Development

Changing sleep pattern (sleep schedule), developmental mobility and cognitive development, interactive learning and communication, media

Changing Sleep Pattern (Sleep Schedule)

At around 9 months of age, it is not unusual for infants who have been sleeping through the night to begin to awaken.

Sample Questions

What changes have you noticed in your baby's sleeping habits? Does she wake up during the night?

Anticipatory Guidance

- This is an age when sleep routines that help your baby gradually relax and get ready for sleep are especially important. The pre-bedtime hour, before the routine begins, should be especially affectionate and nurturing. Disruptions in routine, such as vacations, visitors, or late evenings out, can significantly disturb sleep patterns. Try to avoid these disruptions if possible.
- If your baby is waking in the night, continue to just check on her and settle her back to sleep. This routine can help your baby put herself back to sleep.
- As your baby begins to stand, it is important to lower the mattress in her crib to the lowest level before she learns to stand up in it. Make sure you don't have bumper pads in the crib because she could use them as steps.

Developmental Mobility and Cognitive Development

The infant's increasing mobility and independence, but also her referencing and looking over to see that the parent is still there for protection, are important developmental steps. Parents need to understand their baby's temperament and how the family can adapt to it. If developmental or behavioral concerns exist, a referral to a local Early Intervention Program, often referred to as IDEA Part C, is appropriate to provide parents with education and counseling on strategies they may be able to implement during everyday routines that will support their infant's continuing development.

Sample Questions

How is your baby getting around now? Do you have any concerns about her development or behavior? What have you noticed about changes in your baby's behaviors around you and other people? How does she adapt to new situations, people, and places?

Anticipatory Guidance

- Your baby's gross motor skills, meaning her ability to control her head and body parts and to move around, will rapidly develop during the next 3 months.
- Give your baby opportunities to safely explore. Be there with her so that she can always check to see that you are nearby.
- Sometimes, it's easy to think that your baby can do more than she's really able to do. Be realistic about her abilities at this age and set realistic, nonthreatening, enforceable limits.
- Your baby is eager to interact and play with other people as a way to develop interpersonal relationships. At the same time, at this age, she will show separation anxiety from you and other important caregivers. This anxiety is a sign of her strong attachment to you.
- Pay attention to the way your baby reacts and adapts to new situations and people. These reactions reflect her personality and temperament. To the extent possible, make these situations easy on your baby. For example, if she is a quiet baby who does not like a lot of noise and bustle, explain that to a person meeting her for the first time and ask the person to greet her in a calm and soothing way.

Interactive Learning and Communication

At this age, gestural communication, joint attention, and social referencing are being established. An infant who is not making good eye contact should be closely followed. Encourage parents to engage in interactive, reciprocal play with their infants, as this promotes emotional security as well as language development. This playtime should not be a teaching session, but rather a time to follow the infant's interests and expand the play with simple words. Parents are interested in learning about alternatives to screen time and media entertainment. Interactive entertainment, such as talking, reading, or playing games together or walking in the park, can be reinforced.

Sample Questions

How do you think your baby is learning? How is your baby communicating with you now?

Anticipatory Guidance

- Your baby's way of learning is changing from exploring with her eyes and putting things in her mouth to noticing cause and effect, imitating others, and understanding that objects she cannot see still exist.
- Help your baby develop these skills by playing with simple cause-and-effect toys. Try balls that you can roll back and forth, toy cars and trucks that she can push, and blocks that can be put into a container and dumped out. Songs with clapping and gestures and songs with finger actions will help her learn imitation. Peekaboo and hide-and-seek are great ways to help her understand object permanence, that things and people exist even if she can't see them. It is important to stimulate your child to develop these capacities by interacting with her.
- Your baby will now begin to use gestures, such as pointing, and vocalizations to let you know what she wants. She also will begin to show her preferences more clearly, such as refusing to eat certain foods by clearly turning away. It is important to respond to your baby's efforts to communicate with you by acknowledging her preferences, yet being consistent in your expectations. Using modeling, demonstration, and simple descriptions of what behaviors you want from your baby will work much better than long sentences or a raised voice.

Media

As more families and children have access to, and exposure to, electronic media, it is important to assess for the use of such devices and offer guidance regarding media in the home. Discuss alternatives to infants watching TV. Discourage any TV, computer, tablet, smartphone, or viewing or play for infants and children younger than 18 months. Media use can interfere with the parental interaction with young children that is essential for vocabulary and language development.[9,10]

Sample Questions

How much time each day does your baby spend watching TV or playing on a tablet, smartphone, or other digital device? Is there a TV or other digital media device on in the background while your baby is in the room?

Anticipatory Guidance

- Research shows that babies this age cannot learn information from screens, even though many toys and videos claim to teach babies skills. Babies learn by interacting with caregivers; being read, talked, and sung to; and exploring their environment by grabbing, mouthing, crawling, and cruising. Make special time for this tech-free type of play every day.

- Most babies are starting to eat sitting in high chairs now. Make this an opportunity for face-to-face learning interactions. Don't have the TV on during meals, which distracts babies from learning.

- Starting healthy media habits now is important, because they are much harder to change when children are older.

- Consider making a family media use plan. A family media use plan is a set of rules about media use and screen time that are written down and agreed on by parents. Take into account not only the quantity but the quality and location of media use. Consider TVs, phones, tablets, and computers. Rules should be followed by parents as well as children. The AAP has information on how to make a plan at **www.HealthyChildren.org/MediaUsePlan.**

Priority

Discipline
Parent expectations of child's behavior

Parent Expectations of Child's Behavior

This is an age when the entire family needs to adapt to the increasingly mobile infant. The more consistent parents are in establishing and reinforcing appropriate behavior, the easier it will be for the infant to learn what is, and is not, allowed. Providing parents with appropriate developmental expectations is an important aspect of helping parents come to an agreement on their approaches to parenting.

Sample Questions
What are your thoughts about discipline? How do you and your partner manage your child's behavior? What are your strategies? Do you and other key family members, such as mothers, mothers-in-law, and other elders, agree on ways to manage the baby's environment to support healthy behavior? Have you discussed these issues with your child care provider? How are your other children adapting to the baby as he gets older?

Anticipatory Guidance
- An important aspect of discipline is teaching your child what behaviors you expect. During the first year of life, the parents' primary role is to balance stimulating an infant's natural curiosity with protecting him from harm. During this time, babies learn more by example from what they observe than through what their parents may say to them. Therefore, setting an example of the behaviors you expect of your child is very important.
- Use positive language to describe the behavior that is desired, as often as possible. For example, say, "Time to sit," rather than, "Don't stand." This will give him better direction about the behavior that is desired.
- A critical step in establishing discipline is to limit, "No," to the most important issues. One way to do this is to remove other reasons to say, "No," such as putting dangerous or tempting objects out of reach. Then, when an important issue comes up, such as your baby going toward the stove or radiator, saying, "NO, hot, don't touch," and removing the baby will have real meaning for him.
- Because infants have a natural curiosity about objects they see their parents using, but also a short attention span, distraction and replacing a forbidden object with one that is permissible are excellent strategies for managing your baby's behavior in a positive way.
- Another aspect of discipline is consistency among parents, other family members, and child care providers. It is important to discuss what behaviors are allowed and what behaviors are not allowed. Have this discussion with your partner, family members, and child care provider. Some simple rules for your child can be established, such as saying, "Don't touch," for certain objects.
- Asking siblings to help with the baby to the extent they are able will continue to meet their needs of being involved and feeling they are important members of the family.

Priority

Nutrition and Feeding

Self-feeding, mealtime routines, transition to solid foods (table food introduction), cup drinking; plans for weaning

Self-feeding, Mealtime Routines, Transition to Solid Foods (Table Food Introduction), Cup Drinking

During the next 3 months, infants demonstrate a growing ability to feed themselves. As infants begin to want independence with self-feeding, it is increasingly important for parents to understand the division of responsibility between parent and child with regard to feeding—the parent is responsible for providing a sufficient amount and variety of nutritious foods, and the child is responsible for deciding how much to eat.

The time between the introduction of solid foods and age 9 months is a sensitive period for learning to chew. A gradual exposure to solid textures during this time may decrease the risk of feeding problems, such as rejecting certain textures, refusing to chew, or vomiting.

Sample Questions

How has feeding been going? What is your baby feeding herself? What does your baby eat with her fingers? Has she used a cup? Has your baby received breast milk or other fluids from a bottle or cup?

Anticipatory Guidance

- Try to be patient and understanding as your baby tries new foods and learns to feed herself. Removing distractions, like TV, will help her stay focused on eating. Remember, it may take 10 to 15 tries before your baby will accept a new food.
- As your baby becomes more independent in feeding herself, remember that you are responsible for providing a variety of sufficient nutritious foods, but she is responsible for deciding how much to eat.
- Most 9-month-olds can be on the same eating schedule as the family. This usually means breakfast, lunch, and dinner. The baby also should have a mid-morning, afternoon, and bedtime snack. The amount of food taken at a single feeding may vary and may not be a large amount, but the 3 meals and 2 to 3 snacks help ensure that your baby is exposed to a variety of foods and receives adequate nutrition. Snacks can be an opportunity to try new foods.
- Giving your baby foods of varying textures, including pureed, blended, mashed, finely chopped, and soft lumps, will help her successfully go through the change from gumming to chewing foods. Slowly introducing solid textures during this time may decrease the risk of feeding problems, refusing to chew, or vomiting. Gradually increase table foods. Avoid mixed textures, like broth with vegetables, because they are the most difficult for infants to eat.

■ Encourage your baby to drink from a cup with help. One hundred percent juice may be served as part of a snack, but should be limited to 4 oz per day. Avoid the use of sweetened drinks, such as sodas and artificially flavored "fruit" drinks. These drinks provide calories, but no nutrients.

■ No foods need to be withheld except raw honey and chunks that could cause choking.

Plans for Weaning

The transition from a complete milk diet to a diet of solids and milk continues. Discuss plans for weaning or transitioning from formula to whole milk and from breast or bottle to cup. For babies receiving formula or human milk from a bottle, weaning can be done gradually, substituting 1 bottle with a cup of the liquid. As the infant approaches 12 months of age, most, if not all, bottles can be eliminated.

Because breastfeeding is recommended for the entire first year, weaning is usually delayed to after 12 months. However, some mothers report that their babies appear to be less interested in breastfeeding at around age 9 months. This is often remedied by breastfeeding in a quiet environment free of distraction. Alternatively, pumped human milk or infant formula (NOT cow's milk) may be served from a cup, not a bottle.

Sample Questions
What are your plans for continuing to breastfeed? What questions or concerns do you have?

Anticipatory Guidance
■ Weaning ages vary considerably from child to child. Some are ready to wean earlier than others and will show this by decreasing their interest in breastfeeding as they increase their interest in the foods they see their parents eating.

■ Your baby's best source of nutrition at 9 months of age continues to be breast milk with solid food. Try to continue breastfeeding through the first year of the baby's life, or for as long as both you and your baby want.

■ If your baby is taking formula, it is recommended that it be your baby's major milk source until her first birthday. Whole milk can be introduced after age 1 year.

■ As you begin to wean your baby, consider starting with the least interesting bottle time (perhaps the naptime bottle). Gradually substitute the cup for other bottles.

■ If your baby is used to being held during feeding, hold her while feeding with a cup.

Priority

Safety

Car safety seats; heatstroke prevention; firearm safety; safe home environment: burns, poisoning, drowning, falls

Car Safety Seats

Parents may be tempted to prematurely change their 9-month-old's rear-facing car safety seat to a forward-facing seat as he outgrows the rear-facing–only car safety seat. Remind parents that the rear-facing position offers the best protection for the baby's head, neck, and spine. Death and serious injury are significantly less likely for infants and young children who are rear facing compared with forward facing. Children should ride rear facing to the highest weight or height allowed for rear facing by the manufacturer of their convertible or 3-in-1 seat, until at least age 2 years. These seats have height and weight limits that can accommodate even large toddlers rear facing through the second year of life. Advise parents that it is not dangerous for their baby's feet to touch the vehicle seat back. Lower extremity injuries are extremely rare among rear-facing children in crashes, but are common in forward-facing children, and toddlers are typically quite comfortable with their legs folded or propped up on the seat back.

Remind parents that their own safe driving behaviors (including using seat belts at all times, not driving under the influence of alcohol or drugs, and avoiding use of electronic devices while driving) are important to the health of their children.

Sample Questions

Is your baby fastened securely in the back seat in a rear-facing car safety seat for every ride in a vehicle? Do all members in the family use a seat belt every time they ride in a vehicle?

Anticipatory Guidance

- Never place your baby's car safety seat in the front seat of a vehicle with a passenger air bag because air bags deploy with great force. When it hits a car safety seat, it causes serious injury or death.
- Babies are best protected in the event of a crash when they are in the back seat and in a rear-facing car safety seat. They should be in a 5-point harness at all times.
- Keep your baby's car safety seat rear facing in the back seat of the vehicle until your baby is at least 2 years old. It is preferable to wait even longer, until the baby reaches the highest weight or height allowed by the manufacturer of the rear-facing seat.
- Children who reach the maximum height or weight allowed by their rear-facing–only car safety seat should use a convertible or 3-in-1 seat that is approved for use rear facing to higher weights and heights (up to 50 pounds and 49 inches, depending on the seat). Your baby will be safest if he rides rear facing to the highest weight or height allowed by the manufacturer.

- Your baby should ride in the back seat. The back seat is the safest place to ride until your child is age 13 years.
- Do not start the engine until everyone is buckled in.
- Your own safe driving behaviors are important to the health of your children.
- Use a seat belt at all times, do not drive after using alcohol or drugs, and do not text or use cell phones or other electronic devices while driving.

For information about car safety seats and actions to keep your baby safe in and around cars, visit www.safercar.gov/parents.

Find a Child Passenger Safety Technician: http://cert.safekids.org. Click on "Find a Tech."

Toll-free Auto Safety Hotline: 888-327-4236

Heatstroke Prevention

Each year, an average of 37 children die of heatstroke after being left in cars that become too hot. More than half of the deaths are infants and children younger than 2 years. In most cases, the parent or caregiver forgot the child was in the car, often because there was a change in the usual routine or schedule. Additionally, some children have died while playing in the vehicle or after getting in the vehicle without the caregiver's knowledge. Even very loving and attentive parents can forget a child in the car.

The temperature inside a car can rise to a dangerous level quickly, even when the temperature outside is as low as 60 degrees. Leaving the windows open will not prevent heatstroke. Because children have proportionally less surface area than adults and less ability to regulate internal temperature, their bodies overheat up to 5 times more quickly than adults' bodies.

Sample Question
Every year, children die of heatstroke after being left in a hot car. Would you like to talk about creating a plan so this doesn't happen to you?

Anticipatory Guidance
- Never leave your baby alone in a car for any reason, even briefly.
- Start developing habits that will help prevent you from ever forgetting your baby in the car. Consider putting an item that you need, like your purse, cell phone, or employee ID, in the back seat of the vehicle, so you will see your baby when you retrieve the item before leaving the car.
- Check the back seat before walking away, every time you park your vehicle.

Firearm Safety

Review firearm safety with parents. The AAP recommends that firearms be removed from the places where children live and play. Parents who own firearms may be more receptive to this discussion when firearms are considered along with the other household hazards than when they are the sole focus of a discussion. Children cannot reliably be taught not to handle a firearm. Therefore, if the household where the child resides has a firearm, it is essential that firearms are kept out of the sight and reach of the child.

Sample Questions

Does anyone in your home have a firearm? If so, is the firearm unloaded and locked up? Is the ammunition stored and locked separately from the firearm? Have you considered not owning a firearm because of the danger to your child and other family members?

Anticipatory Guidance

- Homicide and suicide are more common in homes that have firearms. As your baby becomes more active, the potential dangers of a firearm become even greater. The best way to keep your baby safe from injury or death from firearms is to never have a firearm in the home.
- If it is necessary to keep a firearm in your home or if the homes of people you visit have firearms, they should be stored unloaded and locked, with the ammunition locked separately from the firearm.
- A young child's curiosity will always outweigh any lessons about not touching a firearm, so it is essential that you keep firearms far out of the sight and reach of your baby.

Safe Home Environment: Burns, Poisoning, Drowning, Falls

As their baby develops more fine and gross motor skills, it is important to review with the parents how to keep the home environment safe. No home is ever childproof, but parents can initiate changes to make the environment safer. This applies to all homes where the baby spends time, including child care and grandparents' and friends' homes.

Sample Question

Now that your baby can move on his own more, what changes have you made in your home to ensure his safety?

Anticipatory Guidance

- Do not leave heavy objects or containers of hot liquids on tables with tablecloths. Your baby may pull on the tablecloth. Turn handles of pans or dishes so they do not hang over the edge of a stove or table.
- Use appropriate barriers around space heaters, wood stoves, and kerosene heaters.
- Keep electrical cords out of your baby's reach. Mouth burns can result from chewing on the end of a live extension cord or on a poorly insulated wire.
- To prevent poisoning, keep household products, such as cleaners, chemicals, and medicines, locked up and out of your baby's sight and reach. Make sure your baby does not have access to paint chips or chewable surfaces in a home built before 1978 because they may contain lead-based paint. Keep the number of the **Poison Help line (800-222-1222)** posted next to every telephone and saved in your cell phone.

- The kitchen is the most dangerous room for children. A safer place for your baby while you are cooking, eating, or unable to provide your full attention is the play yard, crib, or stationary activity center, or buckled into a high chair.
- Watch your baby constantly whenever he is near water. He can drown in even a few inches of water, including in the bathtub, play pools, buckets, or toilets. A supervising adult should be within an arm's reach, providing "touch supervision," whenever babies are in or around water.
- Do not let young brothers or sisters watch over your infant in the bathtub, house, yard, or playground.
- Empty buckets, tubs, or small pools immediately after you use them.
- To prevent your baby from falling out of a window, keep furniture away from windows and install operable window guards on second- and higher-story windows. Use gates at the top and bottom of stairs.
- Use safety straps to secure bookshelves, dressers, floor lamps, and other tall furniture as well as TVs to the wall. As your baby learns to stand and climb, he could pull the furniture down on himself and be crushed. Even heavy furniture can tip over if not secured to the wall.

References

1. Cohen GJ; American Academy of Pediatrics Committee on Psychosocial Aspects of Child and Family Health. The prenatal visit. *Pediatrics.* 2009;124(4):1227-1232
2. Jones VF; American Academy of Pediatrics Committee on Early Childhood, Adoption, and Dependent Care. Comprehensive health evaluation of the newly adopted child. *Pediatrics.* 2012;129(1):e214-e223
3. Breiding MJ, Basile KC, Smith SG, Black MC, Mahendra R. *Intimate Partner Violence Surveillance: Uniform Definitions and Recommended Data Elements Version 2.0.* Atlanta, GA: National Center for Injury Prevention and Control, Centers for Disease Control and Prevention; 2015. www.cdc.gov/violenceprevention/pdf/intimatepartnerviolence.pdf. Accessed September 15, 2016
4. American Academy of Pediatrics Task Force on Circumcision. Circumcision policy statement. *Pediatrics.* 2012;130(3):585-586
5. American Academy of Pediatrics Task Force on Sudden Infant Death Syndrome. SIDS and other sleep-related infant deaths: updated 2016 recommendations for a safe infant sleeping environment. Pediatrics. 2016;138(5):e20162938
6. Moon RY and American Academy of Pediatrics Task Force on Sudden Infant Death Syndrome. SIDS and other sleep-related infant deaths: evidence base for 2016 updated recommendations for a safe infant sleeping environment. *Pediatrics.* 2016;138(5):e20162940
7. Riordan J, Bibb D, Miller M, Rawlins T. Predicting breastfeeding duration using the LATCH breastfeeding assessment tool. *J Hum Lact.* 2001;17(1):20-23
8. American College of Obstetricians and Gynecologists Committee on Obstetric Practice. Committee Opinion No. 637: marijuana use during pregnancy and lactation. *Obstet Gynecol.* 2015;126(1):234-238
9. American Academy of Pediatrics Council on Communications and Media. Media and young minds. *Pediatrics.* 2016;138(5):e20162591
10. Reid Chassiakos Y, Radesky J, Christakis D, et al., AAP Council on Communications and Media. Children and adolescents and digital media. *Pediatrics.* 2016;138(5):e20162593

Early Childhood Visits

1 Through 4 Years

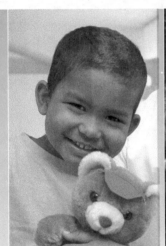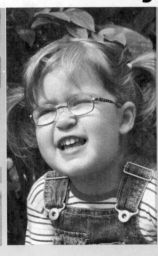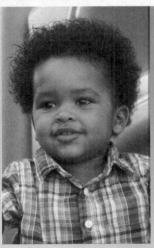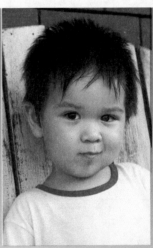

Early Childhood
12 Month Visit

Context

The 12-month-old stands proudly, somewhat bow-legged, belly protruding. Walking, one of the most exciting developmental milestones, occurs around the toddler's first birthday, bringing with it increasing independence. During the first year of life, the infant was rarely in conflict with his environment. He might have been demanding when he cried, he required considerable care, and he changed the balance in the family. However, he spent most of his first year getting to know and trust his parents and his environment. As a toddler, he becomes increasingly competent in acting upon the world around him, all on his own. His world broadens, bringing both excitement and challenge.

Autonomy and independent mobility are developmental achievements of which the parents and toddler are justifiably proud, but the toddler constantly encounters environmental barriers. He cannot go as fast as he would like without tripping, he cannot always reach desired objects, and he can fall and hurt himself. New hazards emerge, such as cups full of hot coffee left on surfaces within reach or stairs without gates. A toddler's parents and other caregivers must watch him constantly to keep him safe.

As the toddler's autonomy, independence, and cognitive abilities increase, he begins to exert his own will. In response, his parents' perceptions of his demands change dramatically, influenced by their own upbringing and childhood experiences. Do the parents understand their toddler's needs and attempt to meet them? The 12-month-old's dramatic struggle for autonomy will test his parents' ability to let go, permit independence, and enjoy aspects of his behavior that are out of their direct control. The toddler's messy attempts to feed himself can be difficult for his parents as they sort out their own desire for order and neatness with his need for self-care.

Fortunately, the toddler is endowed with a social feedback loop to recognize both pleasure and displeasure from significant caregivers. Adults build on this characteristic by providing appropriate responses to a toddler's actions. Adult laughter during a well-played game of peekaboo holds the key to future good times in other interactive games, and turning away, ignoring, or expressing displeasure at a plate of food thrown on the floor, which sends a message that this behavior is not acceptable, helps prevent later disruptive behaviors.

Positive activities, such as cuddling, holding, praising, and firmly enforcing rules about not biting, hitting, and kicking, help the toddler develop emotional expression. Consistency is the keystone for dealing with a 12-month-old, and establishing regular routines is all-important.

Although the toddler's level of activity increases significantly during this period, his rate of weight gain decreases, and struggles over eating arise for many parents. A toddler frequently eats a large amount at one meal and very little at the next. However, hunger guides him and he eats a sufficient amount over time. Not overfeeding is important to help prevent obesity. The key is to offer nutritious foods consistently and not worry about whether all the food is finished each time.

Food should not be a reward for good behavior, nor should food be withheld as a punishment for bad behavior, as it can lead to obesity and it is an ineffective disciplinary technique.

Responding sensitively to the 12-month-old's behavior is a complex task. Some parents who did well with the more dependent, younger infant are less confident of their role now. Toddlers beginning their second year of life thrive when parents accommodate their demands yet maintain a strong parenting presence, including a full measure of patience, enough self-confidence to set limits, the judgment to know which needs are most important, and the ability to realize that their 12-month-old's negative behavior is not directed against them. Physical interaction promotes fun in being active. Reading aloud and singing are positive ways to spend time together and can be worked into the child's daily routines, such as at bedtime or naptime and before mealtime. By letting the child choose the book, the parent can support the child's growing independence and, by reading aloud and naming the pictures, the parent can help the child learn language and satisfy his curiosity about the world. Television (TV) and other digital media should be discouraged at this age.

Parents need to be positive role models for their toddler, both physically (eg, by eating nutritiously, being physically active, wearing seat belts in the car, and reading for pleasure) and emotionally (eg, by being calm and consistent in setting limits and handling tantrums). Parents who enjoy their toddler's growing independence can best provide a stable home base as the toddler's curiosity and mobility carry him into an expanding world.

Children this age may be uncomfortable about being restrained in their activity. The physical examination may be more successfully performed while the child is on a parent's lap or standing on the floor. Speaking directly to the child and taking a playful stance about the examination will make it easier for the child to cooperate. If the child becomes upset, it is a good idea to remind the parent that this reaction is expected at this age. As part of the complete physical examination, perform the noninvasive procedures first, with the eyes, ears, nose, mouth, and abdomen examined last.

Priorities for the 12 Month Visit

The first priority is to attend to the concerns of the parents.

In addition, the Bright Futures Early Childhood Expert Panel has given priority to the following topics for discussion in this visit:

▶ Social determinants of health[a] (risks [living situation and food security; tobacco, alcohol, and drugs], strengths and protective factors [social connections with family, friends, child care and home visitation program staff, and others])

▶ Establishing routines (adjustment to the child's developmental changes and behavior; family time; bedtime, naptime, and teeth brushing; media)

▶ Feeding and appetite changes (self-feeding, continued breastfeeding and transition to family meals, nutritious foods)

▶ Establishing a dental home (first dental checkup and dental hygiene)

▶ Safety (car safety seats, falls, drowning prevention and water safety, sun protection, pets, safe home environment: poisoning)

[a] Social determinants of health is a new priority in the fourth edition of the *Bright Futures Guidelines*. For more information, see the *Promoting Lifelong Health for Families and Communities* theme.

Health Supervision

The *Bright Futures Tool and Resource Kit* contains Previsit Questionnaires to assist the health care professional in taking a history, conducting developmental surveillance, and performing medical screening.

History

Interval history may be obtained according to the concerns of the family and the health care professional's preference or style of practice. The following questions can encourage in-depth discussion:

General Questions

- What are you most proud of since our last visit? (If the parent responds, "Nothing," the clinician should be prepared with a compliment, such as, "You made time for this visit despite your busy schedule.")
- Tell me how things are going at home and how your family is adapting to your 12-month-old.
- What changes have occurred in your family since your last visit? What is the effect of these changes on your family?
- Where are you currently living? Does anyone else care for your child other than you? Do you have any child care needs? Do you feel your child is safe?
- What do you like most about your son/daughter?
- What questions or concerns would you like to share with me about your child?
- What makes you feel hopeful and optimistic?
- What kinds of media does your toddler see (eg, TV, video, cell phone, or other digital media)?

Past Medical History

- Has your child received any specialty or emergency care since the last visit?

Family History

- Has your child or anyone in the family (parents, brothers, sisters, grandparents, aunts, uncles, or cousins) developed a new health condition or died? **If the answer is Yes:** Ascertain who in the family has or had the condition, and ask about the age of onset and diagnosis. If the person is no longer living, ask about the age at the time of death.

Social History

- See the Social Determinants of Health priority in Anticipatory Guidance for social history questions.

Surveillance of Development

Do you or any of your child's caregivers have any specific concerns about your child's development, learning, or behavior?

Clinicians using the *Bright Futures Tool and Resource Kit* Previsit Questionnaires or another tool that includes a developmental milestones checklist, or those who use a structured developmental screening tool, need not ask about these developmental surveillance milestones. *(For more information, see the Promoting Healthy Development theme.)*

Social Language and Self-help

Does your child

- Look for hidden objects?
- Imitate new gestures?

Verbal Language (Expressive and Receptive)

Does she

- Use *Dada* or *Mama* specifically?
- Use 1 word other than *Mama, Dada,* or personal names?
- Follow directions with gestures, such as motioning and saying, "Give me (object)"?

Gross Motor

Does he

- Take first independent steps?
- Stand without support?

Fine Motor

Does she

- Drop an object in a cup?
- Pick up small object with 2-finger pincer grasp?
- Pick up food and eat it?

Review of Systems

The Bright Futures Early Childhood Expert Panel recommends a complete review of systems as a part of every health supervision visit. This review can be done through questions about the following:

Do you have concern about your child's

- Head
  - Shape
- Eyes
  - Cross-eyed
- Ears, nose, and throat
- Breathing
- Stomach or abdomen
  - Vomiting or spitting
  - Bowel movements
- Genitals or rectum
- Skin
- Development
  - Muscle strength, movement of arms or legs, any developmental concerns

Observation of Parent-Child Interaction

During the visit, the health care professional acknowledges and reinforces positive parent-child interactions and discusses any concerns. Observation focuses on

- How does the parent interact with the toddler (eg, anxiously, calmly, reciprocally, in a controlling manner, or inattentively)?
- Does the child check back with the parent visually?
- When the health care professional gives the child a book, does the parent follow the child's gaze?
- Does the child bring an object of interest to show or share with the parent?
- How does the parent react when the health care professional praises the child? How does the parent react to being praised?
- If siblings are in the room, how do they interact with the toddler?
- Does the parent seem positive when speaking about the child?

Physical Examination

A complete physical examination is included as part of every health supervision visit.

When performing a physical examination, the health care professional's attention is directed to the following components of the examination that are important for a child this age:

- **Measure and plot on appropriate World Health Organization (WHO) Growth Chart**
  - Recumbent length
  - Weight
  - Head circumference
  - Weight-for-length

- **Eyes**
  - Assess ocular motility.
  - Examine pupils for opacification and red reflexes.
  - Assess visual acuity using fixate and follow response.

- **Mouth**
  - Observe for dental irregularities like caries, plaque, demineralization (white spots), and staining.

- **Abdomen**
  - Palpate for masses.

- **Neurologic**
  - Observe gait if walking.
  - Observe hand grasp and strength.

- **Genitals**
  - Determine whether testes are fully descended.
  - Determine whether labia are open.

- **Skin**
  - Observe for nevi, café-au-lait spots, birthmarks, or bruising.

Screening

Universal Screening	Action
Anemia	Hematocrit or hemoglobin
Lead (high prevalence area or insured by Medicaid)	Lead blood test
Oral Health (in the absence of a dental home)	Apply fluoride varnish after first tooth eruption and every 6 months.

Selective Screening	Risk Assessment[a]	Action if Risk Assessment Positive (+)
Blood Pressure	Children with specific risk conditions or change in risk	Blood pressure measurement
Hearing	+ on risk screening questions	Referral for diagnostic audiologic assessment
Lead (low prevalence area and not insured by Medicaid)	+ on risk screening questions	Lead blood test
Oral Health	Does not have a dental home	Referral to dental home or, if not available, oral health risk assessment
	Primary water source is deficient in fluoride.	Oral fluoride supplementation
Tuberculosis	+ on risk screening questions	Tuberculin skin test
Vision	+ on risk screening questions	Ophthalmology referral

[a] See the *Evidence and Rationale chapter* for the criteria on which risk screening questions are based.

Immunizations

Consult the Centers for Disease Control and Prevention/Advisory Committee on Immunization Practices (CDC/ACIP) or American Academy of Pediatrics (AAP) Web sites for the current immunization schedule.

CDC National Immunization Program: **www.cdc.gov/vaccines**

AAP *Red Book:* **http://redbook.solutions.aap.org**

Anticipatory Guidance

The following sample questions, which address the Bright Futures Early Childhood Expert Panel's Anticipatory Guidance Priorities, are intended to be used selectively to invite discussion, gather information, address the needs and concerns of the family, and build partnerships. Use of the questions may vary from visit to visit and from family to family. Questions can be modified to match the health care professional's communication style. The accompanying anticipatory guidance for the family should be geared to questions, issues, or concerns for that particular child and family. Tools and handouts to support anticipatory guidance can be found in the *Bright Futures Tool and Resource Kit.*

Priority

Social Determinants of Health

Risks: Living situation and food security; tobacco, alcohol, and drugs

Strengths and protective factors: Social connections with family, friends, child care, home visitation program staff, and others

Risks: Living Situation and Food Security

Parents in difficult living situations or with limited means may have concerns about their access to affordable housing, food, or other resources. Suggest community resources that help with finding quality child care, accessing transportation, or addressing issues such as financial concerns, inadequate means to cover health care expenses, inadequate or unsafe housing, or lack of social support. If the family is having difficulty obtaining sufficient nutritious food, provide information about the Special Supplemental Program for Women, Infants, and Children (WIC), Supplemental Nutrition Assistance Program (SNAP), local food shelves, and local community food programs.

Sample Questions

Tell me about your living situation. Do you have enough heat, hot water, and electricity? Do you have appliances that work? Do you have problems with bugs, rodents, peeling paint or plaster, or mold or dampness?

How are your resources for caring for your child? Do you have enough knowledge to feel comfortable in caring for her? Do you have health insurance? Do you have enough money for food, clothing, and child care?

Within the past 12 months, were you ever worried whether your food would run out before you got money to buy more? Within the past 12 months, did the food you bought not last, and you did not have money to get more?

Have you ever tried to get help for these issues? What happened? What barriers did you face?

Anticipatory Guidance

- If you have problems with any of these things, let me know and I can tell you about community services and other resources that can help you.

Risks: Tobacco, Alcohol, and Drugs

The use of tobacco, alcohol, and other drugs has adverse health effects on the entire family. Focusing on the effect on health is often the most helpful approach and may help some family members with quitting or cutting back on substance use.

Sample Questions

Does anyone in your home smoke? Are you worried about any family members and how much they smoke, drink, or use drugs?

How often do you drink beer, wine, or liquor in your household? Do you, or does anyone you ride with, ever drive after having a drink? Does your partner use alcohol? What kind and for how long?

Are you using marijuana, cocaine, pain pills, narcotics, or other controlled substances? Are you getting any help to cut down or stop your drug use?

Anticipatory Guidance

- A smoke-free environment, in your car, home, and other places where your child spends time, is important. Smoking affects your child by increasing the risk of asthma, ear infections, and respiratory infections.
- **800-QUIT-NOW (800-784-8669); TTY 800-332-8615** is a national telephone helpline that is routed to local resources. Additional resources are available at **www.cdc.gov.**
- Drug and alcohol cessation programs are available in our community and we would like to help you connect to these services.

Strengths and Protective Factors: Social Connections With Family, Friends, Child Care, Home Visitation Program Staff, and Others

Informal and formal supports that promote connections with family and friends continue to be important in the second year of the child's life. Having someone to talk to about parenting issues can help in handling parenting struggles and appreciating the joys of watching their young child grow and develop. Parents also may need help to ensure that they have time away from their toddler to pursue their own interests, have regular time alone to rest, and maintain other important relationships.

During this time, parents also may need extra help from community resources, particularly in finding reliable, high-quality child care and playgroups and accessing reliable information about parenting and child development. Home visiting professionals may continue to visit the family and can be especially helpful in providing knowledge and referral to services that are tailored to the needs of the individual family.

Sample Questions

Who cares for your child other than you? Does a professional visit your home to discuss parenting and your child's health, such as through an early intervention or home visitation program? Have you shared your child's health information with that person? Are you satisfied with the quality of the setting? What activities do you enjoy doing outside of the home? How often do you get together with friends? What things do you do with friends? Do you know parents of children your child's age? Do you need help in finding other community resources, such as a faith-based organization, recreational centers, or volunteer opportunities? How do you reach out to others for help or advice?

Anticipatory Guidance

- Make sure that you discuss your child's medical needs and your feelings about healthy diet, discipline, oral health, physical activity, and media use with all of her caregivers and home visitors.
- Your home visitor can help with issues about your child's health and help you connect to your community.
- Make sure that any environment where your child stays has the same excellent safety standards as your home and that the transportation to and from places outside your home is safe.
- Share any information that we discuss with other caregivers.
- Maintain or expand ties to your community through friends and social, faith-based, cultural, volunteer, and recreational organizations or programs.
- Learn about and consider participating in parent-toddler playgroups and going to activities at the library or other community locations.
- Consider joining a parent education class or parent support group.

Priority

Establishing Routines

Adjustment to the child's developmental changes and behavior; family time; bedtime, naptime, and teeth brushing; media

Adjustment to Child's Developmental Changes and Behavior

A child this age starts to recognize what is permitted, but may try something forbidden. At the same time, he will look back at the parent to test a reaction. This behavior is a normal, positive move toward internalizing rules. Tantrums are more frequent as the child tries to master new skills and struggles with his move toward independence and autonomy. Mention tantrum triggers, like hunger or sleepiness.

Discuss some children's tendency to be clingy sometimes and to go their own ways at other times. Recommend the use of praise to strengthen good behaviors and offer suggestions for how parents might deal with biting, hitting, or other possibly harmful activity. Ask how things are going with any siblings and pets.

Sample Questions

What do you love about your child? How do you reward him? When your child's behavior is troublesome, what do you do? What do you do when he doesn't cooperate? What do the others in your family do? Do you need help in managing your child's behavior? Sometimes raising a child can be frustrating. Does anyone ever get angry with him? What happens then? Do you ever spank him? What helps keep you calm when you are feeling a bit overwhelmed?

Anticipatory Guidance

- Time with family and special caregivers is the best treat you can give your child.
- Try not to punish your child with spanking, shouting, or long explanations. A firm "No!" is the best way to deal with minor irritations, just as "Yes!" is a great way to reward good behavior. You may want to consider a brief time-out. Put the child in his crib or playpen or hold him quietly on your lap for 1 to 2 minutes only, until the undesirable behavior stops.
- Distracting your child with something new that gets her attention and directing the child to a new activity are excellent ways to reduce unwanted behaviors. He wants to be near you and hear your voice—reading aloud to him is a great strategy for this purpose. It is also a way to help him love books.

Family Time

Establishing family traditions is extremely important for establishing a sense of identity within the family and culture. Routines around bedtime and meals, reading together, and playing also are important, even at this young age.

Strong interpersonal relationships are key to developing the emotions of love and well-being and to family growth. At this age, these relationships center on the immediate family and regular caregivers. Warn parents that stranger anxiety reaches a peak in the next few months.

Sample Questions

What do you all do together? What do your child's brothers and sisters do with him? Tell me about your family's traditions, especially your favorite ones. What are some of the new things that your child is doing? How does your child react to changes in his routines or to strangers? What is your child's routine for meals and snacks?

Anticipatory Guidance

- Carve out time for family time each day. Use this time to focus on your child and his brothers and sisters through games, storytelling, reading aloud, pointing and naming, listening to music, laughing, playing, and moving. To minimize your children's exposure to TV, videos, and other forms of media, avoid watching TV or using other digital devices during family time.
- Organized mealtime is another good way to establish a consistent daily routine. Regular times for meals and snacks will protect your toddler against getting too hungry, which will help prevent inappropriate behavior.
- If your child goes to a child care setting, make sure that it, too, has established routines, restricts or limits screen time, and promotes healthy active living and good nutrition.
- At this age, your child may feel anxious around people he does not know. When he meets someone new, allow time for him to warm up. Try to use a consistent child care provider or sitter.

Bedtime, Naptime, and Teeth Brushing

A 1-year-old should be sleeping 12 to 14 hours a day. Bedtime should be at the same time each night and should become a nightly routine. Reading and singing before bedtime are examples of sleep-promoting activities. For both naptime and bedtime, he should be put in the crib awake so that he can make the transition from awake to asleep on his own.

Another important routine to establish during this age is daily tooth brushing twice a day as soon as teeth erupt.

Sample Questions

How are sleeping routines going? Is it difficult getting your child to go to sleep? What time is bedtime? How do you manage naps? How often do you clean your toddler's teeth? How do you clean his teeth?

Anticipatory Guidance

- Establish a nightly bedtime routine that begins with quiet time for your child to relax before bed and ends with your child soothing himself in his own crib. Reading and singing to your child will help him get to sleep. A night-light also can help to reassure and calm your child.
- Toddlers should continue to have at least 1 nap during the day. It is important to establish a regular naptime routine. Make sure to time naps so that your child is tired at bedtime.
- Another important daily routine is teeth brushing or cleaning. Establish a regular time twice each day for this task, such as after breakfast and before bed.

Media

As more families and children have access to and exposure to digital media, it is important to assess for the use of such devices and offer guidance as to what is appropriate for a child at this age. Discuss alternatives to toddlers watching TV. Discourage any TV, computer, tablet, smartphone, or viewing or play for infants and children younger than 18 months. Parents should not put a TV in their child's bedroom.

Sample Questions

How much time each day does your child spend watching TV or playing on a tablet, smartphone, or other digital device? Is there a TV on in the background while your child is playing in the room?

Anticipatory Guidance

- Research shows that toddlers at this age cannot learn information from screens, even though many toys and videos claim to teach them skills. Young children learn by interacting with caregivers; being read to, talked to, and sung to; and exploring their environment (grabbing, mouthing, crawling, and cruising). Make special time for this tech-free type of play every day.
- Make mealtimes an opportunity for face-to-face learning interactions. Don't have the TV on during meals, which distracts babies from eating.
- Starting healthy media habits now is important, because they are much harder to change when children are older. Do not put a TV in your child's bedroom.
- Consider making a family media use plan. A family media use plan is a set of rules about media use and screen time that is written down and agreed upon by parents. Take into account not only the quantity, but the quality and location of media use, including TVs, phones, tablets, and computers. Rules should be followed by parents as well as children. The AAP has information on making a plan at **www.HealthyChildren.org/MediaUsePlan.**

Priority

Feeding and Appetite Changes
Self-feeding, continued breastfeeding and transition to family meals, nutritious foods

Self-feeding

The child should be developing toddler eating skills—biting off small pieces of food, feeding herself, and holding and drinking from a cup. Toddlers learn to like foods by touching, smelling, and mouthing them repeatedly.

Sample Question
How is your child doing with feeding herself during meals and snacks?

Anticipatory Guidance
- Give your toddler a spoon for eating and a cup for drinking. Be sure that they are easy for her small hands to hold.
- Cover your floor and don't worry about messes. Young children learn from experimenting.
- Avoid small, hard foods like peanuts or popcorn, on which your child can choke. Cut any firm, round food, such as hot dogs, raw carrots, grape or cherry tomatoes, or grapes, into thin slices.

Continued Breastfeeding and Transition to Family Meals

Meals can be relaxed, safe, and enjoyable family times. Encourage fine motor skills, such as using a cup or spoon and eating finger foods. Continue to support breastfeeding as long as mutually desired by mother and child. Mothers who breastfeed continue to need support when nursing their child at 12 months of age and beyond. It is now appropriate to switch the child from formula to whole cow's milk. Limit fruit juice (even 100%) to 4 oz total for the day and rely instead on water for hydration. Develop plans to stop bottle-feeding. Bottle-feeding should be used only to provide the toddler with water.

Sample Question
Tell me about mealtime in your home. Tell me about mealtime in your child care setting. What does your child drink?

Anticipatory Guidance

- Include your toddler in family meals by providing a high chair or booster seat at table height placed at a safe distance from the table. Make mealtimes pleasant and companionable. Encourage conversation.
- Whole cow's milk may be introduced by cup, providing up to 16 oz per day. The amount of whole cow's milk intake will increase as breastfeeding diminishes.
- Avoid using raw milk or any milk substitutes that are not equivalent to cow's milk and that do not meet US Department of Agriculture (USDA) standards for milk substitutes. These include beverages such as rice milk, almond milk, or coconut milk.

Nutritious Foods

Now is a good time for parents to establish positive eating patterns for their child by providing healthy foods at regular intervals 5 to 6 times throughout the day, giving appropriate amounts, and emphasizing nutritious foods. Discuss the importance of providing healthy snacks and of minimizing foods and beverages that are high in added sugars and saturated fat and low in nutrients. Remind parents that they are responsible for providing a variety of nutritious foods and that their child is responsible for how much to eat.

Many families wonder whether they should choose organic fruits and vegetables over conventional fruits and vegetables to reduce pesticide exposure in their child's diet. Eating a diet rich in a variety of fruits and vegetables, either conventional or organic, has well-established health benefits. Choosing organic fruits and vegetables can reduce exposures to pesticides in the diet. Mercury in bodies of water like lakes and streams—some of it discharged from industrial plants—can be converted by bacteria into mercury compounds such as methyl mercury. As a result, certain fish, specifically tilefish, shark, swordfish, and king mackerel, can contain high quantities of mercury, which, when consumed, can have a serious negative effect on a young child's developing nervous system.

Sample Questions

How has your child's appetite been? What questions do you have about choosing healthy foods for her? What fruits and vegetables does your child eat? What types of fish does your child eat and how many servings per week? Does your family eat any locally caught fish?

Anticipatory Guidance

- By this time, a toddler will have transitioned from a primarily liquid diet to the family meal. Introducing a wide variety of flavors and textures helps her adjust to this change.
- Your toddler's rate of weight gain will be slower than in the first year. Overall, she may eat less now than when she was an infant. Toddlers also tend to graze. Her appetite will vary; she will eat a lot one time, and not much the next time.
- Include 2- to 3-oz servings of protein, such as eggs, lean meat, chicken, or fish (making sure to remove any bones).
- Let your toddler decide what and how much to eat from an assortment of healthy foods you offer. Trust your child's ability to know when she is hungry and full. If she asks for more, provide a small additional portion. If she stops eating, accept her decision.

- Feed your toddler 5 to 6 times throughout the day (3 meals and 2 or 3 planned snacks). Be sure that your toddler's caregiver or child care center also provides nutritious foods.
- Have healthy snacks on hand, such as
  - Fresh fruit or vegetables, such as apples, oranges, bananas, cucumber, zucchini, and radishes, that are cut in small pieces or thin strips
  - Applesauce, cheese, or small pieces of whole-grain bread or crackers
  - Unflavored yogurt, sweetened with bits of mashed fruit
- Wash fruits and vegetables and eat a variety of fruits and vegetables. Include fish because it has many nutritional benefits, but avoid the 4 kinds that are high in mercury. These are tilefish, shark, swordfish, and king mackerel.

Priority

Establishing a Dental Home
First dental checkup and dental hygiene

First Dental Checkup and Dental Hygiene

Every child should have a dental home, and it should be established soon after the first tooth erupts or by 12 months of age. The dental home must be able to meet the unique needs of each child, including accurate risk assessment for dental diseases and conditions; an individualized preventive dental health program based on risk assessment; anticipatory guidance about growth and development, including teething, finger sucking, or pacifier habits; a plan for responding to emergency dental trauma; comprehensive dental care in accordance with accepted guidelines and periodicity schedules; and referral to other dental specialists when indicated.

Sample Questions
Have you taken your child to a dentist? Tell me about how you care for your child's teeth. What kind of water does your toddler drink? Is it bottle or tap water? Is it fluoridated?

Anticipatory Guidance
- Be sure to take your child to the dentist by 12 months of age or after he gets his first tooth. A dentist will help you keep your child's teeth healthy and will be available in case he ever has an emergency with his teeth, such as a broken tooth or severe pain.
- Brush his teeth with a small smear of fluoridated toothpaste, no more than a grain of rice, twice each day using a soft toothbrush or washcloth.
- If he is still using a bottle, offer only water in the bottle.
- Avoid using beverages and foods with added sugars, such as "fruit"-flavored drinks, candy, or yogurt snacks.

Priority

Safety

Car safety seats, falls, drowning prevention and water safety, pets, sun protection, safe home environment: poisoning

---

Car Safety Seats

Talk with parents to ensure that their child is fastened securely in a car safety seat and that they know to keep their child riding in the rear-facing position as long as possible, at least to age 2 years or when the child reaches the weight or height limit for the rear-facing position in the convertible seat.

Sample Questions

Is your child fastened securely in a rear-facing car safety seat in the back seat every time she rides in a vehicle? Are you having any problems using your car safety seat?

Anticipatory Guidance

- Never place your child's rear-facing safety seat in the front seat of a vehicle with a passenger air bag. The back seat is the safest place for children to ride until your child is 13 years of age.
- The rear-facing position provides the best protection for your child's neck, spine, and head in the event of a crash. For optimal protection, your child should remain in the rear-facing position until she reaches the highest weight or height allowed for use by the manufacturer of a convertible seat or infant-only seat that is approved for use in the rear-facing position to higher weights and heights (up to 40 pounds and 35 inches for rear-facing–only seats and up to 50 pounds and at least 36 inches for convertible seats). Do not switch your child to a forward-facing car safety seat before she is at least 2 years old unless she has reached the manufacturer's weight or height limit for a rear-facing seat.
- Be sure your child's car safety seat is properly installed in the back seat according to the manufacturer's instructions and the vehicle owner's manual. The harness straps should be snug enough that you cannot pinch any webbing between your fingers.

For information about car safety seats and actions to keep your child safe in and around cars, visit www.safercar.gov/parents.

Find a Child Passenger Safety Technician: http://cert.safekids.org. Click on "Find a Tech."

Toll-free Auto Safety Hotline: 888-327-4236

Falls

Never underestimate the ability of a toddler to climb. Parents must be vigilant in preventing injuries from climbing.

Sample Questions

Do you have stair guards and window guards? Where is the mattress positioned in the crib?

Anticipatory Guidance

- Some children can climb out of the crib at this age. Be sure that the crib mattress is on the lowest setting when she is in it.
- Use gates at the top and bottom of stairs and watch your toddler closely when she is on stairs. To prevent children from falling out of windows, keep furniture away from windows and install operable window guards on second- and higher-story windows. Window screens are not effective fall prevention devices.

Drowning Prevention and Water Safety

The child's increased mobility, combined with a heightened curiosity, makes for an extremely dangerous situation around bodies of water. Explain to parents that children can drown in a small amount of water, even in buckets or a few inches of water in a tub.

Children should learn to swim. Swimming programs are not recommended for infants in the first year of life because there is no evidence that they reduce the risk of drowning. Starting in the second year of life, some children may be developmentally ready to start learning swim skills. However, parents should be cautioned that even advanced swimming skills may not prevent drowning.

Sample Questions

Are there swimming pools or other potential water dangers near or in your home? Are you thinking about starting your child in a swimming program?

Anticipatory Guidance

- Watch your toddler constantly whenever she is near water. Your child can drown in even a few inches, including water in the bathtub, play pools, buckets, or toilets. A supervising adult should be within an arm's reach, providing "touch supervision," whenever young children are in or around water.
- Do not let young brothers or sisters watch over your toddler in the bathtub, house, yard, or playground.
- Empty buckets, tubs, or small pools immediately after you use them.
- Be sure that swimming pools in your community, apartment complex, or home have a 4-sided fence with a self-closing, self-latching gate.
- Children should always wear a Coast Guard–approved life jacket when on a boat or other watercraft.
- Swim programs for children this age should include a parent, should emphasize fun and play, should take place in a pool with warm water that is well maintained and clean, and should limit the number of submersions to prevent swallowing water.

Sun Protection

Sun protection now is of increasing importance because of climate change and the thinning of the atmospheric ozone layer. Sun protection is accomplished through limiting sun exposure, using sunscreen, and wearing protective clothing.

Sample Questions

Do you apply sunscreen whenever your child plays outside? Does your child care provider have a sun protection policy? Do you and your child care provider limit outside time during the middle of the day, when the sun is strongest?

Anticipatory Guidance

- Always apply sunscreen with an SPF greater than 15 when your child is outside. Reapply every 2 hours.
- Have your child wear a hat.
- Avoid prolonged time in the sun between 11:00 am and 3:00 pm.
- Wear sun protection clothing for summer.

Pets

Pets can be a source of great joy for children, but should be kept under constant watch when they are around toddlers. Dog and cat bites are particularly common at this age.

Sample Questions

Do you own a pet? How does your child interact with the pet?

Anticipatory Guidance

- Keep your toddler away from animal feeding areas to reduce the risk of both bites and the ingestion of animal food.
- Because children this age are not old enough to understand the difference between playing with and hurting a pet, interactions between them should be supervised at all times. Watch for signs that either your child or your pet is becoming anxious or overexcited.

Safe Home Environment: Poisoning

Injury is the number one cause of toddler morbidity and mortality. The toddler is increasingly mobile and needs protection against common and uncommon hazards. Review all aspects of safety at this visit because safety is one of the most important aspects of care at this age. Make certain that all child care centers and providers are equally committed to excellent safety standards.

If the family lives with other family members or friends, the family may not feel that it has the power to control the environment and may need help in advocating for a safe environment for their child. This can be problematic for families who are living in homeless shelters or other types of temporary or uncertain housing.

Sample Questions

What have you done to childproof your home? The grandparents' homes? The caregiver's home? Do you have cabinet latches? Are tables free of heavy items that your child could pull down on herself? Are heavy furniture and TVs safely anchored? Are electrical outlets covered? Are stairs gated?

How safe do you think your community is? How safe and comfortable do you and your family feel inside your home? Outside your home? How can we help so that your family feels safe? Who else can help your family feel safe?

How often do you let your child's brothers and sisters help you take care of her?

Anticipatory Guidance

- Lock away medications and all cleaning, automotive, laundry, and lawn products out of sight and out of reach. Climbing toddlers can reach even high shelves. Keep emergency phone numbers near every telephone and in your cell phone for rapid dial. The number for the national **Poison Help line** is **800-222-1222.** Call immediately if you have a poisoning emergency. Do not make your child vomit.
- Keep your toddler out of rooms where hot objects may be touched, including hot oven doors, blow-dryers and curling irons, and heaters, or put a barrier around them. Fireplaces can both burn and injure toddlers from falls on the hearth or the glass doors.
- Now that your toddler is crawling and walking, get down on the floor yourself and check for hazards.
- Keep plastic bags, latex balloons, or small objects such as marbles, magnets, and batteries, including button batteries, away from your toddler.
- Be sure there are no dangling telephone, electrical, blind, or drapery cords in your home. Keep all electrical outlets covered. It is best to use cordless window coverings.
- Make sure TVs, furniture, and other heavy items are secure so that your child can't pull them over. Anchor TVs, bookcases, dressers, and cabinets to the wall and put floor lamps behind other furniture.
- Keep sharp objects, such as knives and scissors, out of your toddler's reach.
- Avoid lead sources, especially lead paint on toys, and take-home exposures by people who work with lead. Home renovations in houses built before 1978 also can contaminate house dust and soil with lead. Any renovation to these houses should be done in a lead-safe manner by qualified contractors.
- Never leave young siblings in charge of their baby sister or brother. Allow them to help with daily tasks, like feeding, under the supervision of a responsible adult.

Early Childhood
15 Month Visit

Context

The 15-month-old is a whirlwind of activity and curiosity, with no apparent sense of internal limits. Children this age require constant attention and guidance from parents and caregivers. The child's first tentative steps are now headlong dashes to explore new places. The energy needed to master the challenge of walking now focuses on exploring new horizons. The effect of the dramatic developmental changes at 15 months of age, such as independent mobility, growing self-determination, and more complex cognitive abilities, provides parents with pleasure and delight in the newfound exuberance and determination of their toddler.

With these exciting new developments, the young toddler often forms elevated desires and expectations, as manifested, for example, by a new level of resistance to being dressed, diapered, or put to bed, and a growing desire to explore and do things on her own. These expectations and desires may outstrip her physical abilities, which leads to a new and often displayed emotion—frustration. She gets upset when she is unable to accomplish a task, when she cannot make someone understand her rudimentary communication, and when she cannot do precisely as she wishes. If crying and even screaming fail to elicit the desired response, her protests may escalate to full-blown tantrums or episodes of holding her breath.

The toddler's new mobility, exploratory skills, and exuberance increase her risk of injury. She is likely to run into the street or climb a flight of stairs without a moment's hesitation. Lacking a sense of danger or a fear of falling, the child aged 15 to 18 months will try to scale playground equipment or poke a finger into an electrical socket. Minor injuries may surprise her, but they rarely deter her for long. Her explorations may bring her into contact with dangerous chemicals kept under the sink or medicines in unlocked cabinets if parents are not careful to secure these storage areas.

This critical period of learning for both the parents and the toddler is most productive when parents help their child begin to make healthy choices by serving nutritious foods without pressuring her to eat; offering her the freedom to explore within safe bounds; responding to her needs while limiting her constant demands; encouraging her beginning participation in daily routines, such as feeding herself or offering her a choice between 2 favorite books before bedtime; and learning to cope with their own anger and frustration as they help their toddler master her emotions. At the 15 Month Visit, the health care professional helps parents learn the parenting skills they need to achieve the delicate balancing act of providing a safe and structured environment that also allows their toddler the freedom and independence to learn and explore.

The child at 15 months of age is likely to be wary of the health care professional and balk at the examination. Anxiety connected with the toddler's wariness toward nonfamily members can be lessened if the examination is performed with the child on her parent's lap and the health care professional positioned approximately at eye level with the child. A warming-up phase can be encouraged by initially offering the child a book while speaking with the parent and by starting with the least intrusive aspects of the examination. The tools used in the examination can be made less fearful by first showing them to the child or by modeling their use, such as by putting the measuring tape first around the health care professional's own head, or examining the parent's ear. The child's increasing comfort will be signaled by her giving way to the impulse to explore the new environment of the examination room.

Priorities for the 15 Month Visit

The first priority is to attend to the concerns of the parents.

In addition, the Bright Futures Early Childhood Expert Panel has given priority to the following topics for discussion in this visit:

► Communication and social development (individuation, separation, finding support, attention to how child communicates wants and interests)

► Sleep routines and issues (regular bedtime routine, night waking, no bottle in bed)

► Temperament, development, behavior, and discipline (conflict predictors and distraction, discipline and behavior management)

► Healthy teeth (brushing teeth, reducing caries)

► Safety (car safety seats and parental use of seat belts, safe home environment: poisoning, falls, and fire safety)

Health Supervision

The *Bright Futures Tool and Resource Kit* contains Previsit Questionnaires to assist the health care professional in taking a history, conducting developmental surveillance, and performing medical screening.

History

Interval history may be obtained according to the concerns of the family and the health care professional's preference or style of practice. The following questions can encourage in-depth discussion:

General Questions

- What are you most proud of since our last visit? (If the parent responds, "Nothing," the clinician should be prepared with a compliment, such as, "You made time for this visit despite your busy schedule.")
- What is something funny or wonderful that your child has done lately?
- How would you describe your child's personality these days?
- What things about your child are you most proud of?
- What are your child care needs?
- What questions or concerns do you have about your child?

Past Medical History

- Has your child received any specialty or emergency care since the last visit?

Family History

- Has your child or anyone in the family (parents, brothers, sisters, grandparents, aunts, uncles, or cousins) developed a new health condition or died? **If the answer is Yes:** Ascertain who in the family has or had the condition, and ask about the age of onset and diagnosis. If the person is no longer living, ask about the age at the time of death.

Social History

- What do you find most difficult, challenging, and wonderful about being a parent?
- What major changes or stresses have occurred in your family since your last visit? What is the effect of these changes on your family?

Surveillance of Development

Do you or any of your child's caregivers have any specific concerns about your child's development, learning, or behavior?

Clinicians using the *Bright Futures Tool and Resource Kit* Previsit Questionnaires or another tool that includes a developmental milestones checklist, or those who use a structured developmental screening tool, need not ask about these developmental surveillance milestones. *(For more information, see the Promoting Healthy Development theme.)*

Social Language and Self-help

Does your child

- Imitate scribbling?
- Drink from cup with little spilling?
- Point to ask for something or to get help?
- Look around when you say things like "Where's your ball?" or "Where's your blanket?"

Verbal Language (Expressive and Receptive)

Does he

- Use 3 words other than names?
- Speak in sounds like an unknown language?
- Follow directions that do not include a gesture?

Gross Motor

Does she

- Squat to pick up objects?
- Crawl up a few steps?
- Run?

Fine Motor

Does he

- Make marks with crayon?
- Drop object in and take object out of a container?

Review of Systems

The Bright Futures Early Childhood Expert Panel recommends a complete review of systems as a part of every health supervision visit. This review can be done through questions about the following:

Do you have concern about your child's

- Head
  - Shape
- Eyes
  - Cross-eyed
- Ears, nose, and throat
- Breathing
- Stomach or abdomen
  - Vomiting or spitting
  - Bowel movements
- Genitals or rectum
- Skin
- Development
  - Muscle strength, movement of arms or legs, any developmental concerns

Observation of Parent-Child Interaction

During the visit, the health care professional acknowledges and reinforces positive parent-child interactions and discusses any concerns. Observation focuses on

- What is the emotional tone between parent and child?
- How does the parent support the toddler's need for safety and reassurance in the examination room?
- Does the toddler check back with the parent visually or bring an object to show the parent?
- How do the parent and toddler play with toys (reciprocally, directively, or inattentively)?
- How does the parent react when the health care professional praises the child? How does the parent react to being praised?
- Does the parent notice and acknowledge the child's positive behaviors?
- If siblings are in the room, how do they interact with the toddler?

Physical Examination

A complete physical examination is included as part of every health supervision visit.

When performing a physical examination, the health care professional's attention is directed to the following components of the examination that are important for a child this age:

- **Measure and plot on appropriate WHO Growth Chart**
  - Recumbent length
  - Weight
  - Head circumference
  - Weight-for-length
- **Eyes**
  - Assess ocular motility.
  - Examine pupils for opacification and red reflexes.
  - Assess visual acuity using fixate and follow response.
- **Mouth**
  - Observe for caries, plaque, demineralization (white spots), and staining.
- **Abdomen**
  - Palpate for masses.
- **Skin**
  - Observe for nevi, café-au-lait spots, birthmarks, or bruising.
- **Neurologic**
  - Observe health care professional interaction and stranger avoidance.
  - Observe how the child walks or otherwise moves around the room.

Screening

Universal Screening	Action	
Oral Health (in the absence of a dental home)	Apply fluoride varnish after first tooth eruption and every 6 months.	
Selective Screening	**Risk Assessment[a]**	**Action if Risk Assessment Positive (+)**
Anemia	+ on risk screening questions	Hematocrit or hemoglobin
Blood Pressure	Children with specific risk conditions or change in risk	Blood pressure measurement
Hearing	+ on risk screening question	Referral for diagnostic audiologic assessment
Vision	+ on risk screening questions	Ophthalmology referral

[a] See the *Evidence and Rationale chapter* for the criteria on which risk screening questions are based.

Immunizations

Consult the CDC/ACIP or AAP Web sites for the current immunization schedule.

CDC National Immunization Program: **www.cdc.gov/vaccines**

AAP *Red Book:* **http://redbook.solutions.aap.org**

Anticipatory Guidance

The following sample questions, which address the Bright Futures Early Childhood Expert Panel's Anticipatory Guidance Priorities, are intended to be used selectively to invite discussion, gather information, address the needs and concerns of the family, and build partnerships. Use of the questions may vary from visit to visit and from family to family. Questions can be modified to match the health care professional's communication style. The accompanying anticipatory guidance for the family should be geared to questions, issues, or concerns for that particular child and family. Tools and handouts to support anticipatory guidance can be found in the *Bright Futures Tool and Resource Kit.*

Priority

Communication and Social Development
Individuation, separation, finding support, attention to how child communicates wants and interests

Individuation

This is an age at which parents must encourage their toddler's autonomous behavior, curiosity, sense of emerging independence, and feeling of competence. At the same time, they must provide clear and consistent guidance about appropriate limits of safe and socially acceptable behavior.

Speak positively and honestly about the strengths of the family. Praise the child for being friendly and cooperative. Compliment parents for encouraging their child's autonomy while making sure he is safe and for helping the child through the visit. If siblings are present, compliment them on their strengths as well.

Assess the degree of parental stress in connection with the child's behavior.

Sample Questions
What are some of the new things that your child is doing? How does your child show that he has a will of his own? How do you react?

Anticipatory Guidance
- Whenever possible, allow your child to choose between 2 options, both of which are acceptable to you. For example, let him decide between a banana and peach slices for a snack, or between 2 of his favorite books. Allowing him to make choices in some areas will decrease power struggles in others.
- Allow your child to determine how much of the healthy foods you serve he will eat. Do not continue to feed him if he is not interested.

Separation

Both stranger anxiety and separation anxiety pose frustrating challenges for many parents. Taking the time to explain that they originate in new cognitive gains often helps parents to remain patient with their young toddler.

Sample Question

How does your child react to strangers?

Anticipatory Guidance

- Stranger anxiety and anxiety connected with separation from family members is still common at this age.
- Never make fun of his fear. Do not force him to confront people who scare him, such as Santa Claus or clowns, but gently support and encourage him to explore at his own pace. Accept his fear and speak reassuringly.
- Some children are slow to warm up. They show this by being cautious or withdrawn. Others are outgoing. They show this by being friendly and interactive, or even by being aggressive when they feel anxious or threatened (eg, hitting or biting).

Finding Support

During this time of intense demands by their toddler, parents frequently experience fatigue and frustration in the moment-to-moment effort of providing both support and safe limits. Seeking out opportunities to discuss child-raising issues with other parents can help alleviate stress and give parents new ideas for positive ways to handle difficult moments with their child.

Sample Question

How often do you get out of the house without your child, aside from going to work?

Anticipatory Guidance

- Take some time for yourself and spend some individual time with your partner. Seek support and understanding about being a parent from people you trust.
- If your child has special health care needs, it is even more important to find support from other families like yours. Take time to connect with other families who share your circumstances and can be part of your social and support networks.
- If you feel you are experiencing barriers to taking care of your child, the extensive early childhood service system can help. Ask our office for help with the right referrals.

Attention to How Child Communicates Wants and Interests

15-month-olds usually speak few words, but are able to understand many. Parents need to learn strategies to promote communication and language development. By naming everyday objects, the parent can help the child learn language and satisfy his curiosity about the world. Interactive reading (reading in which parent and child talk together about the text and pictures as well as the parent reading the book to the child) is another important way to stimulate language development. Parents may ask health care professionals about the effects of being raised in a bilingual home. They may be reassured that this situation permits the child to learn both languages simultaneously. Use of multiple languages should be encouraged.

Sample Questions

How does your child communicate what he wants? Who or what does he call by name? What gestures does he use to communicate effectively? For example, does he point to something he wants and then watch to see if you see what he's doing? Does he wave "bye-bye"? What languages do you speak at home? What languages does your child use to communicate his needs? What words does he use?

Anticipatory Guidance

- A child's understanding of how words can be used to share experiences and feelings will be increased by the conversations, songs, verbal games, and books you share with him. Books do not have to be read. You can use simple words to just talk about the pictures and story.
- Help your child learn the language of feelings by using words that describe feelings and emotions.
- Narrate your child's gestures. For example, if he points to a book, say, "You are pointing at a book. Do you want it?"
- Use simple, clear phrases to give your child instructions.
- Encourage your child to repeat words. Respond with pleasure to his attempts to imitate words. Listen to and answer your child's questions.

Priority

Sleep Routines and Issues
Regular bedtime routine, night waking, no bottle in bed

Regular Bedtime Routine, Night Waking, No Bottle in Bed

Reinforce the importance of maintaining naptime and nighttime sleep routines. For toddlers who are still experiencing some night waking or fussing, a review with parents of the toddler's bedtime ritual and sleep history is warranted. Prepare parents for the common reoccurrence of night waking at 18 to 20 months of age. This is normal and is in keeping with the child's new capacity for thinking and remembering both fears and desires. For more difficult and entrenched night waking, a more in-depth assessment and plan may be needed.

Sample Questions
How is your child sleeping? When does she go to sleep? What is your bedtime routine? How many hours a day and night does she sleep?

Anticipatory Guidance
- Continue to put your child to bed at the same time each night. Maintaining a consistent and soothing bedtime routine, in the room where your child will be sleeping, will help prepare her for bedtime.
- Tuck her in when she is drowsy, but still awake.
- Even though they have been sleeping well, some children this age may go through a short period of night waking. If she wakens, do not give her excess attention; a brief visit with reassurance from you is all that is needed for her to return to sleep. Give your child a stuffed animal, blanket, or favorite toy that she can use to help console herself at bedtime, should she wake. Consider using a night-light.
- Do not give her a bottle to sleep with, or bring her into bed with you as a means to get her back to sleep.
- Do not put a TV, computer, tablet, or other form of digital media in your child's bedroom.
- Using media at bedtime to help your child go to sleep actually leads to worse sleep. Instead, use a consistent bedtime routine with quiet songs or stories.

Priority

Temperament, Development, Behavior, and Discipline
Conflict predictors and distraction, discipline and behavior management

Conflict Predictors and Distraction

Some of the trigger points for tantrums and conflict between parent and toddler can be avoided through creative strategies. Encourage parents to check for easily correctable problems that may be based on their child's temperament, hunger, or sleepiness. Often, toddlers will have an identifiable trigger for a problematic behavior that is reinforced by a desired response that is elicited from the parent.

Review with parents whether some conflicts can be avoided by "toddler proofing" the home and by accepting the messiness that usually accompanies the eating and playing of a 15-month-old.

Sample Questions
Does your child have frequent tantrums? What seems to trigger them, and how do you typically respond to them? What kinds of things do you find yourself saying, "No," about? Do you have any questions about what should and should not be allowed for your child?

Anticipatory Guidance
- Modify your child's environment to avoid potential conflicts. For example, keep fragile or expensive items out of the child's play area.
- Distracting your toddler by offering him an alternative activity may prevent needless conflicts or tantrums. Use physical activity, like a game of chase, to distract him. When reading, let him choose the book. Let him control turning the pages.
- Be selective and consistent when using the word *no*. Whenever possible, offer an alternative activity that is more acceptable.
- Be willing to accept minor inconveniences, like messy eating.

Discipline and Behavior Management

Review the effect of temperamental differences on behavior. Discuss parental challenges and goals for discipline and behavior management.

To discipline is to teach. Experienced parents realize the most powerful tool of discipline is to pay attention to the behaviors that they want, and try very hard to avoid paying attention to behaviors that they do not want. Children are rewarded by their parents' attention and will seek even more approval by continuing the desired behavior.

Attention and approval are reinforcing. Withholding approval by ignoring undesired behaviors intends to avoid reinforcement and will ultimately cause the child's behavior to end.

Time-out is a highly organized technique to help parents avoid reinforcement of negative behaviors. Separating the child and parent prevents inadvertently reinforcing negative behaviors. Time-out is not punishment; it is a time to cool down. Sitting with (or holding) an out-of-control child until everybody calms down can be at least as effective as having the child sit in a chair and walking away. Describing feelings—of both parent and child—can help each understand the other.

Sample Questions

What do you do when you become angry or frustrated with your child? How are you and your partner managing your child's behavior? Who else is helping you raise your child? How often do you talk with each other about your child-rearing ideas? How are your approaches similar and how are they different? What do you do when you disagree? How do you stay calm and centered when your child's behavior is challenging? What works well when that happens?

Anticipatory Guidance

- Develop strategies with your partner to consistently manage the power struggles that result from your toddler's need to control his environment.
- Pay attention to your child's behaviors that you like and try to ignore the behaviors you do not like. Avoid using a raised voice or giving a lecture. If you do, you are giving too much attention to the negative behavior.
- Set limits for your toddler by using distraction, gentle restraint, and, when necessary, a brief time-out. Other strategies for managing your toddler's behavior include separating him from the cause of the problem, staying close to him, and sticking to structure and routines.
- Discipline is important for your child. To appropriately discipline is to teach.
- Time-out is an effective technique to avoid paying negative attention. The goal is to not communicate with your child during a time-out to allow time to calm down. Time-outs at this age should be brief— 60 to 90 seconds. An effective time-out technique has 3 components.
  - Use a calm voice, not a raised one.
  - Use as few words as is possible, such as, "Children who hit must do a time-out."
  - End the time-out by looking to the future, such as, "Let's have a hug and go play." Do not recall the negative behavior by saying, "Don't do it again," or by asking for an apology—both are code for "I will pay attention to you again if you do the same negative behavior."
- Teach your toddler not to hit, bite, or use other aggressive behaviors. Model this behavior yourself by not spanking your toddler and by handling conflict with your partner constructively and nonviolently. Spanking increases the chance of physical injury, and your child is unlikely to understand the connection between the behavior and the punishment.
- Make certain that child care personnel use the same consistent discipline measures. Communicate with these caregivers often.

Priority

Healthy Teeth

Brushing teeth, reducing caries

Brushing Teeth

Many children exhibit their independence by demanding to brush their own teeth, but infants and children younger than 4 years may not have the manual dexterity to do so. When a child can tie her shoes, then she has the manual dexterity to brush her own teeth.

Sample Questions

Has your toddler been to the dentist? Who brushes your child's teeth?

Anticipatory Guidance

- Schedule your toddler's first dental visit if it has not already occurred.
- Children this age have not yet developed the hand coordination to brush their own teeth adequately. Brush your child's teeth twice each day (after breakfast and before bed) with a soft toothbrush and a small smear of fluoridated toothpaste, no more than a grain of rice. Allow your child to try brushing on occasion to avoid major conflict over dental hygiene.

Reducing Caries

Early childhood caries is rampant in many populations. Bacterial transmission from parent to child is a primary mechanism for introducing caries-promoting bacteria into children's mouths. Counsel parents on ways to reduce bacterial transmission to their child.

Prolonged exposure to cow's or human milk or fruit juice (even 100%) causes harm to teeth because bacteria in the mouth convert the sugars in milk or juice to acids. The acids attack the enamel and lead to dental caries. The same is true for exposure to foods and beverages containing high amounts of added sugars.

Sample Questions

Does your child take a bottle to bed? If so, what is in the bottle? How many bottles of formula or fruit juice does your child get every day? How much water does your child drink? Did you know that you can do things to prevent your child from developing tooth decay?

Anticipatory Guidance

- Many toddlers develop tooth decay (also called early childhood caries) because bacteria that cause tooth decay can be passed on to your toddler through your saliva when you kiss her or share a cup or spoon. To protect your baby's teeth and prevent decay, make sure you brush and floss your own teeth, don't share utensils, do not chew food and then give to the child, and don't clean her pacifier in your mouth.
- If you are having difficulty weaning your child from the nighttime bottle, do not use formula, milk, or juice in the nighttime bottle. Put only water in the bottle.

EARLY CHILDHOOD
15 MONTH VISIT

Priority

Safety
Car safety seats and parental use of seat belts, safe home environment: poisoning, falls, and fire safety

Car Safety Seats and Parental Use of Seat Belts

Talk with parents to ensure that their child is fastened securely in a car safety seat and that they know to keep their child riding in the rear-facing position as long as possible, at least to age 2 years or when the child reaches the weight or height limit for the rear-facing position in the convertible seat. Reinforce the importance of parents always using a seat belt.

Sample Questions
Is your child fastened securely in a rear-facing car safety seat in the back seat of the car every time he rides in a vehicle? Are you having any problems using your car safety seat? Do you always use your own seat belt?

Anticipatory Guidance
- Never place your child's rear-facing safety seat in the front seat of a vehicle with a passenger air bag. The back seat is the safest place for children to ride until your child is 13 years of age.
- The rear-facing position provides the best protection for your child's neck, spine, and head in the event of a crash. For optimal protection, your child should remain in the rear-facing position until he is 2 years of age or reaches the highest weight or height allowed for rear-facing use by the manufacturer of the convertible car safety seat.
- It is safe for your rear-facing child's feet to touch the vehicle seat in front of him and for his legs to bend or hang over the sides of the seat. Even large toddlers are usually quite comfortable riding in the rear-facing position and are not at risk of foot or leg injuries.
- Be sure your child's car safety seat is properly installed in the back seat according to the manufacturer's instructions and the car owner's manual. There should be no more than a finger's width of space between your child's collarbone and the harness strap.
- Remember that your child's safety depends upon you. Always use your seat belt, too.

For information about car safety seats and actions to keep your child safe in and around cars, visit www.safercar.gov/parents.

Find a Child Passenger Safety Technician: http://cert.safekids.org. Click on "Find a Tech."

Toll-free Auto Safety Hotline: 888-327-4236

Safe Home Environment: Poisoning, Falls, and Fire Safety

Review home safety issues with parents, including poisons, fire, burns, and falling objects. Unintentional injuries are the leading cause of death among young children. Parents must use constant vigilance and regularly review the safety of the home to protect their children from harm.

Sample Questions

When did you last examine your home to be sure that it is safe? Would you like a list of home safety issues to review? What emergency numbers do you have posted near your phone and on your cell phone?

Anticipatory Guidance

- Remove poisons and toxic household products from your home or keep them high and out of sight and reach in locked cabinets. Use safety caps on all medications and lock them away.
- Keep emergency phone numbers near every telephone and in your cell phone for rapid dial. The number for the **Poison Help line** is **800-222-1222.** Call immediately if you have a poisoning emergency. Do not make your child vomit.
- Use gates at the top and bottom of stairs. To prevent children from falling out of windows, keep furniture away from windows and install operable window guards on second- and higher-story windows.
- Make sure that any other caregivers, such as relatives or child care providers, follow these same safety guidelines.

Sample Questions

How do you keep hot liquids out of your toddler's reach? Is your microwave within reach on a counter? Do you have smoke detectors on each floor in the home where your child lives? When did you last change the batteries in the smoke detectors? Do you have a plan for getting everyone out of the house and a meeting place once outside? Do you have a neighbor from whose house you can call the fire department?

Anticipatory Guidance

- Do not leave heavy objects or containers of hot liquids on tables with tablecloths that your child might pull down.
- If your microwave is on a countertop where your toddler might reach it, always stay in the room while it is in use to make sure your child does not open it and remove the hot food or liquid. If you must leave the room while the microwave is on, take your toddler with you.
- Turn pan handles toward the back of the stove. Keep your child away from hot stoves, fireplaces, irons, curling irons, and space heaters.
- Keep small appliances out of reach and keep electrical cords and window covering cords out of your child's reach. It is best to use cordless window coverings.
- Make sure you have a working smoke detector on every level of your home, especially in the furnace and sleeping areas. Test smoke detectors every month. It is best to use smoke detectors that use long-life batteries, but, if you do not, change the batteries at least once a year.
- Develop an escape plan in the event of a fire in your home.
- Keep cigarettes, lighters, matches, and alcohol out of your child's sight and reach.

Early Childhood
18 Month Visit

Context

The 18-month-old requires gentle transitions, patience, consistent limits, and respect. One minute he insists on independence; the next minute he is clinging fearfully to his parent. Much of the energy and drive that were channeled into physical activity are now directed toward more complex tasks and social interaction. Having learned the concept of choice, the toddler becomes assertive about his own wishes. His understanding of language develops rapidly, bringing with it new ways of labeling and remembering his experiences, and a new avenue for understanding the expectations of his parents and for communicating his wants and needs.

Though his communicative and social skills are developing rapidly, an 18-month-old usually still has a quite limited verbal and behavioral repertoire for expressing himself. Thus, the all-purpose exclamation "No!" signals his desire for choice and autonomy, and the seeming defiance and negativism of an 18-month-old are actually assertions of an emerging sense of his own identity. Through this period, he needs to have strong emotional ties to his parents. To venture into the world and test his newfound assertiveness, he must know that he has a safe, emotionally secure place at home. Parents appreciate knowing that the sometimes assertive, sometimes clingy, and sometimes irritable behaviors of their formerly happy and fearless explorer are common in this transitional phase.

The behavior of an 18-month-old may be frustrating at times. Extra patience and a sense of humor can help parents with the tough task of setting limits and then reinforcing them consistently. At the same time, his delight in his own emerging competence and achievements bring a sense of joy and accomplishment to all around him. The 18-month-old lights up a room as he applauds himself and looks around for parental acclaim and reinforcement.

Children typically remain highly resistant to the physical examination at this age. Examining a doll or stuffed animal before examining the child often has a calming effect. To keep the child as comfortable as possible, perform the less-invasive procedures first. Observe, then palpate, the child. Give the child the opportunity to hold the stethoscope or otoscope before it is used. Give the child as many choices as possible about where and how the examination will be conducted (On the parent's lap or on the examination table? Which eye should be examined first?).

Priorities for the 18 Month Visit

The first priority is to attend to the concerns of the parents.

In addition, the Bright Futures Early Childhood Expert Panel has given priority to the following topics for discussion in this visit:

▶ Temperament, development, toilet training, behavior, and discipline (anticipation of return to separation anxiety and managing behavior with consistent limits, recognizing signs of toilet training readiness and parental expectations, new sibling planned or on the way)

▶ Communication and social development (encouragement of language, use of simple words and phrases, engagement in reading, playing, talking, and singing)

▶ Television viewing and digital media (promotion of reading, physical activity and safe play)

▶ Healthy nutrition (nutritious foods; water, milk, and juice; expressing independence through food likes and dislikes)

▶ Safety (car safety seats and parental use of seat belts, poisoning, sun protection, firearm safety, safe home environment: burns, fires, and falls)

Health Supervision

The *Bright Futures Tool and Resource Kit* contains Previsit Questionnaires to assist the health care professional in taking a history, conducting developmental surveillance, and performing medical screening.

History

Interval history may be obtained according to the concerns of the family and health care professional's preference or style of practice. The following questions can encourage in-depth discussion:

General Questions

- What are you most proud of since our last visit? (If the parent responds, "Nothing," the clinician should be prepared with a compliment, such as, "You made time for this visit despite your busy schedule.")
- What's exciting about this stage of development? What do you like most about this age?
- How are things going in your family?
- Let's talk about some of the things you most enjoy about your child.
- What questions or concerns do you have about your child?

Past Medical History

- Has your child received any specialty or emergency care since the last visit?

Family History

- Has your child or anyone in the family (parents, brothers, sisters, grandparents, aunts, uncles, or cousins) developed a new health condition or died? **If the answer is Yes:** Ascertain who in the family has or had the condition, and ask about the age of onset and diagnosis. If the person is no longer living, ask about the age at the time of death.

Social History

- What major changes have occurred in your family since your last visit? Tell me about any stressful events. What is the effect of these changes on your family?
- What are some of the things you find most difficult about your child?

Surveillance of Development

Do you or any of your child's caregivers have any specific concerns about your child's development, learning, or behavior?

Clinicians using the *Bright Futures Tool and Resource Kit* Previsit Questionnaires or another tool that includes a developmental milestones checklist, or those who use a structured developmental screening tool, need not ask about these developmental surveillance milestones. *(For more information, see the Promoting Healthy Development theme.)*

Social Language and Self-help

Does your child

- Engage with others for play?
- Help dress and undress self?
- Point to pictures in book?
- Point to object of interest to draw your attention to it?
- Turn and look at adult if something new happens?
- Begin to scoop with spoon?
- Use words to ask for help?

Verbal Language (Expressive and Receptive)

Does she

- Identify at least 2 body parts?
- Name at least 5 familiar objects, such as ball or milk?

Gross Motor

Does he

- Walk up with 2 feet per step with hand held?
- Sit in small chair?
- Carry toy while walking?

Fine Motor

Does she

- Scribble spontaneously?
- Throw small ball a few feet while standing?

Review of Systems

The Bright Futures Early Childhood Expert Panel recommends a complete review of systems as a part of every health supervision visit. This review can be done through questions about the following:

Do you have concern about your child's

- Head
  - Shape
- Eyes
  - Cross-eyed
- Ears, nose, and throat
- Breathing
- Stomach or abdomen
  - Vomiting or spitting
  - Bowel movements
- Genitals or rectum
- Skin
- Development
  - Muscle strength, movement of arms or legs, any developmental concerns

Observation of Parent-Child Interaction

During the visit, the health care professional acknowledges and reinforces positive parent-child interactions and discusses any concerns. Observation focuses on

- How do the parent and child communicate?
- What are your child care needs?
- If handed a book, does the child show the parent pictures (shared attention)?
- Does the parent speak clearly and in a conversational tone when addressing the child?
- What is the tone of the parent-child interactions and the feeling conveyed? Does the parent notice and acknowledge the child's positive behaviors?
- How does the parent guide the child to learn safe limits?
- Does the parent seem positive when speaking about the child?

Physical Examination

A complete physical examination is included as part of every health supervision visit.

When performing a physical examination, the health care professional's attention is directed to the following components of the examination that are important for a child this age:

- **Measure and plot on appropriate WHO Growth Chart**
  - Recumbent length
  - Weight
  - Head circumference
  - Weight-for-length

- **Neurologic**
  - Observe gait (walking and running), hand control, and arm and spine movement. Note communication efforts.
  - Note behavior (adult-child interaction, eye contact, use of gestures)

- **Eyes**
  - Assess ocular motility.
  - Examine pupils for opacification and red reflexes.
  - Assess visual acuity using fixate and follow response.

- **Mouth**
  - Note number of teeth and observe for caries, plaque, demineralization (white spots), staining, and injury.

- **Abdomen**
  - Palpate for masses.

- **Skin**
  - Observe for nevi, café-au-lait spots, birthmarks, or bruising.

Screening

Universal Screening	Action
Autism	Autism spectrum disorder screen
Development	Developmental screen
Oral Health (in the absence of a dental home)	Apply fluoride varnish after first tooth eruption and every 6 months.

Selective Screening	Risk Assessment[a]	Action if Risk Assessment Positive (+)
Anemia	+ on risk screening questions	Hematocrit or hemoglobin
Blood Pressure	Children with specific risk conditions or change in risk	Blood pressure measurement
Hearing	+ on risk screening questions	Referral for diagnostic audiologic assessment
Lead	If no previous screen or change in risk	Lead blood test
Oral Health	Does not have a dental home	Referral to dental home or, if not available, oral health risk assessment
	Primary water source is deficient in fluoride.	Oral fluoride supplementation
Vision	+ on risk screening questions	Ophthalmology referral

[a] See the *Evidence and Rationale chapter* for the criteria on which risk screening questions are based.

Immunizations

Consult the CDC/ACIP or AAP Web sites for the current immunization schedule.

CDC National Immunization Program: **www.cdc.gov/vaccines**

AAP *Red Book:* **http://redbook.solutions.aap.org**

Anticipatory Guidance

The following sample questions, which address the Bright Futures Early Childhood Expert Panel's Anticipatory Guidance Priorities, are intended to be used selectively to invite discussion, gather information, address the needs and concerns of the family, and build partnerships. Use of the questions may vary from visit to visit and from family to family. Questions can be modified to match the health care professional's communication style. The accompanying anticipatory guidance for the family should be geared to questions, issues, or concerns for that particular child and family. Tools and handouts to support anticipatory guidance can be found in the *Bright Futures Tool and Resource Kit*.

Priority

Temperament, Development, Toilet Training, Behavior, and Discipline

Anticipation of return to separation anxiety and managing behavior with consistent limits, recognizing signs of toilet training readiness and parental expectations, new sibling planned or on the way

Anticipation of Return to Separation Anxiety and Managing Behavior With Consistent Limits

Adaptation to nonparental care may bring a return of separation anxiety. Stranger anxiety may surface.

Assertiveness in exploring the environment and persistence in pursuit of desires are normal developmental features of this age. Balancing support for a child's growing physical and cognitive independence while establishing and maintaining consistent limits is difficult for parents. Taking the time to explain that these changes originate in new cognitive gains often helps parents remain patient with their young toddler.

It is important that family members agree on how best to support the child's emerging independence while maintaining consistent limits. Many communities offer a variety of options to help parents manage their child's behavior during this challenging period. It is important that parents learn about options that are culturally appropriate and affordable.

Sample Questions

What are some of the new things that your child is doing? Who helps you raise your child?

Tell me how you set limits for your child and discipline him. Describe how you and your partner (and other caregivers) work out ways to be consistent in setting limits for him. What have been the most challenging aspects of managing his behavior?

Anticipatory Guidance

- Remember, at this age and for the next 3 to 4 months, your child may be anxious in new situations. Children often cling to parents again as a way to reassure themselves of their secure emotional base.
- Spend time playing with your toddler each day. Focus on activities that he expresses interest in and enjoys. Plan ahead for those situations that have been difficult in the past. Try new approaches, such as doing shopping trips earlier in the day rather than at the end, when everyone is tired.
- Reinforce appropriate actions by praising your toddler for good behavior and accomplishments.
- Learn about and consider participating in parent-toddler playgroups.
- Decide what limits are important to you and your toddler, and try to be realistic and consistent in expectations and discipline.
- Be specific when setting limits and, whenever possible, make agreements with other adult caregivers about limits for your child.
- When your child is engaging in unwanted behavior, use positive directives to tell him what you want him to do instead. Be as consistent as possible when enforcing limits. Remember that the goal is teaching, not punishing.
- Keep time-outs and other disciplinary measures brief, just 1 to 2 minutes, and use them only for troublesome behaviors. Give a warning, then immediately withdraw attention. Do not argue with your child.
- When your child is upset, help him change his focus to another activity, book, or toy. This strategy of distraction and substitution can often calm him.
- Consider attending parent education classes or parent support groups. Many libraries and bookstores also have books and pamphlets about parenting. Your community may even have a parenting advice telephone hotline that can help you.

Recognizing Signs of Toilet Training Readiness and Parental Expectations

Toilet training is part of developmentally appropriate learning. Many parents need guidance about when to begin toilet training. The average age for a child to be toilet trained during the day is approximately 2½ years.

Sample Questions

Have you thought about toilet training? What are your plans for it? Is anyone urging you to toilet train your child?

Anticipatory Guidance

- Wait to start toilet training until your toddler is dry for periods of about 2 hours, knows the difference between wet and dry, can pull his pants up and down, wants to learn, and can indicate when he is about to have a bowel movement.
- It is helpful to read books with your child about using the potty or toilet; to take him into the bathroom with the appropriate-sex parent, if one is in the family, or older sibling to learn the routine; and to praise attempts to sit on the potty or toilet, initially with his clothes on. Many children enjoy a special trip to select "big kid" underwear when they feel ready to stop using diapers during the day.

New Sibling Planned or On the Way

Inquire about any recent or forthcoming changes in the family.

Sample Questions

Are you thinking about having another child? If you are expecting a new baby, how is your health? Are you avoiding alcohol and tobacco? Where are you seeking prenatal care? Do you know what substances should be avoided? Are you taking prenatal vitamins?

Anticipatory Guidance

- If you're expecting a new baby, it's important to prepare your child by reading stories about a family with a new baby, big brothers, or sisters. Enroll your child in a big brother or big sister class at a local hospital to help her know where you will be when the baby is born. Tell her who will care for her while you are having the new baby. Continue to give her lots of love and attention.

- Try not to make any changes or new developmental demands on your toddler close to the time of the new baby's birth. Be prepared for your child to regress in new skills, such as using a cup.

- If you're expecting a new baby, it is important that you continue to concentrate on your health and health habits throughout the pregnancy because you are modeling those behaviors for your toddler.

Priority

Communication and Social Development

Encouragement of language, use of simple words and phrases, engagement in reading, playing, talking, and singing

Encouragement of Language, Use of Simple Words and Phrases, Engagement in Reading, Playing, Talking, and Singing

The development of language and communication during the early childhood years is of central importance to the child's later growth in social, cognitive, and academic domains. Communication is built on interaction and relationships. Health care professionals have the opportunity to educate parents about the importance of language stimulation, including singing songs, reading, and talking to their child. Parent-child play, in which the child takes the lead and the parent is attentive and responsive, elaborating but not controlling, is an excellent technique for enhancing both the parent-child relationship and the child's language development. Because young children are active learners, they find joy in exploring and learning new words.

Parents may ask health care professionals about the effects of being raised in a bilingual home. They may be reassured that this situation permits the child to learn both languages simultaneously. Parents should be encouraged to speak, play, talk, and sing in whatever language they feel most comfortable. What is most important is that the child be exposed to rich, diverse language in any language.

Provide anticipatory guidance about reading aloud at every visit. Look for opportunities to provide children's books at each visit, if they can be made available. The AAP supports the use of Reach Out and Read and other programs for literacy promotion.

Sample Questions

How does your child communicate what she wants? Who or what does she call by name? What gestures does she use to communicate effectively? For example, does she point to something she wants and then watch to see if you see what she's doing? Does she wave "bye-bye"?

Anticipatory Guidance

- Encourage your toddler's language development by reading and singing to her, and by talking about what you both are seeing and doing together. Books do not have to be read. Talk about the pictures or use simple words to describe what is happening in the book. Do not be surprised if she wants to hear the same book over and over. Words that describe feelings and emotions will help your child learn the language of feelings.
- Although play in which your child takes the lead is a wonderful activity, you also will often need to play an active role with your 18-month-old. You may want to make up a story with figures or characters that can be based on an activity you have done together or a book you have read together.
- Ask your child simple questions, affirm her answers, and follow up with simple explanations.
- Use simple, clear phrases to give your child instructions.

Priority

Television Viewing and Digital Media
Promotion of reading, physical activity and safe play

Promotion of Reading, Physical Activity and Safe Play

The AAP recommends that infants and children younger than 18 months not watch TV or use digital media. Having the conversation with parents at this point allows parents to determine how to plan for later media use.

If the parents choose to introduce media at this age, they should ensure that the programs are appropriate and of high quality. Video chat technology can facilitate social connections with relatives. New evidence shows that with parental support, infants and toddlers can engage in joint attention during video chatting.

Families with older children may find it challenging to limit media exposures for their younger child. Explore the reasons behind TV and media use, such as to control behavior, to get the child to sleep, to occupy the child so parents can get things done, or as learning tools. Offer alternatives such as reading, singing, and physical or outdoor activities.

Sample Questions
Does your child watch TV or videos or use other digital media? Does your family video chat with relatives? If yes, how much time each day does your child spend watching TV or playing on a computer, tablet, smartphone, or other digital device? Do you use TV or other screens as a way to calm your child, help him to get to sleep, or keep him occupied if you have something else you must do?

Anticipatory Guidance
- Starting healthy media habits now is important, because bad habits are hard to change when children are older.
- If you choose to introduce digital media at this age, choose high-quality programming or apps, use them together, and limit viewing to less than 1 hour per day. With your help, your child is now old enough to participate in family video chats.
- Parents and caregivers need to be aware of their own media use. Television intended for adults may not be appropriate for a young child in the room.
- Make special time for tech-free play every day to foster development of language, thinking skills, behavior regulation, and attention.
- Research shows that young children this age cannot learn information from screens, even though many toys and videos claim to teach them skills. Children this age learn by interacting with caregivers; being read to, talked to, and sung to; and exploring their environment.

- Do not feel pressure to introduce technology. Interfaces are so intuitive that children quickly figure them out when needed at home or in school. Do not put a TV in your child's bedroom.
- Using TV to calm fussy toddlers doesn't help them learn ways to calm themselves and can lead them to demand media. Use other methods to calm your child, such as distraction, removing them from the trigger, going outside, addressing possible causes of fussiness (such as hunger or tiredness), or reading together.
- Make mealtimes an opportunity for face-to-face learning interactions. Don't have the TV on during meals, which distracts toddlers from eating and interacting with family.

Priority

Healthy Nutrition

Nutritious foods; water, milk, and juice; expressing independence through food likes and dislikes

Nutritious Foods

Meals should be relaxed, safe, and enjoyable family times. Remind parents that they are responsible for providing a variety of nutritious foods and that their child is responsible for how much to eat. Parents can establish positive eating patterns for their child by providing healthy foods at regular intervals throughout the day, giving appropriate amounts, and emphasizing vegetables and fruit and other nutritious foods.

A reduced appetite appropriately accompanies the slower rate of growth of early childhood in contrast with infancy. Parents are often distressed when children eat less than they expected, but food refusal often means their child is not hungry. Parents may fail to realize that by encouraging a child to eat when he is not hungry gives him calories he did not ask for and likely doesn't need. Also, preparing substitute foods only encourages picky eating. Discuss the importance of providing healthy snacks and of minimizing foods and beverages that are high in added sugars and saturated fat and low in nutrients.

Sample Questions

Tell me about mealtime in your home. Tell me about mealtime in your child care setting.

Do you consider your child a healthy eater? Do you provide a variety of vegetables, fruits, and other nutritious foods? What kind of snacks do you serve? Does your child have much food that you would describe as junk food?

How do you feel if your child doesn't eat what you have prepared for him? What do you do?

Anticipatory Guidance

- Offer a variety of healthy foods to your child, especially vegetables and fruits, and include higher protein foods like meat and deboned fish at least 2 times per week.
- Help your child explore new flavors and textures in his food.
- Remember that children this age seldom eat "3 square meals a day," but more likely 1 good meal and multiple smaller meals and snacks.
- When your child refuses something you've prepared, it usually means he is not hungry. It doesn't mean he doesn't like it and wouldn't have it later for a snack.
- Trust your child to determine when he is hungry or full and never encourage him to eat food he did not ask for.
- Your kitchen is not a fast-food restaurant and you don't need to fix another meal if your child refuses what you have already prepared. This only encourages him to be a picky eater.

- Have healthy snacks on hand, such as
  - Fresh fruit or vegetables, such as apples, oranges, bananas, cucumber, zucchini, or radishes, that are cut in small pieces or thin strips
  - Applesauce, cheese, or small pieces of whole-grain bread or crackers
  - Unflavored yogurt, sweetened with bits of mashed fruit

Water, Milk, and Juice

Fluid intake is an important element of nutrition. Water should be provided ad lib at all times and should be regularly offered to children of all ages, with increased attention to water intake in warm or dry environments.

Families may fail to recognize the importance and effect of other fluids to their child's nutrition and it may be useful to remind parents that what we drink contributes protein, fat, and sugar to our daily intake. Milk is an important fluid and protein source and the most accessible source of calcium and vitamin D for children. The fat provided in milk is believed to be of importance until age 2 years, so the introduction of low-fat and fat-free milk should be delayed until the second birthday. Breastfeeding should continue to be supported as long as mutually desired by mother and child. The child will continue to receive benefits, including host defense, through at least 24 months of age. Discuss possible pressure to wean by family or friends. If weaning is desired, discuss appropriate weaning techniques.

Juices demand special attention. The sugar content of all juices demands that juice intake be limited, to reduce the risk of dental caries and limit the intake of sugar calories. Soda or soft drinks, sports drinks, and punches provide many calories of scant nutrient value and should be avoided.

Sample Questions
Does your child drink water every day? How many ounces of milk does your child drink most days? Is it whole milk or lower fat milk? Do you give your child other dairy products like yogurt and cheese every day?

Anticipatory Guidance
- Be sure you always have cool water available to your child, especially on warm days and when your child is physically active.
- Young children should drink 16 to 24 oz of milk each day to help meet their calcium and vitamin D needs. Milk is also an important source of protein for growth.
- Juice is not a necessary drink. If you choose to give juice, limit it to 4 oz daily and always serve it with a meal.
- To protect your child's teeth, don't dilute juice with water and don't allow your child to carry around a bottle, sippy cup, or juice box for drinking over a long period of time.

Expressing Independence Through Food Likes and Dislikes

Food is an area in which toddlers frequently express their newly independent views, especially their likes and dislikes. This is NORMAL.

Sample Question

What does your child do when you offer new foods? Tell me about any concerns you might have about having enough nutritious food for your family.

Anticipatory Guidance

- Your toddler may become more aware and suspicious of new or strange foods, but do not limit the menu to foods she likes. Continue to offer new foods and allow the child to explore at her own pace. Do not force her to eat the food.

- You may have to offer your toddler a new food many times before she accepts it. It often takes repeated exposure to foods before a toddler will enjoy it. Do not give up after a few tries. Parents should not be short-order cooks.

- Let your toddler experiment with a variety of foods from each food group by touching and mouthing them. She can feed herself.

- Allow your child to determine how much of the healthy foods you serve she will eat. Do not continue to feed her if she is not interested.

- A toddler may eat 6 small meals every day or 3 meals with nutritious snacks in between.

Priority

Safety

Car safety seats and parental use of seat belts, poisoning, sun protection, firearm safety, safe home environment: burns, fires, and falls

Car Safety Seats and Parental Use of Seat Belts

Talk with parents to ensure that they know how to securely fasten their child in a car safety seat. Encourage them to keep their child riding in the rear-facing position as long as possible, at least to age 2 years or when the child reaches the weight or height limit for the rear-facing position in the convertible seat. Reinforce the importance of parents always using their seat belt, too.

Sample Questions

How is the car safety seat working? Is your child fastened securely in a rear-facing car safety seat in the back seat every time she rides in a vehicle? Does everyone use a seat belt, booster seat, or car safety seat?

Anticipatory Guidance

- Never place your child's rear-facing safety seat in the front seat of a vehicle with a passenger air bag. The back seat is the safest place for children to ride until your child is age 13 years.
- The rear-facing position provides the best protection for your child's neck, spine, and head in the event of a crash. For optimal protection, your child should remain in the rear-facing position until she is 2 years of age or reaches the highest weight or height allowed for rear-facing use by the manufacturer of the convertible car safety seat.
- It is safe for your rear-facing child's feet to touch the vehicle seat in front of her and for her legs to bend or hang over the sides of the seat. Even large toddlers are usually quite comfortable riding in the rear-facing position and are not at risk of foot or leg injuries.
- Be sure your child's car safety seat is properly installed in the back seat according to the manufacturer's instructions and the car owner's manual. The harness straps should be snug enough that you cannot pinch any webbing between your fingers.
- Do not start your vehicle until everyone is buckled up. Children watch what parents do, so it is important to model safe behaviors for your child.

For information about car safety seats and actions to keep your child safe in and around cars, visit www.safercar.gov/parents.

Find a Child Passenger Safety Technician: http://cert.safekids.org. Click on "Find a Tech."

Toll-free Auto Safety Hotline: 888-327-4236

Poisoning

Confirm with parents that they have important telephone numbers (eg, the national Poison Help line) available in many places in their home and programmed in their cell phones.

Sample Questions

How recently have you examined your home to be sure that it is safe? Do you know the telephone number of the national Poison Help line?

Anticipatory Guidance

- Remove poisons and toxic household products from the home or keep them in locked cabinets. Use safety caps on all medications and lock them away as well. Never refer to medicine as candy. Because children like to mimic what you do, do not take your medicine in front of your child. Check and follow the dosing instructions every time you give your child any medicine.
- Keep emergency phone numbers near every telephone and in your cell phone for rapid dial. The number for the national **Poison Help line** is **800-222-1222.** Call immediately if there is a poisoning emergency. Do not make your child vomit.

Sun Protection

Sun protection now is of increasing importance because of climate change and the thinning of the atmospheric ozone layer. Sun protection is accomplished through limiting sun exposure, using sunscreen, and wearing protective clothing.

Sample Questions

Do you apply sunscreen whenever your child plays outside? Does your child care provider have a sun protection policy? Do you and your child care provider limit outside time during the middle of the day, when the sun is strongest?

Anticipatory Guidance

- Always apply sunscreen with an SPF greater than 15 when your child is outside. Reapply every 2 hours.
- Have your child wear a hat.
- Avoid prolonged time in the sun between 11:00 am and 3:00 pm.
- Wear sun protection clothing for summer.

Firearm Safety

Firearms should be removed from places in which children live and play. If a family does have firearms, they should be stored unloaded and locked in a case, with ammunition stored in a separate locked location. Many young children are killed by firearms each year and most are injured by themselves, a sibling, or a friend.

Sample Questions

Does anyone in your home have a firearm? Does a neighbor, family friend, or any home where your child might play have a firearm? If so, is the firearm unloaded and locked up? Where is the ammunition stored? Have you thought about not owning a firearm because of the danger to children and other family members, since having a firearm in the home increases the risk of firearm injury or death?

Anticipatory Guidance

- The best way to keep your child safe from injury or death from firearms is to never have a firearm in the home.
- If it is necessary to keep a firearm in your home, it should be stored unloaded and locked in a case, with the ammunition locked separately from the firearm.
- Children cannot reliably be taught not to handle a firearm if they find one. Adults must make sure the firearm is completely out of sight and reach of the child.

Safe Home Environment: Burns, Fires, and Falls

The active, climbing toddler challenges parents to provide a safe environment. Highlighting new safety hazards helps parents meet this important responsibility.

Sample Questions

How do you keep hot liquids out of your toddler's reach? Do you have smoke detectors on each floor in the home where your child lives? When did you last change the batteries in the smoke detectors? Do you have a plan for getting everyone out of the house and a meeting place once outside? Do you have a neighbor from whose house you can call the fire department?

Does your child like to climb? What floor in your house or apartment do you live on? Do you have window guards on all windows on the second floor and higher?

Anticipatory Guidance

- Turn pan handles toward the back of the stove. Keep your child away from hot stoves, fireplaces, irons, curling irons, and space heaters.
- Keep small appliances out of reach and keep electrical cords and window covering cords out of your child's reach.
- Make sure you have a working smoke detector on every level of your home, especially in the furnace and sleeping areas. Test smoke detectors every month. It is best to use smoke detectors that use long-life batteries, but, if you do not, change the batteries at least once a year.
- Develop an escape plan in the event of a fire in your home.
- Keep cigarettes, lighters, matches, and alcohol out of your child's sight and reach.
- Do not leave heavy objects or containers of hot liquids on tables with tablecloths that your child might pull down.
- Remember that many toddlers are excellent climbers. Make sure to use gates at the top and bottom of stairs. To prevent children from falling out of windows, keep furniture away from windows and install operable window guards on second- and higher-story windows.

- Secure furniture so that it cannot tip and fall onto your child. Televisions, bookcases, and dressers should be secured to the wall with straps and tall floor lamps should be placed behind furniture where they cannot be pulled down.
- Watch over your toddler closely when she is on stairs.
- When you or other adults are backing the car out of the garage or driving the car forward or backward in the driveway, be certain another adult is holding your child a safe distance away so that she is not run over. All vehicles have blind spots, and the driver may not be able to see her.

Early Childhood
2 Year Visit

Context

The 2-year-old is often spirited, delightful, joyful, carefree, and challenging! She continuously explores her world with glee and frustration. Her emotions can take on the quality of a roller coaster ride, from sheer excitement and happiness to fear, anger, and tantrums. Although families may be frustrated when their 2-year-old cannot communicate her needs successfully, helping the child master the use of language is critical. This is a pivotal time for her social and emotional development and holds many rewards for both the family and the child. The 2-year-old's evolution into early childhood emerges on a day-to-day basis and she needs support and, most of all, patience.

Toddlers at this age are eager to learn, and new discoveries are facilitated by their blossoming skills that prompt many why, what, and how questions. The 2-year-old seems determined to assert her independence, but, when presented with a choice (eg, between apple slices and orange slices), she usually ceases this activity and has a difficult time choosing. After finally making a decision, she often wants to change it.

The 2-year-old enjoys feeding herself, reading a book, and imitating her parents doing household chores. Watching her go through her daily routine is amusing. To fully understand new activities, she tries them repeatedly. What happens when water gets splashed outside the tub? How far will the teddy bear fall down the stairs? What does mud feel like? Sometimes parents find it difficult to realize that curiosity, rather than a rejection of their standards, compels their child's repetitious explorations.

Despite her apparent yearning for independence, the 2-year-old frequently hides behind her parent's legs when approached by other adults. She may develop fears at this age. For the first time, loud sounds, animals, large moving things, and other objects and events that are unpredictable and out of the child's control can appear to be threatening. Fear of the dark may develop as the child struggles with the transition between waking consciousness and sleep. Unexplained events may resonate fearfully with the child's developing imagination (eg, she may develop a fear of going down the drain along with the bathwater, or a fear of thunder and lightning). A transitional object (eg, a blanket or special stuffed animal) helps the child through anxious times, including the transition into sleep. With steady parental support and reassurance, the child gains confidence and gradually overcomes such fears.

The 2-year-old is not yet skilled at interacting with other children and is fiercely attached to her caregivers. Rather than sharing, 2-year-olds engage in parallel play alongside their peers as they learn to be sociable. It is important that adults not expect the child to sit in a circle with other children or listen to a long story. These abilities will develop by the age of 3 years.

At this age, many of the child's actions are still governed by her parents' reactions. She has learned what to do to get her parents to respond, either negatively or positively, and may play one against the other. She will throw tantrums to get her way. Similarly, if her parents overreact when she has difficulty expressing herself clearly, this normal phase of speech development becomes prolonged.

At age 2 years, the child is ready to be taught simple rules about safety and behavior in the family, but she is only beginning to be able to internalize them. It remains essential for parents to ensure the safety of the environment and to continue to adequately supervise their active toddler. Parents who provide gentle reassurance, calmly and consistently maintain limits despite repeated tantrums, and reinforce positive behaviors help their child begin to develop healthy self-confidence and social skills.

Toilet training is often high on the list of priorities that parents have for their 2-year-old. Many, but not all, children this age have the developmental prerequisites to accomplish this major milestone. An essential ingredient to the success of this

endeavor is the child's own desire. Parents often welcome the health care professional's encouragement to recognize the signs of the child's readiness, to develop an approach to training, and to recognize their own limits in effecting this change.

The health care professional should not ask a child this age questions that may be answered with "No." A negative response is a 2-year-old's only way of maintaining a modicum of control. Simple statements addressed to the child are usually more successful, such as, "Now it's time for me to listen to your heart." For many children, the examination may be best accomplished on the parent's lap. Where a choice truly exists, ask the child for help (eg, "Which ear do you want me to look into first?").

Priorities for the 2 Year Visit

The first priority is to attend to the concerns of the parents.

In addition, the Bright Futures Early Childhood Expert Panel has given priority to the following topics for discussion in this visit:

▶ Social determinants of health[a] (risks [intimate partner violence; living situation and food security; tobacco, alcohol, and drugs], strengths and protective factors [parental well-being])

▶ Temperament and behavior (development, temperament, promotion of physical activity and safe play, limits on media use)

▶ Assessment of language development (how child communicates and expectations for language, promotion of reading)

▶ Toilet training (techniques, personal hygiene)

▶ Safety (car safety seats, outdoor safety, firearm safety)

[a] Social determinants of health is a new priority in the fourth edition of the *Bright Futures Guidelines*. For more information, see the *Promoting Lifelong Health for Families and Communities* theme.

Health Supervision

The *Bright Futures Tool and Resource Kit* contains Previsit Questionnaires to assist the health care professional in taking a history, conducting developmental surveillance, and performing medical screening.

History

Interval history may be obtained according to the concerns of the family and health care professional's preference or style of practice. The following questions can encourage in-depth discussion:

General Questions
- What are you most proud of since our last visit? (If the parent responds, "Nothing," the clinician should be prepared with a compliment, such as, "You made time for this visit despite your busy schedule.")
- What's exciting about this stage of development? What do you like most about this age?
- How are things going in your family?
- Let's talk about some of the things you most enjoy about your child. On the other hand, what seems most difficult?
- What major changes have occurred in your family since your last visit? Tell me about any stressful events. What is the effect of these changes on your family?
- What questions or concerns do you have about your child?

Past Medical History
- Has your child received any specialty or emergency care since the last visit?

Family History
- Has your child or anyone in the family (parents, brothers, sisters, grandparents, aunts, uncles, or cousins) developed a new health condition or died? **If the answer is Yes:** Ascertain who in the family has or had the condition, and ask about the age of onset and diagnosis. If the person is no longer living, ask about the age at the time of death.

Social History
- See the Social Determinants of Health priority in Anticipatory Guidance for social history questions.

Surveillance of Development

Do you or any of your child's caregivers have any specific concerns about your child's development, learning, or behavior?

Clinicians using the *Bright Futures Tool and Resource Kit* Previsit Questionnaires or another tool that includes a developmental milestones checklist, or those who use a structured developmental screening tool, need not ask about these developmental surveillance milestones. *(For more information, see the Promoting Healthy Development theme.)*

Social Language and Self-help

Does your child

- Play alongside other children, also called parallel play?
- Take off some clothing?
- Scoop well with a spoon?

Verbal Language (Expressive and Receptive)

Does he

- Use 50 words?
- Combine 2 words into short phrase or sentence?
- Follow 2-step command?
- Name at least 5 body parts, such as nose, hand, or stomach?
- Have speech that is 50% understandable to strangers?

Gross Motor

Does she

- Kick a ball?
- Jump off the ground with 2 feet?
- Run with coordination?
- Climb up a ladder at a playground?

Fine Motor

Does he

- Stack objects?
- Turn book pages?
- Use his hands to turn objects like knobs, toys, and lids?
- Draw lines?

Review of Systems

The Bright Futures Early Childhood Expert Panel recommends a complete review of systems as a part of every health supervision visit. This review can be done through questions about the following:

Does your child have any problems with

- Head
  - Shape
- Eyes
  - Vision
  - Cross-eyed
- Ears, nose, and throat
- Breathing or chest pain
- Stomach or abdomen
  - Nausea or vomiting
  - Bowel movements
- Skin
  - Birthmarks or moles
- Development
  - Muscle strength, movement, or function
  - Language

Observation of Parent-Child Interaction

During the visit, the health care professional acknowledges and reinforces positive parent-child interactions and discusses any concerns. Observation focuses on

- How do the parent and child communicate?
- What is the tone of the interaction and the feelings conveyed?
- Does the parent teach the child the name of a person or object during the visit?
- Does the child feel free to explore the room?
- How does the parent set appropriate limits, if needed?
- Does the parent seem positive when speaking about the child?

Physical Examination

A complete physical examination is included as part of every health supervision visit.

When performing a physical examination, the health care professional's attention is directed to the following components of the examination that are important for a child this age:

- **Measure and plot on appropriate CDC Growth Chart**
  - Standing height (preferred) or recumbent length
  - Weight

- **Calculate and plot on CDC Growth Chart**
  - Body mass index (BMI), if standing height
  - Weight-for-length, if recumbent length

- **Eyes**
  - Assess ocular motility.
  - Examine pupils for opacification and red reflexes.
  - Assess visual acuity using fixate and follow response.

- **Mouth**
  - Observe for caries, plaque, demineralization (white spots), staining, injury, and gingivitis.

- **Abdomen**
  - Palpate for masses.

- **Skin**
  - Observe for nevi, café-au-lait spots, birthmarks, or bruising.

- **Neurologic**
  - Observe running, scribbling, socialization, and ability to follow commands.
  - Assess language acquisition and clarity.

Screening

Universal Screening	Action
Autism	Autism spectrum disorder screen
Lead (high prevalence area or insured by Medicaid)	Lead blood test
Oral Health (in the absence of a dental home)	Apply fluoride varnish every 6 months.

Selective Screening	Risk Assessment[a]	Action if Risk Assessment Positive (+)
Anemia	+ on risk screening questions	Hematocrit or hemoglobin
Blood Pressure	Children with specific risk conditions or change in risk	Blood pressure measurement
Dyslipidemia	+ on risk screening questions	Lipid profile
Hearing	+ on risk screening questions	Referral for diagnostic audiologic assessment
Lead (low prevalence area and not insured by Medicaid)	+ on risk screening questions	Lead blood test
Oral Health	Does not have a dental home	Referral to dental home or, if not available, oral health risk assessment
	Primary water source is deficient in fluoride.	Oral fluoride supplementation
Tuberculosis	+ on risk screening questions	Tuberculin skin test
Vision	+ on risk screening questions	Ophthalmology referral

[a] See the *Evidence and Rationale chapter* for the criteria on which risk screening questions are based.

Immunizations

Consult the CDC/ACIP or AAP Web sites for the current immunization schedule.

CDC National Immunization Program: **www.cdc.gov/vaccines**

AAP *Red Book:* **http://redbook.solutions.aap.org**

Anticipatory Guidance

The following sample questions, which address the Bright Futures Early Childhood Expert Panel's Anticipatory Guidance Priorities, are intended to be used selectively to invite discussion, gather information, address the needs and concerns of the family, and build partnerships. Use of the questions may vary from visit to visit and from family to family. Questions can be modified to match the health care professional's communication style. The accompanying anticipatory guidance for the family should be geared to questions, issues, or concerns for that particular child and family. Tools and handouts to support anticipatory guidance can be found in the *Bright Futures Tool and Resource Kit*.

Priority

Social Determinants of Health

Risks: Intimate partner violence; living situation and food security; tobacco, alcohol, and drugs

Strengths and protective factors: Parental well-being

Risks: Intimate Partner Violence

Children who are exposed to intimate partner violence are at increased risk of adverse mental and physical health outcomes. Intimate partner violence cannot be determined through observation, but is best identified through direct inquiry. Avoid asking about abuse or domestic violence, but use descriptive terms, such as *hit, kick, shove, choke,* or *threaten*. Provide information about the effect of violence on children and about community resources that provide assistance. Recommend resources for parent education or parent support groups.

To avoid causing upset to families by questioning about sensitive and private topics, such as family violence, alcohol and drug use, and similar risks, it is recommended to begin screening about these topics with an introductory statement, such as, "I ask all patients standard health questions to understand factors that may affect the health of their child as well as their own health."

Sample Questions

Because violence is so common in so many people's lives, I've begun to ask about it. I don't know if this is a problem for you, but many children I see have parents who have been hurt by someone else. Some are too afraid or uncomfortable to bring it up, so I've started asking about it routinely. Do you always feel safe in your home? Has your partner, or another significant person in your life, ever hit, kicked, or shoved you, or physically hurt you or the baby? Are you scared that you or other caregivers may hurt the baby?

Do you have any questions about your safety at home? What will you do if you feel afraid? Do you have a plan? Would you like information on where to go or who to contact if you ever need help?

Anticipatory Guidance

- If you feel unsafe in your home, seek help in moving your children and yourself to a safe place.
- One way that I and other health care professionals can help you if your partner, or another significant person in your life, is hitting or threatening you is to support you and provide information about local resources that can help you.
- You can also call the toll-free **National Domestic Violence Hotline** at **800-799-SAFE (7233).**

Risks: Living Situation and Food Security

Parents in difficult living situations or with limited means may have concerns about their access to affordable housing, food, or other resources. Provide information and referrals, as needed, for community resources that help with finding quality child care, accessing transportation, or addressing issues such as financial concerns, or inadequate or unsafe housing. If the family is having difficulty obtaining sufficient nutritious food, provide information about WIC, SNAP, local food shelves, and local community food programs. Public health agencies can be excellent sources of help because they work with all types of community agencies and family needs.

Pesticides are often used in a variety of products for the control of pests both in indoor and outdoor environments. They may affect children's health in a variety of ways. Thousands of cases of pesticide poisoning are still reported to US poison control centers every year.

Sample Questions

Tell me about your living situation. Do you live in an apartment or a house? Is permanent housing a worry for you? Do you have the things you need to take care of your child? Does your home have enough heat, hot water, electricity, working appliances? Do you need help paying for health insurance?

Within the past 12 months, were you ever worried whether your food would run out before you got money to buy more? Within the past 12 months, did the food you bought not last, and you did not have money to get more?

Have you ever tried to get help for these issues? What happened? What barriers did you face?

Do you use any pesticides on your pets?

Anticipatory Guidance

- Community agencies are available to help you with concerns about your living situation.
- If you need financial assistance to help pay for health care expenses, ask about resources or referrals to the state Medicaid programs or other state assistance and health insurance programs.
- Programs and resources are available to help you and your child. You may be eligible for the WIC food and nutrition program, or housing or transportation assistance programs. Several food programs, such as the Commodity Supplemental Food Program and SNAP, the program formerly known as Food Stamps, can help you. If you are breastfeeding and eligible for WIC, you can get nutritious food for yourself and support from peer counselors.
- Avoid, or use the least toxic, pesticides on pets. Keep pets clean and wash pets' bedding frequently to keep away fleas.

Risks: Tobacco, Alcohol, and Drugs

The use of tobacco, alcohol, and other drugs has adverse health effects on the entire family. Focusing on the effect on health is often the most helpful approach and may help some family members with quitting or cutting back on substance use.

Sample Questions

Does anyone in your home smoke? Are you worried about any family members and how much they smoke, drink, or use drugs?

How often do you drink beer, wine, or liquor in your household? Do you, or does anyone you ride with, ever drive after having a drink? Does your partner use alcohol? What kind and for how long?

Are you using marijuana, cocaine, pain pills, narcotics, or other controlled substances? Are you getting any help to cut down or stop your drug use?

Anticipatory Guidance

- A smoke-free environment, in your car, home, and other places where your child spends time, is important. Smoking affects your child by increasing the risk of asthma, ear infections, and respiratory infections.
- **800-QUIT-NOW (800-784-8669);** TTY **800-332-8615** is a national telephone helpline that is routed to local resources. Additional resources are available at **www.cdc.gov.**
- Drug and alcohol cessation programs are available in our community and we would like to help you connect to these services.

Strengths and Protective Factors: Parental Well-being

Parental well-being is a key component of healthy family functioning. Congratulate the parents on their own preventive and health-promoting practices, such as using seat belts, avoiding tobacco, eating a nutritious diet, being physically active, and following appropriate health screening advice.

The lives of families with young children are usually filled with changes, such as employment, housing, and sometimes new siblings. Inquire about any recent or forthcoming changes in the family.

Acknowledge that other parents and children may be living in the household and those children may not be siblings (eg, they may be cousins or children of friends). This may present challenges as the parent may not be the only adult to intervene when situations arise. Opportunities for parents to discuss potential solutions to stressful situations can promote parental resilience and help parents stay connected to family and friends.

Sample Questions

Tell me about your own health and mood. How often do you take time for yourself? How often do you and your partner spend time together? What activities do you do together as a family? What's one of the things you do with your child or family that you really enjoy? How can you find more time to do that really enjoyable thing? Who helps you with your child? Do you have someone to turn to if you need to talk about problems?

Anticipatory Guidance

- Because your role as parents requires both physical and emotional energy, you must take care of yourselves so you can care for your child.
- It's important for you to maintain your friendships and family connections. Consider reaching out to the parents of children your child's age.
- Create opportunities for your family to share time together and for family members to talk and play with your toddler. Family mealtimes and time off from work are ideal opportunities.
- Keep family outings relatively short and simple. Lengthy activities tire your toddler and may lead to irritability or a tantrum.
- Spend individual time with each child in your family as often as you can.
- Acknowledge conflicts between siblings. Whenever possible, attempt to resolve conflicts without taking sides. For example, if a conflict arises about a toy, the toy can be put away. Do not expect your toddler to share his toys.
- Allow older children to have toys and other objects that they do not have to share with the toddler. Give them a storage space that the toddler cannot reach.
- Do not allow hitting, biting, or other aggressive behavior. Brief time-outs are a good way to tell your toddler these behaviors are not appropriate.

Priority

Temperament and Behavior
Development, temperament, promotion of physical activity and safe play, limits on media use

Development

The parent or caregiver has the best understanding of the child and can provide much useful information about the child's development at this stage. Discuss with parents their expectations about their child's understanding and behavior. A child at age 2 years still has limited abilities to internalize rules for behavior. Allowing the child to make choices among acceptable alternatives, redirecting and setting sensible limits, praising the child for being good, and giving smiles and encouragement all work better than punishment.

Through positive approaches and interactions with the child, parents and caregivers can nurture good behavior, self-confidence, and a desire to learn and explore.

Sample Questions
What are some of the new things that your child is doing? What do you and your partner enjoy most about your child? What seems to be most difficult? Do you have special times that you set aside to be with your child?

Anticipatory Guidance
- Praise your child for good behavior and accomplishments.
- Spend individual time with your child, playing with her, reading to her, hugging or holding her, taking walks, painting, going to the zoo or library, and doing puzzles together. Focus on activities that she expresses interest in and enjoys.
- Listen to and respect your child.
- Appreciate your child's investigative nature, and avoid excessively restricting her explorations. Guide her through fun learning experiences.
- Play helps children learn to solve problems, such as how to get toys upright when they fall over.
- Give your child opportunities to assert herself. Encourage self-expression. Let your child play music, dance, and paint.
- Help your child express such feelings as joy, anger, sadness, fear, and frustration.
- Promote a sense of competence and control by inviting your child to make choices limited to 2 equally acceptable options when possible. For example, allow her to choose between 2 kinds of fruit when picking out a snack.
- Allow your child to determine how much of the healthy foods you serve she will eat. Do not continue to feed her if she is not interested.
- It is important to let your child know how you would like her to act or respond. This is equally important to using time-outs to let your child know she chose a response that was not appropriate. In the long run, positive reinforcement for desired behavior is more effective in teaching children than negative consequences for undesired behavior.

Temperament

Discuss with the parent typical variations in children's behavioral styles, including such temperamental qualities as general activity level, sensitivity or reactivity to changes in the environment, tendency to approach or withdraw in new situations, adaptability to change in routine, intensity of response, and the predominance of a positive or negative mood, especially in social situations.

Sample Question

How does your child act around family members?

Anticipatory Guidance

- Your child varies in how she reacts to different situations and she will quickly learn the different ways in which her parents and other family members respond to her actions and requests. Encourage family members to be consistent, patient, and respectful in how they respond to her. Being around adults who care for them helps stimulate children's brains and makes learning easier.

Promotion of Physical Activity and Safe Play

The main ideas behind promoting physical activity at this age are to be physically active in a safe environment and to establish a lifelong habit of being active, both as an individual and as a family. Children this age enjoy playing independently, but have not yet developed the skills necessary to interact with other children.

Sample Questions

Tell me about your child's typical play. What kind of physical activities does your child enjoy? What types and amounts of physical activity does your child enjoy when she's with other caregivers, such as at child care and with other family members? How does your child act around other children? If your child is in group child care, how does she do with the other children? Are your child care arrangements working for your family and for your child?

Anticipatory Guidance

- Encourage free play for up to 60 minutes per day.
- Engage in guided interactive play with your child several times a day, 5 to 10 minutes each time.
- Enjoy being physically active as a family, such as by walking, hiking, and playing tag.
- Make sure that other caregivers also make time for physical activity with your child.
- To make exercise fun, give your child age-appropriate play equipment, from balls to plastic bats. Let your child choose what to play with.
- Encourage your child to play with other children, but do not expect her to share the play or toys yet. Two-year-olds enjoy playing among, not with, other children. Your child may be physically aggressive toward other children.

Limits on Media Use

The AAP recommends that children older than 2 years limit TV and digital media use to no more than 1 hour of high-quality programming per day. In addition to educational shows being too stimulating, many e-readers and "educational" apps are more distracting than educational because of the extra features programmed into their design to keep children engaged. Review that even interactive media cannot teach language or other important skills at this age.

If a child watches TV, parents should ensure that the programs are appropriate. Many cartoon shows are violent, soap operas often feature issues that are inappropriate for young children, and talk shows and sporting events are overwhelming for many young children. Even educational shows can be too stimulating for young minds.

Sample Questions

Does your child watch TV or videos or use other digital media? If so, what TV shows does your child watch? How much time each day does your child spend watching TV or playing on a tablet, a smartphone, or other digital device? Is there a TV on in the background while your child is playing in the room? Do you use TV or other screens as a way to calm your child, help her to get to sleep, or keep her occupied if you have something else you must do?

Anticipatory Guidance

- Research shows that young children this age cannot learn information from screens, even though many toys and videos claim to teach them skills. Children this age learn by interacting with caregivers; being read to, talked to, and sung to; and exploring their environment.
- At this young age, media viewing can hinder the development of language, thinking skills, behavior regulation, and attention. Make special time for tech-free type of play every day.
- If there are times when you or your caregiver cannot actively engage in play with your child, encourage unstructured, unplugged play. This encourages her to think innovatively, problem-solve, and develop reasoning skills.
- Make mealtimes an opportunity for face-to-face learning interactions. Don't have the TV on during meals, which distracts toddlers from eating and interacting with family.

EARLY CHILDHOOD
2 YEAR VISIT

Priority

Assessment of Language Development
How child communicates and expectations for language, promotion of reading

---

How Child Communicates and Expectations for Language

A 2-year-old is rapidly developing language skills and he experiences joy in reciprocal communication. This is a time to assess how the child communicates and to set expectations with the parents about their child's language development. Parents are keen observers of the child's behavior and often correctly identify sensory problems.

Sample Questions
How does your child communicate what he wants? What do you think your child understands? How well do you think your child hears and sees? If your child uses 2 languages, how intelligible is he in each?

Ask the Child
"What's that?" (pointing to a picture); "Which one is the ___?" (in a book); "Give me the ___." (from among several objects).

Anticipatory Guidance
- Don't use baby talk.
- Two-year-olds should begin using 2-word sentences or phrases, such as, "Want milk," "Have book," and "Go home."
- Two-year-olds also should be able to follow simple 1- or 2-step commands, such as, "Pick up the doll and bring it to me."
- Encourage your child's language development also by singing songs to him and by talking about what you both are seeing and doing together.
- Many children struggle to respond quickly at this age, so talk and question slowly so that your child has the opportunity to respond without pressure. Praise all efforts to respond, and repeat what is said in an affirming way.
- If you need to have your child look at you before you know he is listening to you, let us know. Hearing problems are important to identify early and are more common in children with many ear infections.
- If you notice your child squinting, holding books very close to his face, or failing to look at things you are pointing out to him, let us know. He may have a vision problem.

Promotion of Reading

Children this age begin to take a definite interest in words and wordplay. Books are fun and reading is a fun activity to share. They may ask to read the same book over and over. Reading every day will help establish reading as a lifelong pleasurable habit.

Sample Question

Do you or other caregivers sit down and read with your child every day?

Anticipatory Guidance

- Read to your child every day. Ask your child to point to pictures of objects, animals, or people on the page. If the story is familiar, pause every now and then for your child to insert a phrase or sound to help tell the story or to finish a familiar sentence or phrase.
- Many toddlers love the same story over and over. This is normal, and repetition is good. It helps build important language skills.
- Reading and storytelling do not have to be a huge project. Even sitting together for a short, 3-minute story will promote reading.
- Even if you or your caregiver has reading challenges, looking at a book and pointing to pictures and asking questions about what is going on is still reading.

Priority

Toilet Training
Techniques, personal hygiene

Techniques

Toilet training is part of developmentally appropriate learning. Each child progresses through toilet training differently and parents need to understand signs of readiness and how to support and encourage their child during this process. Explain that many children do not achieve even partial toilet training before the age of 3 years or complete daytime dryness until the age of 4 years.

Explore family attitudes about toilet training, including parental experiences and expectations.

Sample Question
How is your child's toilet training progressing?

Anticipatory Guidance
- Encourage toilet training when your child is dry for about 2 hours at a time, knows the difference between wet and dry, can pull her pants up and down, wants to learn, and can tell you when she is about to have a bowel movement. Do not pressure or punish, and avoid friction. Be supportive, give your child an active role, and keep the learning process fun. Praise or reward child for cooperation and success.
- Here are some ways to help your child be successful. Make sure she has easy access to a potty chair, dress her in easy-to-remove pants, establish a daily routine to place her on the potty every few hours, give underwear as a special present for reinforcement, and provide a relaxed environment by reading or singing songs while she is on the potty.
- Children use the toilet more frequently than adults, often up to 10 times a day. Plan for frequent toilet breaks when traveling with your child, even if you are out for a short time.

Personal Hygiene

This is a good time for parents to help their child establish good personal hygiene habits, especially hand-washing. Modeling these behaviors yourself can reinforce the teaching.

Sample Questions

Does your child wash her hands after toileting? Before eating?

Anticipatory Guidance

- Help your child wash her hands after diaper changes or toileting and before eating. Make sure to wash your own hands often.
- Clean potty chairs after each use.
- Teach your child to sneeze and cough into her shoulder. Teach your child to wipe her nose with a tissue and then wash her hands.
- Soap and water is sufficient for cleaning your child's toys.
- If your child is in child care, provide personal items, such as blankets, cups, combs, and brushes, for individual use.

Priority

Safety
Car safety seats, outdoor safety, firearm safety

Car Safety Seats

Talk with parents to ensure that they know how to securely fasten their child in a car safety seat. Adults should model car safety by always using a seat belt themselves.

When the child reaches 2 years of age, his parents may choose to turn his car safety seat forward facing. However, it is even better to continue to ride in the rear-facing position as long as the child has not reached the weight or height limit for the rear-facing position in his convertible seat. Parents should read and follow the manufacturer's instructions for switching a seat from rear facing to forward facing.

Sample Questions
How is the car safety seat working? Is your child fastened securely in a car safety seat in the back seat every time he rides in a vehicle? Does everyone use a seat belt, booster seat, or car safety seat?

Anticipatory Guidance
- Be sure that the car safety seat is properly installed in the back seat according to the manufacturer's instructions and the vehicle owner's manual. The harness straps should be snug enough that you cannot pinch any webbing between your fingers.
- The back seat is the safest place for children to ride until your child is age 13 years.
- Do not start your vehicle until everyone is buckled up. Children watch what parents do, so it is important for you to model safe behaviors by always wearing your seat belt.

For information about car safety seats and actions to keep your child safe in and around cars, visit www.safercar.gov/parents.

Find a Child Passenger Safety Technician: http://cert.safekids.org. Click on "Find a Tech."

Toll-free Auto Safety Hotline: 888-327-4236

Outdoor Safety

The young toddler is beginning to play outside as well as inside. This new opportunity for physical activity introduces new hazards. Outdoor safety should be tailored to the local environment where the child lives (rural versus urban hazards). Reinforce the importance of safety in physical activities, such as always using a bike helmet. Modeling is the best way to ensure that a child develops lifelong safe behaviors. Building safe habits at an early age is easier than trying to introduce them when your child is older.

Sample Questions

Would you like a list of outdoor health and safety tips for your toddler? Does your child wear a bike helmet when he rides his tricycle?

Anticipatory Guidance

- When your toddler is playing outside, make sure he stays within fences and gates and remember to watch him closely.
- Backyard swimming pools, hot tubs, or spas need to be completely fenced on 4 sides to separate them from the house and yard with a self-closing and self-latching gate.
- Carefully supervise your child when he is using playground equipment, and make sure that the surface under play equipment is soft enough to absorb a fall.
- Keep your toddler away from moving machinery, lawn mowers, overhead garage doors, driveways, and streets.
- Young children should never be left unsupervised in or around vehicles. A parked car is not a safe place to play; lock cars when they are parked so your toddler cannot get in.
- When you or other adults are backing out of the garage or driving the car forward or backing in the driveway, be certain another adult is holding your child so that he is not run over. All vehicles have blind spots and the driver may not be able to see him.
- If a child is missing, check the pool or spa first, and then the car.
- Be sure that your child wears a helmet approved by the Consumer Product Safety Commission (CPSC) when riding on a tricycle, in a towed bike trailer, or in a seat on an adult's bicycle. Wear a helmet yourself. Make sure everyone's helmets fit properly according to the manufacturer's instructions.

Firearm Safety

Firearms should be removed from places in which children live and play. If a family does have firearms, they should be stored unloaded and locked in a case, with ammunition stored in a separate locked place. Many young children are killed by firearms each year and most are injured by themselves, a sibling, or a friend.

Sample Questions

Does anyone in your home have a firearm? Does a neighbor, family friend, or any home where your child might play have a firearm? If so, is the firearm unloaded and locked up? Where is the ammunition stored? Have you thought about not owning a firearm because of the danger to children and other family members?

Anticipatory Guidance

- The best way to keep your child safe from injury or death from firearms is to never have a firearm in the home.
- If it is necessary to keep a firearm in your home, it should be stored unloaded and locked in a case, with the ammunition locked separately from the firearm.
- Children cannot reliably be taught not to handle a firearm if they find one. Adults must make sure the firearm is completely out of sight and reach of the child.

Early Childhood
2½ Year Visit

Context

At age 2½, significant advances in all developmental trajectories are readily observable. Compared with the 2-year-old, the motor coordination (gross and fine) of a child at age 2½ years is much improved. The child now can walk on tiptoes and can jump with both feet. He modulates his movement, speeding up and slowing down as he desires, negotiating turns while running, and coming to a sudden stop. His finger movements are now better differentiated from whole-hand movements. For example, he is more able to manage puzzle pieces and string beads, and put snapblocks together.

A strong incentive for the health care professional to see children routinely at age 2½ years is the opportunity to check on the child's development of language and social communication. Where the 2-year-old is typically just starting the process of creatively joining a few words in combination, the 2½-year-old uses a wide variety of short phrases of 3 and 4 words (many, if not most, of which are understandable to family members). Vocabulary has expanded dramatically, and the child often accompanies his actions with short, verbal descriptions, such as, "Me make it go," and "I take my coat off." At age 2½ years, children typically enjoy the playful use of words, including rhyming games and simple songs with rhythm and accompanying movement, and the child's pleasure in such interactions with others becomes an important measure of his social development. As at age 2 years, receptive language usually develops well in advance of expressive abilities and makes for new receptivity to book reading and stories. Children this age like stories that tell about everyday activities, such as getting dressed, playing with toys, eating meals with the family, and bedtime. He likes to hear the same story read to him over and over, and often insists on it being read the same way each time.

Play behaviors also have become more elaborate at age 2½ years. The child this age enjoys acting out the behaviors seen in other family members, such as feeding a dolly, talking on the phone, or sweeping the floor. A new sense of order, sometimes repetitive and perfectionistic, emerges at this age, as shown in the child's interest in lining up toys or placing crayons in a specific color order. In social situations, play with peers continues to be more often parallel than collaborative. Yet, with some play activities that have an easily recognized theme and sequence of actions (eg, the tea party), 2½-year-olds delight in independent play with peers.

This age is often the time when parents begin to consider what sort of early education experience will be best for their child. The 2½ Year Visit is an ideal time to review the child's developmental readiness, behavioral style, and parental goals for such a placement, and to support parents in their efforts to determine the best programmatic match for their child.

Priorities for the 2½ Year Visit

The first priority is to attend to the concerns of the parents.

In addition, the Bright Futures Early Childhood Expert Panel has given priority to the following topics for discussion in this visit:

▸ Family routines (day and evening routines, enjoyable family activities, parental activities outside the family, consistency in the child's environment)

▸ Language promotion and communication (use of simple words and reading together)

▸ Promoting social development (play with other children, giving choices, limits on television and media use)

▸ Preschool considerations (readiness for early childhood programs and playgroups, toilet training)

▸ Safety (car safety seats, outdoor safety, water safety, sun protection, fires and burns)

Health Supervision

The *Bright Futures Tool and Resource Kit* contains Previsit Questionnaires to assist the health care professional in taking a history, conducting developmental surveillance, and performing medical screening.

History

Interval history may be obtained according to the concerns of the family and the health care professional's preference or style of practice. The following questions can encourage in-depth discussion:

General Questions

- What new things is your child doing now? Tell me about your child. How would you describe his personality these days? What are his favorite things, activities, people?
- What do you enjoy and dislike the most about this age?
- What questions or concerns do you have about your child today?

Past Medical History

- Has your child received any specialty or emergency care since the last visit?

Family History

- Has your child or anyone in the family (parents, brothers, sisters, grandparents, aunts, uncles, or cousins) developed a new health condition or died? **If the answer is Yes:** Ascertain who in the family has or had the condition, and ask about the age of onset and diagnosis. If the person is no longer living, ask about the age at the time of death.

Social History

- How are you and your family doing these days?

Surveillance of Development

Do you or any of your child's caregivers have any specific concerns about your child's development, learning, or behavior?

Clinicians using the *Bright Futures Tool and Resource Kit* Previsit Questionnaires or another tool that includes a developmental milestones checklist, or those who use a structured developmental screening tool, need not ask about these developmental surveillance milestones. *(For more information, see the Promoting Healthy Development theme.)*

Social Language and Self-help

Does your child

- Urinate in a potty or toilet?
- Spear food with a fork?
- Wash and dry hands?
- Engage in imaginary play, such as with dolls and toys?
- Try to get you to watch by saying, "Look at me!"

Verbal Language (Expressive and Receptive)

Does she

- Use pronouns correctly?
- Explain the reasons for things, such as needing a sweater when it's cold?
- Name at least 1 color?

Gross Motor

Does he

- Walk up steps, alternating feet?
- Run well without falling?

Fine Motor

Does she

- Copy a vertical line?
- Grasp crayon with thumb and fingers instead of fist?
- Catch large balls?

Review of Systems

The Bright Futures Early Childhood Expert Panel recommends a complete review of systems as a part of every health supervision visit. This review can be done through questions about the following:

Does your child have any problems with

- Head
  - Shape
- Eyes
  - Vision
  - Cross-eyed
- Ears, nose, and throat
- Breathing or chest pain
- Stomach or abdomen
  - Nausea or vomiting
  - Bowel movements
- Skin
  - Birthmarks or moles
- Development
  - Muscle strength, movement, or function
  - Language

Observation of Parent-Child Interaction

During the visit, the health care professional acknowledges and reinforces positive parent-child interactions and discusses any concerns. Observation focuses on

- How actively do the parent and child communicate with each other?
- Does the child use questions and phrases at an appropriate age level?
- If given a book, do the child and the parent look at it together, discuss it, and interact?
- How well does the parent calm the child during the visit?

Physical Examination

A complete physical examination is included as part of every health supervision visit.

When performing a physical examination, the health care professional's attention is directed to the following components of the examination that are important for a child this age:

- **Measure and plot on appropriate CDC Growth Chart**
    - Standing height (preferred) or recumbent length
    - Weight

- **Calculate and plot on CDC Growth Chart**
    - BMI, if standing height
    - Weight-for-length, if recumbent length

- **Eyes**
    - Assess ocular motility.
    - Examine pupils for opacification and red reflexes.
    - Assess visual acuity using fixate and follow response.

- **Abdomen**
    - Palpate for masses.

- **Skin**
    - Observe for nevi, café-au-lait spots, birthmarks, or bruising.

- **Neurologic**
    - Observe coordination, language acquisition and clarity, and socialization.
    - Assess vocalizations.

Screening

Universal Screening	Action	
Development	Developmental screen	
Oral Health (in the absence of a dental home)	Apply fluoride varnish every 6 months.	

Selective Screening	Risk Assessment[a]	Action if Risk Assessment Positive (+)
Anemia	+ on risk screening questions	Hematocrit or hemoglobin
Blood Pressure	Children with specific risk conditions or change in risk	Blood pressure measurement
Hearing	+ on risk screening questions	Referral for diagnostic audiologic assessment
Oral Health	Does not have a dental home	Referral to dental home or, if not available, oral health risk assessment
	Primary water source is deficient in fluoride.	Oral fluoride supplementation
Vision	+ on risk screening questions	Ophthalmology referral

[a] See the *Evidence and Rationale chapter* for the criteria on which risk screening questions are based.

Immunizations

Consult the CDC/ACIP or AAP Web sites for the current immunization schedule.

CDC National Immunization Program: **www.cdc.gov/vaccines**

AAP *Red Book:* **http://redbook.solutions.aap.org**

Anticipatory Guidance

The following sample questions, which address the Early Childhood Expert Panel's Anticipatory Guidance Priorities, are intended to be used selectively to invite discussion, gather information, address the needs and concerns of the family, and build partnerships. Use of the questions may vary from visit to visit and from family to family. Questions can be modified to match the health care professional's communication style. The accompanying anticipatory guidance for the family should be geared to questions, issues, or concerns for that particular child and family. Tools and handouts to support anticipatory guidance can be found in the *Bright Futures Tool and Resource Kit.*

Priority

Family Routines

Day and evening routines, enjoyable family activities, parental activities outside the family, consistency in the child's environment

Day and Evening Routines

Mealtimes are part of a family's routine that enhances a child's language, math, and motor skills as well as promotes communication and other socialization abilities. Consistent evening and bedtime routines help young children transition from the active daytime to a good night's sleep.

Sample Questions

What meals does your child eat with the family? What types of evening and bedtime routines do you use at home? How consistently do you follow these routines?

Anticipatory Guidance

- Family meals are an excellent way to support language and social development in the young child. Eat together as often as possible—it doesn't matter which meal.
- In the hour before bedtime, try not to use digital media, play vigorously, or do other stimulating activities with your child. Quiet evening activities will help your child recognize that bedtime is coming and smooths the way to the bedtime routine and settling in early for high-quality sleep. A good night's sleep is essential to good daytime behavior and to preventing tantrums. Do not place a TV, computer, or other digital media device in your child's room. This is an important way you can establish healthy sleep and healthy media habits.

Enjoyable Family Activities

Routine participation in activities as a family (eg, physical activities and going to museums or the park) helps build family togetherness.

Sample Questions

Tell me about how you have fun with your family. What activities do you and your family participate in together?

Anticipatory Guidance

- Reading to your child at least once a day is a habit that both of you will grow to look forward to. Pick books with simple stories that your child can understand, and try to find ones that reflect your culture and interests.
- Encourage family exercise, such as walking, swimming, or bicycling (with helmets).
- Expand your child's experiences by visiting museums, zoos, and other educational centers. Take advantage of programs designed for young children, such as library programs for toddlers and seasonal community events.

Parental Activities Outside the Family

Parents need to reconnect regularly with friends and personal interests and work beyond the family.

Sample Questions

What kinds of things do you do outside the family? If you work outside of the home, where do you work?

Anticipatory Guidance

- Try some activities outside the family. Being with friends helps reduce stress, gives you pleasure, and rewards your efforts.
- Sometimes parents of toddlers find themselves making new friends with the parents of other toddlers and enjoying the informal support of others who have many of the same challenges and interests.

Consistency in the Child's Environment

Consistent guidance, regular playful experiences during the day, and clear limits about bedtime all help a child develop a sense of security and self-control. As children develop more effective language skills, they and their parents experience increasing pleasure in talking together. Parents and caregivers build their child's self-esteem by noting and encouraging efforts to master emerging skills. Each new skill is a rudiment for a more advanced skill, so skills beget skills. Having all the child's caregivers use a consistent supportive approach to helping the child participate in these routines and begin to achieve this self-control is critical.

Sample Question

How well do you and your family agree on routines, limits, and discipline for your child?

Anticipatory Guidance

- Reach agreement with all family members on how best to support your child's emerging independence while maintaining consistent limits.

Priority

Language Promotion and Communication
Use of simple words and reading together

Use of Simple Words and Reading Together

At 2½ years of age, children vary considerably in their spoken language skills. Most, however, are already speaking in short, complete sentences. They typically are forming 3- to 4-word sentences, most of which should be understandable to family members.

Speech tends to be unidirectional at this age, with the child most often asserting his needs and desires and describing his activities.

Sample Questions

Is your child speaking in sentences? How frustrated does he become when others cannot understand what he is saying? Does he enjoy having stories read to him? Does he enjoy participating with you in songs, rhymes, and games involving rhythm and movement, such as "Itsy, Bitsy Spider"?

Anticipatory Guidance

- Read books together every day. Reading aloud will help him be ready for preschool, and then for school.
- At this age, children typically are able to follow the story line of simple books, and they may ask you to read the same book again and again.
- Take your child to the library and its story time regularly.
- Young children process spoken language more slowly than adults. Be sure to give your toddler plenty of time to respond when you say something to him.
- When your child is speaking, listen attentively. If necessary, clarify what he means, using the right words. For example, if he says, "Me want milk," you can correct him and say, "I think you mean, 'I want milk.'"

Priority

Promoting Social Development

Play with other children, giving choices, limits on television and media use

Play With Other Children

Children this age should feel comfortable and engaged when playing side by side with peers and older children. Play helps to set the stage for the development of strong social relationships in later life. However, their capacity for cooperative, reciprocal play is still quite limited.

If the child is not yet in a child care or preschool program, parents should be encouraged to help organize playdates or a regular playgroup to help promote the child's social development.

Sample Questions

How often does your child play with other children? How do these playtimes go?

Anticipatory Guidance

- Provide opportunities for your toddler to play with other toddlers near your child's age. Be sure to supervise these times, because your child is not ready to share or play cooperatively.
- Having 2 of each toy is a good way to avoid battles over toys. If you have a close friend whose child plays with yours, consider purchasing the same toys for your children.

Giving Choices

- At this age, children usually enjoy initiating actions and decisions, and the frequent upsets and frustrations experienced by the 2-year-old are usually decreasing by 2½ years. At the same time, they definitely need and appreciate consistent parental guidance about safe, acceptable behavior and limits.

Sample Questions

Does your child enjoy making independent decisions about what to eat and wear or where to play? What are some of the new things that your child is doing?

Anticipatory Guidance

- Offering toddlers limited choices between 2 equally acceptable options helps build your child's independence. Having more than 2 options to choose from is overwhelming and frustrating for your toddler. Once your child decides, confirm the choice and move along.
- Continue to follow daily routines for eating, sleeping, and playing.

Limits on Television and Media Use

The AAP recommends that children older than 2 limit TV and digital media to no more than 1 hour of quality programming per day. If a child watches TV or plays with computer games or other media activities, parents should ensure that the programs are appropriate.

Sample Questions

How much time does your child spend watching TV or using Internet-connected devices, such as computers or tablets? What programs and activities does she watch or do?

Anticipatory Guidance

- Limit screen time to no more than 1 hour each day. Screen time is not a replacement for singing, talking, and reading together—screen time should always be less than personal time together with your child.

- Monitor the types of shows and computer activities your child watches or does. Look for media choices that are educational and teach good values, such as empathy, tolerance, and how to get along with others.

- When you watch TV with your child, make it interactive. Ask questions about what is happening on the program and what your child thinks will happen next.

- Starting healthy media habits now is important, because they are a lot harder to change when children are older. Consider making a family media use plan. This plan is a set of rules about media use and screen time that is written down and agreed upon by all family members. Take into account not only the quantity but the quality and location of media use. Consider TVs, phones, tablets, and computers. Rules should be followed by parents as well as children. The AAP has information on how to make a plan at **www.HealthyChildren.org/MediaUsePlan.**

Priority

Preschool Considerations

Readiness for early childhood programs and playgroups, toilet training

Readiness for Early Childhood Programs and Playgroups

Discuss the child's developmental readiness for an early care and education program. In determining the appropriateness of the match between child and program, have parents review the features of the program (eg, duration of care, size of group, and type and closeness of supervision), temperamental qualities of the child, goals and philosophy of the program, and the family's goals for the child. For children with special health care needs who are receiving services under the Individuals with Disabilities Education Act Part C, ensure that the family is working with the family service coordinator to transition the child's services to Part B. This transition needs to occur before the child's third birthday.

Sample Questions

What are your plans for child care or preschool in the year ahead? Do you need help locating or selecting a quality early education experience for your child?

Anticipatory Guidance

- Child care and preschool settings offer young children the opportunity to develop social skills with other children on a daily basis. They also help children learn skills that will help them make the transition to kindergarten. If you need help in selecting a program, let me know and I can provide information and resources that can help you.
- If you choose not to enroll your child in child care or preschool, visit a teacher's store or bookstore to look at books for ideas about preparing your child for the transition to school. Provide your child with frequent, regular times to play with children his age.

Toilet Training

Full "toilet independence" may be a requirement for attendance at preschool or child care programs. This usually is not achieved before the child is at a developmental age of 2½ years. Children 2½ years and older who are not yet toilet trained are likely to respond best to an approach that includes encouragement, with respect for the child's own decision and determination to succeed.

Sample Question

Where do things stand with toilet training?

Anticipatory Guidance

▪ Use an approach that encourages your child to make the decision to use the potty. Do not force, punish, or shame him for accidents or reluctance to try. Instead, use praise for all efforts and interest, offer choices about trying the potty, and read stories about potty training with your toddler.

▪ Here are some ways to help your child be successful. Dress him in easy-to-remove pants, establish a daily routine, place him on the potty every 1 to 2 hours, and provide a relaxed environment by reading or singing songs while he is on the potty.

Priority

Safety

Car safety seats, outdoor safety, water safety, sun protection, fires and burns

Car Safety Seats

Talk with parents to ensure that they know how to securely fasten their child in a car safety seat. Adults should model car safety by always using a seat belt themselves.

Sample Questions

How is the car safety seat working for you? Is your child fastened securely in a car safety seat in the back seat every time she rides in a vehicle? Does everyone use a seat belt, booster seat, or car safety seat?

Anticipatory Guidance

- Be sure your child's car safety seat is properly installed in the back seat according to the manufacturer's instructions and your vehicle owner's manual. The harness straps should be snug enough that you cannot pinch any webbing between your fingers.
- The back seat is the safest place for children to ride until your child is age 13 years.
- Do not start your vehicle until everyone is buckled up. Children watch what parents do, so it is important for you to model safe behaviors by always wearing your seat belt.

For information about car safety seats and actions to keep your child safe in and around cars, visit www.safercar.gov/parents.

Find a Child Passenger Safety Technician: http://cert.safekids.org. Click on "Find a Tech."

Toll-free Auto Safety Hotline: 888-327-4236

Outdoor Safety

Unintentional injury is the number one cause of death among young children. Because the urge to explore and learn is so strong, and young children do not have good judgment, parents must use constant vigilance and regularly review the safety of the environment to protect their young child from harm.

Sample Question

Would you like a list of outdoor health and safety considerations for your toddler?

Anticipatory Guidance

- When your toddler is playing outside, make sure she stays within fences and gates and that you or an adult supervisor is watching her closely.

- Carefully supervise your child when she is using playground equipment, and make sure that the surface under play equipment is soft enough to absorb a fall.

- Keep your toddler away from moving machinery, lawn mowers, overhead garage doors, driveways, alleys, and streets. Driveways are not a safe place to play.

- Be sure that your toddler wears a helmet that is approved by the CPSC when riding in a seat on an adult's bicycle or on a tricycle. Wear a helmet yourself.

- Teach your toddler to ask permission before approaching dogs, especially if the dogs are unknown or are eating.

Water Safety

Parents still must supervise their child closely to ensure her safety around water. All children require constant supervision by an adult whenever they are near water. Swim lessons do not provide drown-proofing at any age and children may not be developmentally ready for formal swimming lessons at this age. However, parents may choose to start their child in swimming lessons depending on the child's readiness and frequency of exposure to water.

Sample Questions

Are there swimming pools or other potential water dangers near your home? Does your child enjoy swimming?

Ask the Child

Do you like swimming?

Anticipatory Guidance

- Watch your toddler constantly whenever she is near water, including bathtubs, play pools, buckets and the toilet. A supervising adult should be within an arm's reach, providing "touch supervision," whenever young children are in or around water.

- Do not expect young brothers or sisters to supervise your toddler in the bathtub, house, or yard.

- Empty buckets, tubs, or small pools immediately after use.

- Be sure that swimming pools in your community apartment complex or home have a 4-sided fence with a self-closing, self-latching gate.

- Swim programs for children this age should include a parent, should emphasize fun and play, should take place in a pool with warm water that is well maintained and clean, and should limit the number of submersions to prevent swallowing water.

- Children and adults should always wear a properly fitted US Coast Guard–approved life jacket at all times when boating.

Sun Protection

Sun protection now is of increasing importance because of climate change and the thinning of the atmospheric ozone layer. Sun protection is accomplished through limiting sun exposure, using sunscreen, and wearing protective clothing.

Sample Questions

Do you apply sunscreen whenever your child plays outside? Does your child care provider have a sun protection policy? Do you and your child care provider limit outside time during the middle of the day, when the sun is strongest?

Anticipatory Guidance

- Always apply sunscreen with an SPF greater than 15 when your child is outside. Reapply every 2 hours.
- Have your child wear a hat.
- Avoid prolonged time in the sun between 11:00 am and 3:00 pm.
- Wear sun protection clothing for summer.

Fires and Burns

Young children require constant supervision around fires. They are fascinated by fire and its colors. They also may play with matches in an attempt to imitate parents who smoke. When playing, they often forget safety rules and can easily run into grills, stoves, and open fires.

Sample Questions

Where are the smoke detectors located in the home where your child lives? When did you last change the batteries in the smoke detectors? What is your plan for getting everyone out of the house and to a meeting place once outside? Do you have a neighbor from whose house you can call the fire department?

Anticipatory Guidance

- Make sure you have a working smoke detector on every level of your home, especially in the furnace and sleeping areas. Test smoke detectors every month. It is best to use smoke detectors that use long-life batteries, but, if you do not, change the batteries at least once a year.
- Develop an escape plan in the event of a fire in your home.
- Install a carbon monoxide detector/alarm, certified by Underwriters Laboratories, in the hallway near every separate sleeping area of the home.
- Put matches well out of sight and reach of your child, or keep them in a locked cabinet.
- Watch your child closely when you are near a hot grill, the stove, or an open fire. Place a barrier around open fires, fire pits, or campfires.
- Do not leave irons and curling irons plugged in.

Early Childhood
3 Year Visit

Context

Around her third birthday, a very self-determined individualist makes her presence known. Her successes or failures at controlling the world around her will influence her behavior. As she makes her own simple choices, she is able to learn consequences and is beginning to develop a sense of right and wrong. She looks forward to something pleasant or perceives an encounter as disagreeable. Unpredictable behavior still reigns, and "benign" lying is extremely common. She can decide whether to stand her ground, talk her way out of situations, or avoid interactions in which she feels insecure.

Speech and motor activity are now focused on investigating or modifying the environment. The 3-year-old has developed understandable speech—a major achievement. She can now negotiate with her parents (eg, "Story first and then nap."). She also makes choices, deciding between green and blue socks or between playing ball or riding a tricycle outside. Body shape has developed from the protuberate abdomen of the baby and toddler into the well-proportioned child's body. Awareness of gender differences has begun to emerge, in terms of both physical differences and society's expectations. Most children at age 3 years can easily state, "I am a girl," or "I am a boy." Her physical abilities have improved as well, giving her better control over what her hands are touching or where her feet take her. With her greater quickness

and agility come new safety concerns (resulting in the need, for instance, to teach new rules and cautions around cars and streets).

At this age, the child's increasingly well-developed capacity to communicate her interests, desires, and preferences opens up a new world of social interaction. With children her age, language provides a new means for discovering mutual interests. At home, she proudly shows her ability to independently carry out activities of everyday living, such as feeding, bathing, dressing, and toileting. These activities still require supervision even though she wants to do it "all by myself." Food selection, for example, should remain a parental decision with minimal deviation allowed from the family's meals and food choices.

Including the child in interactions within the family, asking the child for opinions, and allowing the child to contribute to discussions within the family encourage her self-esteem and reinforce her special place in the family. Family transitions often occur during this year, including pregnancy or birth of a sibling and the progression into a preschool or other educational setting. These transitions call for additional support and education by the health care professional. This is also an opportunity to suggest to parents that they enroll their child in a structured preschool experience no later than age 4 years.

Priorities for the 3 Year Visit

The first priority is to attend to the concerns of the parents.

In addition, the Bright Futures Early Childhood Expert Panel has given priority to the following topics for discussion in this visit:

► Social determinants of health[a] (risks [living situation and food security; tobacco, alcohol, and drugs], strengths and protective factors [positive family interactions, work-life balance])

► Playing with siblings and peers (play opportunities and interactive games, sibling relationships)

► Encouraging literacy activities (reading, talking, and singing together; language development)

► Promoting healthy nutrition and physical activity (water, milk, and juice; nutritious foods; competence in motor skills and limits on inactivity)

► Safety (car safety seats, choking prevention, pedestrian safety and falls from windows, water safety, pets, firearm safety)

[a] Social determinants of health is a new priority in the fourth edition of the *Bright Futures Guidelines.* For more information, see the *Promoting Lifelong Health for Families and Communities theme.*

Health Supervision

The *Bright Futures Tool and Resource Kit* contains Previsit Questionnaires to assist the health care professional in taking a history, conducting developmental surveillance, and performing medical screening.

History

Interval history may be obtained according to the concerns of the family and the health care professional's preference or style of practice. The following questions can encourage in-depth discussion:

General Questions

- What are you most proud of since our last visit? (If the parent responds, "Nothing," the health care professional should be prepared with a compliment, such as, "You made time for this visit despite your busy schedule.")
- What is something funny or wonderful that your child has done lately?
- What changes have occurred in your family since your last visit?
- How are you feeling as a parent?
- What types of opportunities does your child have to interact with peers?
- What questions or concerns would you like to share with me about your child?

Past Medical History

- Has your child received any specialty or emergency care since the last visit?

Family History

- Has your child or anyone in the family (parents, brothers, sisters, grandparents, aunts, uncles, or cousins) developed a new health condition or died? **If the answer is Yes:** Ascertain who in the family has or had the condition, and ask about the age of onset and diagnosis. If the person is no longer living, ask about the age at the time of death.

Social History

- See the Social Determinants of Health priority in Anticipatory Guidance for social history questions.

Surveillance of Development

Do you or any of your child's caregivers have any specific concerns about your child's development, learning, or behavior?

Clinicians using the *Bright Futures Tool and Resource Kit* Previsit Questionnaires or another tool that includes a developmental milestones checklist, or those who use a structured developmental screening tool, need not ask about these developmental surveillance milestones. (*For more information, see the Promoting Healthy Development theme.*)

Social Language and Self-help

Does your child

- Enter bathroom and urinate by herself?
- Put on coat, jacket, or shirt by herself?
- Eat independently?
- Engage in imaginative play?
- Play in cooperation and share?

Verbal Language (Expressive and Receptive)

Does he

- Use 3-word sentences?
- Speak in words that are 75% understandable to strangers?
- Tell you a story from a book or TV?
- Compare things using words like *bigger* or *shorter*?
- Understand simple prepositions, such as *on* or *under*?

Gross Motor

Does she

- Pedal a tricycle?
- Climb on and off couch or chair?
- Jump forward?

Fine Motor

Does he

- Draw a single circle?
- Draw a person with head and 1 other body part?
- Cut with child scissors?

Review of Systems

The Bright Futures Early Childhood Expert Panel recommends a complete review of systems as a part of every health supervision visit. This review can be done through questions about the following:

Does your child have any problems with

- Head
  - Shape
  - Headaches
- Eyes
  - Vision
  - Cross-eyed
- Ears, nose, and throat
- Breathing or chest pain
- Stomach or abdomen
  - Nausea or vomiting
  - Bowel movements
- Skin
  - Birthmarks or moles
- Development
  - Muscle strength, movement, or function
  - Language

Observation of Parent-Child Interaction

During the visit, the health care professional acknowledges and reinforces positive parent-child interactions and discusses any concerns. Observation focuses on

- How do the parent and the child communicate?
- How much of the communication is verbal? Nonverbal?
- Does the parent speak clearly in a conversational tone with the child?
- Does the parent give the child choices (eg, "Do you want to sit or stand?")?
- Does the parent encourage the child's cooperation during the visit?
- Does the parent notice and acknowledge the child's positive behaviors?
- Does unacceptable behavior elicit gentle, but firm limit setting from the parent?

EARLY CHILDHOOD
3 YEAR VISIT

Physical Examination

A complete physical examination is included as part of every health supervision visit.

When performing a physical examination, the health care professional's attention is directed to the following components of the examination that are important for a child this age:

- **Measure and compare with norms for age, sex, and height**
  - Blood pressure

- **Measure and plot on appropriate CDC Growth Chart**
  - Height
  - Weight

- **Calculate and plot on appropriate CDC Growth Chart**
  - BMI

- **Eyes**
  - Assess ocular motility.
  - Examine pupils for opacification and red reflexes.
  - Assess visual acuity using fixate and follow response.

- **Mouth**
  - Observe for caries, plaque, demineralization (white spots), staining, injury, and gingivitis.

- **Skin**
  - Observe for nevi, café-au-lait spots, birthmarks, or bruising.

- **Neurologic**
  - Observe language acquisition and speech clarity.

- **Abdomen**
  - Palpate for masses.

Screening

Universal Screening	Action
Vision	Objective measure with age-appropriate visual acuity measurement using HOTV or LEA symbols. Instrument-based measurement may be used for children who are unable to perform acuity testing.
Oral Health (in the absence of a dental home)	Apply fluoride varnish every 6 months.

Selective Screening	Risk Assessment[a]	Action if Risk Assessment Positive (+)
Anemia	+ on risk screening questions	Hematocrit or hemoglobin
Hearing	+ on risk screening questions	Referral for diagnostic audiologic assessment
Lead	If no previous screen and + on risk screening questions or change in risk	Lead blood test
Oral Health	Does not have a dental home	Referral to dental home or, if not available, oral health risk assessment
	Primary water source is deficient in fluoride.	Oral fluoride supplementation
Tuberculosis	+ on risk screening questions	Tuberculin skin test

[a] See the *Evidence and Rationale chapter* for the criteria on which risk screening questions are based.

Immunizations

Consult the CDC/ACIP or AAP Web sites for the current immunization schedule.

CDC National Immunization Program: **www.cdc.gov/vaccines**

AAP *Red Book:* **http://redbook.solutions.aap.org**

Anticipatory Guidance

The following sample questions, which address the Bright Futures Early Childhood Expert Panel's Anticipatory Guidance Priorities, are intended to be used selectively to invite discussion, gather information, address the needs and concerns of the family, and build partnerships. Use of the questions may vary from visit to visit and from family to family. Questions can be modified to match the health care professional's communication style. The accompanying anticipatory guidance for the family should be geared to questions, issues, or concerns for that particular child and family. Tools and handouts to support anticipatory guidance can be found in the *Bright Futures Tool and Resource Kit*.

Priority

Social Determinants of Health

Risks: Living situation and food security; tobacco, alcohol, and drugs

Strengths and protective factors: Positive family interactions, work-life balance

Risks: Living Situation and Food Security

Parents in difficult living situations or with limited means may have concerns about their access to affordable housing, food, or other resources. Suggest community resources that help with finding quality child care, accessing transportation, or addressing issues such as financial concerns, inadequate resources to cover health care expenses, inadequate or unsafe housing, limited food resources, or lack of social support.

Sample Questions

Tell me about your living situation. Do you have enough heat, hot water, and electricity? Do you have appliances that work? Do you have problems with bugs, rodents, peeling paint or plaster, or mold or dampness?

How are your resources for caring for your child? Do you have enough knowledge to feel comfortable in caring for him? Do you have health insurance? Do you have enough money for food, clothing, and child care?

Within the past 12 months, were you ever worried whether your food would run out before you got money to buy more? Within the past 12 months, did the food you bought not last, and you did not have money to get more?

Have you ever tried to get help for these issues? What happened? What barriers did you face?

Anticipatory Guidance

- If you have problems with any of these things, let me know and I can tell you about community services and other resources that can help you.
- If you need financial assistance to help pay for health care expenses, ask about resources or referrals to the state Medicaid programs or other state assistance and health insurance programs.
- Programs and resources are available to help you and your family. You may be eligible for housing or transportation assistance programs. Several food programs, such as the Commodity Supplemental Food Program and SNAP, the program formerly known as Food Stamps, can help you.

Risks: Tobacco, Alcohol, and Drugs

The use of tobacco, alcohol, and other drugs has adverse health effects on the entire family. Focusing on the effect on health is often the most helpful approach and may help some family members with quitting or cutting back on substance use.

Sample Questions

Does anyone in your home smoke? Are you worried about any family members and how much they smoke, drink, or use drugs?

How often do you drink beer, wine, or liquor in your household? Do you, or does anyone you ride with, ever drive after having a drink? Does your partner use alcohol? What kind and for how long?

Are you using marijuana, cocaine, pain pills, narcotics, or other controlled substances? Are you getting any help to cut down or stop your drug use?

Anticipatory Guidance

- A smoke-free environment, in your car, home, and other places where your child spends time, is important. Smoking affects your child by increasing the risk of asthma, ear infections, and respiratory infections.
- **800-QUIT-NOW (800-784-8669);** TTY **800-332-8615** is a national telephone helpline that is routed to local resources. Additional resources are available at **www.cdc.gov.**
- Drug and alcohol cessation programs are available in our community and we would like to help you connect to these services.

Bright Futures Guidelines for Health Supervision of Infants, Children, and Adolescents

EARLY CHILDHOOD
3 YEAR VISIT

Strengths and Protective Factors: Positive Family Interactions

Healthy family interactions are the foundation of a positive family environment and healthy child development. Noticing and acknowledging positive child behaviors and praising the child's efforts to help around the house help build healthy family interactions. Remind parents that this process also involves creating realistic expectations for acceptable behavior by the child. Discuss consistent limits that are realistic and consistent with the child's developmental level. Frustration and anger are common reactions of both children and parents and can be handled constructively by all family members.

In some situations, it can be helpful to engage parents in a discussion about their experiences as children to help them gain insight into why they parent their children as they do and to help them learn alternative strategies if they tend to use unhelpful or maladaptive strategies.

Sample Questions

Has anything changed at home since your last visit? Tell me how family members show affection for one another? Anger? Describe what you do together as a family. How often do you do these things?

Ask the Child

Who loves you? How do you know? What do you do when you are really mad? What do your parents do? What do you like to do best with your parents?

Anticipatory Guidance

- Show affection in your family.
- Discuss and name emotions like love and sadness.
- Notice and acknowledge your child's positive behaviors. Reward these behaviors with your attention.
- Handle anger constructively in your family by settling disputes with respectful discussion, exercise, or time alone to cool down.
- Don't allow your child to hit, bite, or use other violent behavior. Stop it immediately and use a time-out or change your child's attention to something positive.
- Reinforce limits and appropriate behavior. Enlist all caregivers in efforts to be consistent in expectations and discipline.
- To resolve conflicts, use time-outs or remove the source of conflict.
- Give your child opportunities to make choices, such as what clothes to wear, books to read, what games/activities to play, and places to go.
- Set realistic and developmentally appropriate expectations. Keep instructions and tasks simple and easy to follow.
- Don't be surprised if you talk, act, and think in the same ways your parents did when you were a child. After all, that was your primary experience. You can use this awareness to think about how you want to come across to your own children. What did you like about your parents' style and how would you like to be different?

612

Strengths and Protective Factors: Work-Life Balance

In many families, both parents work full-time or part-time, or are thinking about going back to work.

Remind parents about the importance of carving out special time with their child and note that it is key to a young child's development. Time alone for parents also is valuable. Encourage working parents to maintain family time and to do activities together.

Sample Questions

If you, your partner, or both of you work outside the home, how does that work affect you and your family? Who helps you? Who takes care of your children? How much time does it allow for family activities and what are those activities?

Anticipatory Guidance

- Take time to care for yourself and spend time alone with your partner. Find one or more good, reliable babysitters.
- Create opportunities for your family to share focused time together and for family members to talk, read, and play with your child. This could be as simple as reading a book or taking a short walk together. Point out to your child that this is your special time together.

EARLY CHILDHOOD 3 YEAR VISIT

Priority

Playing With Siblings and Peers
Play opportunities and interactive games, sibling relationships

Play Opportunities and Interactive Games

Playtime with peers provides valuable opportunities to learn social skills that are important to a successful transition to school. By this age, children are able to play interactive games with peers as they begin to learn about taking turns. Encourage parents whose children are not in preschool to arrange playdates for their child. Adults should supervise closely to facilitate interactions, prevent conflicts, and mediate when conflicts occur.

Sample Questions
What are some of the new things that your child is doing? What do you and your partner enjoy most about him these days? What seems most difficult? Tell me about your child's typical play. How does your child interact with children his age? At child care or otherwise? Does he engage in imaginative play with other children? How does he do with sharing?

Ask the Child
What is your favorite toy?

Anticipatory Guidance
- Encourage your child to play with his favorite toys creatively. Toys should be appropriate for his age.
- Expect your child to engage in increasingly elaborate fantasy play, using dolls, toy animals, blocks, vehicles of transport, and other toys, on his own and with others. Dressing up in play clothing is often a favorite activity.
- As often as you can, spend time alone with your child, doing something you both enjoy.
- Provide opportunities for your child to safely explore the world around him.
- If your child is not in child care or preschool, make sure he has opportunities to play with other children.
- Encourage interactive games with peers and help him understand the importance of taking turns.

Sibling Relationships

Siblings play a special role in the socialization and development of self-esteem in the young child. Many parents require advice on how to help their children develop good relationships with each other and how to constructively handle sibling rivalry.

Sample Questions

How do your children get along with one another? How are you preparing your child for the birth of a new baby?

Ask the Child

What do you like to do best with your brothers and sisters?

Anticipatory Guidance

- Help your children develop good relationships with each other. Acknowledge conflicts between siblings and, whenever possible, try to resolve them without taking sides.
- Spend some individual time with each child in your family.

**EARLY CHILDHOOD
3 YEAR VISIT**

Priority

Encouraging Literacy Activities

Reading, talking, and singing together; language development

Reading, Talking, and Singing Together

Encourage interactive reading (reading in which parent and child talk together about the text and pictures as well as the parent reading the book to the child) every day and provide specific advice for parents with no or low literacy. Gaining an awareness of syllables and sounds (phonological awareness) is an important readiness activity for early literacy.

Sample Questions

How often are you able to read to your child? How do you include your child in reading books? Do you and your child have library cards? Do you attend events at your public library? Does he like to draw or do crafts? Play games? How about music? How often do you sing spontaneously or while you are listening to music that others can hear? Do you include your child in the singing or dance movements?

Ask the Child

What is your favorite book? What do you like to do?

Anticipatory Guidance

- Encourage your child's language development and awareness of sounds by reading books, singing songs, and playing rhyming games. Look for ways to practice reading wherever you go, like reading STOP signs or items in stores.
- When taking your child to the grocery store, identify fruits and vegetables by name, color, and shape.
- Use books as a way to talk together. You don't always have to read the text to your child. You can just look at the pictures and talk about the story. Let your child "tell" part of the story.
- Call attention to new words and use them again in a different context.
- Children like rhythm and stories that are found in nursery rhymes, poems, and songs. No matter the quality of your voice, your child likes to be sung to and can remember many songs through the rhythm and repetition. The personal joy emitted by the singer, good or bad, also is contagious and will be transmitted to your child and the home environment.

Language Development

Language continues to develop rapidly at this age. Children should be using plurals, pronouns, sentences of 3 words, and short paragraphs. Speech is understandable to others 75% of the time. The child also should be able to name most common objects, know gender differences, and understand 2-step instructions, such as, "Pick up your doll and put it on the chair."

Sample Questions

How does your child tell you what she wants? What do you think your child understands? What languages does your family speak at home? How well do family members understand your child's speech?

Anticipatory Guidance

- Encourage your child to talk with you about her preschool, friends, experiences, and observations.

Priority

Promoting Healthy Nutrition and Physical Activity
Water, milk, and juice; nutritious foods; competence in motor skills and limits on inactivity

Water, Milk, and Juice

Fluid intake is an important element of nutrition. Water should be provided ad lib at all times and should be regularly offered to children of all ages, with increased attention to water intake in warm or dry environments.

Families may fail to recognize the importance and effect of other fluids to their child's nutrition and it may be useful to remind parents that what we drink contributes protein, fat, and sugar to our daily intake. Milk is an important fluid and protein source and the most accessible source of calcium and vitamin D for children. Juices demand special attention. The sugar content of all juices demands that juice intake be limited, to reduce the risk of dental caries and limit the intake of sugar calories. Soda or soft drinks, sports drinks, and punches provide many calories of scant nutrient value and should be avoided.

Sample Questions
Does your child drink water every day? How many ounces of milk does your child drink most days? Is it whole milk or lower fat milk? Do you give your child other dairy products like yogurt and cheese every day?

Anticipatory Guidance
- Be sure you always have cool water available to your child, especially on warm days and when your child is physically active.
- Young children should drink 16 to 24 oz of low-fat or fat-free milk or fortified soy beverage each day to help meet their calcium and vitamin D needs. Milk is also an important source of protein for growth.
- Avoid using raw milk or any milk substitutes that are not equivalent to cow's milk and that do not meet USDA standards for milk substitutes. These include beverages such as rice milk, almond milk, or coconut milk.
- Juice is not a necessary drink. If you choose to give juice, limit it to 4 oz daily and always serve it with a meal.
- To protect your child's teeth, don't dilute juice with water and don't allow your child to carry around a sippy cup or juice box for drinking over a long period of time.

Nutritious Foods

Meals should be relaxed, safe, and enjoyable family times. Remind parents that they are responsible for providing a variety of nutritious foods and that their child is responsible for how much to eat. Parents can establish positive eating patterns for their child by providing healthy foods at regular intervals throughout the day, giving appropriate amounts, and emphasizing vegetables and fruit and other nutritious foods.

A reduced appetite associated with a slower rate of growth continues at this stage of early childhood. Parents are often distressed when children eat less than they expected, but food refusal often means their child is not hungry. Parents may fail to realize that by encouraging a child to eat when he is not hungry gives him calories he did not ask for and likely doesn't need. Also, preparing substitute foods only encourages picky eating. Discuss the importance of providing healthy snacks and of minimizing foods and beverages that are high in added sugars and saturated fat and low in nutrients.

Sample Questions

Tell me about mealtime in your home. Tell me about mealtime in your child care setting.

Do you consider your child a "healthy eater"? Do you provide a variety of vegetables, fruits, and other nutritious foods? What kind of snacks do you serve? Does your child have much food that you would describe as junk food?

How do you feel if your child doesn't eat what you have prepared for him? What do you do?

Anticipatory Guidance

- Offer a variety of healthy foods to your child, especially vegetables and fruits, and include protein foods like meat and deboned fish at least 2 times per week.
- Help your child explore new flavors and textures in his food.
- Remember that children this age seldom eat "3 square meals a day," but more likely 1 larger meal and multiple smaller meals and snacks.
- When your child refuses something you've prepared, it usually means he is not hungry. It doesn't mean he doesn't like it and wouldn't have it later for a snack.
- Trust your child to determine when he is hungry or full and never encourage him to eat calories he did not ask for.
- Your kitchen is not a fast-food restaurant and you don't need to fix another meal if your child refuses what you have already prepared. This only encourages him to be a picky eater.
  - Have healthy snacks on hand, such as
    - Fresh fruit or vegetables, such as apples, oranges, bananas, cucumber, zucchini, or radishes, that are cut in small pieces or thin strips
    - Applesauce, cheese, or small pieces of whole-grain bread or crackers
    - Unflavored yogurt, sweetened with bits of mashed fruit

Competence in Motor Skills and Limits on Inactivity

By this age, many children have practiced running, jumping, and marching, and have begun to gallop. Children need to play every day; it is their "job." Preschool-aged children learn from watching others and mimicking their movements when they play, and adult guidance can improve their fitness (stability, agility, balance, and coordination). Adults can help their child master physical activity skills by demonstrating ways to move their bodies, how to move around and through objects, and how to confidently learn spatial relationships.

Children should not be inactive for more than 60 minutes at a time, except when sleeping. Counsel parents to limit screen time to no more than 1 hour per day of educational, nonviolent programming with adult supervision. Children should not have media devices (eg, TV, computers, phones, tablets) in their bedrooms, as these devices interfere with sleep and adults are less able to supervise media viewing in this setting.

Talk with parents of children with special health care needs (whether physically or cognitively delayed) to ensure that they have opportunities to be physically active.

Sample Questions

Tell me about what you and your child enjoy doing together each day. If your child is in child care or preschool, what types of physical activity are offered daily? How much time does your child spend watching TV or videos each day? How much time does he spend playing on a computer, phone, or tablet device? Does he have a TV or other device in his bedroom?

Ask the Child

Let me see how fast you can run. What are your favorite games? Do you like to play inside or outside?

Anticipatory Guidance

- Create opportunities for your family to share time and be physically active together.
- Limit all forms of screen time to no more than 1 hour total per day. Do not allow media devices in your child's bedroom because they interfere with sleep and you are less able to supervise their viewing time.
- Monitor the TV programs your child watches. Be aware that many commercials strongly influence even young children to want things that are not healthy for them. Look for media choices that are educational and teach good values, such as empathy, tolerance, and how to get along with others.
- When you allow your child to watch TV, try to watch it together and make it interactive. Ask questions about what is happening on the program and what your child thinks will happen next.
- Starting healthy media habits now is important, because they are a lot harder to change when children are older. Consider making a family media use plan. This plan is a set of rules about media use and screen time that is written down and agreed upon by all family members. Take into account not only the quantity but the quality and location of media use. Consider TVs, phones, tablets, and computers. Rules should be followed by parents as well as children. The AAP has information on how to make a plan at **www.HealthyChildren.org/MediaUsePlan.**

Priority

Safety

Car safety seats, choking prevention, pedestrian safety and falls from windows, water safety, pets, firearm safety

Car Safety Seats

Talk with parents to ensure that they and their child's caregivers know how to securely fasten their child in a car safety seat. Adults should model car safety by always using a seat belt themselves.

In the past year, the parents may have chosen to turn the child's car safety seat forward facing. However, it is even better to continue to ride in the rear-facing position as long as the child has not reached the weight or height limit for the rear-facing position in his convertible seat. Parents should read and follow the manufacturer's instructions for switching a seat from rear facing to forward facing.

Sample Questions

Is your child buckled securely in a car safety seat in the back seat every time he rides in a vehicle? Are you having any problems using your car safety seat?

Ask the Child

Where do you sit when you ride in the car? Do you have a special seat?

Anticipatory Guidance

- The back seat is the safest place for children to ride until age 13 years.
- Continue to use a size-appropriate rear-facing or forward-facing car safety seat that is properly installed in the back seat according to the manufacturer's instructions and the vehicle owner's manual.
- Most 3-year-olds are not tall enough or don't weigh enough to ride safely in a booster seat. It is safest for a child to ride in a car safety seat with a 5-point harness until the child reaches the manufacturer's limit for weight or height.

For information about car safety seats and actions to keep your child safe in and around cars, visit www.safercar.gov/parents.

Find a Child Passenger Safety Technician: http://cert.safekids.org. Click on "Find a Tech."

Toll-free Auto Safety Hotline: 888-327-4236

Choking Prevention

The 3-year-old is able to eat a wide variety of foods. However, he still may have immature chewing and swallowing skills. It is important to continue cutting high-risk foods, like grapes or hot dogs, into small pieces. Other foods that cannot easily be cut into small pieces, like globs of peanut butter, marshmallows, and chewing gum, should be avoided. Children should always be seated and supervised while eating any foods.

Sample Questions

What finger foods do you give your child? Do you continue to cut foods such as grapes and hot dogs into small pieces?

Anticipatory Guidance

- It is important to continue to cut foods such as grapes and hot dogs into small pieces.
- The size of your child's airway still makes these foods high-risk for choking.
- Seated and supervised is a safe meal.

Pedestrian Safety and Falls From Windows

Unintentional injury is the number one cause of death among young children. Because the urge to explore and learn is so strong, and young children do not have a developed sense of good judgment, parents must use constant vigilance and regularly review the safety of the environment to protect them from harm.

Remind parents about the importance of installing operable window guards on all windows on the second floor and higher. Window screens alone are not adequate guards.

Sample Questions

Who watches your child when you cannot? Does your child play in a driveway or close to the street? What floor in your house or apartment do you live on? Do you have window guards on all windows on the second floor and higher?

Ask the Child

When you play outside, who watches you? Who watches you when your parents are gone?

Anticipatory Guidance

- Never leave your child alone in the car, house, or yard.
- Do not allow young brothers or sisters to watch over your child.
- Supervise all outdoor play. Driveways and streets are not safe places to play. Your child is not ready to cross the street alone.
- Remember that many young children are excellent climbers. To prevent children from falling out of windows, keep furniture away from windows and install operable window guards on second- and higher-story windows.

Water Safety

Parents still must supervise their child closely to ensure his safety around water. All children require constant supervision by an adult whenever they are near water. Swim lessons do not provide drown-proofing at any age. However, parents may choose to start their child in swimming lessons depending on the child's readiness and frequency of exposure to water.

Sample Question

Are there swimming pools or other potential water dangers near or in your home?

Anticipatory Guidance

- Provide "touch supervision" any time your toddler is in or near water, even small play swimming pools. This means that a parent or responsible adult is within an arm's reach of the child at all times.
- Be sure that swimming pools in your community, apartment complex, or home have a 4-sided fence that completely separates the pool from the house and the yard with a self-closing, self-latching gate.
- Children should always wear a properly fitted US Coast Guard–approved life jacket when on a boat or other watercraft. Simple blow-up water wings do NOT prevent drowning.
- If a child is missing, check the pool or spa first. Consider learning CPR.

Pets

Pets can be a source of great joy for children, but should be kept under constant watch when they are around young children. Dog and cat bites are particularly common at this age.

Sample Questions

Do you own a pet or animals? How does your child get along with your pet or animals?

Anticipatory Guidance

- Pets are a great source of fun and help to develop a child's sense of responsibility. Educate your child on animal safety to avoid bite and scratch injury. Teach your toddler to ask permission before petting or playing with a dog, and help him learn to be gentle with all types of pets.

Firearm Safety

Young children are curious about everything, including firearms, and have no concept of the consequences of firing a weapon. Firearms should be removed from places in which children live and play. If it is necessary to keep a firearm in the home, it should be stored unloaded and locked, with the ammunition locked separately from the firearm.

Sample Question

Is there a firearm in your home or in the homes where your child might play or go for child care?

Anticipatory Guidance

- Remember that young children simply do not understand how dangerous firearms can be, despite your warnings. They cannot be taught not to handle a firearm if they find one. The best way to keep your child safe from injury or death from firearms is to never have a firearm in your home.

- Children this age are naturally curious and will get into everything! Just as you need to keep medications, cleaning solutions, and insecticides out of children's reach, loaded firearms should never be anywhere where your child can get to them. If it is necessary to keep a firearm in your home, it should be stored unloaded and locked, with the ammunition locked separately from the firearm.

- Ask if there are firearms in homes where your child plays. If so, make sure they are stored unloaded and locked, with the ammunition locked separately, before allowing your child to play in the home.

Early Childhood
4 Year Visit

Context

Rapidly developing language skills, combined with an insatiable curiosity, enlarge the world of the 4-year-old and give him a sense of independence. Able to dress and undress himself and maintain bowel and bladder control (although he may not be dry at night), the 4-year-old feels grown up beyond his years. Although his thinking remains self-focused, he is sensitive to the feelings of others. He identifies such emotions as joy, happiness, sadness, anger, anxiety, and fear, in others as well as himself. Now he plays collaboratively and he has budding friendships with his peers.

Talkative and animated, the 4-year-old is a delightful conversationalist, able to tell an involved story or relate a recent experience, often interrupting a conversation as if it were not occurring. He frequently demands to know why, what, when, and how. Lying or failing to take responsibility for his actions is common. His seemingly boundless energy and increased motor skills find release in group games and physical activities, such as running, climbing, swinging, sliding, and jumping. Yet, he also needs opportunities to rest and play quietly by himself. Imaginative play, including make-believe and dress up, reflect the fantasy and magical thinking of this age. Media use (eg, TV, computers, cell phones, and tablets) and even educational videos may hold a strong appeal for this new fascination with fantasy and may hold excessive power over his time and attention unless limited by parents and child care providers. Parents should choose and preview age-appropriate media choices, co-view, and monitor content, time, and behavior related to media use.

Because 4-year-olds are curious about their own bodies and those of the opposite sex, genital exploration is typical at this age. Modesty and a desire for privacy also begin to emerge. Every culture considers sexual behaviors and explorations in different ways. The health care professional must attempt to gain an understanding of the cultural norms of the child's family when addressing the topic of sexuality. In some cultures, an open discussion of this topic is inappropriate. That belief must be respected, but cautiously explored to ensure the child's safety. To help them address culturally specific issues, especially sensitive issues like sexuality, health care practices should employ staff from the communities served whenever possible and should ask employees to learn about the cultural beliefs of the community.

Some children are gender nonconforming, gender variant, or transgender and it may manifest at this age. By this age, some children will identify themselves as a gender different from the gender they were assigned. Children who have gender identities that differ from their assigned sex may start to display distress if faced with conflicting expectations from adults about how they should act or dress.

The child enjoys and looks forward to the social and learning opportunities at preschool. Argumentative behavior with peers can present a problem at preschool or during play, but the 4-year-old can learn to be assertive without being aggressive. Making allowances for the appropriateness of the match between the child and the program, the 4-year-old's experiences in the early education and child care settings provide an important measure of his social development and his developing readiness for elementary school.

The 4-year-old is a terrific companion who responds well to praise and clearly stated rules. However, his family also may find his behavior frustrating and challenging at times. He is still trying to understand how and why things work as they do and he is interested in seeing the consequences of his actions on family members. How many times will his parents say, "No," before they get angry? How far off the sidewalk can he stray before they chase after him? How many toys can he take before his sister protests? In his efforts to learn about appropriate social interaction and expected behavior in the family, he frequently tests the limits of his parents and siblings.

With the parent in the room, reassure the child at the beginning of the physical examination through talking and through touch. The child should be able to discuss the function of the eyes and ears, relate recent and past memories, or relate how to take a bath, and he may want to listen with your stethoscope. The examination may flow easily from head to toe. Talking about the physical findings is instructive to the child and parent and demystifies the office visit. The child at 4 years of age often participates in the examination to a much greater degree than at past visits. Speaking to the child about what is being examined and how, and including the child in conversation about his ears, eyes, muscles, and other body parts, successfully engages the 4-year-old's curiosity and gains his cooperation.

Priorities for the 4 Year Visit

The first priority is to attend to the concerns of the parents.

In addition, the Bright Futures Early Childhood Expert Panel emphasizes the following topics for discussion at this visit:

▶ Social determinants of health[a] (risks [living situation and food security; tobacco, alcohol, and drugs; intimate partner violence; safety in the community], strengths and protective factors [engagement in the community])

▶ School readiness (language understanding and fluency, feelings, opportunities to socialize with other children, readiness for structured learning experiences, early childhood programs and preschool)

▶ Developing healthy nutrition and personal habits (water, milk, and juice; nutritious foods; daily routines that promote health)

▶ Media use (limits on use, promoting physical activity and safe play)

▶ Safety (belt-positioning car booster seats, outdoor safety, water safety, sun protection, pets, firearm safety)

[a] Social determinants of health is a new priority in the fourth edition of the *Bright Futures Guidelines*. For more information, see the *Promoting Lifelong Health for Families and Communities theme.*

Health Supervision

The *Bright Futures Tool and Resource Kit* contains Previsit Questionnaires to assist the health care professional in taking a history, conducting developmental surveillance, and performing medical screening.

History

Interval history may be obtained according to the concerns of the family and the health care professional's preference or style of practice. The following questions can encourage in-depth discussion:

General Questions

- What are you most proud of about your child? (If the parent responds, "Nothing," the clinician should be prepared with a compliment, such as, "You made time for this visit despite your busy schedule.")
- Tell me about his abilities and what he most likes and dislikes these days.
- How is your child doing at home, preschool, or child care?
- What questions or concerns do you have about him? His health? His ability to get along with other people?
- How are things going for your family?
- How are things going for your child?
- What changes have occurred in your family over the past year?

Past Medical History

- Has your child received any specialty or emergency care since the last visit?

Family History

- Has your child or anyone in the family (parents, brothers, sisters, grandparents, aunts, uncles, or cousins) developed a new health condition or died? **If the answer is Yes:** Ascertain who in the family has or had the condition, and ask about the age of onset and diagnosis. If the person is no longer living, ask about the age at the time of death.

Social History

- See the Social Determinants of Health priority in Anticipatory Guidance for social history questions.

Surveillance of Development

Do you or any of your child's caregivers have any specific concerns about your child's development, learning, or behavior?

Clinicians using the *Bright Futures Tool and Resource Kit* Previsit Questionnaires or another tool that includes a developmental milestones checklist, or those who use a structured developmental screening tool, need not ask about these developmental surveillance milestones. *(For more information, see the Promoting Healthy Development theme.)*

Social Language and Self-help

Does your child

- Enter the bathroom and have a bowel movement by himself?
- Brush teeth?
- Dress and undress without much help?
- Engage in well-developed imaginative play?

Verbal Language (Expressive and Receptive)

Does she

- Answer questions like "What do you do when you are cold?" or "…when you are sleepy?"
- Use 4-word sentences?
- Speak in words that are 100% understandable to strangers?
- Draw pictures you recognize?
- Follow simple rules when playing board or card games?
- Tell you a story from a book?

Gross Motor

Does he

- Skip on 1 foot?
- Climb stairs, alternating feet, without support?

Fine Motor

Does she

- Draw a person with at least 3 body parts?
- Draw simple cross?
- Unbutton and button medium-sized buttons?
- Grasp pencil with thumb and fingers instead of fist?

Review of Systems

The Bright Futures Early Childhood Expert Panel recommends a complete review of systems as a part of every health supervision visit. This review can be done through questions about the following:

Does your child have any problems with

- Head
  - Headaches
- Eyes
  - Vision
  - Cross-eyed
- Ears, nose, and throat
- Breathing or chest pain
- Stomach or abdomen
  - Nausea or vomiting
  - Bowel movements
- Skin
  - Birthmarks or moles
- Development
  - Muscle strength, movement, or function
  - Language

Observation of Parent-Child Interaction

During the visit, the health care professional acknowledges and reinforces positive parent-child interactions and discusses any concerns. Observation focuses on

- How do the parent and the child communicate?
- Does the parent allow the child to answer the health care professional's questions directly, or does the parent intervene?
- Does the child separate from the parent for the weighing and measuring and the physical examination?
- Does the child dress and undress himself?
- Does the parent pay attention to the child's behavior, verbally correcting unacceptable behavior?
- How do the parent, the 4-year-old, and any siblings interact? Does the parent pay attention to all of the children?
- If child is offered 2 or more books to choose from, does the parent advise and encourage, and then let the child choose?

Physical Examination

A complete physical examination is included as part of every health supervision visit.

When performing a physical examination, the health care professional's attention is directed to the following components of the examination that are important for a child this age:

- **Measure and compare with norms for age, sex, and height**
  - Blood pressure

- **Measure and plot on appropriate CDC Growth Chart**
  - Height
  - Weight

- **Calculate and plot on appropriate CDC Growth Chart**
  - BMI

- **ENT**
  - Nasal stuffiness

- **Teeth**
  - Observe for white spots and gum inflammation.

- **Skin**
  - Observe for rashes or bruises.

- **Eyes**
  - Assess ocular motility.
  - Examine pupils for opacification and red reflexes.

- **Abdomen**
  - Palpate for masses.

- **Neurologic**
  - Assess fine and gross motor skills: Draw a picture. A formal assessment of the motor system is indicated at this age.
  - Observe language acquisition, speech fluency and clarity, thought content, and abstraction; articulation difficulties.

Screening

Universal Screening	Action
Hearing	Audiometry
Oral Health (in the absence of a dental home)	Apply fluoride varnish every 6 months.
Vision	Objective measure with age-appropriate visual acuity measurement using HOTV or LEA symbols. Instrument-based measurement may be used for children who are unable to perform acuity testing.

Selective Screening	Risk Assessment[a]	Action if Risk Assessment Positive (+)
Anemia	+ on risk screening questions	Hematocrit or hemoglobin
Dyslipidemia	+ on risk screening questions and not previously screened with normal results	Lipid profile
Lead	If no previous screen and + on risk screening questions or change in risk	Lead blood test
Oral Health	Does not have a dental home	Referral to dental home
	Primary water source is deficient in fluoride.	Oral fluoride supplementation
Tuberculosis	+ on risk screening questions	Tuberculin skin test

[a] See the *Evidence and Rationale chapter* for the criteria on which risk screening questions are based.

Immunizations

Consult the CDC/ACIP or AAP Web sites for the current immunization schedule.

CDC National Immunization Program: **www.cdc.gov/vaccines**

AAP *Red Book:* **http://redbook.solutions.aap.org**

Anticipatory Guidance

The following sample questions, which address the Bright Futures Early Childhood Expert Panel's Anticipatory Guidance Priorities, are intended to be used selectively to invite discussion, gather information, address the needs and concerns of the family, and build partnerships. Use of the questions may vary from visit to visit and from family to family. Questions can be modified to match the health care professional's communication style. The accompanying anticipatory guidance for the family should be geared to questions, issues, or concerns for that particular child and family. Tools and handouts to support anticipatory guidance can be found in the *Bright Futures Tool and Resource Kit.*

Priority

Social Determinants of Health

Risks: Living situation and food security; tobacco, alcohol, and drugs; intimate partner violence; safety in the community

Strengths and protective factors: Engagement in the community

Risks: Living Situation and Food Security

Parents in difficult living situations or with limited means may have concerns about their access to affordable housing, food, or other resources. Provide information and referrals, as needed, for community resources that help with finding quality child care, accessing transportation, or addressing issues such as financial concerns, inadequate or unsafe housing, or limited food resources. Public health agencies can be excellent sources of help because they work with all types of community agencies and family needs. Facilitate referrals.

Sample Questions

Tell me about your living situation. Do you live in an apartment or a house? Is permanent housing a worry for you? Do you have the things you need to take care of your child? Does your home have enough heat, hot water, electricity, working appliances? Do you need help paying for health insurance?

Within the past 12 months, were you ever worried whether your food would run out before you got money to buy more? Within the past 12 months, did the food you bought not last, and you did not have money to get more?

Have you ever tried to get help for these issues? What happened? What barriers did you face?

Anticipatory Guidance

- Community agencies are available to help you with concerns about your living situation.
- If you need financial assistance to help pay for health care expenses, ask about resources or referrals to the state Medicaid program or other state assistance and health insurance programs.
- Programs and resources are available to help you and your family. You may be eligible for housing or transportation assistance programs. Several food programs, such as the Commodity Supplemental Food Program and SNAP, the program formerly known as Food Stamps, can help you.

Risks: Tobacco, Alcohol, And Drugs

The use of tobacco, alcohol, and other drugs has adverse health effects on the entire family. Focusing on the effect on health is often the most helpful approach and may help some family members with quitting or cutting back on substance use.

Sample Questions

Does anyone in your home smoke? Are you worried about any family members and how much they smoke, drink, or use drugs?

How often do you drink beer, wine, or liquor in your household? Do you, or does anyone you ride with, ever drive after having a drink? Does your partner use alcohol? What kind and for how long?

Are you using marijuana, cocaine, pain pills, narcotics, or other controlled substances? Are you getting any help to cut down or stop your drug use?

Anticipatory Guidance

- A smoke-free environment, in your car, home, and other places where your child spends time, is important. Smoking affects your child by increasing the risk of asthma, ear infections, and respiratory infections.
- **800-QUIT-NOW (800-784-8669); TTY 800-332-8615** is a national telephone helpline that is routed to local resources. Additional resources are available at **www.cdc.gov.**
- Drug and alcohol cessation programs are available in our community and we would like to help you connect to these services.

**EARLY CHILDHOOD
4 YEAR VISIT**

Risks: Intimate Partner Violence

Children who are exposed to intimate partner violence are at increased risk of adverse mental and physical health outcomes. Intimate partner violence cannot be determined through observation, but is best identified through direct inquiry. When inquiring, avoid asking about abuse or domestic violence. Instead, use descriptive terms, such as *hit, kicked, shoved, choked,* and *threatened.*

To avoid causing upset to families by questioning about sensitive and private topics, such as family violence, alcohol and drug use, and similar risks, it is recommended to begin screening about these topics with an introductory statement, such as, "I ask all patients standard health questions to understand factors that may affect health of their child and their health."

Because of the sensitivity of the topic and the desirability of avoiding distress to a receptive child, it may be necessary to have this conversation with the parent alone. Alternatively, some health care professionals prefer to use a written screen to assess for potential intimate partner violence. Either approach may help increase disclosure and minimize increasing risk of violence in the family.

Provide information on the effect of intimate partner violence on children and describe community resources that provide assistance. Recommend resources and support groups. Many states have laws that require all cases of intimate partner violence to be reported when a child is in the home.

Sample Questions

Because violence is so common in many people's lives, I've begun to ask about it. I don't know if violence is a problem for you, but many children I see have parents who have been hurt by someone else. Some are too afraid or uncomfortable to bring it up, so I've started asking about it routinely. Do you always feel safe in your home? Has your partner or ex-partner ever hit, kicked, or shoved you, or physically hurt you or your child? Are you scared that your partner or someone else may try to hurt you or your child? What will you do if you feel this way? Do you have a plan? How do you handle the feeling? Would you like information about who to contact or where to go if you need help?

Anticipatory Guidance

- If you feel unsafe in your home, seek help in moving your children and yourself to a safe place.
- One way that I and other health care professionals can help you if your partner is hitting or threatening you is to support you and provide information about local resources that can help you.
- You can also call the toll-free **National Domestic Violence Hotline** at **800-799-SAFE (7233).**

Risks: Safety in the Community

Parents should know the adults with whom their children will come in contact. Parents should keep their children away from any adult or older child they think may be dangerous.

Sample Questions

How safe do you feel in your community? Do you or other trusted adults watch over your child when she is in the neighborhood? How cautious is your child around strangers? Who do you turn to if you have concerns about your child's safety?

Anticipatory Guidance

- Explain to your child that certain parts of the body (those areas normally covered by a bathing suit) are private and should not be touched by others without her permission.
- Use correct terms for all body parts, including the genitals. A 4-year-old may repetitively use words related to bodily elimination functions and can be gently reminded that these words are best used in private, if at all.
- Anticipate your child's normal curiosity about her body and the differences between boys and girls.
- People who abuse children are often persons whom other members of the family may consider to be trustworthy. Teach your child rules for how to be safe with all adults, using these 3 principles: (1) no adult should tell a child to keep secrets from parents, (2) no adult should express special interest in the private parts, and (3) no adult should ask a child for help with the adult's own private parts.

Strengths and Protective Factors: Engagement in the Community

As children begin to spend more time outside the home in preschool, neighborhood, and playground activities, and developmentally enjoy playing with other children, the safety of the environment becomes critical. An environment where young children are physically and emotionally safe enhances the efforts of the family to support their child's healthy development. Talk with the parents about available high-quality community programs and experiences for their child.

Sample Questions

What activities do you participate in outside of the home? What help do you need in finding other community resources, such as a faith-based group, recreational centers, or volunteer opportunities? What help do you need in finding safe places in your community where your child can play and participate in activities? Do you know parents of other children? Tell me about family or friends you enjoy spending your free time with. Can you go to them when you have a problem?

Anticipatory Guidance

- Maintain or expand ties to your community through social, faith-based, cultural, volunteer, and recreational organizations or programs.
- Participate in community projects that provide opportunities for physical activity for the whole family, such as walkathons, community cleanup day, or a community garden project.
- Find out what you can do to make your community safe.
- Advocate for and participate in a neighborhood watch program.
- Advocate for adequate housing and for safe play spaces and playgrounds.

Priority

School Readiness

Language understanding and fluency, feelings, opportunities to socialize with other children, readiness for structured learning experiences, early childhood programs and preschool

Language Understanding and Fluency

A 4-year-old best understands explanations that are short and to the point, and that refer to the direct experiences of the child.

As children develop speech and language skills, they often experience normal disfluencies, such as repetitions of whole words, false starts and revisions in sentences, or stuttering. Most children outgrow stuttering. Indications for speech evaluation include stuttering for more than 6 months and no improvement during this time. Referral may be appropriate if the parent describes the child as struggling to get words out and showing signs of distress about difficulties with speaking.

Sample Questions

What do you think your child understands? For example, can he understand concepts of "same" and "different"? Does he understand 2- or 3-step instructions?

How does your child communicate what he wants and knows? Can he speak clearly enough so that strangers understand him almost 100% of the time? Does he use the past as well as the present tense? Does he use sentences of 4 words and short paragraphs? Can he describe a recent experience? Does he like to sing?

Ask the Child

Do you have a favorite storybook that you like to hear? What music or songs do you like? Do you like to dance?

Anticipatory Guidance

- Because children this age ask many questions, it is easy to offer too much information. It is best to keep answers short, simple, and factual.
- Help your child develop his language skills by encouraging him to talk with you about his preschool, friends, experiences, or observations.
- Read together daily and ask your child questions about the stories.
- Provide plenty of time for your child to tell stories or respond to questions. Hurrying a child's response increases stuttering.
- Allow children to finish sentences and thoughts, do not interrupt, speak in a relaxed tone, and pause before responding.
- Sing together and play music often.

Feelings

At 4 years, children are very sensitive. They wear their feelings on their sleeves and are easily encouraged or hurt by what people say or do to them.

Sample Questions

How does your child act around others? Is he generally happy and active? What do you do when he is sad or upset? Has his personality or predominant mood changed much since he was younger?

Anticipatory Guidance

- Watching your child interact with other children provides a valuable window into his social understanding and skills.
- Listen to and always treat your child with the respect you offer a fellow adult. Insist that all family members treat one another with respect and model respectful behavior for your children.
- Model apologizing if you are wrong or have hurt someone's feelings. Help your child apologize for hurting others' feelings, too. Praise him when he demonstrates sensitivity to the feelings of others.
- Reassure your children that nothing is wrong with strong emotions. Help your child express such feelings as joy, anger, sadness, fear, and frustration. Letting him know that strong emotions are normal can decrease his stress and help him calm down. Remind your children that strong emotions are not problems, but what we do about them can be.
- Learning to handle emotions appropriately is the beginning of learning healthy coping styles. Teach him how to cope with strong emotions by using healthy distractions like exercise, singing, dancing, drawing, and avoiding unhealthy distractions like eating or watching TV.

Opportunities to Socialize With Other Children

At this age, children spend increasing amounts of time with peers and begin enjoying participating in a group environment. Learning to interact with other children helps to build strong social skills.

Sample Questions

How interested is your child in other children? How confident is he socially and emotionally? Who are his special playmates?

Ask the Child

Who do you like to play with? Do you have a favorite friend?

Anticipatory Guidance

- Praise your child for his cooperation and accomplishments.
- As often as you can, spend time alone with your child doing something you both enjoy.
- Provide opportunities for your child to play with other children in playgroups, preschool, or other community activities.

EARLY CHILDHOOD
4 YEAR VISIT

Readiness for Structured Learning Experiences

Readiness for a structured learning experience is a lengthy process that begins at birth. Advise parents about ways to prepare their child for a successful transition to school. Early literacy skills are emerging as children show interest in letters and play with sounds, making rhymes of real and nonsense words.

Sample Questions

How is your child learning and getting ready for school? What thoughts have you had about starting her in school in the year ahead? Do you need help in finding and signing up for educational opportunities for your child?

Anticipatory Guidance

- Read interactively with your child. Reading with your child is important to help him enjoy reading and be ready for school.
- As your child shows interest in words, engage him by pointing out letters, particularly the ones that begin his name, such as, "It's a T like in Taylor!" and playing with sounds by making rhymes of real and nonsense words, such as, "oodles and boodles of noodles and foodles."
- Enlarge your child's experiences through trips and visits to parks and other places of interest. Take him often to the library. Ask whether he can get a library card, and let him choose books that interest him.

Early Childhood Programs and Preschool

High-quality early care and education programs, whether they be Head Start, preschool, Sunday school, or a community program or child care center, have a positive effect on a child's socialization, school readiness, health, and ultimate success in life. Encourage parents to become actively involved in their child's preschool or child care program and to talk with their child about her activities and experiences at school. If your state has free, state-funded prekindergarten, discuss this option with parents.

Sample Questions

How happy are you with your preschool or child care arrangements? What does your child care provider or teacher say about your child? On most days, does she seem happy to go? How many other children are in her class and how is she coping socially?

Ask the Child

What do you like to do best at child care/preschool?

Anticipatory Guidance

- Visit your child's preschool or other child care program. You can learn a lot about what really goes on at the program if you arrive unannounced.
- Become actively involved in your child's preschool or care program, and ensure good communication between you and the program.
- You may be eligible for free, state-funded prekindergarten. If you are interested, I can give you information.
- Show interest in your child's preschool or child care activities. Talk to your child about his daily activities and what he's learning.
- If your child is in child care, continue to provide personal items, such as blankets, clothing, combs, and brushes, for his own use.

Priority

Developing Healthy Nutrition and Personal Habits
Milk, water, and juice; nutritious foods; daily routines that promote health

Milk, Water, and Juice

Fluid intake is an important element of nutrition. Water should be provided ad lib at all times and should be regularly offered to children of all ages, with increased attention to water intake in warm or dry environments.

Families may fail to recognize the importance and effect of other fluids to their child's nutrition and it may be useful to remind parents that what we drink contributes protein, fat, and sugar to our daily intake. Milk is an important fluid and protein source and is the most accessible source of calcium and vitamin D for children.

Juices demand special attention. The sugar content of all juices demands that juice intake be limited, to reduce the risk of dental caries and limit the intake of sugar calories. Soda or soft drinks, sports drinks, and punches provide many calories of scant nutrient value and should be avoided.

Sample Questions
Does your child drink water every day? How many ounces of milk does she drink most days? Is it whole milk or lower fat milk? Do you give your child other dairy products like yogurt and cheese every day?

Anticipatory Guidance
- Be sure your child always has cool water available, especially on warm days and when she is physically active.
- Young children should drink 16 to 24 oz of low-fat or fat-free milk each day to help meet their calcium and vitamin D needs. Milk is also an important source of protein for growth.
- Juice is not a necessary drink. If you choose to give juice, limit it to 4 oz daily and always serve it with a meal.
- To protect your child's teeth, don't dilute juice with water and don't allow her to carry around a sippy cup or juice box for prolonged consumption.

Nutritious Foods

Meals should be relaxed, safe, and enjoyable family times. Remind parents that they are responsible for providing a variety of nutritious foods and that their child is responsible for how much to eat. Parents can establish positive eating patterns for their child by providing healthy foods at regular intervals throughout the day, giving appropriate amounts, and emphasizing vegetables and fruit and other nutritious foods.

A reduced appetite associated with a slower rate of growth continues at this stage of early childhood. Parents are often distressed when children eat less than they expected, but food refusal often means their child is not hungry. Parents may fail to realize that by encouraging a child to eat when she is not hungry gives her calories she did not ask for and likely doesn't need. Also, preparing substitute foods only encourages picky eating. Discuss the importance of providing healthy snacks and of minimizing foods and beverages that are high in added sugars and saturated fat and low in nutrients.

Sample Questions

Tell me about mealtime in your home. Tell me about mealtime in your child care setting.

Do you consider your child a "healthy eater"? Do you provide a variety of vegetables, fruits, and other nutritious foods? What kind of snacks do you serve? Does your child have much food that you would describe as junk food? How do you feel if your child doesn't eat what you have prepared for her? What do you do?

Anticipatory Guidance

- Offer a variety of healthy foods to your child, especially vegetables and fruits, and include higher protein foods like meat and deboned fish at least 2 times per week.
- Help your child explore new flavors and textures in her food.
- Remember that children this age seldom eat "3 square meals a day," but more likely 1 good meal and multiple smaller meals and snacks.
- When your child refuses something you've prepared, it usually means she is not hungry. It doesn't mean she doesn't like it and wouldn't have it later for a snack.
- Trust your child to determine when she is hungry or full and never encourage her to eat food she did not ask for.
- Your kitchen is not a fast-food restaurant and you don't need to fix another meal if your child refuses what you have already prepared. This only encourages her to be a picky eater.
- Have healthy snacks on hand, such as
  - Fresh fruit or vegetables, such as apples, oranges, bananas, cucumber, zucchini, or radishes, that are cut in small pieces or thin strips
  - Applesauce, cheese, or small pieces of whole-grain bread or crackers
  - Unflavored yogurt, sweetened with bits of mashed fruit

Daily Routines That Promote Health

The 4-year-old typically enjoys being recognized as being "big enough" to assume greater independence in daily routines, like getting dressed and washing hands. Helping with household chores is particularly rewarding. Learning simple cooking skills, like stirring ingredients in a bowl, will enhance food acceptance.

Nightmares and night terrors are common at this age. Discuss the parents' approach to sleep disturbances. Family stresses and TV viewing habits should be evaluated in children with sleep disturbances.

Sample Questions

How is she sleeping at night? Does she still require a nap on most days? Are you encouraging her to take a more active role in daily routines connected with mealtimes, cleanliness, and help around the house?

Ask the Child

What do you like to eat? Are you getting good at brushing your teeth and washing your hands? Can you fasten your own seat belt?

Anticipatory Guidance

- Create a calm bedtime ritual that includes reading or telling stories to promote language development and pre-reading skills and to help your child sleep peacefully.
- A poor appetite or limited food preference is not a major concern if your child's growth rate has been normal. Create a pleasant atmosphere at mealtimes by turning off the TV and having table conversation that includes your child. Focus the conversation away from how much or even which of the foods the child is eating. Talk about where the food comes from, how others might cook the same food, and any other ideas that stimulates your child's natural curiosity. Allow your child to stop eating when full even if that means leaving food on her plate.
- Be sure that your child brushes her teeth twice a day with a pea-sized amount of fluoridated toothpaste. She should spit out the toothpaste after brushing, but not rinse her mouth with water. Supervise tooth brushing each time.

Priority

Media Use

Limits on use, promoting physical activity and safe play

Limits on Use

Inappropriate and excessive media use has been associated with attention problems, impaired sleep, school difficulties, and obesity. It also has been shown to increase violence in children, create conflicts over purchase of advertised products, and decrease time for physically active play.

Judicious use of educational media can improve school readiness in children, but children should spend no more than 1 hour total a day watching or using any type of media. They should not have a TV or digital device in their bedrooms. Parents should preview media content and monitor use and content. The TV should be turned off during mealtimes.

Explore the reason or motivations behind media use. Many preschoolers need help learning self-regulation skills (how to calm down, handle strong emotions, and control their bodies), and giving them a device may seem like an easy way to keep them calm during difficult moments, but does not teach them more internal ways of regulating themselves. Excessive media use is associated with worse behavioral regulation in the long-term, so it should be discouraged as the main way parents use to keep children calm. Parents can offer alternative approaches, such as avoiding tantrum triggers, using time-outs or calm-down time, teaching breathing or sensory regulation techniques, or teaching them to learn the words for their emotions. Discuss that media use at bedtime actually leads to worse sleep habits, less sleep, and school problems. Parents can offer alternative approaches, such as a bedtime routine or reading books in bed.

Sample Questions

What digital media devices do your children use, such as handheld devices, video games, digital toys, TV, or computers? Does your child have a TV in his bedroom? Does your child have a computer or tablet in his bedroom?

Ask the Child

What is your favorite TV show or computer? Why do you like it?

Anticipatory Guidance

- At this age, preschool-aged children can learn things like language, early literacy, and early math skills from well-designed educational TV and apps. Content is very important, and many educational shows have good messages about positive behaviors and friendship. However, children need other experiences, too, such as unstructured play alone and with peers, time outdoors, and hands-on learning to develop all parts of their brain, including more complicated skills such as executive functioning and social skills.

- Limit TV and video viewing and use of other media devices to no more than 1 hour per day. Do not allow digital devices in your child's bedroom because they interfere with sleep and you are less able to supervise your child's viewing time.

- Consider the reasons why you allow your child to watch TV or play video games. Is it to control his behavior or help him get to sleep? Unfortunately, media doesn't actually help children regulate their behavior or sleep better. Using other approaches, such as calm down time, breathing techniques, learning words to describe their emotions, and quiet bedtime routines, are a better option.

- Starting healthy media habits now is important, because they are a lot harder to change when children are older. Consider making a family media use plan. This plan is a set of rules about media use and screen time that is written down and agreed upon by all family members. Take into account not only the quantity but the quality and location of media use, including TVs, phones, tablets, and computers. Rules should be followed by parents as well as children. This kind of plan can help you preserve special face-to-face time during family routines, such as meals, playtime, and bedtime. You may even want to designate some parts of your home as media-free. The AAP has information on how to make a plan at **www.HealthyChildren.org/MediaUsePlan.**

- Supervise any Internet use so that you can teach your child skills to help him stay safe.

Promoting Physical Activity and Safe Play

Unless a child has a developmental delay, he should be able to run, hop, march, and gallop, and try to jump by this age. He should also be able to balance on 1 foot and cross the midline (right hand to left side; left foot in front of right foot).

Sample Questions

Does your child play with other children? Does he play outdoors as well as indoors? Is your community safe for him to play outdoors?

Ask the Child

Let me see you hop. What else do you like to do when you play?

Anticipatory Guidance

- Encourage your child to be active in many ways, including running, marching, and jumping. Praise him for his ability to do these activities.

- As often as possible, be physically active as a family. Go on walks, play in the park or on a safe street, or ride bikes. Use this time to help your child get to know his community.

- Make sure your child has plenty of opportunity for active play at child care or preschool.

Priority

Safety

Belt-positioning car booster seats, outdoor safety, water safety, sun protection, pets, firearm safety

Belt-Positioning Car Booster Seats

At this age, children are best protected in a car safety seat with a 5-point harness. However, some large 4-year-olds may start to outgrow the manufacturer's weight or height limit for a seat with a harness. Most forward-facing car safety seats have weight limits of 65 pounds or more and height limits of 49 inches or more. Children should ride in car safety seats with 5-point harnesses as long as possible. When the child has outgrown the car safety seat with a harness, she should ride in a belt-positioning booster seat in the back seat. Adults should model car safety by always using a seat belt themselves.

Sample Question

Is your child fastened securely in a car safety seat or belt-positioning booster seat in the back seat every time she rides in a vehicle?

Ask the Child

Where do you sit when you ride in the car? Do you have a special seat?

Anticipatory Guidance

- Continue to use a size-appropriate forward-facing car safety seat that is properly installed in the back seat according to the manufacturer's instructions and the vehicle owner's manual until your child reaches the highest weight or height allowed by the manufacturer, her shoulders are above the top harness slots, or her ears come to the top of the car safety seat. When she reaches one of these limits, consider whether she is mature enough for the greater flexibility of movement allowed by a belt-positioning booster seat. If not, use a forward-facing seat with a harness with a higher weight limit or a travel vest. Many 4-year-olds are not tall enough or do not weigh enough to ride safely in a booster seat.
- The back seat is the safest place for children to ride until your child is age 13 years.

For information about car safety seats and actions to keep your child safe in and around cars, visit www.safercar.gov/parents.

Find a Child Passenger Safety Technician: http://cert.safekids.org. Click on "Find a Tech."

Toll-free Auto Safety Hotline: 888-327-4236

Outdoor Safety

Young children lack the cognitive and neurologic maturity, skills, and knowledge needed to safely cross the street. They have not developed neurologically enough to have the skills to see cars in their peripheral vision, localize sounds, and judge vehicle distance and speed. In general, children are not ready to cross the street alone until they are at least 10 years old. Parents must use constant vigilance and regularly review the safety of the environment to protect their young child from harm.

Sample Questions

Where does your child play when she goes outdoors? Who watches your child when you cannot?

Ask the Child

When you play outside, who watches you? Who watches you when your parents are gone?

Anticipatory Guidance

- Never leave your child alone when she is outside.
- Supervise all outdoor play. Streets and driveways are not safe places to play. Your child is not ready to cross the street alone.

Water Safety

Parents still must supervise their child closely to ensure her safety around water. All children require constant supervision by an adult whenever they are near water. However, parents may choose to start their child in swimming lessons depending on the child's readiness and frequency of exposure to water. Parents should be cautioned that even advanced swimming skills may not prevent drowning.

Sample Questions

What are your plans to teach your child about swimming? Do you use life jackets?

Anticipatory Guidance

- Be sure that swimming pools in your community, apartment complex, or home have a 4-sided fence that completely separates the pool from the house and the yard with a self-closing, self-latching gate.
- Do not rely on water wings to keep your child safe in the water. Use a properly fitted life jacket every time your child is on a boat or other watercraft.
- Children need to learn how to swim. By this age, children can start to learn swimming skills. However, parents should be mindful that swimming ability does not provide drown-proofing and that even strong swimmers can drown.

Sun Protection

Sun protection now is of increasing importance because of climate change and the thinning of the atmospheric ozone layer. Sun protection is accomplished through limiting sun exposure, using sunscreen, and wearing protective clothing.

Sample Questions

Do you apply sunscreen whenever your child plays outside? Does your child care provider have a sun protection policy? Do you and your child care provider limit outside time during the middle of the day, when the sun is strongest?

Anticipatory Guidance

- Always apply sunscreen with an SPF greater than 15 when your child is outside. Reapply every 2 hours.
- Have your child wear a hat.
- Avoid prolonged time in the sun between 11:00 am and 3:00 pm.
- Wear sun protection clothing for summer.

Pets

Pets can be a source of great joy for children, but should be kept under constant watch when they are around young children. Dog and cat bites are particularly common at this age.

Sample Questions

Do you have any pets or are there pets in your neighborhood that may come into contact with your child? Dogs, cats? How have you advised your child to act around unfamiliar dogs?

Anticipatory Guidance

- Make certain that your child knows to avoid stray animals and to treat household pets gently and lovingly.

Firearm Safety

Young children are curious about everything, including firearms, and have no concept of the consequences of firing a weapon. Firearms should be removed from places in which children live and play. If it is necessary to keep a firearm in the home, it should be stored unloaded and locked, with the ammunition locked separately from the firearm.

Sample Question

Is there a firearm in your home or in the homes where your child might play or go for child care?

Anticipatory Guidance

- The best way to keep your child safe from injury or death from firearms is to never have a firearm in the home.
- Remember that young children simply do not understand how dangerous firearms can be, despite your warnings. Children cannot be taught not to handle a firearm if they find one.
- Children this age are naturally curious, and will get into everything! Just as you need to keep medications, cleaning solutions, and insecticides out of children's reach, loaded firearms should never be anywhere where the child can get to them. If it is necessary to keep a firearm in your home or where your child plays or goes to preschool, it should be stored unloaded and locked, with the ammunition locked separately from the firearm.

Middle Childhood Visits

5 Through 10 Years

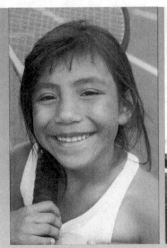
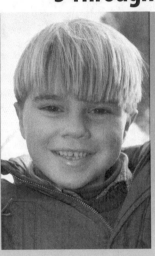
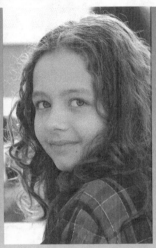
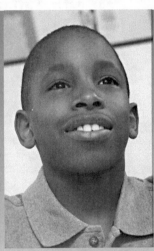

Middle Childhood
5 and 6 Year Visits

Context

As the middle childhood stage begins, boys and girls are growing steadily and their physical competence continues to increase. Their improved language and communication skills match social competence to physical ability. They are prepared to move out of home care and child care or preschool. At this age, they are ready for school.

Starting school is a major milestone for the 5- or 6-year-old and her family. As she prepares to enter kindergarten or elementary school, key developmental issues emerge, such as her readiness for school and her ability to separate from her parents. The 5-year-old who has attended preschool or has been in child care out of the home may be able to separate from her parents more easily than the child who has stayed at home. Most 6-year-olds will have attended kindergarten and acquired the social skills necessary for learning in a full-day, first-grade setting. By observing how the child responds to new situations, the parents, teacher, and health care professional can anticipate how temperament and experience may affect school readiness and competence. The 5 and 6 Year Visits permit observation of the child's ability to follow directions, as well as her language skills, maturity level, and motor ability.

Starting school brings new opportunities, challenges, and rules for children. School activities require increased ability to function in a group setting, which requires greater impulse control and social skills. Children are expected to obey rules, get along with others, and avoid disruptive behavior. Paying attention to teachers and other adults can be difficult for some children. Acquiring skills in listening, reading, and math excites some children and challenges others. Children entering kindergarten will have many opportunities to make friends, conquer new tasks, and meet other families. They may go on school field trips or participate in after-school activities. They will need to adjust to school routines, such as eating at school with self-service lunches or designated times for lunch and snacks. Most will manage these new challenges gracefully, while others will struggle to learn appropriate behaviors during these transitions. Parents should listen to their child's feelings, encourage her, and praise her efforts and accomplishments.

A child's progress in school is an important factor in her development at this age. School-based assessments and report cards are used to track her progress. A child with special health care needs, with disabilities or developmental delay, may qualify for an Individualized Education Program (IEP) or a Section 504 Plan. If she received services through her community's early childhood special education services program, inquiry regarding transition from this program to kindergarten is appropriate. The goal is always to have the child in the least restrictive environment that also promotes academic, social, and emotional success.

Not every child is immediately successful in the school experience. Adjustment difficulties, anxiety, or psychosocial stressors must be addressed. Children who present with learning, academic, or behavioral problems and symptoms of inattention, hyperactivity, or impulsivity should be evaluated for attention-deficit/hyperactivity disorder (ADHD) and for anxiety and learning disability[1] as well as for prenatal alcohol and other exposures associated with attention problems. Federal education law requires school systems to evaluate children who are experiencing learning or developmental difficulties. Some families may need help finding individuals who can help them advocate for the exact services they need.

Each family will have its own perspective on how their child is performing in school. A child will perform best if she feels there is consistency between the expectations of the school and her family regarding educational performance and behavior at school. Some teaching styles may not be the best fit for some children (eg, an overly nurturing teacher may not have firm expectations that some children need and an overly rigid teacher might not provide the flexibility and support needed for other children, especially those who are anxious). In addition, parents sometimes need help in understanding the significance of particular academic struggles. The concept of a learning disability or learning difference may not make sense within certain cultural beliefs about health or abilities. It is essential to identify areas of strength and weakness so that interventions can be put in place early for any areas of vulnerability.

Families who are newly immigrated may not understand the US educational system and may need guidance about what to expect and how they can be involved in supporting their child in school. A language mismatch can be an added barrier between the teacher and parent communication. It may be helpful to have a parent advocate present at educational meetings. If English is not spoken at home, health care professionals should assess the child's exposure to English and what resources are needed to support the important learning tasks ahead. Health care professionals will support multilingual or bilingual language development.

It is developmentally appropriate for 5- and 6-year-olds to spend increasing amounts of time with friends and others outside the home. Parents should meet these new friends and their families. Parents need to encourage their child's friendships and respect the growing influence of peers. Rules and behavioral expectations will vary among families, especially across cultures. As children this age acquire new experiences, they normally begin to test whether the rules can change now that they are older. Some rules can be loosened, but others must be maintained in the interest of sustaining appropriate behavior, providing emotional security and personal safety, and promoting moral upbringing.

Many children younger than 5 years have been exposed to the digital world. The 5-year-old is often fascinated by the online world and her ability to become involved with it. With emerging reading and fine motor skills, some will become skilled with the computer and the Internet. However, children this age and throughout childhood still need strong and frequent parental supervision and monitoring to ensure that they are not exposed to inappropriate materials. Parents may consider getting child-specific browsers and setting up a favorite's toolbar so the child can go only to approved Web sites. Parents also should use an Internet safety tool to limit access to content, Web sites, and activities. It is always important to balance computer and online time with active play. Setting limits on sedentary activities can help children remain active and healthy.

Certain hazards, such as matches, cigarette lighters, gas stoves, and fireplaces, often fascinate 5- and 6-year-olds. This is especially true for children who tend to be impulsive. Thus, parents should remember to keep matches, lighters, and cigarette and e-cigarette paraphernalia out of reach, and to remind children that these items are not toys. Parents should be cautioned specifically about the dangers of keeping firearms in the home and informed of the importance of keeping all firearms

MIDDLE CHILDHOOD
5 AND 6 YEAR VISITS

locked up, with the ammunition locked separately and the keys in a place their child cannot access. It is critical that children continue to use appropriate car safety seats and booster seats.

By her sixth birthday, a child is eager to act independently, but she is not yet able to consistently make good decisions. She likes to climb trees or fire escapes and play in the yard or on the sidewalk with other children, but she is still learning about safety. Children must learn to be safe at home, at school, on the playground, and in the neighborhood. Families will need to continue to set appropriate boundaries and other limits while encouraging and promoting their child's growing independence. Before she is ready to start exploring the community on her own, she must be able to remember and understand safety rules well enough to interpret them and adapt them for different situations. Children need frequent reminders on rules for interacting with and avoiding strangers, as well as instructions on telephone numbers to call for help in case of emergencies. At this age, most children are riding bicycles or using skates and may be learning to use skateboards and to swim. Parents need to teach their child, and frequently review, the safety rules for playing on the playground, riding a bicycle in the neighborhood, and engaging in other recreational activities. Children this age are not yet ready to cross the street alone, and adult supervision also is needed for swimming and other water sports. A child's bicycle should be suited to her ability level and adjusted to her size. She should always wear an approved helmet and protective equipment when riding a bike, skateboarding, skating, or playing in organized sports. Parents need to model this behavior.

The child's community affects safety concerns because the setting and seasonal climate determine common activities and risks. Traffic crashes and playing around cars are health risks for the young

child. Children living in poverty may have limited access to appropriate play areas or activities, and may be out in the neighborhood playing in unsafe venues. Families with limited economic resources may be able to find places in the community (eg, community centers, public clinics, children's hospitals) where they can receive help in obtaining low-cost bike helmets, car safety seats, and other safety equipment.

Newly found skills generate interest in testing physical prowess. How fast can she run? How far can she throw? As she learns how her body works, the 5- and 6-year-old gains the confidence and skills needed to enjoy physical activities or to participate in individual or team sports. A team sport focused on skill building and learning sportsmanlike behavior, rather than winning or keeping score, is a good way to encourage further engagement in physical activities. Parents should be sure that coaches' demands are reasonable. For children who are from cultures where gender roles and modesty issues preclude girls from participating in typical sports activities, opportunities for cooperation and physical development can be found in activities such as ethnic dance groups, scouting, or same-sex physical activities that are arranged by the cultural community.

As the child's cognitive skills continue to develop, her ability to understand and communicate becomes more sophisticated. At this age, health care professionals can talk directly with the child about her family, friends, and excitement or fears about going to school and becoming more independent. This provides an opportunity for the health care professional to develop a partnership directly with the child and to encourage her to assume responsibility for her clothes, toys, or other belongings; selected chores; and good health habits. These responsibilities will help promote autonomy, independence, and a sense of competence.

Priorities for the 5 and 6 Year Visits

The first priority is to attend to the concerns of the parents.

In addition, the Bright Futures Middle Childhood Expert Panel has given priority to the following topics for discussion in the 5 and 6 Year Visits:

▶ Social determinants of health[a] (risks [neighborhood and family violence, food security, family substance use], strengths and protective factors [emotional security and self-esteem, connectedness with family])

▶ Development and mental health (family rules and routines, concern for others, respect for others; patience and control over anger)

▶ School (readiness, established routines, school attendance, friends; after-school care and activities, parent-teacher communication)

▶ Physical growth and development (oral health [regular visits with dentist, daily brushing and flossing, adequate fluoride, limits on sugar-sweetened beverages and snacks], nutrition [healthy weight; increased vegetable, fruit, whole-grain consumption; adequate calcium and vitamin D intake; healthy foods at school], physical activity [60 minutes of physical activity a day])

▶ Safety (car safety, outdoor safety, water safety, sun protection, harm from adults, home fire safety, firearm safety)

---

[a] Social determinants of health is a new priority in the fourth edition of the *Bright Futures Guidelines*. For more information, see the *Promoting Lifelong Health for Families and Communities* theme.

Health Supervision

The *Bright Futures Tool and Resource Kit* contains Previsit Questionnaires to assist the health care professional in conducting history taking, developmental surveillance, and medical screening.

History

Interval history may be obtained according to the concerns of the family and the health care professional's preference or style of practice. The following questions can encourage in-depth discussion:

General Questions for the Parent

- Tell me something your child does that makes you proud.
- What are your concerns about your child's behavioral, physical well-being, or special health care needs?
- Do you have any concerns about your child's development or learning (eg, walking, talking, drawing, or writing her name or ABCs)?
- Do you have any concerns about your child starting school? What concerns do you have about her social or academic experience?
- Please share any concerns about your child's mood or behavior (eg, attention, hitting, temper, worries, not participating in play with others, irritability, mood, or activity level).

Past Medical History

- Has your child received any specialty or emergency care since the last visit?

Family History

- Has your child or anyone in the family, such as parents, brothers, sisters, grandparents, aunts, uncles, or cousins, developed a new health condition or died? **If the answer is Yes:** Ascertain who in the family has or had the condition, and ask about the age of onset and diagnosis. If the person is no longer living, ask about the age at the time of death.

Social History

- See the Social Determinants of Health priority in Anticipatory Guidance for social history questions.

Questions for the Child

- Do you think you are healthy?
- What do you mean when you say you are "healthy"?
- Tell me something you're really good at.

Surveillance of Development

Children Transitioning to Kindergarten

Starting school is a major milestone for child and family. Parents may have concerns about their child's readiness for this big step. Although many parents tend to focus on the child's knowledge of the alphabet, numbers, or drawing skills as evidence of school readiness, teachers are most concerned about the child's language skills and social readiness to separate from parents easily and get along with other children.

The child with special health care needs transitions from early childhood special education services to the classroom setting. The child's IEP should be revised before this move, and the health care professional should discuss appropriate changes with the family.

Children Currently Attending School

Adjustment to new school experiences are both the measure and the endpoint of developmental accomplishment. Health care professionals may measure school success by parent and child report or by review of the child's most recent report card. The health care professional must be alert for diagnoses such as ADHD and learning disorders. For children with special health care needs, it is important for the health care professional to review a copy of the IEP, Section 504 Plan, or any special accommodations.

Do you or any of your child's caregivers have any specific concerns about your child's development, learning, or behavior?

- A 5- or 6-year-old
  - Balances on 1 foot, hops, and skips
  - Is able to tie a knot, has mature pencil grasp, can draw a person with at least 6 body parts, prints some letters and numbers, and is able to copy squares and triangles
  - Has good articulation, tells a simple story using full sentences, uses appropriate tenses and pronouns, can count to 10, and names at least 4 colors
  - Follows simple directions, is able to listen and attend, and undresses and dresses with minimal assistance

Review of Systems

The Bright Futures Middle Childhood Expert Panel recommends a complete review of systems as a part of every health supervision visit. This review can be done through questions about the following:

Does your child have any problems with

- Regular or frequent headaches or dizziness
- Eyes or vision
- Ears or hearing
- Nose or throat
- Breathing problems or pains in chest
- Belly aches or pains, throwing up, problems with urine or bowel movements
- Rashes
- Muscle aches, injury, or other problems

Observation of Parent-Child Interaction

- Do the parent and child speak to one another respectfully?
- Does the parent seem to share positives or encourage and be supportive of the child?
- Does the parent allow the child to talk with the health care professional and not interrupt?
- Does the parent engage the child in an age-appropriate manner?

Physical Examination

A complete physical examination is included as part of every health supervision visit.

Respect the child's privacy by using appropriate draping during the examination. Ask siblings to wait in the waiting room if possible.

When performing a physical examination, the health care professional's attention is directed to the following components of the examination of importance to the child at this age:

- **Measure and compare with norms for age, sex, and height**
  - Blood pressure
- **Measure and plot on appropriate Centers for Disease Control and Prevention (CDC) Growth Chart**
  - Height
  - Weight
- **Calculate and plot on appropriate CDC Growth Chart**
  - Body mass index (BMI)
- **Eyes**
  - Perform ocular motility assessment.
- **Mouth**
  - Observe for caries, gingival inflammation, malocclusion.
- **Neurodevelopment**
  - Observe fine and gross motor skills and gait.

Screening — 5 Year

Universal Screening	Action
Hearing	Audiometry
Oral Health (in the absence of a dental home)	Apply fluoride varnish every 6 months.
Vision	Objective measure with age-appropriate visual acuity measurement using HOTV or LEA symbols. Instrument-based measurement may be used for children who are unable to perform acuity testing.

Selective Screening	Risk Assessment[a]	Action if Risk Assessment Positive (+)
Anemia	+ on risk screening questions	Hematocrit or hemoglobin
Lead	If no previous screen and + on risk screening questions or change in risk	Lead blood test
Oral Health	Does not have a dental home	Referral to dental home
	Primary water source is deficient in fluoride.	Oral fluoride supplementation
Tuberculosis	+ on risk screening questions	Tuberculin skin test

[a] See the *Evidence and Rationale chapter* for the criteria on which risk screening questions are based.

Screening — 6 Year

Universal Screening	Action
Hearing	Audiometry
Vision	Objective measure with age-appropriate visual-acuity measurement using HOTV or LEA symbols, Sloan letters, or Snellen letters

Selective Screening	Risk Assessment[a]	Action if Risk Assessment Positive (+)
Anemia	+ on risk screening questions	Hematocrit or hemoglobin
Dyslipidemia	+ on risk screening questions and not previously screened with normal results	Lipid profile
Lead	If no previous screen and + on risk screening questions or change in risk	Lead blood test
Oral Health	Does not have a dental home	Referral to dental home
	Primary water source is deficient in fluoride.	Oral fluoride supplementation
Tuberculosis	+ on risk screening questions	Tuberculin skin test

[a] See the *Evidence and Rationale chapter* for the criteria on which risk screening questions are based.

Immunizations

Consult the CDC/Advisory Committee on Immunization Practices (ACIP) or American Academy of Pediatrics (AAP) Web sites for the current immunization schedule.

CDC National Immunization Program: **www.cdc.gov/vaccines**

AAP *Red Book:* **http://redbook.solutions.aap.org**

Anticipatory Guidance

The following sample questions, which address the Bright Futures Middle Childhood Expert Panel's Anticipatory Guidance Priorities, are intended to be used selectively to invite discussion, gather information, address the needs and concerns of the family, and build partnerships. Use of the questions may vary from visit to visit and from family to family. Questions can be modified to match the health care professional's communication style. The accompanying anticipatory guidance for the family should be geared to questions, issues, or concerns for that particular child and family. Tools and handouts to support anticipatory guidance can be found in the *Bright Futures Tool and Resource Kit*.

Priority

Social Determinants of Health

Risks: Neighborhood and family violence, food security, family substance use

Strengths and protective factors: Emotional security and self-esteem, connectedness with family

Risks: Neighborhood and Family Violence

Children in families that are affected by poverty, neighborhood violence, or family violence are dealing with a level of stress that affects their current and future health. For example, families in difficult living situations may have concerns about their ability to provide a safe environment for their child.

Questions on this topic can be sensitive. The health care professional can identify these issues in a supportive and non-blaming way and help the parents formulate steps toward solutions. A referral to community resources or federal assistance programs may be a useful first step.

Children need a safe environment at home to thrive—free of violence and toxic stress. Likewise, they need to feel safe at school, on their way to and from school and, if possible, in their community. Bullying, teasing, and feeling left out can interfere with normal development and school performance. Assist parents in being observant for signs of bullying and ostracism. Children with disabilities and other special health care needs are at increased risk of bullying. *(For more information on this topic, see the Bullying section of the Promoting Mental Health theme.)*

Sample Questions

Are there frequent reports of violence in your community? Do you think your child is safe in the neighborhood? Has he ever been injured in a fight? Has your child been bullied or hit by others? Has he demonstrated bullying or aggression toward others?

Anticipatory Guidance

- Bullying or a suspicion of bullying should always be immediately discussed with your child's teacher and guidance counselor. If this is happening in a community-based program, talk to the responsible adult who is leading the program.
- Teach your child nonviolent conflict-resolution techniques.

For the Child

- Talk to your parent or another grown-up you trust if anyone bullies or hurts you or makes you feel scared. If you see another child being bullied, tell an adult.

Risks: Food Security

Families with limited means may have concerns about their ability to acquire sufficient food. The need for adequate calories and nutritious food choices during this period of steady growth and development and increasingly independent food decision-making makes food security a critical issue in middle childhood. If the family is having difficulty obtaining nutritious food, provide information about the Supplemental Nutrition Assistance Program (SNAP), the Commodity Supplemental Food Program, local food shelves, and local community food programs.

Sample Questions

Within the past 12 months, did you worry that your food would run out before you got money to buy more? In the past 12 months, did the food you bought just not last and you didn't have money to buy more?

Anticipatory Guidance

- Community programs, like food banks and food pantries, are available to help you and your family. You also may be eligible for food and nutrition assistance, or programs like SNAP, which used to be called Food Stamps, can help you.

Risks: Family Substance Use (Tobacco, E-cigarettes, Alcohol, Drugs)

Exposure to tobacco smoke remains an important environmental risk. Encourage parents to keep their home and vehicles smoke-free, as well as free from vapor from e-cigarettes. Becoming familiar with community and online resources for quitting smoking allows health care professionals to refer parents who are interested in quitting.

Worrying about a family member with a substance use or mental health problem also may be a source of significant stress.

Sample Questions

Does anyone who lives with your child smoke or use e-cigarettes? Does anyone smoke or use e-cigarettes in your home or vehicle? If so, who? Is there anyone in your child's life whose alcohol or drug use concerns you?

Anticipatory Guidance

- Exposure to secondhand smoke greatly increases the risk of heart and lung diseases in your child. For your health and your child's health, please stop smoking if you are a smoker, and insist that others not smoke around your child.

- Exposure to vapor from e-cigarettes also may be harmful. For your child's health, please don't use e-cigarettes—also called vaping—around your child, especially indoors or inside cars.

- It's not always possible, but, when you can, avoid spending time in places where people are smoking cigarettes or using e-cigarettes.

- If you are ever interested in quitting smoking, please talk to me. **800-QUIT-NOW (800-784-8669);** TTY **800-332-8615** is a national telephone helpline that is routed to local resources. Additional resources are available at **www.cdc.gov.** I can also refer you to local or online resources.

- If you are worried about any family members' drug or alcohol use problems, you can talk with me.

Strengths and Protective Factors: Emotional Security and Self-esteem

Identifying strengths and providing feedback to families about what they are doing well helps provide a comprehensive and balanced view of the child's health and well-being. For families living in difficult circumstances, such strengths may help protect the child from, or reduce the degree of, negative health outcomes. Parents need to know that they can positively influence the healthy development of their child no matter what difficulties or problems exist. Anticipatory guidance provides parents with ideas about opportunities they can give their child, such as the chance to become good at things, begin to make independent decisions, have social connections, and do things for others.

Parents can help make their child feel secure by giving hugs, participating in activities together, and listening without interrupting. Children with warm, nurturing parents are more likely to have high self-esteem. Hypercritical parents who have unrealistically high expectations, and uninvolved parents who do not encourage their children to achieve and to try new experiences, can damage their child's self-esteem. Protective factors for any child include having at least one supportive adult in their life.

Self-esteem is a key feature of a fulfilling life and has an enormous influence on mental health. Children develop a positive sense of self if they think they are making a contribution. Words of encouragement are important and provide energizing motivation. Help parents think about how they can encourage their child to be responsible by modeling responsibility themselves, keeping promises, showing up on time, and completing tasks on time.

Sample Questions

How happy is your child? Do you feel he has good self-confidence?

Ask the Child

Tell me about some of the things you are good at doing. What are some of the things that make you happy?

Anticipatory Guidance

- Encourage competence, independence, and self-responsibility in all areas by not doing everything for your child, but by helping him do things well himself, and by supporting him in helping others.

- Show affection and pride in your child's special strengths and praise appropriately and liberally.

Strengths and Protective Factors: Connectedness With Family

One of the most important protective factors and a component of healthy child development is the ability to form caring and supportive relationships with family. At home, this involves a relationship characterized by both warm supportive interactions with parents and guardians combined with clear expectations and an opportunity for children to begin to gain the skills necessary for problem-solving.

Sample Questions
How are you getting along as a family? What do you do together?

Anticipatory Guidance
- Spend time with your child. Express willingness for questions and discussion. Make time every day to talk, such as at mealtimes, bedtime, and drive time, and do things you both enjoy.

Priority

Development and Mental Health

Family rules and routines, concern for others, respect for others; patience and control over anger

Family Rules and Routines, Concern for Others, Respect for Others

Family routines create a sense of safety and security for the child. Assigning regular household chores helps teach a sense of responsibility in the child and helps her feel as though she is an essential part of the family.

Parents should provide a balance of privileges and responsibility. Children can earn more privileges when they follow directions and demonstrate responsibilities. Making conversation, rather than watching television (TV) or playing electronics, the priority at mealtimes can build family togetherness and provides an opportunity to teach respect for others.

Parents should encourage self-discipline and impulse control, as well as concern for others. These are important skills to model.

Sample Questions

What are some of the family routines you have at home? What chores is your child responsible for at home? How do you acknowledge her when she is being good? How do you discipline her? How do you and your partner or other caregiver handle discipline? Are you and your partner as unified as possible in your expectations and rules? Is she kind? Does she show respect for others?

Ask the Child

What regular jobs do you have at home? What family traditions do you enjoy? What happens in your house if your dad or mom doesn't approve of something you're doing?

Anticipatory Guidance

- Promote a sense of responsibility in your child by assigning chores and expecting them to be done. For all children, including children with special health care needs, chores should be determined by what is needed and what is appropriate for the child's ability. Visual reminders may help your child follow through on expectations. Parents need to be consistent and follow through with appropriate consequences if expectations are not met.

- Human nature is to speak up when rules are being broken or behavior is not appropriate, yet "catching our kids being good" may shape outcomes more than any restrictions or discipline. Being clear on expectations is essential.

- Teach your child the difference between right and wrong. The goal of discipline is to teach appropriate behavior and self-control, not to be mean and cruel in response to wrongdoing. Punishment should be viewed as a teaching moment. Spanking and other physical punishments convert a teaching moment to an angry moment that makes your child afraid and fails to teach about the unwanted behavior.

- It is important to set aside time to connect with your child one-on-one. Allowing your child to direct some activities for a few minutes strengthens the parent-child bond, which, in turn, makes it easier to implement fair discipline.
- Show appropriate affection in your family.
- Listen to and respect your child as well as your partner. Don't interrupt; model and teach concern and respect for others. Serve as a positive ethical and behavioral role model.

For the Child
- Chores are an important part of being in a family. You help make things go well at home and learn new skills you can be proud of. If you need a break from a chore, talk about it with your parents.

Patience and Control Over Anger

Children depend on their parents to help them learn the skills of appropriate expression of emotions and frustrations. Parents model appropriate responses and respect by their own behavior as they interact with family members. Providing children with routine guidance is key, including appropriate consequences that are not physically punitive.

Healthy development includes learning to handle frustration and express emotions appropriately. Parents can help by setting reasonable limits, providing opportunities for their child to share her worries and concerns, and listening to her ideas about possible solutions. Parents are the most important role models in these critical areas.

Sample Questions
How does your child handle angry feelings?

Ask the Child
What things make you sad? Angry? Scared? How do you handle these feelings? Are you more likely to share them or keep them to yourself? Do you talk to your parents about your concerns?

Anticipatory Guidance
- Try to help your child see that she wants to treat others as she wants to be treated. Model anger management by talking about the ways that you handle your own frustrations and your anger and what you have learned about letting off steam in positive ways. Help your child think through a difficult situation. Talk about what choices she has, what are the good and bad choices, and what might come next depending on what choice she makes.
- Help your child manage anger and resolve conflicts without violence or destruction of property. Do not allow hitting, biting, throwing, destroying, or other violent behavior.
- Encourage self-discipline and impulse control in your child by modeling these behaviors and by praising her efforts at self-control.

For the Child
- Everyone gets angry at times, but it's never OK to hit, bite, or kick another person or to throw or break something. Better ways to deal with feeling angry are to talk about what has upset you with the person who made you angry, get outside and run or play hard, or just walk away from the person who is making you angry. Sometimes waiting a little while, then talking about the problem, allows everyone to cool off.

Priority

School

Readiness, established routines, school attendance, friends; after-school care and activities, parent-teacher communication

Readiness, Established Routines, School Attendance, Friends

Starting school is a major milestone for the 5- or 6-year-old and his family, bringing new opportunities and challenges. Children who have attended preschool or K through 4 programs may easily separate from parents compared to children who stayed home for the early childhood years. The 5 and 6 Year Visits permit observations of the child's readiness for school (ability to follow directions, language skills, maturity level, and motor ability). The health care professional should use these visits to discuss school issues, such as the ability to transition, routines related to school, school attendance, friends, maturity, management of disappointments, fears, parent-teacher communication, and after-school care and activities.

Sample Questions

Did your child attend a preschool program? Tell me about his preschool experiences. Do you have any concerns about your child's school experience?

Ask the Child

Are you excited about starting school? What do you like best about school? Tell me about your friends at school.

Anticipatory Guidance

- A child who arrives at school fed and rested is ready to learn. Help your child have a healthy breakfast every morning before school, and establish bedtime routines on school nights so that he gets at least 10 to 11 hours of sleep.
- Talk about new opportunities, friends, and activities at school. Tour your child's school with him and meet his teacher.
- Make it a priority to attend back-to-school nights, parent-teacher meetings, and other school functions. These will give you a chance to get to know your child's teacher and become familiar with the school so you can talk more knowledgeably with your child about his experiences at school.
- Stresses or changes in the family, such as a parent not being available, a loss in the family, or family violence, can contribute to poor school performance. If you are experiencing these kinds of stresses, you can talk with me about ways to help your child cope with them.
- If you enroll your child in an after-school program or hire a caregiver for the after-school period, be sure your child is in a safe environment. Talk with caregivers about their attitudes and behavior about discipline. Do not let them discipline your child by hitting or spanking him.
- After-school activities, such as sports teams, social activities, clubs, and extracurricular activities, place a big demand on children's time. Be cautious to not overschedule your child. Children need unstructured time as well as structured activities.

After-school Care and Activities, Parent-Teacher Communication

If learning or behavioral problems have been identified, talk to the parents about obtaining educational evaluations for special education services and transition from Early Education services to classroom services. An office-based psychosocial assessment may be useful. Determine whether newly immigrated families understand the local educational system, which may be very different from that of their country of origin. Check whether any language barriers exist to parent or caregiver interactions with the school.

Sample Questions

Is there anything the teacher or school should know related to any special needs your child may have? Are you concerned about learning or behavioral factors that may require additional evaluations?

Does your child receive any special educational services at school, such as an Individual Educational Program, or IEP; Section 504 Plan; or other special services? What does your child do after school?

Anticipatory Guidance

- If your child has special health care needs, maintain an active role in the IEP process. We would like a copy of the current IEP for your child's health record.

Priority

Physical Growth and Development

Oral health (regular visits with dentist, daily brushing and flossing, adequate fluoride, limits on sugar-sweetened beverages and snacks), nutrition (healthy weight; increased vegetable, fruit, whole-grain consumption; adequate calcium and vitamin D intake; healthy foods at school), physical activity (60 minutes of physical activity a day)

Oral Health (Regular Visits With Dentist, Daily Brushing and Flossing, Adequate Fluoride, Limits on Sugar-Sweetened Beverages and Snacks)

By ages 5 and 6 years, the child already should have an established dental home. She should have regularly scheduled visits with her dentist at least twice each year. She also should receive a fluoride supplement if the fluoride level in community water supplies (at home and at school) is low. Assure parents that fluoride is safe and effective at preventing decay.

Sample Questions

How many times a day does your child brush her teeth? Does she floss every day? Has your child lost any teeth?

For Parents of Children With Special Health Care Needs

Does your child need help brushing her teeth? Do you use any special oral health equipment, such as a mouth prop to keep her mouth open, to complete this task?

Ask the Child

Do you brush and floss your teeth every day? How many times? When do you brush your teeth? Do you have any loose teeth?

Anticipatory Guidance

- Be sure that your child brushes her teeth for 2 minutes, twice a day, with a pea-sized amount of fluoridated toothpaste, and flosses once a day with your help. Enjoy sharing this time with your child as you allow her to brush and floss her own teeth first. Then you take a turn to get the teeth thoroughly brushed and flossed. At this age, children will not get their teeth clean by themselves.
- Your child should be seeing a dentist regularly. This is called having a dental home. If your child doesn't have a dental home, we can help you find one.
- Stress the importance to your child about taking care of her permanent teeth, which will start to come in both in the front and in the back of her mouth.
- Limit your child's consumption of sweetened beverages and snacks with lots of sugar, such as candy. Prolonged contact with the teeth can increase the chance of cavities.

For the Child

- It is important to brush your teeth for at least 2 minutes, twice a day, and to floss at least once a day, especially when your new teeth come in, because they are the teeth you'll have forever.
- Let your mom, dad, or other adult help you with your brushing and flossing until you get really good at it.

Nutrition (Healthy Weight; Increased Vegetable, Fruit, Whole-Grain Consumption; Adequate Calcium and Vitamin D Intake; Healthy Foods at School)

Discuss healthy weight by using a BMI chart to show the child and her family how her height and weight compare with those of other children of the same sex and age. If the child's BMI is greater than the 85th percentile, it is appropriate to begin more in-depth counseling on nutritious food choices and physical activity. Note that some children between the 85th and 94th percentiles are healthy and do not have chronic disease risk factors.

As children aged 5 and 6 years begin to broaden their experiences beyond home, they are increasingly expected to make their own choices about what to eat (eg, school lunch, snacks at a friend's house). This is a time when the overall quality of many children's eating patterns begins to decline. It is, therefore, a good time to counsel families about appropriate food choices that promote nutritional adequacy and to reinforce the positive nutrition habits established earlier. Ensuring sufficient calcium and vitamin D intake can be a particular concern, especially if the child does not consume dairy products. Supplementation with these nutrients can be considered. Fortified orange juice typically has calcium and vitamin D. Soy milk generally has both, but that is not always true for other products marketed as "milks" (eg, almond, rice, coconut, hemp). Families should be encouraged to check the package label to be sure. Not all yogurt has vitamin D.

Provide guidance or a referral if the family needs nutrition information, counseling, or assistance for cultural, religious, or financial reasons. For children with special health care needs, ensure that nutrition and physical activity are incorporated into the IEP.

Sample Questions
What concerns do you have about your child's eating, such as getting her to drink enough milk and eat vegetables and fruits? What does your child usually eat for snacks? How often does she drink sweetened beverages?

Ask the Child
What vegetables and fruits did you eat yesterday? How many sweet beverages, such as soda, fruit drinks, or sports drinks, do you drink each day? How many glasses of milk did you drink yesterday? What do you eat for breakfast?

Anticipatory Guidance
- Choose healthy eating behaviors.
  - Every day, give your child a healthy breakfast. Research shows that eating breakfast helps children learn and behave better at school.
  - Help your child recognize and respond to hunger and fullness cues.
  - Eat together as a family. Make mealtimes pleasant and companionable; encourage conversation and turn off the TV.
  - Be a role model for your child with your own healthy eating behaviors.
- Make nutritious foods and drinks the usual options at home for meals and snacks. These include vegetables; fruits; whole grains; lean protein, such as meat, fish, poultry, eggs, beans and peas, legumes, nuts and seeds; and low-fat and nonfat dairy.

- Limit foods and drinks that are high in calories, saturated fat, salt, added sugars, and refined grains, and low in nutrients. These include ice cream, baked goods, salty snacks, fast foods, pizza, and soda and other sweetened beverages.
- Limit juice to 4 to 6 oz of 100% fruit juice each day.
- Make sure your child gets dairy foods and calcium- and vitamin D–containing foods and beverages each day. Children aged 4 to 8 years need 12 to 16 oz of low-fat or fat-free milk each day plus an additional serving of low-fat yogurt and cheese. If your child doesn't drink milk or consume other dairy products, then let's talk about alternatives. These can include foods and beverages that are fortified with calcium and vitamin D (like some orange juices and cereals).

For the Child

- Eating breakfast helps you learn better and feel better at school, so always eat something healthy for breakfast.
- Pay attention to what your body tells you. Eat when you feel hungry and stop eating when you feel satisfied.
- Vegetables and fruits are an important part of healthy eating. Ask your parents to let you help choose vegetables and fruits at the store and to help prepare them for meals and snacks.
- Be sure to drink fat-free or low-fat milk at least 2 times a day. Three times a day is better. You can eat cheese or yogurt, too.
- Try not to have drinks that have lots of sugar, such as sodas, fruit drinks, and sports drinks. The healthiest drinks are milk and water; try to drink only them.

Physical Activity (60 Minutes of Physical Activity a Day)

Encourage parents to support their children in being physically active and to be physically active together as a family. Current recommendations state that children should be physically active for at least 60 minutes each day. Encourage the parents of children with special health care needs to allow their children to participate in regular physical activity or cardiovascular fitness within the limits of their medical conditions. Adaptive physical education can be part of a child's IEP.

Emphasize the importance of safety equipment when the child participates in physical activity. Help families identify appropriate community activities for their child (eg, Boys & Girls Clubs, 4-H, community centers, parks, and faith-based programs).

The time a child is using media or the Internet is time she is not being physically active. Counsel regarding media time expenditure and Internet safety.

Sample Questions

How much physical activity does your child get every day? Do you and your child participate in physical activities together? Are you physically active yourself? How much recreational screen time does your child spend each weekday? How about on weekends? Does your child have a TV or Internet-connected device in her bedroom? What is your child's usual bedtime on school nights and on nonschool nights? Does your child have trouble going to sleep or does she wake up during the night?

Ask the Child

How often during the day do you play actively? Do you play together with your family? How much time each day do you spend watching TV or using a computer or other devices, such as a tablet or smartphone?

Anticipatory Guidance

- Encourage your child to be physically active for at least 60 minutes total every day. It doesn't have to happen all at once, but can be split up into several periods of activity over the course of the day.
- Be a role model by being physically active yourself. Find physical activities your family can enjoy together and incorporate them into your daily lives.
- Identify activities your child can do indoors to be physically active.
- Children this age can learn reading, science, and math skills from computers, and may be using computers and other Internet-connected media in school. However, they need other experiences such as unstructured play alone and with peers, time outdoors, physical activity, and hands-on learning. These kinds of activities help them develop all parts of their brain, including more complicated skills such as executive functioning and social skills.
- Do not allow your child to sleep with any electronic device in her bedroom, including phones or tablets.
- In order to balance your child's needs for physical activity, sleep, school activities, and unplugged time, consider making a family media use plan to balance these important health behaviors and media use time in your child's day. The family media use plan is an online tool that you and your child can fill out together. The tool prompts you and your child to enter daily health priorities such as an hour for physical activity, 8 to 11 hours of sleep, time for homework and school activities, and unplugged time each day for time with family and independently. You and your child can then view the time left over and decide on rules around daily screen time for your child. The AAP has information on making a plan at **www.HealthyChildren.org/MediaUsePlan.**
- Take into account not only the quantity but the quality and location of media use. Consider TVs, phones, tablets, and computers. Rules should be followed by parents as well as children. Construct it so that it suits your families' media needs, but also helps you preserve face-to-face time during family routines such as meals, playtime, and bedtime. Times or locations in the house can be designated as media-free.
- Children learn more from educational media when you watch a show or use an app with them and talk about it afterwards.
- Supervise your child's Internet use so that you can teach her how to use it safely and how to avoid inappropriate content.
- If your child is using media excessively, find out why. Is she having trouble with friends or social skills? Some children seek solitary activities if they are struggling with friendships. Encourage your child to find activities that interest her, or seek help through the school.
- Most children this age need an average of 10 to 11 hours of sleep each night. Create a regular and consistent sleep schedule and bedtime routine.
- Help your child get to sleep each night by making her bedroom dark, cool, and quiet and avoiding caffeinated drinks. Reading a book in bed is a better option than using media. Media use before bedtime actually leads to worse sleep habits, less sleep, and school problems.

For the Child

- It's a good idea to be active often during the day.
- Turn off your TV and video games. Get up and play instead.

▪ Don't eat in front of a screen.

Priority

Safety

Car safety, outdoor safety, water safety, sun protection, harm from adults, home fire safety, firearm safety

Car Safety

Car safety is a critical area to address because many deaths at this age are caused by crashes involving vehicles when child passengers are inadequately restrained. It is safest to continue using a seat with a 5-point harness until the child reaches the weight or height limit of the seat. When the child has outgrown the car safety seat, he should use a belt-positioning booster seat until the seat belt fits well, usually between the ages of 8 and 12 years and when he is about 4 feet 9 inches tall. The seat belt fits properly when the lap belt lies low across the hips and upper thighs, the shoulder belt lies across the middle of the chest and shoulder, and the child is tall enough to sit all the way back with his knees bent comfortably at the edge of the seat without slouching forward. The back seat is the safest place for all children to ride until age 13 years. Assist families who cannot afford appropriate car safety seats by connecting them with community resources. It is especially important for children with behavioral problems or special health care needs to continue using seats with 5-point harnesses to the highest possible weights or heights; some may benefit from using restraints designed for children with special health care needs (**www.preventinjury.org**).

Sample Questions
Does your child always use a car safety seat or belt-positioning booster seat securely fastened in the back seat of a vehicle?

Ask the Child
What type of seat do you sit in when you ride in a car? Do you sit in the back seat?

Anticipatory Guidance
▪ Be sure the vehicle lap and shoulder belt are positioned across your child in the car safety seat or the belt-positioning booster seat in the back seat of the vehicle. Your child should use a car safety seat or a booster seat until the lap belt can be worn low and flat across his hips and upper thighs and the shoulder belt can be worn across his chest and shoulder rather than the face or neck, and he can bend at the knees while sitting against the vehicle seat back. This usually happens when your child is between 8 and 12 years old and at about 4 feet 9 inches tall. The back seat is the safest place for all children younger than 13 years to ride.

For the Child
▪ Always sit in your car seat or booster seat and ride in the back seat of the car because that is where you are safest.

For information about car safety seats and actions to keep your child safe in and around cars, visit www.safercar.gov/parents.

Find a Child Passenger Safety Technician: http://cert.safekids.org. Click on "Find a Tech."

Toll-free Auto Safety Hotline: 888-327-4236

Outdoor Safety

Young children lack the neurologic maturity, skills, and knowledge needed to safely cross the street. They have not developed neurologically to have the skills to see cars in their peripheral vision, localize sounds, and judge vehicle distance and speed, and, in general, are not ready to cross the street alone until age 10 or older. To protect their young child from harm, parents must use constant vigilance and regularly review the safety of the environment. Parents often overestimate the cognitive and sensory integration of young children and need advice on how to teach and provide adequate supervision for injury prevention. Riding bikes safely and pedestrian safety are other issues of importance for counseling parents.

At this age, children will begin to participate in team sports and engage in other physical activities. Reinforce with the parents and the child the importance of always wearing protective gear (eg, helmet, mouth guard, eye protection, and knee and elbow pads).

Sample Questions
What have you done to prepare your child for crossing the street on the way to school or for taking a school bus?

Does your child use safety equipment when doing any outdoor activity, like biking or skating?

Ask the Child
Do you always wear a helmet when biking, skating, or doing other outdoor activities?

Anticipatory Guidance
- Begin to teach your child safe street habits. Teach your child to stop at the curb, and then look to the left, to the right, and back to the left again. Teach your child never to cross the street without a grown-up. Teach your child to walk, not run, when crossing the street.
- Teach your child where to wait for the school bus and make sure an adult is always supervising when the children are getting on and off the bus.
- Be sure your child always wears appropriate safety equipment when doing any outdoor activity, like biking or skating.
- Make sure your child wears a properly fitted, approved helmet every time he rides a bike or does any other wheeled activity. Never let your child ride in the street. Your child is too young to ride in the street safely.

For the Child
- Being active is good for you, but being safe while being active is just as important. One of the best ways to protect yourself is to wear the right safety equipment, especially a helmet, every time you go biking or skating.

Water Safety

An adult should supervise whenever children are in or near water.

Sample Questions

Does your child know how to swim? Does he know how to stay safe around water?

Ask the Child

Do you know how to swim? What rules do your parents have about swimming?

Anticipatory Guidance

- Teach your child to swim if he has not yet learned.
- Do not let your child play around any water (lake, stream, pool, or ocean) unless an adult is watching. Even if your child knows how to swim, never let him swim alone. NEVER let your child swim in any fast-moving water.
- Teach your child to never dive into water unless an adult has already checked the depth of the water.
- When on any boat, be sure your child is wearing an appropriately fitting, US Coast Guard–approved life jacket.
- Be sure that swimming pools in your community, apartment complex, or home have a 4-sided fence with a self-closing, self-latching gate.

For the Child

- Swimming lessons are an important way to become safe in the water. Ask your parents about learning to swim.
- Never swim without an adult around.
- Always wear a life jacket in a boat.

Sun Protection

Sun protection now is of increasing importance because of climate change and the thinning of the atmospheric ozone layer. Sun protection is accomplished through limiting sun exposure, using sunscreen, and wearing protective clothing.

Sample Questions

Do you apply sunscreen whenever your child plays outside? Do you limit outside time during the middle of the day, when the sun is at its strongest?

Ask the Child

Do you always use sunscreen?

Anticipatory Guidance

- Always apply sunscreen with an SPF greater than 15 when your child is outside. Reapply every 2 hours.
- Encourage your child to wear a hat.
- Avoid prolonged time in the sun between 11:00 am and 3:00 pm.

For the Child

- Always wear sunscreen and a hat when you are outside.
- Try not to be outside in the sun too long between 11:00 am and 3:00 pm, when it is really easy to get a sunburn.

Harm From Adults

As children now spend increasing amounts of time with other adults, parents should discuss personal safety in a manner that is informative and empowering without provoking unnecessary anxiety.

Because most sexual abuse and misuse occurs within the family, safety messages must focus on privacy, autonomy, and avoiding being abused and not just on the risks from strangers. Children with special health care needs are at increased risk of being abused.

Sample Questions

Have you talked to your child about ways to avoid sexual abuse?

Ask the Child

What are your "privates"? Why do we call them that? What would you do if a grown-up made you scared? Who could you tell? Who would help you?

Anticipatory Guidance

- Teach your child that it is never OK for an adult to tell a child to keep secrets from parents, to express interest in private parts, or to ask a child for help with his or her private parts.

For the Child

- We call the parts of your body that are usually under a bathing suit privates because we keep them covered and because you are the only one in charge of them. That is why I asked your permission before I checked your privates.
- It is never OK for an older child or an adult to show you his or her private parts, to ask you to show your privates, to touch you there, to scare you, or to ask you not to tell your parents about what he or she did with you. Always get away from the person as quickly as possible and tell your parent or another adult right away.

Home Fire Safety

Home fire safety is best achieved with prevention (teaching children not to play with matches or lighters), protection (smoke alarms), and planning (reaction and escape).

Sample Questions

Where are the smoke alarms in your home? (**Probe for multiple locations.**) *Do you have carbon monoxide detectors/alarms in your home? Do you have an emergency escape plan in case of fire and does your child know what to do in case the alarm rings?*

Ask the Child

What should you do if a fire starts in your home? What should you do if your clothes catch on fire?

Anticipatory Guidance

- Install smoke alarms on every level in your house, especially in furnace and sleeping areas, and test the alarms every month. It is best to use smoke alarms that use long-life batteries; change the batteries once a year when the clock changes in the spring or fall.
- Install a carbon monoxide detector/alarm, certified by Underwriters Laboratories (known as UL), on every level of your home and in the hallway near every separate sleeping area of the home.
- Make an escape plan in case of fire in your home. Your fire department can tell you how. Teach your child what to do when the smoke alarm rings. Practice what you and your child would do if you had a fire.
- Keep all matches and lighters out of reach of children.

For the Child

- Never play with matches or lighters or let others do so.
- If your clothes catch on fire, don't run. Stop, drop, and roll.

Firearm Safety

Discuss firearm safety in the home and danger to family members and children. Homicide and completed suicide are more common in homes in which firearms are kept. The evidence is clear that the safest home for children is one without firearms. If it is necessary to keep a firearm, it should be stored unloaded and locked, with the ammunition locked separately from the firearm.

At this age, children lack the maturity or cognitive capacity to reliably follow advice concerning firearms. They cannot reliably be taught not to handle a firearm if they find one. The health care professional's guidance should be addressed to the parents.

Sample Questions

If there is a firearm in your home? Is it unloaded and locked up? Where is the ammunition stored? Have you considered not owning a firearm because it poses the danger to children and other family members?

Anticipatory Guidance

- The best way to keep your child safe from injury or death from firearms is to never have a firearm in your home.
- If it is necessary to keep a firearm in your home, keep it unloaded and in a locked place, with ammunition locked separately. Keep the key where children cannot have access.
- Ask if there are firearms in homes where your child plays. If so, make sure they are stored unloaded and locked, with the ammunition locked separately, before allowing your child to play in the home.
- Remember that young children simply do not understand how dangerous firearms can be, despite your warnings.

Middle Childhood
7 and 8 Year Visits

Context

Now bigger, increasingly interactive, and involved with friends, the prepubertal, emotionally developing 7- and 8-year-old uses his growing cognitive strengths and communication skills to plot a developmental trajectory toward mature independence and autonomy. His newly formed superego, or conscience, allows the understanding of rules, relationships, and social mores. During this age period, moral development progresses. Experiences with school and social activities and separation from parents and family foster individuation. Coping skills develop, supporting the child's social activities, friendships outside the family, and school and community competencies. This process continues into young adulthood.

At 7 or 8 years of age, a child begins to look outside the family for new ideas and activities. Opportunities for formal after-school activities, such as scouts, team sports, and arts activities, are beginning to be readily available, and children these ages spend an increasing amount of time away from the family. A 7- or 8-year old's peer group grows in importance as he identifies with children of the same gender who have similar interests and abilities. He may have a best friend, a milestone in interpersonal development. The child may encounter beliefs and practices in his peer group that differ from those of his family. He will try to make sense of these differences and may begin to experience some conflict between the beliefs and values at home and those of his peers. The growing influence of peers may present a challenge to the family.

A 7- or 8-year-old has family responsibilities, such as making his own bed, picking up his clothes, setting the table, and helping with meals. These responsibilities can help him develop a sense of personal competence. His sense of accomplishment and pride helps him become confident in attempting activities that require increased responsibility.

By 8 years, a child is able to use logic and can focus on multiple aspects of a problem. Busy with school projects and book reports, and creating collections that reflect his interests in sports, animals, or other topics, he wants to learn how things work and he has many questions about the world around him. He also is beginning to recognize that others' viewpoints may differ from his own.

School performance remains a functional marker of a child's development and accomplishments across all developmental domains (social and emotional, communicative, cognitive, and physical). By now, a child should have completed the transition to the classroom setting. During this age period, behaviors necessary for learning, such as cooperation and attention, are demonstrated. Success or difficulty in these areas may affect self-esteem in positive or negative ways. School attendance is necessary for learning. It is important to discuss and address poor attendance.

If the child has a special health care need or a disability, the health care professional should be concerned with how well the child is coping, given the new developmental, social, and environmental demands of becoming older. A child with special health care needs may be on a different or similar developmental trajectory when compared with age and classroom peers. Cultural and family values and beliefs about the cause of the special health care needs and expectations for individuals with illnesses and disabilities will influence both current adjustments and planning for future transitions.

For children with special health care needs and for children receiving supplemental or special education services, a review of services with parents is appropriate. Parents should be asked to provide a copy and discuss their child's IEP or Section 504 Plan for in-classroom accommodations. These documents should be checked for accurate attention to medical comorbidities, for appropriate accommodations, and for comprehensive approaches to learning. The parents may choose to have a parent advocate present with them for school meetings, as parents are sometimes not aware of what services their child might be entitled to receive. The role of, and evidence-based information on, the use of psychotropic medications may need to be reviewed. Children with special health care needs should have a shared plan of care that is developed in conjunction with the parents and shared with the school nurse and after-school caregivers. The shared plan of care should address any chronic medications, emergency medications, alterations of diet or activity, and signs of a worsening health condition. *(For more information on this topic, see the Promoting Health for Children and Youth With Special Health Care Needs theme.)*

Children from cultures other than the predominant one of their community may continue to struggle with individuality and assimilation. By ages 7 and 8 years, a child living in linguistically isolated households (defined by the Census Bureau as those in which no one >14 years speaks English at least "very well") may be taking on responsibilities beyond those typical for his age in dealing with family needs. He is required to be a bridge between the family and unfamiliar school, neighborhood, or social services. For example, he may need to serve as an interpreter for adults in communicating with the school, with agencies, or on issues such as keeping the electricity on in the house. These are weighty tasks for a 7- or 8-year-old. The health care professional should ask about these situations and be mindful not to allow the child to be exploited and placed in circumstances for which he is not developmentally prepared. When possible, a certified medical interpreter should be responsible for interpreting medical, legal, and social interactions.

Health supervision visits with a child of 7 or 8 years of age provide an opportunity for the health care professional to talk directly with the child and build a trusting relationship with him. As the child continues to grow and develop, he will need to feel comfortable asking questions and discussing concerns with the health care professional if he is to begin to assume personal responsibility for his health.

The child is now cementing health habits, including those related to nutrition, physical activity, oral health, and safety. This visit provides an excellent opportunity to foster self-responsibility for positive health behaviors. The child needs to eat a variety of nutritious foods, participate in physical activities, brush his teeth twice a day, limit screen time, and make safety a priority by, for example, using a booster seat and seat belt when riding in a vehicle and by wearing a helmet when biking. Parents continue to be role models for their children in health behaviors. Many health care professionals will now note the importance of not smoking or drinking alcohol. For parents who do smoke, education about secondhand smoke, even from exposure on clothes, is important. Support for smoking cessation should be offered.

A discussion of the initiation of puberty and value of ongoing sexuality education within the family is appropriate at this age and developmental stage.

MIDDLE CHILDHOOD
7 AND 8 YEAR VISITS

Puberty may have begun in some girls. Pubertal onset is marked by breast development and can occur as early as ages 7 and 8 years for girls.

Children this age are still naive when it comes to the digital world. They may have little understanding of how the online world works, even if virtual worlds and massively multiplayer online games are common online hangouts with friends. Children this age still need parental supervision and monitoring to ensure that they are not exposed to inappropriate materials. Parents should use Internet safety tools and filtering software to limit access to content, Web sites, and activities. Parents should be present to help their children navigate outside the filters for homework assignment when necessary. Education must be given concerning the risks of sharing personal information and talking with strangers over the Internet.

Priorities for the 7 and 8 Year Visits

The first priority is to attend to the concerns of the parents.

In addition, the Bright Futures Middle Childhood Expert Panel has given priority to the following topics for discussion in the 7 and 8 Year Visits:

▶ Social determinants of health[a] (risks [neighborhood and family violence, food security, family substance use, harm from the Internet], strengths and protective factors [emotional security and self-esteem, connectedness with family and peers])

▶ Development and mental health (independence, rules and consequences, temper problems and conflict resolution; puberty and pubertal development)

▶ School (adaptation to school, school problems [behavior or learning issues], school performance and progress, school attendance, Individualized Education Plan or special education services, involvement in school activities and after-school programs)

▶ Physical growth and development (oral health [regular visits with dentist, daily brushing and flossing, adequate fluoride, avoidance of sugar-sweetened beverages and snacks], nutrition [healthy weight, adequate calcium and vitamin D intake, limiting added sugars intake], physical activity [60 minutes of physical activity a day, screen time])

▶ Safety (car safety, safety during physical activity, water safety, sun protection, harm from adults, firearm safety)

---

[a] Social determinants of health is a new priority in the fourth edition of the *Bright Futures Guidelines*. For more information, see the *Promoting Lifelong Health for Families and Communities* theme.

Health Supervision

The *Bright Futures Tool and Resource Kit* contains Previsit Questionnaires to assist the health care professional in conducting history taking, developmental surveillance, and medical screening.

History

Interval history may be obtained according to the concerns of the family and the health care professional's preference or style of practice. The following questions can encourage in-depth discussion:

General Questions for the Parent

- Tell me something your child does that makes you proud.
- What are your concerns about your child's behavioral, physical well-being, or special health care needs?
- Do you have any concerns about your child's development or learning? How is your child enjoying school? What concerns do you have about his social or academic experience? Are you concerned about your child's friendships? Bullying?
- Please share any concerns you may have about your child's mood or behavior (eg, attention, hitting, temper, worries, not participating in play with others, irritability, mood, or activity level)?

Past Medical History

- Has your child received any specialty or emergency care since the last visit?

Family History

- Has your child or anyone in the family, such as parents, brothers, sisters, grandparents, aunts, uncles, or cousins, developed a new health condition or died? **If the answer is Yes:** Ascertain who in the family has or had the condition, and ask about the age of onset and diagnosis. If the person is no longer living, ask about the age at the time of death.

Social History

- See the Social Determinants of Health priority in Anticipatory Guidance for social history questions.

Questions for the Child

- What would you like to discuss about your health today?
- Tell me something you're really good at.

Surveillance of Development

As children move into the second and third grades, issues of inattention, hyperactivity, and impulsiveness can interfere with the learning of complex concepts as well as with fitting into most school environments. Aggressive and oppositional behaviors may become maladaptive behaviors rather than behaviors of adjustment to the expectations and demands of school. Demanding learning tasks may reveal learning disabilities.

School performance deficits are assessed in light of the child's previous developmental and social history. Sorting among the issues created by parent and cultural expectations and the "goodness of fit" of the child with teacher and school expectations is challenging, but of critical importance to the child's well-being. School failure has significant negative effect on a child's self-esteem and confidence. Therefore, the nature of problems revealed in excessive absences, truancy, or poor school performance needs to be identified as soon as possible. Assessments may include sensory screening, psychosocial screening, and referrals for the assessment and diagnosis of learning disabilities and mental disorders so that appropriate treatments can begin.

For children with special health care needs and for children receiving supplemental or special education services, a review of services with parents is appropriate. It is helpful for parents to provide a copy of their child's IEP or Section 504 Plan for discussion. Review these documents carefully for accurate attention to medical comorbidities, appropriate accommodations for the child's special needs, and for comprehensive approaches to learning.

Do you or any of your child's caregivers have any specific concerns about your child's development, learning, or behavior?

A 7- or 8-year-old

- Demonstrates social and emotional competence (including self-regulation)
- Engages in healthy nutrition and physical activity behaviors
- Forms caring, supportive relationships with family members, other adults, and peers

Review of Systems

The Bright Futures Middle Childhood Expert Panel recommends a complete review of systems as a part of every health supervision visit. This review can be done through questions about the following:

Do you have any problems with

- Regular or frequent headaches or dizziness
- Eyes or vision
- Ears or hearing
- Nose or throat
- Breathing problems or pains in chest
- Belly aches or pains, throwing up, problems with urine or bowel movements
- Rashes, sunburns
- Muscle aches, injury, or other problems

Observation of Parent-Child Interaction

- Do the parent and child speak to one another respectfully?
- Does the parent seem to be supportive of the child?
- Does the parent allow the child to talk with the health care professional and not interrupt?
- Do both the parent and the child ask questions?
- Does the parent engage the child in an age-appropriate manner?

Physical Examination

A complete physical examination is included as part of every health supervision.

Respect the child's privacy by using appropriate draping during the examination. Ask siblings to wait in the waiting room, if possible.

When performing a physical examination, the health care professional's attention is directed to the following components of the examination of importance to the child at this age:

- **Measure and compare with norms for age, sex, and height**
  - Blood pressure
- **Measure and plot on appropriate CDC Growth Chart**
  - Height
  - Weight
- **Calculate and plot on appropriate CDC Growth Chart**
  - BMI
- **Mouth**
  - Observe for caries, gingivitis, and malocclusion.
- **Breasts and genitalia**
  - Assess for sexual maturity rating.
- **Musculoskeletal**
  - Observe hip, knee, and ankle function and gait.

Screening—7 Year

Universal Screening	Action	
None		

Selective Screening	Risk Assessment[a]	Action if Risk Assessment Positive (+)
Anemia	+ on risk screening questions	Hematocrit or hemoglobin
Hearing	+ on risk screening questions	Audiometry
Oral Health	Primary water source is deficient in fluoride.	Oral fluoride supplementation
Tuberculosis	+ on risk screening questions	Tuberculin skin test
Vision	+ on risk screening questions	Objective measure with age-appropriate visual-acuity measurement using HOTV or LEA symbols, Sloan letters, or Snellen letters

[a] See the *Evidence and Rationale chapter* for the criteria on which risk screening questions are based.

Screening—8 Year

Universal Screening	Action	
Hearing	Audiometry	
Vision	Objective measure with age-appropriate visual-acuity measurement using HOTV or LEA symbols, Sloan letters, or Snellen letters	

Selective Screening	Risk Assessment[a]	Action if Risk Assessment Positive (+)
Anemia	+ on risk screening questions	Hematocrit or hemoglobin
Dyslipidemia	+ on risk screening questions and not previously screened with normal results	Lipid profile
Oral Health	Primary water source is deficient in fluoride.	Oral fluoride supplementation
Tuberculosis	+ on risk screening questions	Tuberculin skin test

[a] See the *Evidence and Rationale chapter* for the criteria on which risk screening questions are based.

Immunizations

Consult the CDC/ACIP or AAP Web sites for the current immunization schedule.

CDC National Immunization Program: **www.cdc.gov/vaccines**

AAP *Red Book:* **http://redbook.solutions.aap.org**

Anticipatory Guidance

The following sample questions, which address the Bright Futures Middle Childhood Expert Panel's Anticipatory Guidance Priorities, are intended to be used selectively to invite discussion, gather information, address the needs and concerns of the family, and build partnerships. Use of the questions may vary from visit to visit and from family to family. Questions can be modified to match the health care professional's communication style. The accompanying anticipatory guidance for the family should be geared to questions, issues, or concerns for that particular child and family. Tools and handouts to support anticipatory guidance can be found in the *Bright Futures Tool and Resource Kit*.

Priority

Social Determinants of Health

Risks: Neighborhood and family violence (bullying, fighting), food security, family substance use (tobacco, e-cigarettes, alcohol, drugs), harm from the Internet

Strengths and protective factors: Emotional security and self-esteem, connectedness with family and peers

Risks: Neighborhood and Family Violence (Bullying, Fighting)

Children in families that are affected by poverty, neighborhood violence, or family violence are dealing with a level of stress that affects their current and future health. For example, families in difficult living situations may have concerns about their ability to provide a safe environment for their child.

Questions on this topic can be sensitive. The health care professional can identify these issues in a supportive and non-blaming way and help the parents formulate steps toward solutions. A referral to community resources or federal assistance programs may be a useful first step.

Fighting and bullying can occur in school and neighborhood settings. These behaviors may indicate the presence of conduct disorders in bullies or may co-occur with problems of depression or anxiety in both bullies and children who are bullied. *(For more information on this topic, see the Bullying section of the Promoting Mental Health theme.)* Family violence includes physical attacks and sexual coercion. Children can benefit from a discussion of safety in all these aspects.

Sample Questions

Are there frequent reports of violence in your community or school? Is your child involved in that violence? Do you think she is safe in the neighborhood? Has your child ever been injured in a fight? Has she been bullied or hit by others? Has your child demonstrated bullying or aggression toward others? Have you talked to her about violence and how to be safe?

Ask the Child

Have you ever been involved with a group who did things that could have gotten them into trouble? What do you do when someone tries to pick a fight with you? What do you do when you are angry? Have you been in a physical fight in the past 6 months? Do you know anyone in a gang? Have you ever been touched in a way that made you feel uncomfortable or that was unwelcome? Have you ever been touched on your private parts against your wish or without your permission?

Anticipatory Guidance

- Teach your child nonviolent conflict-resolution techniques.
- Talk to your child about your family's expectations for time with friends.
- Make sure your child knows she can call you if she ever needs help. Be prepared to step in and help if needed.

For the Child

- Talk to your parent, another trusted adult (such as a teacher), or me if anyone bullies, stalks, or abuses you or makes you feel unsafe. If you see another child being bullied, tell an adult.
- Learn to manage conflict nonviolently. Walk away if you can.

Risks: Food Security

The need for adequate calories and nutritious food choices during this period of steady growth and development and increasingly independent food decision-making makes food security a critical issue in middle childhood. If the family is having difficulty obtaining nutritious food, provide information about SNAP, the Commodity Supplemental Food Program, local food shelves, and local community food programs.

Sample Questions

Within the past 12 months, did you worry that your food would run out before you got money to buy more? In the past 12 months, did the food you bought just not last and you didn't have money to buy more?

Anticipatory Guidance

- Programs and resources are available to help you and your family. You may be eligible for food and nutrition assistance through programs like SNAP, which used to be called Food Stamps. Food banks, food pantries, and community food programs can also help.

Risks: Family Substance Use (Tobacco, E-cigarettes, Alcohol, Drugs)

Exposure to tobacco smoke remains an important environmental risk. Encourage parents to keep their home and vehicles smoke-free, as well as free of vapor from e-cigarettes. Becoming familiar with community and online resources for quitting smoking allows health care professionals to refer parents who are interested in quitting.

Worrying about a family member with a substance use or mental health problem also may be a source of significant stress.

Sample Questions
Does anyone who lives with your child smoke or use e-cigarettes? Does anyone smoke or use e-cigarettes in your home or vehicle? If so, who? Is there anyone in your child's life whose alcohol or drug use concerns you?

Anticipatory Guidance
- Exposure to secondhand smoke greatly increases the risk of heart and lung diseases in your child. For your health and your child's health, please stop smoking if you are a smoker, and insist that others not smoke around your child.
- Exposure to vapor from e-cigarettes also may be harmful. For your child's health, please don't use e-cigarettes around your child, especially indoors or inside cars.
- It's not always possible, but when you can, avoid spending time in places where people are smoking cigarettes or using e-cigarettes.
- If you are ever interested in quitting smoking, please talk to me. **800-QUIT-NOW (800-784-8669);** TTY **800-332-8615** is a national telephone helpline that is routed to local resources. Additional resources are available at **www.cdc.gov.** I can also refer you to local or online resources.
- If you are worried about any family members' drug or alcohol use problems, you can talk with me.

For the Child
- Don't try cigarettes or e-cigarettes. They are bad for your lungs and heart, and your skin and teeth. Walk away from kids who offer you cigarettes, e-cigarettes, alcohol, or drugs.

Risks: Harm From the Internet

Internet safety is similar to neighborhood safety. Younger children never play outside unsupervised or leave the yard. More mature children will be allowed to go to known safe places like a playground, but are not allowed to wander into inappropriate or unsafe areas. Internet use should parallel safe play outdoors. Younger children should only be online supervised, and, with increasing maturity, limited browsing can be permitted. Information about safe Internet use can be found at **www.HealthyChildren.org.**

Sample Questions
How much do you know about your child's Internet use? For example, what sites is she visiting, what games is she playing, who is she talking to, and how much time is she spending on the computer? Do you have rules for the Internet? Have you installed an Internet filter?

Ask the Child
What would you do if you came to an Internet site that you thought wasn't a good idea or that scared you?

Anticipatory Guidance

- Your family computer should be in a place where you can easily observe your child's use.
- Check the Internet history regularly to be sure you approve of your child's Internet choices.
- Just as you monitor your child's activity in the neighborhood and community, it is important to be aware of her Internet use. A safety filter allows some parental supervision.

For the Child

- It is important to go online only when your parents say it's OK. Never go to Internet sites unless you know they are good choices.
- Never chat online unless you tell your parents. No one should ever make you feel scared online.
- Do not give your personal information, like your full name or address or phone number on a Web site unless your parents say it is OK.

Strengths and Protective Factors: Emotional Security and Self-esteem

Identifying strengths and providing feedback to families about what they are doing well helps provide a comprehensive and balanced view of the child's health and well-being. For families living in difficult circumstances, such strengths may help protect the child from, or reduce the degree of, negative health outcomes. Parents need to know that they can positively influence the healthy development of their child no matter what difficulties or problems exist. Anticipatory guidance provides parents with ideas about how to give their child opportunities to become good at things, to begin to make independent decisions, to have social connections, and to do things for others.

Parents can help make their child feel secure by giving hugs, participating in activities together, and listening without interrupting during family discussions. Children with warm, nurturing parents are more likely to have high self-esteem. Hypercritical parents who have unrealistically high expectations, and uninvolved parents who do not encourage their children to achieve and to try new experiences, can damage their child's self-esteem. Protective factors for any child include having at least one supportive adult in their life.

Self-esteem is a key feature of a fulfilling life and has an enormous influence on mental health. Children develop a positive sense of self if they think they are making a contribution. Words of encouragement are important and provide energizing motivation. Help parents think about how they can encourage their child to be responsible by modeling responsibility themselves, keeping promises, showing up on time, and completing tasks on time.

Sample Questions

How happy is your child? Do you feel your child has good self-confidence?

Ask the Child

Tell me about some of the things you are good at doing. What are some of the things that make you happy?

Anticipatory Guidance

- Encourage competence, independence, and self-responsibility in all areas by not doing everything for your child, but by helping her do things well herself, and by supporting her in helping others.
- Show affection and pride in your child's special strengths and use appropriate praise liberally.

Strengths and Protective Factors: Connectedness With Family and Peers

One of the most important protective factors and a component of healthy development is the ability to form caring and supportive relationships with family, other adults, and peers. At home, this involves a relationship characterized by warm supportive interactions with parents and guardians combined with clear expectations and an opportunity for children to begin to gain the skills necessary for independent decision-making. Children this age also can benefit from feeling they can contribute to planning family activities and helping out when needed. Children are more likely to make healthy choices if they stay connected with family members and if clear rules and limits are set.

Sample Questions

How are you getting along as a family? What do you do together? What responsibilities does your child have at home? What are your expectations?

Ask the Child

How do you get along with your family? What do you like to do together?

Anticipatory Guidance

- Spend time with your child. Express willingness for questions and discussion. Develop a pattern of communication and support her as an independent person. Make time every day, such as at mealtimes, bedtime, drive time, or check-in time, to talk about lots of things.
- Discuss your child's responsibilities in the family and how they change with age.
- Clearly communicate rules and expectations.
- Get to know your child's friends.

For the Child

- Spend time with family members. Help out at home.

Priority

Development and Mental Health

Independence, rules and consequences, temper problems and conflict resolution; puberty and pubertal development

Independence, Rules and Consequences, Temper Problems and Conflict Resolution

Healthy development includes progress in emotional and relational domains. Self-regulation is an important task to master. Children this age now learn to handle frustration and express emotions appropriately. Parents can help by setting reasonable limits (or reasonable consequences for not following family rules), providing opportunities for their child to share his worries and concerns and listening to his ideas about possible solutions. Having appropriate responsibilities at home builds a sense of competence as well. Parents are the most important role models in these critical areas.

Sample Questions

What are your child's favorite activities? What concerns and worries has your child shared with you? What types of discipline do you use most often? Does it work? What responsibilities does your child have at home, such as helping care for younger siblings, helping prepare meals together, or raking an elderly neighbor's leaves? What are the consequences if he does not carry out his responsibilities? Are tantrums a frequent problem for your child? How does he deal with frustration? Is he kind? Is he honest?

Ask the Child

What new things have you tried in the past year? Do you think your family rules are fair? Tell me the last really fun thing you did. How are you sleeping? Do you have any worries? Who do you usually talk to about your worries and things that made you mad?

Anticipatory Guidance

- Establish family expectations and reasonable consequences for not following family rules.
- Provide opportunities for your child to share his worries and concerns. If you are concerned that these worries and concerns are interfering with your child's ability to function well, please talk with me about it.
- Help your child begin to solve problems by asking for his ideas.
- Having appropriate responsibilities at home builds a sense of competence.
- Encourage competence, independence, and self-responsibility in all areas by not doing everything for your child, but by helping him do things well himself, and by supporting him in helping others.
- Be a positive role model for your child in terms of activities, values, attitudes, and morality.
- Do not hit, shake, or spank your child or permit others to do so. Instead, talk with your child about establishing reasonable consequences for breaking the rules, and follow through with the agreed-upon consequences each time a rule is broken.

- If you live in an area where corporal punishment is allowed in schools, you have the right to say that your child may not be spanked and that you should be consulted anytime the school might use spanking.

For the Child

- Everyone has worries. The best way to deal with these feelings is to talk with someone who listens well and who will help you learn how to deal with them in good ways. Often, just talking about worries helps them go away, but if they don't, let your parents, me, or another adult you trust know so that we can help you with your worries.
- Everyone has things that make them mad. These feelings don't feel good. It is OK to have them, but when you're mad, it's not OK to hurt yourself or someone else or to break or damage something. The best way to deal with angry feelings is to talk with someone who listens well and who will help you learn how to deal with these feelings in good ways.

Puberty and Pubertal Development

Puberty includes dramatic changes in physical, emotional, and cognitive aspects of development.

Parents from various cultural and religious backgrounds may differ in their opinions about puberty. Explore their beliefs and respect them, while also explaining that their child's curiosity about this issue is normal.

Sample Question

What have you told your child about how to care for his changing body?

Ask the Child

Do you know what puberty is? Has anyone discussed with you how your body will change during the time called puberty?

Anticipatory Guidance

- Answer questions simply and honestly at a level appropriate to your child's understanding. If your child receives family life education at school or in the community, discuss the information with him.

For the Child

- Lots of changes happen to you and your body during puberty, and some of those changes can be surprising or hard to figure out. It's always OK to ask your parent or another adult you trust if you have any concerns or worries.
- Even embarrassing questions can be important ones. It's OK to talk about your body's development.

Priority

School

Adaptation to school, school problems (behavior or learning issues), school performance and progress, school attendance, Individualized Education Program or special education services, involvement in school activities and after-school programs

Adaption to School, School Problems (Behavior or Learning Issues), School Performance and Progress, School Attendance, Individualized Education Program or Special Education Services, Involvement in School Activities and After-school Programs

School is a regular part of the daily activities for the child at 7 and 8 years of age. Most waking hours are now spent at school and in extracurricular activities. Children this age display behaviors necessary for learning, such as cooperation and attention. After-school activities, such as scouts, team sports, and the arts, are some of the possible opportunities for engaging children in school and community activities. These should be balanced with adequate unstructured time for children to play and explore.

Sample Questions

How is your child doing in school? Is she enjoying school? What types of activities is your child doing after school? What concerns do you have about your child's school experience? Has she had many absences? Does she receive any special educational services such as an IEP, a Section 504 Plan, or other special services at school?

Ask the Child

What do you like best about school? Tell me about your friends at school. What are your favorite activities to do after school?

Anticipatory Guidance

- A child who arrives at school fed and rested is healthy and ready to learn. Help your child have a healthy breakfast every morning before school, and establish bedtime routines on school nights so that she gets at least 10 to 11 hours of sleep.
- Academic or learning difficulties can become evident in children this age. If your child is not doing well in school, talk with her teacher about possible reasons and what can be done to identify and address the problem. If you have any concerns about her vision, hearing, attention, or other stresses that may be bothering her, let's talk about them.
- If your child is anxious about going to school, talk with her about her worries. Try to obtain a complete picture of what is happening, and when and where. Consider the possibility that she is being bullied by another child. Contact your child's teacher and the principal to seek their assistance.

- If your child has special health care needs, maintain an active role in the IEP process. Bring a copy of the IEP to each visit here with me.
- After-school activities, such as sports teams, social activities, clubs, and extracurricular activities, place increased demands on children's time. Try not to overschedule your child with too many extracurricular activities. Children need unstructured time as well as structured activities.

Priority

Physical Growth and Development

Oral health (regular visits with dentist, daily brushing and flossing, adequate fluoride, avoidance of sugar-sweetened beverages and snacks), nutrition (healthy weight, adequate calcium and vitamin D intake, limiting added sugars intake), physical activity (60 minutes of physical activity a day, screen time)

Oral Health (Regular Visits With Dentist, Daily Brushing and Flossing, Adequate Fluoride, Avoidance of Sugar-Sweetened Beverages and Snacks)

By ages 7 and 8 years, a child already should have an established dental home with regularly scheduled visits with his dentist at least twice each year. He also should receive a fluoride supplement if the fluoride level in community water supplies (at home and at school) is low. Assure parents that fluoride is safe and effective at preventing tooth decay. If the child plays contact sports, he should wear protective mouth guards as appropriate.

Sample Questions

How many times a day does your child brush his teeth? Does he floss once a day? Do you help your child brush and floss his teeth? How often does your child see the dentist? Does he take a fluoride supplement pill? Does your child consume sugar-sweetened snacks and drinks? Does your child wear a mouth guard when playing contact sports?

Ask the Child

Do you brush and floss your teeth every day? How many times? Do you always wear a mouth guard when you play contact sports?

Anticipatory Guidance

- Your child already should be seeing a dentist regularly. This is called having a dental home. If your child does not have a dental home, we can help you find one.
- Be sure that your child brushes his teeth for 2 minutes, twice a day, with a pea-sized amount of fluoridated toothpaste, and flosses once a day. Make this task enjoyable. Take turns. Allow him to brush and floss his own teeth first and then you take a turn to get his teeth thoroughly brushed and flossed.
- Every child needs fluoride supplementation. If your community water system is not fluoridated, he will need a supplement.
- Limit your child's consumption of sweetened drinks and snacks. Prolonged contact with the teeth can increase the chance of the teeth getting cavities.

For the Child

- To protect your teeth from getting cavities, it is important to brush your teeth for at least 2 minutes, twice a day, and to floss at least once a day.
- If you are playing contact sports, always wear a mouth guard to protect your teeth.

Nutrition (Healthy Weight, Adequate Calcium and Vitamin D Intake, Limiting Added Sugars Intake)

Discuss healthy weight by using the BMI chart to show a child and his parents how his height and weight compare to those of other children of the same sex and age. If the child's BMI is greater than the 85th percentile, it is appropriate to begin more in-depth counseling on nutritious food choices and physical activity.

Counsel all families about appropriate food choices to promote nutritional adequacy and reinforce positive nutrition habits. Ensuring sufficient calcium and vitamin D intake can be a particular concern, especially if the child does not consume dairy products. Supplementation with these nutrients can be considered. Fortified orange juice typically has calcium and vitamin D. Soy milk generally has both, but that is not always true for other products marketed as "milks" (eg, almond, rice, coconut, hemp). Families should be encouraged to check the package label to be sure. Not all yogurt has vitamin D.

Guidance or a referral is appropriate if the family needs nutrition help because of cultural, religious, or financial reasons. For children with special health care needs, ensure that nutrition and physical activity are incorporated into the IEP.

Sample Questions

What do you think of your child's weight and growth over the past year? What concerns, if any, do you have about your child's eating, such as getting him to drink enough milk and eat vegetables and fruits? How often does he drink sweetened beverages, such as soda, sport drinks, or juice drinks? How often does he drink or eat dairy foods, such as milk, cheese, or yogurt? How often do you eat together as a family?

Ask the Child

How many sweetened beverages do you drink each day? Do you drink milk? How many times a week do you eat breakfast? What vegetables and fruits do you eat?

Anticipatory Guidance

- Choose healthy eating behaviors.
  - Every day, give your child a healthy breakfast. Research shows that eating breakfast helps children learn and behave better at school.
  - Help your child recognize and respond to hunger and fullness cues.
  - Eat together as a family. Make mealtimes pleasant and companionable; encourage conversation and turn off the TV.
  - Be a role model for your child with your own healthy eating behaviors.
- Make nutritious foods and drinks the usual options at home for meals and snacks. These include vegetables; fruits; whole grains; lean protein, such as meat, fish, poultry, eggs, legumes, nuts and seeds; and low-fat and nonfat dairy products.
- Limit foods and drinks that are high in calories, saturated fat, salt, added sugars, and refined grains, and low in nutrients. These include ice cream, baked goods, salty snacks, fast foods, pizzas, and soda and other sweetened beverages.
- Limit juice to 4 to 6 oz of 100% fruit juice each day.

- Make sure your child gets dairy foods and calcium- and vitamin D–containing foods and beverages each day. Children aged 4 to 8 years need 12 to 16 oz of low-fat or fat-free milk each day plus an additional serving of low-fat yogurt and cheese. If your child doesn't drink milk or consume other dairy products, then let's talk about alternatives. These can include foods and beverages that are fortified with calcium and vitamin D (like some orange juices and cereals).

For the Child

- Eating healthy foods is important to helping you do well in school and being physically active.
- Pay attention to what your body tells you. Eat when you feel hungry and stop eating when you feel satisfied.
- Dairy foods are important for strong bones and teeth. Be sure to drink at least 3 glasses of milk each day. You can also eat yogurt instead of drinking milk.

Physical Activity (60 Minutes of Physical Activity a Day, Screen Time)

All children should be able to participate in some type of physical activity daily. Current recommendations state that children should be physically active for at least 60 minutes a day. Encourage parents of a child with special health care needs to allow him to participate in regular physical activity or cardiovascular fitness within the limits of his medical, developmental, or physical condition.

Emphasize the importance of safety equipment when the child participates in physical activity.

This is the age when children may become involved in organized sports. Encourage parents to check out programs before enrolling their children (eg, rules about all children playing, coaching training/certification). Children who do not participate in organized sports should still be encouraged to find individual ways to be physically active (eg, dancing, skating, biking).

The time a child is using media or the Internet is time he is not being physically active. Counsel regarding media time expenditure and Internet safety.

Sample Questions

How much physical activity does your child get every day? How much recreational screen time does your child spend each weekday? How about on weekends? Does your child have a TV or Internet-connected device in his bedroom? Is your child involved in a sports program? What is your child's usual bedtime on school nights and on nonschool nights? Does your child have trouble going to sleep or does he wake up during the night?

Ask the Child

How often are you physically active outside of school? How much time each day do you spend watching TV or playing on the computer or with other devices that are connected to the Internet?

Anticipatory Guidance

- Encourage your child to be physically active for at least 60 minutes total every day. It doesn't have to be all at once. Find physical activities that your family enjoys. Include physical activity in your daily lives.

- Do not allow your child to sleep with any electronic device in his bedroom, including phones or tablets.

- In order to balance your child's needs for physical activity, sleep, school activities, and unplugged time, consider making a family media use plan to balance these important health behaviors and media use time in your child's day. The family media use plan is an online tool that you and your child can fill out together. The tool prompts you and your child to enter daily health priorities such as an hour for physical activity, 8 to 11 hours of sleep, time for homework and school activities, and unplugged time each day for time with family and independently. You and your child can then view the time left over and decide on rules around daily screen time for your child. The AAP has information on making a plan at **www.HealthyChildren.org/MediaUsePlan.**

- Take into account not only the quantity but the quality and location of media use. Consider TVs, phones, tablets, and computers. Rules should be followed by parents as well as children. Construct it so that it suits your families' media needs, but also helps you preserve face-to-face time during family routines such as meals, playtime, and bedtime. Times or locations in the house can be designated as media-free.

- Children this age can learn reading, science, and math skills from computers, and may be using computers and other Internet-connected media in school. However, they need other experiences such as unstructured play alone and with peers, time outdoors, physical activity, and hands-on learning. These kinds of activities help them develop all parts of their brain, including more complicated skills such as executive functioning and social skills.

- Children learn more from educational media when you watch a show or use an app with them and talk about it afterwards.

- Supervise your child's Internet use so that you can teach him how to use it safely and how to avoid inappropriate content.

- If your child is using media excessively, find out why. Is he having trouble with peer relationships or social skills? Some children seek solitary activities if they are struggling with friendships. Encourage your child to find activities that interest him, or seek help through the school.

- Getting enough sleep every night is important for your child's health. Using media before bedtime to get to sleep actually leads to worse sleep habits, less sleep, and school problems. Suggest a quiet bedtime routine or reading in bed instead.

For the Child

- It's a good idea to be physically active several times every day.
- Turn off your TV and video games. Get up and play instead.
- Don't eat in front of a screen.

Priority

Safety
Car safety, safety during physical activity, water safety, sun protection, harm from adults, firearm safety

Car Safety

Remind parents of the ongoing importance of automobile and bicycle safety. Children should use belt-positioning booster seats until the seat belt fits well. This means that the lap belt lies low across the hips and upper thighs, the shoulder belt lies across the middle of the chest and shoulder, and the child is tall enough to sit all the way back with knees bent comfortably at the edge of the seat without slouching forward. This usually happens when the child is between the ages of 8 and 12 years and about 4 feet 9 inches tall. The back seat is the safest place for children to ride until age 13 years. Stress the need for parental modeling of safe behaviors by wearing their own seat belts.

Sample Questions
Does everyone in the family always wear a seat belt?

Ask the Child
What type of seat do you sit in when you are in the car? Do you sit in the back seat every time you ride in the car? Do you always wear your seat belt?

Anticipatory Guidance
- Continue to use a belt-positioning booster seat with the lap and shoulder safety belt until the lap/shoulder belt fits. This means the lap belt can be worn low and flat across the hips and upper thighs, the shoulder belt can be worn across the shoulder rather than the face or neck, and your child can bend at the knees while sitting against the vehicle seat back. This usually happens when your child is between the ages of 8 and 12 years and at about 4 feet 9 inches tall.
- The back seat is the safest place for children younger than 13 years to ride.

For the Child
- Always sit up and stay buckled in your booster seat and ride in the back seat of the car because that is where you are safest.

For information about booster seats and actions to keep your child safe in and around cars, visit www.safercar.gov/parents.

Toll-free Auto Safety Hotline: 888-327-4236

Safety During Physical Activity

Reinforce the importance of safety in sports and other physical activities, emphasizing the need for wearing protective gear (eg, helmet, mouth guard, eye protection, and knee and elbow pads).

Children and adolescents younger than 16 years should not drive or ride an all-terrain vehicle.

Sample Questions

Do you enforce the use of helmets? Do you always wear helmets yourself?

Ask the Child

Do you always wear a helmet when biking, skating, or doing other outdoor activities?

Anticipatory Guidance

- Make sure your child always wears a helmet while riding a bike. Now is the time to teach your child "rules of the road." Be sure she knows the rules and can use them.
- Watch your child ride her bike. See if she is in control of the bike. See if your child uses good judgment. Your 8-year-old is not old enough to ride at dusk or after dark. Make sure your child brings in the bike when the sun starts to set.
- Make sure your child also always wears a helmet and other protective equipment when skating, riding a scooter, or doing other outdoor activities.

For the Child

- Being active is good for you, but being safe while being active is just as important. One of the best ways to protect yourself is to wear the right safety equipment, especially a helmet, when you are biking, skating, or doing other outdoor activities.

Water Safety

Drowning is a leading cause of death in this age group. An adult should actively supervise whenever children are in or near water. Swimming is a skill that everyone needs; children should at least learn basic water survival skills.

Sample Questions

Does your child know how to swim?

Ask the Child

Do you know how to swim? What rules do your parents have about swimming?

Anticipatory Guidance

- Teach your child to swim. Knowing how to swim does not make children drown-proof, so, even if your child knows how to swim, never let her swim alone.
- Do not let your child play around any water (lake, stream, pool, or ocean) unless an adult is watching. NEVER let your child swim in any fast-moving water.
- Teach your child to never dive into water unless an adult has already checked the depth of the water.

- When on any boat or other watercraft, be sure your child is wearing an appropriately fitting, US Coast Guard–approved life jacket. Children are more likely to wear a life jacket if adults are wearing them as well. Be a role model; wear your life jacket, too.
- Be sure that swimming pools in your community, apartment complex, or home have a 4-sided fence with a self-closing, self-latching gate.

For the Child

- Swimming lessons are an important way to become comfortable in the water. Ask your parents about learning to swim.
- Never swim without an adult around.

Sun Protection

Sun protection now is of increasing importance because of climate change and the thinning of the atmospheric ozone layer. Sun protection is accomplished through limiting sun exposure, using sunscreen, and wearing protective clothing.

Sample Questions

Do you apply sunscreen whenever your child plays outside? Do you limit outside time during the middle of the day, when the sun is strongest?

Ask the Child

Do you always use sunscreen?

Anticipatory Guidance

- Always apply sunscreen with an SPF greater than 15 when your child is outside. Reapply every 2 hours.
- Encourage your child to wear a hat.
- Avoid prolonged time in the sun between 11:00 am and 3:00 pm.

For the Child

- Always wear sunscreen and a hat when you are outside.
- Try not to be outside in the sun too long between 11:00 am and 3:00 pm, when it is really easy to get a sunburn.

Harm From Adults

As children now spend more time with other children and families, parents must help their children develop safe play habits. Play should be supervised by a responsible adult aware of children's activities and available in case of problems.

Parents should discuss personal safety in a manner that is informative and empowering without provoking unnecessary anxiety. Child sexual abuse prevention requires that children have knowledge and age-appropriate skills to keep themselves safe.

Sample Questions

Do you know your child's friends? Their families? Does your child know how to get help in an emergency if you are not present? Does your child have a backup plan if you are not home when she gets there after school? Have you discussed with your child ways to prevent sexual abuse?

Ask the Child

Do you know what to do if you get home and Mom or Dad is not there? What would you do if you felt unsafe at a friend's house? What would you do if a grown-up made you scared? Who could you tell? Who would help you? Has anyone ever touched you in a way that made you feel uncomfortable? Has anyone ever tried to harm you physically?

Anticipatory Guidance

- Teach your child that the safety rules at home apply at other homes as well.
- Be sure that your child is supervised in a safe environment before and after school and at times when school is out.
- Anticipate providing less direct supervision as your child demonstrates more maturity.
- Be sure your child understands safety rules for the home, including emergency phone numbers, and that she knows what to do in case of a fire or other emergency. Teach your child how to dial 911.
- Help your child to understand it is always OK to ask to come home or call you if she is not comfortable at someone else's house.
- Teach your child that it is never OK for an adult to tell a child to keep secrets from parents, to express interest in private parts, or to ask a child for help with his or her private parts.

For the Child

- Don't open the door to anyone you don't know. It's best not to have friends over unless your parents give you permission for them to be there.
- Be sure you play safe wherever you play. Every family should have the same safety rules.
- It's always OK to ask a grown-up for help if you are scared or worried. And it's OK to ask to go home and be with your Mom or Dad.
- We call the parts of your body that are usually under a bathing suit "privates" because we keep them covered and because you are the only one in charge of them. That is why I asked your permission before I checked your privates.

- It is never OK for an older child or an adult to show you his or her private parts, to ask you to show your privates, to touch you there, to scare you, or to ask you not to tell your parents about what he or she did with you. Always get away from the person as quickly as possible and tell your parent or another adult right away.

Firearm Safety

Discuss firearm safety in the home and the danger of firearms to family members and children. Homicide and completed suicide are more common in homes in which firearms are kept. The evidence is clear that the safest home for children is one without firearms. If it is necessary to keep a firearm, it should be stored unloaded and locked, with the ammunition locked separately from the firearm.

Children this age are curious. Because firearms can lead to serious injury or death, parents cannot rely on their own children, no matter how well-behaved or well taught they are, to avoid handling a weapon that they find. At this age, children still lack the maturity or cognitive capacity to reliably follow advice concerning firearms.

Sample Questions

If there is a firearm in your home, is it unloaded and locked up? Where is the ammunition stored? Have you considered not owning a firearm because it poses a danger to children and other family members?

Ask the Child

What would you do if you saw a firearm?

Anticipatory Guidance

- If it is necessary to keep a firearm in your home, it should be stored unloaded and locked, with the ammunition locked separately from the firearm. Keep the key where children cannot have access.
- Remember that children simply do not understand how dangerous firearms can be, despite your warnings.

For the Child

- Adults are supposed to keep their firearms away from children. If you see a firearm that is unlocked, don't touch it, but do tell your parent right away.

Middle Childhood
9 and 10 Year Visits

Context

By ages 9 to 10 years, puberty may have begun in some children. Pubertal onset is marked by breast development at about ages 7 and 8 years for girls, and by testicular enlargement at about age 9 and 10 for boys. These changes are accompanied by a growth spurt. Individual differences are noted with pubertal onset. This is an opportunity for the health care professional to learn about family and cultural beliefs about puberty and about how the family's cultural and religious values will guide the discussion of sexuality and the physical changes of puberty.

By this age, the child has become a member of a peer group. Most of her friends are the same gender, and these friends have assumed great importance in her life. The child's growing independence from the family is now more apparent.

Parents can acknowledge the child's desire for independence by offering her opportunities to earn privileges by demonstrating her responsibility (eg, parents may identify appropriate chores, while allowing the child to decide when to complete them and the consequences if the chores are not completed). The value placed on independence and how it is defined is determined by culture, the economic realities of the family, and the safety of the general environment. In some families, conflict arises if the parents misinterpret this normal realignment of allegiance toward peers as a rejection of family values, past support, and guidance.

Supporting and enhancing the child's self-esteem and self-confidence are critical during this period, and enhance resiliency. Children who feel good about themselves are better equipped to withstand negative peer pressure than children who have a lot of self-doubt. Families need to spend time with their child, talking with her, showing affection, and praising her efforts and accomplishments. Parents or caregivers who are depressed and feel alienated and unaccepted may have difficulty providing such emotional support. The health care professional can help by identifying the child's strengths and promoting communication between the child and her family. In some cultures, it is deemed inappropriate to praise children, and parents will have alternative approaches to enhance their child's sense of competence and self-esteem. It is important to have this discussion with parents in the context of the family's culture.

School performance indicates the child's accomplishments across all developmental domains (social and emotional, communicative, cognitive, and physical). Inquire about school success. It may be of value to review the child's most recent report card. Increasing requirements for autonomy and self-motivation may lead to academic deterioration for children who functioned well with supervised and structured academic tasks. The health care professional can explore whether the child is having any academic or social problems, whether she gets along with teachers and peers, and whether she is participating in extracurricular activities or clubs. At this age, many children become involved in a variety of outside activities, including sports, music, scouting, and community or faith-based activities. A child can easily become overscheduled, and parents need to balance enriching activities with sufficient downtime and family time.

Children 9 and 10 years of age are technologically savvy. Smart phones, tablets, computers, video games, e-mail, texting, and social media are part of their daily lives. However, children this age still need supervision, and parents must be clear that use of these devices will be monitored and that they will be checking for inappropriate pictures and texts. Parents should discuss Internet safety, responsibilities, and rules of the cyberworld with their child. Parents should use Internet safety tools to limit access to undesirable content, Web sites, and activities. In addition, parents should balance computer and media time with active time. Children need to be physically active throughout the day with limited sedentary time.

Injury prevention should be emphasized during this stage of development. The 9- or 10-year-old may begin to engage in dangerous risk-taking behaviors (eg, dares, drinking, smoking, inhaling, or gang involvement). If the peer group includes older children, the child may encounter pressure to perform acts and take risks for which she is not developmentally prepared. Some families do not recognize that these behaviors can start this young. Recognizing and discussing this possibility may help parents teach their children about dealing with peer pressure.

Parents need to know their children's friends and the friends' parents. For parents and caregivers with limited English proficiency, supervising their child in the broader community can be a challenge. Health care professionals can help provide connections to supports in the community that will enhance the parents' role. Children this age should still be in environments where appropriate adult supervision exists so as to limit opportunities for experimentation with cigarettes, e-cigarettes, alcohol and other drugs, and other developmentally inappropriate activities. The amount of unsupervised time and the incidence of drug use are directly related.

The health care professional may want to meet alone with the child or the child may want to meet alone with the health care professional. It may be most appropriate to give the child the choice. At this age, some children may feel a need to have a parent close by during the visit to help describe any individual or family concerns, while others may feel they are preteen-agers and should be seen without parental supervision. However, the health care professional may need the parents to verify and expand some of the child's answers. Cultural norms should be taken into account in making this decision.

Priorities for the 9 and 10 Year Visits

The first priority is to attend to the concerns of the parents.

In addition, the Bright Futures Middle Childhood Expert Panel has given priority to the following topics for discussion in this visit:

▶ Social determinants of health[a] (risks [neighborhood and family violence, food security, family substance use, harm from the Internet], strengths and protective factors [emotional security and self-esteem, connectedness with family and peers])

▶ Development and mental health (temper problems, setting reasonable limits, friends; sexuality [pubertal onset, personal hygiene, initiation of growth spurt, menstruation and ejaculation, loss of baby fat and accretion of muscle, sexual safety])

▶ School (school attendance, school problems [behavior or learning], school performance and progress, transitions, co-occurrence of middle school and pubertal transitions)

▶ Physical growth and development (oral health [regular visits with dentist, daily brushing and flossing, adequate fluoride, avoidance of sugar-sweetened beverages and snacks], nutrition [healthy weight, disordered eating behaviors, importance of breakfast, limits on saturated fat and added sugars, healthy snacks], physical activity [60 minutes of physical activity a day, after-school activities])

▶ Safety (car safety, safety during physical activity, water safety, sun protection, knowing child's friends and their families, firearm safety)

---

[a] Social determinants of health is a new priority in the fourth edition of the *Bright Futures Guidelines.* For more information, see the *Promoting Lifelong Health for Families and Communities* theme.

Health Supervision

The *Bright Futures Tool and Resource Kit* contains Previsit Questionnaires to assist the health care professional in conducting history taking, developmental surveillance, and medical screening.

History

Interval history may be obtained according to the concerns of the family and the health care professional's preference or style of practice. The following questions can encourage in-depth discussion:

General Questions for the Parent

- Tell me something your child does that makes you proud.
- What concerns do you have about your child's physical well-being or special health care needs?
- Do you have any concerns about your child's development or learning?
- Do you have any concerns about your child's weight, eating behaviors, physical activity level, or sleep patterns?
- Tell me about any concerns you may have about your child's mood or behavior (eg, attention, hitting others, temper, worries, not having good friends, irritability, mood, or activity level)?

Past Medical History

- Has your child received any specialty or emergency care since the last visit?

Family History

- Has your child or anyone in the family, such as parents, brothers, sisters, grandparents, aunts, uncles, or cousins, developed a new health condition or died? **If the answer is Yes:** Ascertain who in the family has or had the condition, and ask about the age of onset and diagnosis. If they are no longer living, ask about their age at the time of death.

Social History

- See the Social Determinants of Health priority in Anticipatory Guidance for social history questions.

Questions for the Child

- What would you like to talk about today?
- Do you have any questions about your health? Your body? Or how your body is changing?
- Tell me something you're really good at.
- What do you do to help others?

Surveillance of Development

School performance is a functional marker of a child's development and accomplishments across all developmental domains (social and emotional, communicative, cognitive, and physical). Increasing requirements for autonomy and self-motivation sometimes lead to academic deterioration for children who functioned well with supervised and structured academic tasks.

The child's intellectual abilities as well as learning problems become more apparent during this period of the child's development. Many learning problems become evident in the later elementary school years, as expectations for class performance increase. School failure, poor school attendance, or new struggles require investigation, as they frequently indicate an unrecognized learning disability, ADHD, or the effect of stressors, such as family dysfunction and divorce, bullying at school, or depression in the child or parent. Some children and parents also become apprehensive about the transition to middle school.

For children and youth with special health care needs and for children receiving supplemental or special education services, a review of services with parents is appropriate. It is helpful for parents to provide a copy of their child's IEP or Section 504 Plan for discussion. Review these documents carefully for accurate attention to medical comorbidities, appropriate accommodations for the child's special needs, and comprehensive approaches to learning. Also, review medications that may need to be administered during the school day, including psychotropic medications, and ensure completion of appropriate school forms.

Do you or any of your child's caregivers have any specific concerns about your child's development, learning, or behavior?

A 9- or 10-year-old

- Demonstrates social and emotional competence (including self-regulation)
- Engages in healthy nutrition and physical activity behaviors
- Uses independent decision-making skills (including problem-solving skills)
- Forms caring and supportive relationships with family members, other adults, and peers
- Displays a sense of self-confidence and hopefulness

Review of Systems

The Bright Futures Middle Childhood Expert Panel recommends a complete review of systems as a part of every health supervision visit. This review can be done through questions about the following:

Do you have any problems with

- Regular or frequent headaches or dizziness
- Eyes or vision
- Ears or hearing
- Nose or throat
- Breathing problems or chest pains
- Belly aches or pains, throwing up, problems with urine or bowel movements
- Rashes, moles, birthmarks, or sunburns
- Muscle aches, injury, or other problems

For Girls

- Have you started your periods?

Observation of Parent-Child Interaction

- Do both parent and child ask questions?
- Does the parent allow the child to communicate with you directly?
- Does the parent interfere with your interaction with the child?
- Does the parent dismiss the child? Is disrespectful of the child?

Physical Examination

A complete physical examination is included as part of every health supervision.

Respect the child's privacy by using appropriate draping during the examination. If possible, ask siblings to wait in the waiting room.

When performing a physical examination, the health care professional's attention is directed to the following components of the examination of importance to the child at this age:

- **Measure and compare with norms for age, sex, and height**
  - Blood pressure
- **Measure and plot on appropriate CDC Growth Chart**
  - Height
  - Weight
- **Calculate and plot on appropriate CDC Growth Chart**
  - BMI
- **Skin**
  - Signs of self-injury, such as cutting
- **Breasts and genitalia**
  - Assess for sexual maturity rating.
- **Spine**
  - Examine the back.

Screening—9 Year

Universal Screening	Action	
Dyslipidemia (once between the 9 Year and 11 Year Visits)	Lipid profile	

Selective Screening	Risk Assessment[a]	Action if Risk Assessment (+)
Anemia	+ on risk screening questions	Hematocrit or hemoglobin
Hearing	+ on risk screening questions	Audiometry
Oral Health	Primary water source is deficient in fluoride.	Oral fluoride supplementation
Tuberculosis	+ on risk screening questions	Tuberculin skin test
Vision	+ on risk screening questions	Objective measure with age-appropriate visual-acuity measurement using HOTV or LEA symbols, Sloan letters, or Snellen letters

[a] See the *Evidence and Rationale chapter* for the criteria on which risk screening questions are based.

Screening—10 Year

Universal Screening	Action	
Dyslipidemia (once between the 9 Year and 11 Year Visits)	Lipid profile	
Hearing	Audiometry	
Vision	Objective measure with age-appropriate visual-acuity measurement using HOTV or LEA symbols, Sloan letters, or Snellen letters	

Selective Screening	Risk Assessment[a]	Action if Risk Assessment Positive (+)
Anemia	+ on risk screening questions	Hematocrit or hemoglobin
Oral Health	Primary water source is deficient in fluoride.	Oral fluoride supplementation
Tuberculosis	+ on risk screening questions	Tuberculin skin test

[a] See the *Evidence and Rationale chapter* for the criteria on which risk screening questions are based.

Immunizations

Consult the CDC/ACIP or AAP Web sites for the current immunization schedule.

CDC National Immunization Program: **www.cdc.gov/vaccines**

AAP *Red Book:* **http://redbook.solutions.aap.org**

Anticipatory Guidance

The following sample questions, which address the Bright Futures Middle Childhood Expert Panel's Anticipatory Guidance Priorities, are intended to be used selectively to invite discussion, gather information, address the needs and concerns of the family, and build partnerships. Use of the questions may vary from visit to visit and from family to family. Questions can be modified to match the health care professional's communication style. The accompanying anticipatory guidance for the family should be geared to questions, issues, or concerns for that particular child and family. Tools and handouts to support anticipatory guidance can be found in the *Bright Futures Tool and Resource Kit.*

Priority

Social Determinants of Health

Risks: Neighborhood and family violence (fighting, bullying), food security, family substance use (tobacco, e-cigarettes, alcohol, drugs), harm from the Internet

Strengths and protective factors: Emotional security and self-esteem, connectedness with family and peers

Risks: Neighborhood and Family Violence (Fighting, Bullying)

Children in families that are affected by poverty and neighborhood or family violence are dealing with a level of stress that affects their current and future health. For example, families in difficult living situations may have concerns about their ability to provide a safe environment for their child.

Questions on this topic can be sensitive. The health care professional can identify these issues in a supportive and non-blaming way and help the parents formulate steps toward solutions. A referral to community resources or federal assistance programs may be a useful first step.

Fighting and bullying behaviors can indicate the presence of conduct disorders in bullies or may co-occur with problems such as substance use, depression, or anxiety. *(For more information on this topic, see the Bullying section of the Promoting Mental Health theme.)* Family violence includes physical attacks and sexual coercion. Children can benefit from a discussion of safety in all these aspects.

Sample Questions

Are there frequent reports of violence in your community or school? Is your child involved in that violence? Do you think he is safe in the neighborhood? Has your child ever been injured in a fight? Has he been bullied or hit by others? Has your child demonstrated bullying or aggression toward others? Have you talked to him about violence and how to be safe?

Ask the Child

Have you ever been involved with a group who did things that could have gotten them into trouble? What do you do when someone tries to pick a fight with you? What do you do when you are angry? Have you been in a physical fight in the past 6 months? Do you know anyone in a gang?

Have you felt excluded or not a part of any group of friends? Do you sometimes get left out of things? How does that make you feel? What concerns do you have about being bullied, teased, or hurt physically?

Have you ever been touched in a way that made you feel uncomfortable or that was unwelcome? Have you ever been touched on your private parts against your wish or without your permission?

Anticipatory Guidance

- Be sensitive to the effect on your child of any stresses or changes in the family, such as a parent not being available, a loss in the family, or family violence.
- Teach your child nonviolent conflict-resolution techniques.
- Talk to your child about your family's expectations for time with friends.
- Make sure your child knows he can call you if he ever needs help. Be prepared to step in and help if needed.
- If your child is anxious about going to school, try to obtain a complete picture of what is happening, and when and where. Contact your child's teacher and the principal to seek their assistance. Talk with your child about the possibility that he is being bullied by another child.

For the Child

- Talk to your parent; another trusted adult, such as a teacher; or me if anyone bullies, stalks, or abuses you or threatens your safety. If you see another child being bullied, tell an adult.
- Learn to manage conflict nonviolently. Walk away if you can.

Risks: Food Security

Food security is a critical issue during this age because of increased calorie needs that result from the beginning of the adolescent growth spurt. If the family is having difficulty obtaining nutritious food, provide information about SNAP, the Commodity Supplemental Food Program, local food shelves, and local community food programs.

Sample Questions

Within the past 12 months, did you worry that your food would run out before you got money to buy more? In the past 12 months, did the food you bought just not last and you didn't have money to buy more?

Anticipatory Guidance

- Programs and resources are available to help you and your family. You may be eligible for food and nutrition assistance through programs like SNAP, which used to be called Food Stamps. Food banks, food pantries, and community food programs can also help.

Risks: Family Substance Use (Tobacco, E-Cigarettes, Alcohol, Drugs)

Exposure to tobacco smoke remains an important environmental risk. Encourage parents to keep their home and vehicles smoke-free, as well as free from vapor from e-cigarettes. Becoming familiar with community and online resources for quitting smoking allows health care professionals to refer parents who are interested in quitting. Refer parents who smoke and request assistance in quitting to community resources for smoking cessation.

Tobacco, alcohol, and drugs are new risks for children as they approach middle school. Children need clear messages about the dangers of substance use. Worrying about a family member with a substance use or mental health problem also may be a source of significant stress.

Sample Questions

Is smoking, alcohol, or drug use a concern in your family? Is your child exposed to substance use? Does your child spend time with anyone who smokes or uses e-cigarettes?

Ask the Child

Do any of your friends smoke, use or vape e-cigarettes, drink alcohol or beer, or use drugs? Will you ever smoke, use e-cigarettes, drink alcohol, or use drugs?

Anticipatory Guidance

- Exposure to secondhand smoke greatly increases the risk of heart and lung diseases in your child. Exposure to vapor from e-cigarettes also may be harmful. It's not always possible, but, when you can, avoid spending time in places where people are smoking cigarettes or using e-cigarettes.
- Children are constantly exposed to smoking, drinking, and drug-use behaviors through TV and other media. They need clear messages that substance use is substance misuse.
- If alcohol is used in the home, its use should be appropriate and discussed with your child.
- If you or anyone in the house smoke or use e-cigarettes, try to quit. If quitting is not possible, discuss the difficulty of addiction with your child.
- If you are ever interested in quitting smoking, please talk to me. **800-QUIT-NOW (800-784-8669);** TTY **800-332-8615** is a national telephone helpline that is routed to local resources. Additional resources are available at **www.cdc.gov.** I can also refer you to local or online resources.
- If you are worried about any family members' drug or alcohol use problems, you can talk with me.

For the Child

- Don't try cigarettes or vape e-cigarettes. They are bad for your lungs and heart, and your skin and teeth.
- Don't drink alcohol or use drugs, inhalants, anabolic steroids, or diet pills. Smoking marijuana and other drugs can hurt your lungs. Alcohol and other drugs are bad for your brain's development.
- Walk away from kids who offer you cigarettes, e-cigarettes, alcohol, or drugs.

Risks: Harm From the Internet

Internet safety is similar to neighborhood safety. Younger children should never play outside unsupervised or leave the yard. More mature children may be allowed to go to known safe places like a playground, but should not be allowed to wander into inappropriate or unsafe areas. Internet use should parallel safe play outdoors. Younger children should only be online supervised, and, with increasing maturity, limited browsing can be permitted. Information about safe Internet use can be found at **www.HealthyChildren.org.**

Sample Questions

How much do you know about your child's Internet use? For example, what sites is he visiting, what games is he playing, who is he talking to, and how much time is he spending on the computer? Do you have rules for the Internet? Have you installed an Internet filter?

Ask the Child

What would you do if you came to an Internet site that you thought wasn't a good idea or that scared you?

Anticipatory Guidance

- Your family computer should be in a place where you can easily observe your child's use.
- Check the Internet history regularly to be sure you approve of your child's Internet choices.
- Just as you monitor your child's activity in the neighborhood and community, it is important to be aware of his Internet use. A safety filter allows some parental supervision.

For the Child

- It is important to go online only when your parents say it's OK. Never go to Internet sites unless you know they are good choices.
- Never chat online unless you tell your parents. No one should ever make you feel scared online.
- Do not give your personal information, like your full name or address or phone number, on a Web site unless your parents say it is OK.

Strengths and Protective Factors: Emotional Security and Self-esteem

In concert with identifying risk factors, providing anticipatory guidance about strengths and protective factors for all children is a critical component of surveillance of developmental tasks. Identifying strengths and providing feedback to families about what they are doing well helps provide a comprehensive and balanced view of the child's health and well-being. For families living in difficult circumstances, such strengths may help protect the child from, or reduce the degree of, negative health outcomes. Parents need to know that they can positively influence the healthy development of their child no matter what difficulties or problems exist. Anticipatory guidance provides parents with ideas about opportunities they can give their child, such as the chance to become good at things, begin to make independent decisions, have social connections, and do things for others.

Parents can help make their child feel secure by giving hugs, participating in activities together, and listening without interrupting during family discussions. Children with warm, nurturing parents are more likely to have high self-esteem. Hypercritical parents who have unrealistically high expectations, and uninvolved parents who do not encourage their children to achieve and to try new experiences, can damage their child's self-esteem. Protective factors for all children include having at least one supportive adult in their life.

Self-esteem is a key feature of a fulfilling life and has an enormous influence on mental health. Children develop a positive sense of self if they think they are making a contribution.

Sample Questions

How happy is your child? Do you feel he has good self-confidence? Does your child have a chance to do things for others at home, at school, or in the community?

Ask the Child

Tell me about some of the things you are good at doing. What are some of the things that make you happy?

Anticipatory Guidance

- Provide opportunities for your child to try out new interests and develop friendships with other children by participating in group activities, such as classes, sports teams, music lessons, community activities, and faith-based and after-school activities. Having a chance to develop skills in things he likes to do besides schoolwork is important.
- Give him a chance to help others out at home or as a family in your neighborhood or community.

For the Child

- Think about new things you are interested in besides schoolwork. Talk with your parents about trying one out.
- Help your parents plan some family activities that would be both fun and inexpensive. Mix in some new things you might all enjoy together.

Strengths and Protective Factors: Connectedness With Family and Peers

One of the most important protective factors and a component of healthy development is the ability to form caring and supportive relationships with family, other adults, and peers. At home, this involves a relationship characterized by warm supportive interactions with parents and guardians combined with clear expectations and an opportunity for children to begin to gain the skills necessary for independent decision-making. Children this age also can benefit from feeling that they can contribute to planning family activities and helping out when needed. Children are more likely to make healthy choices if they stay connected with family members and if clear rules and limits are set. Note that friendships and relationships with peers will begin to be increasingly important to the child. This shift can be difficult for parents to deal with, but it is an important time to continue to cement family relationships. This effort will pay off later because close family ties are an important protective, risk-reducing factor in adolescence. Asking parents whether they understand their child's world and daily life is particularly important for immigrant parents and families.

Sample Questions

How are you getting along as a family? What do you do together? Tell me what you know about your child's world and daily life? What responsibilities does your child have at home? What are your expectations?

Ask the Child

How do you get along with your family? What do you like to do together? Tell me about your friends in the neighborhood and at school.

Anticipatory Guidance

- Spend time with your child. Express willingness for questions and discussion. Develop a pattern of communication and support him as an independent person. Make time every day, such as at mealtimes, bedtime, drive time, or check-in time, to talk about lots of things.
- Discuss your child's responsibilities in the family and how they change with age.
- Clearly communicate rules and expectations.
- Words of encouragement are important and provide energizing motivation.
- Family activities don't have to be expensive to be fun for children this age. Family picnics, playing or walking in a park, or a trip to the library can be enjoyable, especially if the child can help plan the outing.
- You can encourage your child to be responsible by modeling responsibility yourself, by keeping promises, showing up on time, and completing tasks on time.
- Get to know your child's friends and encourage him to make good decisions about choosing friends.

For the Child

- Spend time with family members. Help out at home.
- How to make friends and keep them is an important life skill.

Priority

Development and Mental Health

Temper problems, setting reasonable limits, friends; sexuality (pubertal onset, personal hygiene, initiation of growth spurt, menstruation and ejaculation, loss of baby fat and accretion of muscle, sexual safety)

Temper Problems, Setting Reasonable Limits, Friends

Healthy development includes learning to handle frustration and express emotions appropriately and to make good decisions. Parents can help by setting reasonable limits, providing opportunities for their child to express opinions respectfully, and offering solutions to selected problems. This helps the child have a good opinion of herself and feel competent. The ability to handle and recover from stressors develops into the important quality of resiliency. Friendships are an important component of the child's social development. Parents can help guide their children to make good choices of whom to spend time with.

Sample Questions

Has your child experienced any recent stresses in the family or school? How do you discipline her? How often do you share a clear "no use" message about alcohol, tobacco, and other drugs? What are your household rules and the consequences for not observing them? How respectful of others do you think your child is?

Ask the Child

What are some of the things that make you sad? Angry? Frustrated? Worried? How do you handle those feelings? How do your parents or other adults help you or make it more difficult when you get upset or angry? Do they let you cool off before you talk about problems? How do your parents discipline you? What do you and your friends like to do together? What do you do when your friends pressure you to do things you don't want to do? If you said, "No," what do you think your friends would do?

Anticipatory Guidance

- Anticipate the emergence of early adolescent behaviors, including the pervasive influence of peers, a change in the communication between you and your child, sudden challenges to parental rules and authority, conflicts over issues of independence, refusal to participate in some family activities, moodiness, and a new desire to take risks.
- Your child is beginning to get a sense of right and wrong. Reinforce this sense by praising her good choices. Be sure to point out your children's strengths and unique talents.
- Assign age-appropriate chores, including responsibility for personal belongings and for some household or yard tasks. If you say that there will be consequences if chores are not completed, then follow up. Use age-appropriate consequences.

- Encourage your child to develop a sense of responsibility and independence. Help your child set achievable goals to take pride in herself. As these strengths develop, acknowledge them by allowing your child new privileges. Talk to your child about the importance of being able to trust her and how this will be tied to privileges.
- Provide personal space at home, even if limited, for your child.
- Encourage developmentally appropriate decision-making. Help her think about consequences before acting. Require her to follow rules, control anger, respect others, and have patience.
- Your child is now better able to talk about her thoughts and feelings. Help her do this in a constructive way. Encourage concern for others and helping people in need.
- Be a positive ethical and behavioral role model. If you made a mistake, then admit it, ask for forgiveness, and use this as a teachable moment.
- Help your child learn appropriate and respectful behavior. Reinforce the importance of respectful behavior toward others.
- Handle anger constructively in the family. Do not allow either physical or verbal violence; encourage compromise. Do not permit yourself or others to use corporal punishment.
- Supervise your child's activities with peers. Encourage your child to bring friends into your home and help them feel welcome.

For the Child
- Talking with a safe and trusted adult is an important way to handle anger, disappointment, and worry.
- Good friends are important. They never ask you to do harmful or scary things; they want what is best for you. If you find that a good friend has become a bad friend, try talking with her. If that person is unwilling to change, stop spending time with her. Kids can get in trouble by being around peers who make poor decisions.
- Everyone gets angry. It's normal. Here are some ways you can cope if you're angry with someone else. You can avoid getting defensive by catching yourself when you feel your frustrations mounting. Calm yourself and acknowledge the importance of the other person's point of view and your willingness to compromise. Listen without interrupting, repeat your understanding of what the issues are, and show your desire to understand the other person.
- It's normal to have up moods and down moods, but, if you feel sad or anxious most of the time, enjoy very few things, or find yourself wishing you were dead, we should talk about it. Almost everyone worries at times about how they look, how others are accepting them, and whether they are developing normally.
- Every person has to decide whether to try alcohol, drugs, cigarettes, e-cigarettes, and sex. Chances are, you know at least some of the dangers of trying each of these, but there are many more dangers you likely don't know or don't want to think about. It's not enough to just say, "No." If you really mean "No!" to any one of these choices, you need to clearly say why you feel that way.
- Do not write or text anything or take pictures of anything that you would not want displayed on a bulletin board. Inappropriate texting and photography can be against the law.

Sexuality (Pubertal Onset, Personal Hygiene, Initiation of Growth Spurt, Menstruation and Ejaculation, Loss of Baby Fat and Accretion of Muscle, Sexual Safety)

At ages 9 and 10 years, children enter a stage of rapid sexual development. They are aware of sexual themes and content in media. It is essential to give children access to accurate and culturally appropriate information on sexual development and sexuality from multiple sources, including home, school, and health care professionals.

Parents are encouraged to engage their children in an ongoing conversation about sexual development. Questions can be answered simply, and additional discussion should be welcomed.

Sample Questions

How well do you and your partner agree on how to talk with your child about issues related to sexual development and sexuality? Have you had discussions with your child about sex? Do you talk to her about your values and attitudes about appropriate modesty and privacy? Does your child know any gay men or lesbian women? How about children brought up by same-sex couples? How would you respond if your child asked you about this topic? Do you convey an attitude of accepting differences in others?

Ask the Child

What questions do you have about the way your body is developing? Have you ever been pressured to touch someone in a way that made you feel uncomfortable? Has anyone ever tried to touch you in a way that made you feel uncomfortable? Has anyone ever said inappropriate things to you about your body?

Anticipatory Guidance

- Encourage your child to ask questions. Answer them at a level appropriate to her understanding. Discuss these issues even if sexual activity seems unlikely.
- Be prepared to answer questions about sexuality and to provide concrete examples of the types of behavior that are not acceptable to you.
- Teach your child the importance of delaying sexual behavior. Make sure you convey an attitude that home is a place where it is safe to talk about these values.
- If your child receives family life education at school or in the community, discuss the information and review materials with her.
- Teach your child that it is never OK for an adult to tell a child to keep secrets from parents, to express interest in private parts, or to ask a child for help with his or her private parts.

For the Child

- **For boys and girls**
  - Around age 8 or 9, you will notice your body starting to change. Some of the first things that happen are that you develop body odor, and the skin on your face becomes oilier and may break out in pimples or acne. You will need to bathe every day, use deodorant, and wash your face well in the morning and at night.

- **For girls**
  - The next changes you will notice are that your breasts will start to get bigger. It's normal for one side to be bigger than the other at first. As your breasts grow, you may be more comfortable wearing a bra.
  - Hair will grow on your underarms and pubic area, becoming thicker, darker, and curlier over time. You also will start to grow taller at a very fast rate. This is called the growth spurt. Now is a good time to have pads available to use in your underwear when your periods start. Pads are also called sanitary napkins. Your periods generally start about a year after you see underarm and pubic hair.
  - Girls can have their first period, or menses, as early as 10, but usually by 13. Every girl is different. Periods often come at unpredictable times at first, but they eventually will come about once every 4 weeks. A small amount of blood, sometimes more brown in color than red, will come from your vagina and appear on your underwear. Use the pads to catch the blood. Change your pad every few hours and wrap the used pad in toilet paper or place it in a small paper bag to be put in the trash can. Most pads cannot be flushed down toilets. Always wash your hands after changing your pad.

- **For boys**
  - The next change you will notice is that your testicles will begin to grow larger. Hair will grow on your underarms and pubic area, becoming thicker, darker, and curlier over time. Soon, your penis will become longer and wider and your testicles will continue to grow. You also will start to grow taller at a very fast rate. This is called the growth spurt. Your voice will also start to crack and deepen as your larynx or voice box grows longer. You may find a wet, sticky discharge, called an ejaculation, on your pajama bottoms in the morning. This is called a wet dream. Ejaculations are not the same as passing urine. Ejaculations contain sperm and a special fluid. This happens because of strong surges of hormones that occur while you sleep.

- **For boys and girls**
  - It is never OK for an older child or an adult to show you his or her private parts, to ask you to show your "privates," to touch you there, to ask you to touch them, to scare you, or to ask you not to tell your parents about what he or she did with you. Always get away from the person as quickly as possible and tell your parent or another adult right away.

Priority

School

School attendance, school problems (behavior or learning), school performance and progress, transitions, co-occurrence of middle school and pubertal transitions

School Attendance, School Problems (Behavior or Learning), School Performance and Progress, Transitions, Co-occurrence of Middle School and Pubertal Transitions

At this age, the child is expected to display self-confidence, with a sense of mastery and pride in school and extracurricular activities. The 9- to 10-year-old is expected to participate in group activities, understand and adhere to most rules at school, and assume reasonable responsibility for his schoolwork. Probe for academic or learning difficulties. Reinforce the strengths of the child and parents with comments such as, "I'm so pleased that you are making good progress with math."

This age period also may be associated with transitions, as the child may move to more independent learning environments (eg, middle school), and some children may begin to experience pubertal transitions as well.

Sample Questions

What issues about your child's school experience would you like to discuss? Has he had many absences? Do you have any concerns about your child moving up to middle school with more independence for his learning? What extracurricular activities does your child participate in?

If the child has an IEP or is receiving special services: *How are things going with the special services your child is getting at school?*

Ask the Child

How is school going? What are some of the things you are good at doing in school? What are your favorite activities to do after school?

Anticipatory Guidance

- A child who arrives at school fed and rested is ready to learn. Help your child have a healthy breakfast every morning before school and establish bedtime routines on school nights so that he gets at least 10 to 11 hours of sleep.

- Children this age are making transitions in a new school building, such as getting a locker and having classes in multiple classrooms. They're also having to organize their time to meet assignments from a number of different teachers. If your child is not doing well in school, talk with his teacher about possible reasons and what can be done to identify and address the problem. Ask the teacher about tutoring or an evaluation of his learning abilities.

- Children in this age group become more independent in their schoolwork. Praise your child's efforts in school. Show interest in his school performance, but be careful to praise only genuine accomplishments.

- Set routine times for homework, and provide a well-lit, quiet space for your child to do his work. Remove distractions such as the TV or electronic devices. Homework and school activities often require computers and Internet access, so be sure to carefully monitor for safe and appropriate computer and Internet use.

- After-school activities, such as sports teams, social activities, clubs, and extracurricular activities, place increased demands on children's time. Be careful to not sign up your child for too many extracurricular activities. Children need unstructured time as well as structured activities.

- With the different rates of pubertal development, there will be much more variety in height and stage of development among age mates in middle school that may result in new concerns, especially for children who are either developing earlier or later than average.

Priority

Physical Growth and Development

Oral health (regular visits with dentist, daily brushing and flossing, adequate fluoride, limits on sugar-sweetened beverages and snacks), nutrition (healthy weight, disordered eating behaviors, importance of breakfast, limits on saturated fat and added sugars, healthy snacks), physical activity (60 minutes of physical activity a day, after-school activities)

Oral Health (Regular Visits With Dentist, Daily Brushing and Flossing, Adequate Fluoride, Limits on Sugar-Sweetened Beverages and Snacks)

By ages 9 and 10 years, a child should have an established dental home. She should have regularly scheduled visits with her dentist at least twice each year. She also should receive a fluoride supplement if the fluoride level in community water supplies (at home and at school) is low. Assure parents that fluoride is safe and effective at preventing decay.

A child who participates in contact sports should wear a protective mouth guard.

Sample Questions

Who is your child's regular dentist? Is the water you drink fluoridated? Has your dentist prescribed fluoride pills? Does your child drink a lot of soda or sports drinks? Is your child involved in physical activities, such as contact sports, that could potentially result in dental injuries? How would you handle a dental emergency?

Ask the Child

Do you brush and floss your teeth every day? Are you wearing a mouth guard when you play contact sports? How often do you drink soda or sports drinks?

Anticipatory Guidance

- Be sure that your child brushes her teeth for 2 minutes, twice a day, with a fluoridated toothpaste and flosses once a day. At this age, your child may be in a hurry while brushing. Supervise her and help as needed.
- By the time your child is 9 or 10 years old, she already should be seeing a dentist regularly. This is called a dental home. She should see the dentist at least twice a year. If your child does not have a dental home, we can help you find one.
- Give your child fluoride supplements if your community water doesn't have fluoride.
- Limit your child's consumption of sweetened beverages and snacks. Prolonged contact with the teeth can increase the chance of getting cavities.
- If your child plays contact sports, make sure she wears a mouth guard to prevent dental injuries.

For the Child

- To keep your teeth healthy, it is important to brush your teeth for at least 2 minutes, twice a day, and to floss at least once a day. Do not hurry through your brushing.
- If you are playing contact sports, always wear a mouth guard to protect your teeth.

Nutrition (Healthy Weight, Disordered Eating Behaviors, Importance of Breakfast, Limits on Saturated Fat and Added Sugars, Healthy Snacks)

Children this age may be at increased risk of overweight or obesity. Carefully assess BMI and discuss results with parents. During this age, children begin skipping breakfast. Eating breakfast has been shown to improve academic performance and children who eat breakfast tend to have lower BMIs. Often, a child will eat snacks and not be hungry at mealtimes. This habit may lead to unhealthy eating practices.

Ensuring sufficient calcium and vitamin D intake can be a particular concern, especially if the child does not consume dairy products. Supplementation with these nutrients can be considered. Fortified orange juice typically has calcium and vitamin D. Soy milk generally has both, but that is not always true for other products marketed as "milk" (eg, almond, rice, coconut, hemp). Families should be encouraged to check the package label to be sure. Not all yogurt has vitamin D.

In addition, at this age, girls begin to think of dieting and weight loss. Evaluate the child's risk of severe dieting or tendencies toward disordered eating.

Sample Questions

Do you have any concerns about your child's weight?

Do you have any concerns about her eating behaviors or food intake, such as getting her to drink enough milk and eat vegetables and fruits, or hearing her talk about dieting? How often does she drink sugar-sweetened beverages such as soda, sports drinks, or fruit drinks? How often do you have a family meal together?

Ask the Child

What concerns do you have about your weight? How do you feel about how you look? How often have you cut back on how much you eat or tried a diet to lose weight? What vegetables and fruits did you eat yesterday? Did you eat breakfast this morning? How often do you drink sugar-sweetened beverages, such as soda, sports drinks, or fruit drinks?

Anticipatory Guidance

- Choose healthy eating behaviors.
  - Every day, give your child a healthy breakfast. Research shows that eating breakfast helps children learn and behave better at school.
  - Help your child recognize and respond to hunger and fullness cues.
  - Eat together as a family. Make mealtimes pleasant and companionable; encourage conversation, turn off the TV, and discourage use of portable electronics, such as smartphones or handheld devices, at the dinner table.
  - Be a role model for your child by your own healthy eating behaviors.

- Make nutritious foods and drinks the usual options at home for meals and snacks. These include vegetables, fruits, whole grains, lean protein, such as meat, fish, poultry, eggs, beans and peas, legumes, nuts and seeds, and low-fat and nonfat dairy.
- Limit foods and drinks that are high in calories, saturated fat, salt, added sugars, and refined grains, and low in nutrients. These include ice cream, baked goods, salty snacks, fast foods, pizza, and soda and other sweetened beverages.
- Sports drinks are high in sugar and should only be used after vigorous exercise lasting more than 1 hour, but even after an hour of exercise, a sports drink or juice may give your child more calories than she just burned off with exercise. Energy drinks are potentially dangerous and should not be consumed by children of any age.
- Limit juice to 4 to 6 oz of 100% fruit juice each day.
- Make sure your child gets dairy foods and calcium- and vitamin D–containing foods and beverages each day. Children aged 9 and 10 years need 20 to 24 oz of low-fat or fat-free milk each day plus an additional serving of low-fat yogurt and cheese. If your child doesn't drink milk or consume other dairy products, then let's talk about alternatives. These can include foods and beverages that are fortified with calcium and vitamin D (like some orange juices and cereals).
- Beware of dangers of dieting for weight loss.
- If you are considering offering dietary or sports supplements to your child, please discuss these plans with me to make sure they are safe and really will help her.

For the Child

- I am happy to answer your questions and explain your weight and height measurements. The key to good health is a balance between the calories you take in from foods and the calories your body burns in carrying out its normal activities and in physical activity.
- Pay attention to what your body tells you. Eat when you feel hungry and stop eating when you feel satisfied.
- Eating a healthy breakfast every day is especially important and helps you do better in school.
- Every day, try to eat vegetables, fruit, whole-grain breads and cereals, low-fat or fat-free dairy products, and lean meats. Drink low-fat or fat-free milk or water instead of soda and sugared drinks. If you choose foods that are high in fat or sugar, have a small portion instead of a large one, or share your portion with someone else.
- Weight loss is almost never a good idea while your body is rapidly growing in puberty. If you are considering going on a diet to lose weight, let's talk about it first.
- If you are considering taking dietary or sports supplements, please discuss these plans with me to make sure they are safe and really will help you reach your goals.

Physical Activity (60 Minutes of Physical Activity a Day, After-school Activities)

All children should participate in some type of physical activity whether in a group or an individual setting. Current recommendations state that children should be physically active for at least 60 minutes a day. Encourage children to find individual ways to be physically active (eg, dancing, skating, biking). Talk to parents of children with special health care needs about the benefits and risks associated with physical activity. Emphasize the importance of safety equipment when the child participates in physical activity. Backyard trampolines should be discouraged, as it is not possible to make them safe.

At this age, children become involved in organized sports. Educate parents about appropriate sports for age and ability. Discuss with the family the attributes of a quality program and coaching. Encourage parents to check out programs before enrolling their children (eg, rules about all children playing, coaching training or certification).

Sample Questions

Do you have concerns about your child's physical activity level, either too much or too little? What is your child's usual bedtime on school nights and on nonschool nights? Does she have trouble going to sleep or does she wake up during the night? How much recreational screen time does your child spend each weekday? How about on weekends? Does your child have a TV or Internet-connected device in her bedroom?

Ask the Child

Tell me about the physical activities you do inside and outside of school. How often do you do them? How much time do you spend watching TV or using devices that are connected to the Internet?

Anticipatory Guidance

- Encourage your child to be physically active for at least 60 minutes total every day. Support your child's sport and physical activity interests, and be active with your child.
- Do not allow your child to sleep with any electronic device in her bedroom, including phones or tablets.
- In order to balance your child's needs for physical activity, sleep, school activities, and unplugged time, consider making a family media use plan to balance these important health behaviors and media use time in your child's day. The family media use plan is an online tool that you and your child can fill out together. The tool prompts you and your child to enter daily health priorities such as an hour for physical activity, 8 to 11 hours of sleep, time for homework and school activities, and unplugged time each day for time with family and independently. You and your child can then view the time left over and decide on rules around daily screen time for your child. The AAP has information on making a plan at **www.HealthyChildren.org/MediaUsePlan.**
- Take into account not only the quantity but the quality and location of media use. Consider TVs, phones, tablets, and computers. Rules should be followed by parents as well as children. Construct it so that it suits your families' media needs, but also helps you preserve face-to-face time during family routines such as meals, playtime, and bedtime. Times or locations in the house can be designated as media-free.
- Supervise your child's Internet use so that you can teach her how to use it safely, how to avoid inappropriate content, and what to do if she comes across inappropriate content.

- If your child is using media excessively, find out why. Is she having trouble with peer relationships or social skills? Some children seek solitary activities if they are struggling with friendships. Encourage your child to find activities that interest her, or seek help through the school.
- Getting enough sleep every night is important for your child's health. Using media before bedtime to get to sleep actually leads to worse sleep habits, less sleep, and school problems. Suggest avoiding media in the hour before bedtime, developing a quiet bedtime routine, or reading in bed instead.

For the Child

- Try to get at least 1 hour of moderate-to-vigorous exercise every day. Vigorous activity makes you breathe hard and sweat. Find ways to become more active, such as walking or biking instead of riding in a car. Take the stairs, not elevators. Be active with your friends to increase the fun. Being physically active every day helps you feel good and focus on your schoolwork.
- It helps to plan times each day that are dedicated to a physical activity you enjoy. Make activity part of your routine, rather than an exception.

Priority

Safety

Car safety, safety during physical activity, water safety, sun protection, knowing child's friends and their families, firearm safety

Car Safety

A child should use a booster seat until the seat belt fits properly, which means the lap belt can be worn low and flat across the hips and upper thighs, the shoulder belt can be worn across the shoulder rather than the face or neck, and the child can bend at the knees while sitting against the vehicle seat back (usually between the ages of 8 and 12 years and at about 4 feet 9 inches tall).

The back seat is the safest place for children younger than 13 years to ride.

Sample Questions

Does everyone in the family use a seat belt?

Ask the Child

Do you use a booster seat or seat belt every time you ride in the car? Do you sit in the back seat every time you ride in the car?

Anticipatory Guidance

■ Do not start your vehicle until everyone's seat belt is buckled.

For the Child

■ The back seat of the car is still the safest place for you to sit until you are at least 13 years of age.

■ Using a booster seat or wearing a seat belt every time you get in the car is the best way to protect yourself from injury and death in a crash.

For information about booster seats and actions to keep your child safe in and around cars, visit www.safercar.gov/parents.

Toll-free Auto Safety Hotline: 888-327-4236

Safety During Physical Activity

Reinforce the importance of safety in sports and other physical activities, emphasizing the need for wearing protective gear (helmet, mouth guard, eye protection, and knee and elbow pads).

Sample Questions

Do you enforce the use of helmets? Do you model this behavior?

Ask the Child

How often do you wear a helmet and protective gear when biking, skating, or doing other outdoor activities?

Anticipatory Guidance

- Make sure your child always wears a helmet and other protective equipment when biking, skating, or doing other outdoor activities.

For the Child

- Being active is good for you, but being safe while being active is just as important. One of the best ways to protect yourself is to wear the right safety equipment, especially a helmet when you are biking, skating, or doing other outdoor activities.

Water Safety

An adult should actively supervise children when they are near water.

Sample Questions

Does your child know how to swim?

Ask the Child

Do you know how to swim? What rules do your parents have about swimming?

Anticipatory Guidance

- Make sure your child is taught to swim.
- Do not let your child play around any water, including lakes, streams, pools, or the ocean, unless an adult is watching. Even if your child knows how to swim, never let him swim alone. NEVER let your child swim in any fast-moving water.
- Teach your child to never dive into water unless an adult has already made sure the water is deep enough for diving.
- When on any boat or other watercraft, be sure your child is wearing an appropriately fitting, US Coast Guard–approved life jacket.
- Be sure that swimming pools in your community, apartment complex, or home have a 4-sided fence with a self-closing, self-latching gate.

For the Child

- Swimming lessons are an important way to become comfortable in the water. Ask your parents about learning to swim.
- Never swim without an adult around.

Sun Protection

Sun protection now is of increasing importance because of climate change and the thinning of the atmospheric ozone layer. Sun protection is accomplished through limiting sun exposure, using sunscreen, and wearing protective clothing. Reinforce the continuing importance of using sunscreen on your child when he is outside.

Sample Questions

Do you apply sunscreen whenever your child plays outside? Do you limit outside time during the middle of the day when the sun is strongest?

Ask the Child

Do you always use sunscreen?

Anticipatory Guidance

- Always apply sunscreen with an SPF greater than 15 to your child when your child is outside. Reapply every 2 hours.
- Encourage your child to wear a hat.
- Avoid prolonged time in the sun between 11:00 am and 3:00 pm.

For the Child

- Always wear sunscreen and a hat when you are outside.
- Try not to be outside in sun too long between 11:00 am and 3:00 pm, when it is really easy to get a sunburn.

Knowing Child's Friends and Their Families

As their children are now spending increasing amounts of time with other children and families, parents must help their children develop safe play habits. Play should be supervised by a responsible adult who is aware of children's activities and available in case of problems.

Sample Questions

Do you know your child's friends? Their families? Does your child know how to get help in an emergency if you are not present?

Ask the Child

What would you do if you felt unsafe at a friend's house?

Anticipatory Guidance

- Teach your child that the safety rules at home apply at other homes as well.
- Help your child understand it is always OK to ask to come home or call his parent if he is not comfortable at someone else's house.

For the Child

- Be sure you play safe wherever you play. Every family should have the same safety rules.
- It's always OK to ask a grown-up for help if you are scared or worried. And it's OK to ask to go home and be with your Mom or Dad.

Firearm Safety

The safest home is one without a firearm. A firearm kept in the home is far more likely to kill or injure someone known to the family than to kill or injure an intruder. A firearm kept in the home triples the risk of homicide. The risk of completed suicide also is far more likely if a firearm is kept in the home.

Evidence shows that programs designed to teach children to avoid contact with firearms are not effective in overcoming the child's innate curiosity and social pressure to handle firearms. At this age, children still lack the maturity or cognitive capacity to reliably follow advice concerning firearms.

Sample Questions

Who, among family members and friends, owns a weapon or firearm? Have you considered not owning a firearm because it poses a danger to children and other family members?

Ask the Child

What have your parents taught you about firearms and what not to do with them?

Anticipatory Guidance

- Homicide and completed suicide are more common in homes that have firearms. The best way to keep your child safe from injury or death from firearms is to never have a firearm in the home.
- If it is necessary to keep a firearm in your home, it should be stored unloaded and locked, with the ammunition locked separately from the firearm. Keep the key where children cannot have access.
- Ask if there are firearms in homes where your child plays. If so, make sure they are stored unloaded and locked, with the ammunition locked separately, before allowing your child to play in the home.
- Talk to your child about firearms in school or on your streets. Find out if your child's friends carry firearms.

For the Child

- Adults are supposed to keep their firearms away from children. If you see a firearm that is unlocked, don't touch it, but tell your parent right away.
- If you are starting to hunt with adults in your family, learn how to use firearms and hunting knives safely, and use them only under adult supervision.

References

1. Wolraich M, Brown L, Brown RT, et al; American Academy of Pediatrics Subcommittee on Attention-Deficit/Hyperactivity Disorder, Steering Committee on Quality Improvement Management. ADHD: clinical practice guideline for the diagnosis, evaluation, and treatment of attention-deficit/hyperactivity disorder in children and adolescents. *Pediatrics.* 2011;128(5):1007-1022
2. Biro FM, Galvez MP, Greenspan LC, et al. Pubertal assessment method and baseline characteristics in a mixed longitudinal study of girls. *Pediatrics.* 2010;126(3):e583-e590
3. Herman-Giddens ME, Steffes J, Harris D, et al. Secondary sexual characteristics in boys: data from the Pediatric Research in Office Settings Network. *Pediatrics.* 2012;130(5):e1058-e1068

Adolescence Visits

11 Through 21 Years

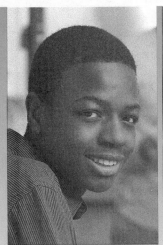
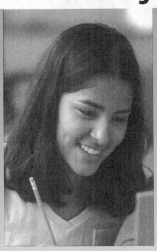
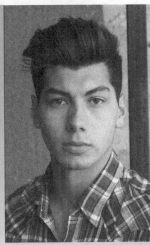
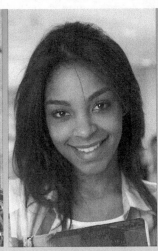

Early Adolescence
11 Through 14 Year Visits

Context

The early adolescent is embarking on a journey of remarkable transitions and transformations—physically, cognitively, emotionally, and socially—and the pace at which he experiences these physical and emotional changes varies widely. The onset of puberty is one indicator that the adolescent phase of life is beginning. Puberty typically manifests itself visibly with breast development at about age 9 or 10 years for girls, and testicular enlargement for boys at about age 11 years. Many youth have some degree of pubertal developmental as they enter early adolescence. Breast development occurs about 1 year earlier in girls of normal weight who are non-Hispanic African American or Mexican American than it does in girls of normal weight who are non-Hispanic white.[1] These changes are accompanied by a growth spurt. For girls, the maximal growth rate is reached about 6 to 12 months before menarche. Boys have a later growth spurt and, during their growth spurt, have a greater peak height velocity[1] than girls. Other physical changes also become apparent. The skin of both boys and girls becomes oily as apocrine glands begin to secrete. Secondary sex characteristics (ie, female breasts, characteristics of male genitalia, and pubic hair) develop, notable changes in body fat and musculature occur, and a boy's voice begins to change. Many of these physical changes are more closely associated with the stage of sexual maturity than with chronological age. The average age for menarche is between 12 and 13 years. The American Academy of Pediatrics (AAP) and the American College of Obstetricians and Gynecologists recommend that health care professionals view the menstrual cycle as a "vital sign"[2] and include education about the normal timing and characteristics of menstruation and other pubertal markers as an important component of health supervision for young girls and their parents.

Puberty, perhaps the key developmental milestone of early adolescence, is an important focus for all cultures. Health care professionals should seek to understand the meaning of it in the cultures of the families they serve.

Early adolescents with special health care needs can experience puberty at the usual time or they can have an earlier or delayed onset of pubertal change based on their health condition. All children should receive appropriate education about the changes of puberty and what to expect for themselves and classmates.[3] Recent studies have shown that the age of onset of puberty is decreasing in both girls and boys.[4-6] These changes have implications both medically, in determining who requires evaluation for premature puberty, and socially, as some adolescents, especially girls, may have difficulties because of a mismatch between their physical appearance, chronological age, and psychological maturity.

Along with the physical changes of puberty, the early adolescent's cognitive abilities are developing. As he matures, he develops an increased capacity for logical, abstract, and idealistic thinking. Schooling shifts from the emotionally secure environment of elementary school, where students have only a single teacher and the same classmates, to the more challenging social environment of middle school and high school, with intense course work, multiple teachers, multiple groups of classmates, and rising expectations for academic and social advancement. These academic demands provide many opportunities for the early adolescent to explore his burgeoning interests and for his sense of achievement and self-esteem to blossom. They also can unmask a previously undiagnosed learning disorder or attention-deficit problems, or can affect the adolescent's ability to cope, which, in turn, can lead to depression and other mental health issues. As academic work increases in complexity, parents may feel challenged and unsure about how to help. These issues can be even more difficult for the youth with special health care needs, who may be challenged physically, cognitively, or socially to engage in school activities and fit in with his peers.

Socially, the early adolescent experiences dramatic changes over relatively few years as he matures. He needs to belong to a peer group and he desires the independence or freedom to do what he wants and with whom he wants. However, these changes do not occur at the same time or at the same pace among all youth. In an attempt to keep pace with individual physical changes that can outpace or lag behind that of his friends, a young adolescent often will use clothing (eg, designer T-shirts), accessories (eg, body piercing or tattoos), and hairstyles (eg, color rinses) as a way to fit in with peers. The youth with special health care needs experiences the same social changes, although his reactions may be influenced by the nature of his condition and the level of acceptance of his condition by friends, family, and community (eg, stigma of being human immunodeficiency virus positive or having a very obvious physical difference).

For many, early adolescence can be a difficult time socially. Parents and educators must remain alert and take extra steps to ensure inclusion as social networks form and re-form, and activities sometimes take place in geographically dispersed parts of the community. The age at which an adolescent can obtain a driver's license varies from state to state, so he may have to walk, ride his bike, use public transportation, or depend upon others, including other friends, to drive him to such popular hangouts as shopping malls, movie theatres, music concerts, and parks. Parental monitoring remains critical to ensure that young adolescents remain safe while gradually becoming more independent.

As the early adolescent matures, he spends time without adult supervision both at home and away. This freedom presents opportunities to mature in new responsibilities and develop strong decision-making skills. Indeed, many early adolescents begin babysitting other children, including their younger siblings. This new freedom presents challenges because of the attractions of risky behaviors. The temptation to experience something that one believes is pleasurable or "cool" or that builds status is hard to resist if the youth lacks insight to the consequences, has poor negotiation skills, and has ample opportunity to experiment. Brain research demonstrates that the neurologic structures that underlie the functions of controlling impulses and making decisions are still maturing during adolescence.[7-9] Discretion and decision-making is further inhibited under the influence of alcohol or drugs. As a social creature, the adolescent enjoys being with his friends, having fun, and going places. Shored up by the power and energy of his peer group, the early adolescent may shun caution to satisfy his curiosity. If he is eager to impress a new friend or a crush, a naive, uninitiated youth may feel overly confident about engaging in risky behavior. The introduction and proliferation of new social media technologies have made the social interactions of early adolescence more complicated than in previous generations, with issues such as lack of privacy, bullying, and sexting adding layers of complexity and difficulty to the daily life of the young adolescent.

The adolescent's relationships with his parents and other adults may begin to change during the early stages of this period. In some families, an orderly progression to independent decision-making can be noted. For many young people, however, mood swings and attempts at independence can trigger volatile arguments and challenges to rules. Occasional arguments with parents are common. Authoritative (accepting, firm, and democratic) parents who have a balanced approach with unconditional love combined with clear boundaries (family rules, limits, and expectations) and consistent enforcement of discipline build a strong protective bond between themselves and their adolescent. Research data consistently show that authoritative parents have adolescents who are less depressed, enter into risk-taking behaviors at later ages, and succeed better academically than parents who use authoritarian (strong parental control with low warmth and little youth input) approaches.[10] Having a positive relationship with parents, engagement in school and community activities, and a sense of spirituality are major assets associated with positive youth development.[11] *(For more information on this topic, see the Promoting Lifelong Health for Families and Communities, Promoting Healthy Development, and Promoting Family Support themes.)*

An adolescent from a background that differs from the majority population may have to juggle the demands and values of his family and community culture with the demands and values of the mainstream culture. In families who have immigrated, this tension may be exacerbated because the youth may speak English better than his parents, and may be more engaged in the predominant social environment. This role reversal is particularly difficult during the adolescent years when the youth needs support and guidance and when parents need to

be able to assert their ability to protect and guide the youth. As the adolescent works to establish his identity, dealing with being bicultural can be confusing and stressful.

The early adolescent also may experience a variety of unexpected dramatic personal changes, such as parental divorce or death, or family relocation. These events, coming on top of the other emotional, social, and academic pressures that are typically experienced during early adolescence, will require the youth to develop mature coping mechanisms. Family members and other adults play an essential role in helping the early adolescent develop coping mechanisms, and these personal challenges provide opportunities for emotional growth, leading to increased resiliency (a trait that will prove valuable throughout adolescence and into adulthood).

Similarly, an adolescent who identifies as lesbian, gay, bisexual, transgender, or questioning may face unique challenges with regard to family or mainstream culture, and this may trigger stress. Research demonstrates these youth report lower levels of protective factors, such as family connectedness and adult caring, than their peers.[12] Yet it has been demonstrated that family acceptance has the strongest overall influence on positive health outcomes for youth who are lesbian, gay, bisexual, transgender, or questioning.[13]

Health behaviors and lifestyle habits that are formed in adolescence often continue into adulthood. Therefore, early adolescence is a key period for engaging the adolescent's active participation in a variety of health-promoting and risk-reducing behaviors, such as healthy eating, daily physical activity, and avoiding substance use, and for supporting family connectedness and promoting healthy sexuality. *(For more information on this topic, see the Promoting Lifelong Health for Families and Communities and Promoting Healthy Development themes.)* Parents who also practice these behaviors reinforce their child's willingness and ability to promote their own healthy lifestyles. Health care professionals should be sensitive to the patient's concerns about his body image and the emergence of disordered patterns of eating, from anorexia nervosa to obesity. Evaluating the level of body satisfaction and practices that the adolescent uses to maintain body weight (eg, dieting or binge eating and physical activity patterns) will help the health care professional recognize early symptoms of eating disorders or patterns that promote unhealthy body weight.

As children transition into early adolescence, attention should be paid to the issue of sleep hygiene. Although studies have shown that 8 to 10 hours of sleep are recommended,[14] only about 20% of adolescents receive that amount of sleep, and most adolescents average only 7 to 7½ hours of sleep per night. This sleep deficit increases throughout the adolescent years, despite the fact that most adolescents do some catch-up on weekends. One study shows that sixth graders average approximately 8½ hours of sleep per night, while 12th graders average approximately 7 hours per night.[15] A phase delay in circadian rhythm that begins in early puberty and the use of both traditional and new media and the early start times of junior and senior high school are all considered to be contributors to the general sleep deficit in the adolescent

years. Later start time for school has been shown to be an effective countermeasure to chronic sleep loss. Because decreased school performance, as well as a possible increase in depression and other mental health issues and health risk behaviors, has been associated with lack of appropriate sleep, this becomes an important area of attention in the health and well-being of adolescents.[16] The family and environmental conditions that can pose a risk to a child's health or that can act as protective factors and contribute to a child's healthy development continue to be important during adolescence. However, these risks and strengths typically manifest themselves in different ways to reflect the adolescent's growing maturity.

Health care routines also change according to the adolescent's development and his unique cultural circumstances. Beginning with the Early Adolescence Visits, many health care professionals conduct the first part of the medical interview with the parent in the examination room and then spend time with the adolescent alone. This approach helps the early adolescent build a unique relationship with his health care professional, promotes confidence and full disclosure of health information, and enhances self-management. When this approach is explained within the context of healthy adolescent development, parents usually support it.

Priorities for the 11 Through 14 Year Visits

The first priority is to address the concerns of the adolescent and the parent.

In addition, the Bright Futures Adolescence Expert Panel has given priority to the following additional topics for discussion in the 4 Early Adolescence Visits.

The goal of these discussions is to determine the health care needs of the youth and family that should be addressed by the health care professional. The following priorities are consistent throughout the Early Adolescence Visits. However, the questions used to effectively obtain information and the anticipatory guidance provided to the youth and family can vary.

Although each of these issues is viewed as important, they may be prioritized by the individual needs of each patient and family. The goal should be to address issues important to this age group over the course of multiple visits. The issues are

▶ Social determinants of health[a] (risks [interpersonal violence, living situation and food security, family substance use], strengths and protective factors [connectedness with family and peers, connectedness with community, school performance, coping with stress and decision-making])

▶ Physical growth and development (oral health, body image, healthy eating, physical activity and sleep)

▶ Emotional well-being (mood regulation and mental health, sexuality)

▶ Risk reduction (pregnancy and sexually transmitted infections; tobacco, e-cigarettes, alcohol, prescription or street drugs; acoustic trauma)

▶ Safety (seat belt and helmet use, sun protection, substance use and riding in a vehicle, firearm safety)

---

[a] Social determinants of health is a new priority in the fourth edition of the *Bright Futures Guidelines*. For more information, see the *Promoting Lifelong Health for Families and Communities theme.*

Health Supervision

The *Bright Futures Tool and Resource Kit* contains Previsit Questionnaires to assist the health care professional in taking a history, conducting developmental surveillance, and performing medical screening.

History

Interval history, including a review of systems, can be obtained according to the health care professional's preference or style of practice. In most cases, the youth will be alone at the visit. In some situations, especially if the youth has a special health care need, he may be accompanied by a parent or guardian. Some clinicians use the HEEADSSS (Home, Education, Eating Activities, Drugs, Sexuality, Suicide, Safety) or SSHADESS (Strengths, School, Home, Activities, Drugs, Emotions/Eating/Depression, Sexuality, Safety) mnemonics to help organize the questions for their youth patients.[17,18] The following questions may encourage in-depth discussion to determine changes in health status that would warrant further physical or emotional assessment:

General Questions for the Youth

- How do you stay healthy?
- What are you good at?
- What do you do to help others?
- Who are the important adults in your life?
- What are your responsibilities at home and at school?
- What do you and your friends like to do together?
- What health problems, concerns, or questions do you have?

General Questions for the Parent

- What questions do you have about your child's physical well-being, growth, or pubertal development?
- Tell me something your child does really well.
- What questions or concerns do you have about your child's emotional well-being, feelings, behavior, or learning?
- What have you and your child discussed about feelings and behaviors that are contributing to his emotional well-being and a healthy lifestyle?
- What have you and your child discussed about avoiding risky behaviors? Does your child have any behaviors that you are concerned about?

Past Medical History

- Has your child received any specialty or emergency care since the last visit?

Family History

- Has your child or anyone in the family, such as parents, brothers, sisters, grandparents, aunts, uncles, or cousins developed a new health condition or died? **If the answer is Yes:** Ascertain who in the family has or had the condition, and ask about the age of onset and diagnosis. If the person is no longer living, ask about the age at the time of death.

Social History

- See the Social Determinants of Health priority in Anticipatory Guidance for social history questions.

Surveillance of Development

The developmental tasks of early adolescence can be addressed by asking specific questions, through information obtained in the medical examination, by observation, and through general discussion. The following areas can be assessed to understand the developmental health of the youth. A goal of this assessment is to determine whether the youth is developing in an appropriate fashion and, if not, to provide information, assistance, or intervention. In the assessment, determine whether the youth is making progress on the following developmental tasks[19]:

- Forms caring and supportive relationships with family members, other adults, and peers
- Engages in a positive way with the life of the community
- Engages in behaviors that optimize wellness and contribute to a healthy lifestyle
  - Engages in healthy nutrition and physical activity behaviors
  - Chooses safety (wearing bike helmets, using seat belts, avoiding alcohol and drugs)
- Demonstrates physical, cognitive, emotional, social, and moral competencies (including self-regulation)
- Exhibits compassion and empathy
- Exhibits resiliency when confronted with life stressors
- Uses independent decision-making skills (including problem-solving skills)
- Displays a sense of self-confidence, hopefulness, and well-being

Review of Systems

The Bright Futures Adolescence Expert Panel recommends a complete review of systems as a part of every health supervision visit. This review can be done through the following questions:

Do you have any problems with

- Regular or frequent headaches or dizziness
- Fainting or passing out
- Eyes or vision
- Ears or hearing
- Nose or throat
- Breathing problems or chest pains
- Belly aches or pains, throwing up, problems with bowel movements
- Painful urination or other urine problems
- Rashes, moles, sunburn
- Muscle aches, injury, or other problems
- Fatigue

For Girls
- Have you had your first period?
  - If so, when was your last period?
  - Do you have any problems with your periods?
  - Do you have any itching, burning, or discharge in your vaginal area?

Observation of Parent-Youth Interaction

The parent or guardian of the early adolescent often accompanies the youth to the visit, but the health care professional will spend some time with the youth alone during each Early Adolescence Visit. The health care professional can observe parent-youth interactions, including

- How comfortably do the youth and parent interact, both verbally and nonverbally?
- Who asks and answers most of the questions?
- Does the youth express an interest in managing his own health issues (including youth with special health care needs)?

Cultural norms and values shape parent-youth interactions. To accurately interpret observations, the health care professional should learn about the norms and expectations of the populations served. Different cultures have different norms about how youth and adults interact and whether youth speak directly to adults or offer their own opinions in front of adults.

In addition to observation, the health care professional can help guide the parent and the youth's interaction to encourage the youth's participation in his health decisions. For example, if the parent is answering all the questions, then the health care professional can redirect questions straight to the youth with wording such as, "What are your thoughts on what we are discussing?"

Physical Examination

A complete physical examination is included as part of every health supervision visit.

When performing a physical examination, the health care professional's attention is directed to the following components of the examination that are important for youth aged 11 through 14 years. Use of a chaperone is advised, especially when performing sensitive parts of the examination.[20]

- **Measure and compare with norms for age, sex, and height**
  - Blood pressure
- **Measure and plot on appropriate Centers for Disease Control and Prevention (CDC) Growth Chart**
  - Height
  - Weight
- **Calculate and plot on appropriate CDC Growth Chart**
  - Body mass index (BMI)
- **Skin**
  - Inspect for acne, acanthosis nigricans, atypical nevi, piercings, and signs of abuse or self-inflicted injury.
- **Spine**
  - Examine the back and spine to detect deformities, including scoliosis.
- **Breast**

  FEMALE
  - Perform visual inspection or palpation, and assess for sexual maturity rating.

  MALE
  - Observe for gynecomastia.

- **Genitalia**

  FEMALE
  - Perform visual inspection for sexual maturity rating.
  - A pelvic examination may be clinically warranted, based on specific problems.

  MALE
  - Perform visual inspection and palpate testicles for sexual maturity rating.
  - Examine testicles for hydrocele, hernias, varicocele, or masses.

Screening

Universal Screening	Action
Depression: Adolescent (beginning at 12 Year Visit)	Depression screen[a]
Dyslipidemia (once between 9 Year and 11 Year Visits)	Lipid profile
Hearing (once between 11 Year and 14 Year Visits)	Audiometry, including 6,000 and 8,000 Hz high frequencies
Tobacco, Alcohol, or Drug Use	Tobacco, alcohol, or drug use screen
Vision (12 Year Visit)	Objective measure with age-appropriate visual-acuity measurement using HOTV or LEA symbols, Sloan letters, or Snellen letters

Selective Screening	Risk Assessment[b]	Action if Risk Assessment Positive (+)
Anemia	+ on risk screening questions	Hematocrit or hemoglobin
Dyslipidemia	+ on risk screening questions and not previously screened with normal results	Lipid profile
HIV	+ on risk screening questions	HIV test[c]
Oral Health	Primary water source is deficient in fluoride.	Oral fluoride supplementation
STIs		
▶ Chlamydia	Sexually active girls	Chlamydia test
	Sexually active boys + on risk screening questions	
▶ Gonorrhea	Sexually active girls	Gonorrhea test
	Sexually active boys + on risk screening questions	
▶ Syphilis	Sexually active and + on risk screening questions	Syphilis test
Tuberculosis	+ on risk screening questions	Tuberculin skin test

continued

Screening *(continued)*

Selective Screening	Risk Assessment[b]	Action if Risk Assessment Positive (+)
Vision (11, 13, and 14 Year Visits)	+ on risk screening questions	Objective measure with age-appropriate visual-acuity measurement using HOTV or LEA symbols, Sloan letters, or Snellen letters

Abbreviations: HIV, human immunodeficiency virus; STI, sexually transmitted infection; USPSTF, US Preventive Services Task Force.

[a] If depression screen is positive, further evaluation should be considered during the Bright Futures Health Supervision Visit. Suicide risk and the presence of firearms in the home must be considered. Disorders of mood are further discussed in the *Anticipatory Guidance section* of this visit.

[b] See *Evidence and Rationale chapter* for the criteria on which risk screening questions are based.

[c] Adolescents should be screened for STIs per recommendations in the current edition of the AAP *Red Book: Report of the Committee on Infectious Diseases.* Additionally, all adolescents should be screened for HIV according to the USPSTF recommendations (**www.uspreventiveservicestaskforce.org/uspstf/uspshivi.htm**) once between the ages of 15 and 18, making every effort to preserve confidentiality of the adolescent. Those at increased risk of HIV infection should be tested for HIV and reassessed annually.

Immunizations

Consult the CDC/Advisory Committee on Immunization Practices (ACIP) or AAP Web sites for the current immunization schedule.

CDC National Immunization Program: **www.cdc.gov/vaccines**

AAP *Red Book:* **http://redbook.solutions.aap.org**

Anticipatory Guidance

The following sample questions, which address the Bright Futures Adolescent Expert Panel's Anticipatory Guidance Priorities for this visit, are intended to be used selectively to invite discussion, gather information, address the needs and concerns of the family, and build partnerships. Use of the questions may vary from visit to visit. Questions can be modified to match the health care professional's communication style. Any anticipatory guidance for the family should be geared to questions, issues, or concerns for that particular adolescent and family.

During the early adolescent years, a primary focus of discussion should be with the youth, without dismissing the concerns or questions of the parent. For this reason, questions should first be directed to the youth and then to the parent. Similarly, guidance should first be given to the youth, and then to the parent or guardian as needed. Tools and handouts to support anticipatory guidance can be found in the *Bright Futures Tool and Resource Kit. (For more information on this topic, see the introduction to the visits.)*

Priority

Social Determinants of Health

Risks: Interpersonal violence (fighting, bullying), living situation and food security, family substance use (tobacco, e-cigarettes, alcohol, drugs)

Strengths and protective factors: Connectedness with family and peers, connectedness with community, school performance, coping with stress and decision-making

Risks: Interpersonal Violence (Fighting, Bullying)

Youth in families that are affected by poverty, intimate partner violence, or neighborhood violence are dealing with a level of stress that affects the youth's current and future health. The health care professional can identify these issues in a supportive and non-blaming way and help the youth (and her parents, if appropriate) formulate steps toward solutions, or make referrals to appropriate community services.

Fighting and bullying behaviors can indicate the presence of conduct disorders or may co-occur with problems of substance use, depression, or anxiety. *(For more information on this topic, see the Bullying section of the Promoting Mental Health theme.)* Youth who identify as lesbian, gay, bisexual, transgender, or questioning experience high rates of bullying. Interpersonal violence includes physical attacks and sexual coercion. Cyberbullying also is a concern. Young adolescents can benefit from a discussion of safety in all these aspects.

Sample Questions

Ask the Youth

Have you ever been involved with a group who did things that could have gotten them into trouble? What do you do when someone tries to pick a fight with you? What do you do when you are angry? Have you been in a physical fight in the past 6 months? Do you know anyone in a gang? Have you ever been touched in a way that made you feel uncomfortable or that was unwelcome? Have you ever been touched on your private parts against your wish or without your consent? Has anyone ever forced you to have sex? Are you in a relationship with a person who threatens you physically or hurts you? Do you feel safe at home? Do you feel you have been bullied on the Internet or through social media?

Ask the Parent

Are there frequent reports of violence in your community or school? Is your child involved in that violence? Do you think she is safe in the neighborhood? Has your child ever been injured in a fight? Has she been bullied or hit by others? Has she demonstrated bullying or aggression toward others? Have you talked to your child about dating violence and how to be safe?

Anticipatory Guidance

For the Youth

- Confide in your parents or guardians; health care professionals, including me; or other trusted adults (such as teachers) if anyone bullies, stalks, or abuses you or threatens your safety in person, on the Internet, or through social media. If you see another person being bullied, tell an adult.
- Learn to manage conflict nonviolently. Walk away if necessary.
- Avoid risky situations. Avoid violent people. Call for help if things get dangerous.
- When dating, or in any situations related to sexual behavior, remember that, "No," means NO. Saying, "No," is OK.
- Healthy dating relationships are built on respect, concern, and doing things both of you like to do.

For the Parent

- Teach your child nonviolent conflict-resolution techniques.
- Talk to your child about Internet safety and avoiding cyberbullying.
- Talk to your child about your family's expectations for time with friends and rules about dating.
- Make sure your child knows she can call you if she ever needs help. Be prepared to step in and help if needed.

Risks: Living Situation and Food Security

Families in difficult living situations or with limited resources may have concerns about their ability to acquire adequate housing and sufficient food. Questions on this topic, especially those directed to the youth, can be sensitive. If the family has housing difficulties, refer the family to community housing resources.

Increased caloric needs during the adolescent growth spurt make food security a critical issue in early adolescence. If the family is having difficulty obtaining nutritious food, provide information about the Special Nutrition Assistance Program (SNAP), the Commodity Supplemental Food Program, local food shelves, and local community food programs.

Sample Questions

Ask the Parent

Tell me about your living situation. Do you have enough heat, hot water, and electricity? Do you have appliances that work? Do you have problems with bugs, rodents, or peeling paint or plaster? In the past 12 months, did you worry that your food would run out before you got money to buy more? In the past 12 months, did the food you bought not last and you did not have money to buy more?

Anticipatory Guidance

For the Parent

- The people at community agencies have expertise in housing issues and can get you the help you need. Would you like me to help you get in touch with them?
- Community food and nutrition programs and resources, like food banks, food pantries, and community food programs, are available to help you and your family. You also may be eligible for programs like SNAP, the program formerly known as Food Stamps.

Risks: Family Substance Use (Tobacco, E-cigarettes, Alcohol, Drugs)

Exposure to tobacco smoke remains an important environmental risk. Although the long-term health effects of e-cigarettes have not yet been established, exposure to secondhand vapor from them likely carries health risks. Youth with family members and peers who use e-cigarettes (also called vaping) are more likely to begin using these devices themselves, and youth who use e-cigarettes are more likely to start using conventional cigarettes.

Worrying about a family member with a substance use or mental health problem may be a source of significant stress.

Sample Questions

Ask the Youth

Does anyone in your house or other places where you spend a lot of time smoke cigarettes or vape with e-cigarettes?

Ask the Parent

Is there anyone in your child's life whose alcohol or drug use concerns you?

Anticipatory Guidance

For the Youth

- It's not always possible, but, when you can, avoid spending time indoors or in cars where people are smoking cigarettes or vaping with e-cigarettes.
- If someone in your family smokes, they have probably tried to stop many times. Nicotine from cigarettes and e-cigarettes is one of the most addicting drugs we know. That's why it's so hard to quit. That's also why your family and I don't want you to start using tobacco or e-cigarettes.
- If you are worried about any family members' drug or alcohol use problems, you can talk with me.

Strengths and Protective Factors: Connectedness With Family and Peers

In concert with identifying risks, providing anticipatory guidance about protective factors and strengths for all youth is a critical component of surveillance of adolescent developmental tasks. Identifying strengths and providing feedback to youth (and families, when appropriate) about what they are doing well helps provide a comprehensive and balanced view of the young person's health and well-being. Often, youth and parents can build on these strengths when they make plans about how to deal with the challenges of chronic health conditions or a needed behavior change, such as better nutrition or more physical activity. For youth and families living in difficult circumstances, such strengths may help protect the youth from, or reduce the degree of, negative health outcomes. The more developmental assets or strengths youth have, the less likely they are to engage in risky health behaviors. All youth and parents need to know that they can positively influence healthy development no matter what difficulties or problems exist. Anticipatory guidance provides parents with ideas about opportunities they can give their child, such as the chance to become good at things, begin to make independent decisions, have social connections, and do things for others.

One of the most important protective factors and a component of healthy adolescent development is the ability to form caring and supportive relationships with family, other adults, and peers. At home, this involves a relationship characterized by warm supportive interactions with parents combined with clear expectations and an opportunity for young teens to begin to gain the skills necessary for independent decision-making. Youth also benefit from feeling they can contribute to planning family activities and helping out when needed. Young people are more likely to make healthy choices if they stay connected with family members and if clear rules and limits are set. Remind parents that although their child's friends are becoming increasingly important to her, they should not underestimate their own ability to positively influence her opinions and decisions. This shift in the balance can be difficult for parents to deal with, but it is an important time to continue to cement family relationships. This effort will pay off later because close family ties are an important protective, risk-reducing factor in middle and late adolescence. Connection to parents and other responsible adults is associated with a reduced number of risk behaviors. Asking parents whether they understand their child's world and daily life is particularly important for immigrant parents and families.

Sample Questions

Ask the Youth

How do you get along with your family? What do you like to do together? How closely connected do you feel to your family's cultural and faith life? Which adult do you feel most closely connected with? What rules do you have at home? What happens if you break the rules?

Ask the Parent

How are you getting along as a family? What do you do together? Tell me what you know about your child's world and daily life. What responsibilities does she have at home? What are your expectations? Do you regularly praise your child when she does something good?

Anticipatory Guidance

For the Youth

- This is an important time to stay connected with your parents. You might not always agree on everything, but work with your family to solve problems, especially around difficult situations or topics.
- Spend time with family members. Help out at home.
- Follow your family rules, such as for curfews and riding in a car (eg, who you accept rides from and whether the driver has been drinking or doing drugs).
- How to make friends and keep them is an important life skill.

For the Parent

- Spend time with your child. Express willingness for questions and discussion. Develop a pattern of communication and support her as an independent person. Make time every day to talk at mealtime, bedtime, drive time, or check-in time about a lot of things, not just about difficult or unpleasant topics.
- Discuss youth responsibilities in the family and how they change with age.
- Clearly communicate rules and expectations.
- Get to know your child's friends and encourage her to make good decisions about choosing friends.
- Discuss your expectations for dress, friends, media, and activities, and supervise your child.

Strengths and Protective Factors: Connectedness With Community

Youth who take part in activities that interest them are more confident, manage their time better, and do better in school than those who do not. These activities can nurture strengths and assets that will help an early adolescent successfully navigate this developmental stage. Living in a community or neighborhood that is safe, with positive community norms and opportunities for engagement and participation, is a protective factor in adolescent development.

Sample Questions

Ask the Youth

What are your interests outside of school? What do you like to do after school or on weekends? Do you have a chance to help others out at home or at school or in your community?

Ask the Parent

What does your child do after school or on weekends? What activities does she enjoy?

Anticipatory Guidance

For the Youth

- This is a good time to start figuring out your interests. Art, drama, mentoring, volunteering, construction, gardening, and individual and organized sports are only a few possibilities. Consider learning new skills that can be helpful to your friends, family, or community, such as lifesaving CPR or peer mentoring. Consider being part of a youth organization, such as 4-H or Big Brothers, Big Sisters.

For the Parent

- Provide opportunities for your child to find activities, other than academics, that truly interest her, especially if she is struggling academically.
- Help your child see things from another person's point of view, becoming more aware of other peoples' situations in your community.

Strengths and Protective Factors: School Performance

An opportunity to develop academic competence in school also is a strength and protective factor for youth; school performance **and** engagement with school personnel and activities are key. The transition from elementary school to middle school and then to high school is an exciting time because it brings new experiences and responsibilities and increased freedom. It also has its difficult moments, as youth grapple with new social and academic situations and challenges. Success in school is associated with a reduced number of risky behaviors and it increases positive social relationships. Poor academic achievement may be a sign of depression, anxiety, attention, or learning problems. Chronic absenteeism, which is frequently defined as missing at least 10% of school days, is a very frequent problem, especially in areas of poverty, either rural or urban. Among states that currently measure it, rates across a state range from about 11% on the low end to as high as 24%. Chronic absenteeism is a leading harbinger of dropping out of school, regardless of reason. Rates start to increase during middle school. Emphasizing to parents and to patients the importance of attending school every day is extremely important.[21]

Sample Questions

Ask the Youth

How are you doing in school? What do you enjoy at school? What is your favorite subject? Are you having particular difficulty with any subjects? Do you get any therapies in school or extra help with any particular subjects?

Ask the Parent

Is your child getting to school on time? How is your child doing in school? Is she completing her homework? How are her grades? Has she missed more than 2 days of school in any month?

Anticipatory Guidance

For the Youth

- Take responsibility for getting your homework done and getting to school on time.
- If you are having any difficulty at school, talk with your parent or another trusted adult about it.

For the Parent

- Emphasize the importance of school.
- Praise positive efforts.
- Recognize success and achievements.
- Monitor and guide your child as she assumes more responsibility for her schoolwork.
- Many youth need help with organization and setting priorities as they transition through middle school and into high school.
- Encourage reading by helping your child find books and magazines about subjects that interest her.
- Have her bring a book when you know she'll be waiting somewhere or in a situation requiring patience.

Strengths and Protective Factors: Coping With Stress and Decision-making

The ability to solve problems, make good decisions, and cope with stress is an important skill for youth. Health care professionals can support parents in helping their children set priorities, manage stress, and make progress toward goals.

Sample Questions

Ask the Youth

Do you worry a lot or feel overly stressed out? What stresses or worries you? What do you do to feel better when you are stressed?

Ask the Parent

Do you think your child worries too much or appears overly anxious? How do you help your child cope with stress? How do you teach her to make decisions and solve problems?

Anticipatory Guidance

For the Youth

- Everyone has stress in their lives, such as school deadlines or occasional difficulties with friends. It's important for you to figure out how to deal with stress in the ways that work best for you. If you would like some help with this, I would be happy to give you some ideas.

For the Parent

- Involve your child in family decision-making, as appropriate, to give her experience with solving problems and making decisions.
- Encourage your child to think through solutions rather than giving her all the answers.

Priority

Physical Growth and Development
Oral health, body image, healthy eating, physical activity and sleep

Oral Health

The value of brushing the teeth with fluoridated toothpaste extends to all ages. Fluoride is beneficial because it remineralizes tooth enamel and inhibits bacterial growth, thereby preventing caries. Flossing daily is important to prevent gum disease. Youth should have regularly scheduled visits with their dentist at least twice each year. They also should receive a fluoride supplement if the fluoride level in community water supplies (at home and at school) is low.

Sample Questions

Ask the Youth
How often do you brush your teeth? When was your last dental visit? Do you play contact sports? If so, do you wear a mouth guard?

Ask the Parent
When was the last time your child had a dental visit? Do you have trouble getting dental care?

Anticipatory Guidance

For the Youth
- Brush your teeth twice daily with fluoridated toothpaste and floss every day.
- Limit soda and other sweetened beverages, sport drinks, and energy drinks.
- Limit the frequency of between-meal snacks.
- If you chew gum, make sure that it is sugarless gum.
- Use a mouth guard for all contact sports.

For the Parent
- Help your child establish a daily oral health routine of brushing and flossing.
- Continue dental appointments twice a year or according to the individual schedule for your child that is set within his dental home.
- Give your child a fluoride supplement if recommended by your dentist.

Body Image

Many young adolescents going through puberty develop a vastly enhanced sensitivity to their physical appearance, how it is changing, and how it compares with their peers and with the idealized body image portrayed in the media. Health care professionals can evaluate patient concerns about body image and the emergence of disordered patterns of eating, from anorexia to obesity. Evaluating the level of body satisfaction and practices that the adolescent uses to maintain body weight will help the health care professional recognize early symptoms of eating disorders or patterns that promote unhealthy weight.

Sample Questions

Ask the Youth

How do you feel about the way you look? Do you feel that you weigh too little? Weigh too much? Just right? How much would you like to weigh? Are you teased about your weight? Are you doing anything to change your weight? What kinds of things are you doing?

Ask the Parent

Do you have any questions or concerns about your child's nutrition, weight, or physical activity? Does he talk about getting fat or dieting to lose weight?

Anticipatory Guidance

For the Youth

- Manage your weight through eating healthy foods and being physically active every day. One of the most important ways to stay healthy is to balance calorie intake from foods and calorie output through physical activity.

For the Parent

- Support a healthy weight in your child by emphasizing a balance between eating healthy foods and being physically active every day.
- Support your child's evolving self-image by commenting on the positive things he does or has learned rather than on his physical appearance only.

Healthy Eating

As the early adolescent begins to take responsibility for what he eats, his parents can support this decision-making by providing healthy foods at home and opportunities for him to participate in food shopping and meal preparation. This can help the young person learn how to make healthy food choices (eg, foods lower in saturated fat and added sugars) in other situations, such as in school and restaurants. Eating family meals together provides parents with an opportunity to model healthy eating behaviors and promote communication. Advocating for offering healthy food choices in school cafeterias, vending machines, snack bars, school stores, and other venues that offer food and beverages to students also can be an important strategy.

Adequate calcium and vitamin D intake is an important concern for early adolescents, who are experiencing their growth spurts and need calcium to support optimal bone growth. Educate parents and youth on ways to ensure sufficient calcium and vitamin D intake through daily choices of low-fat or fat-free milk and milk products, such as yogurt and cheese. Supplementation can be considered for youth who cannot consume calcium-containing foods. Fortified orange juice typically has calcium and vitamin D. Soy milk generally has both, but families should be encouraged to check the package label. Not all yogurt has vitamin D.

Sample Questions

Ask the Youth

Which meals do you usually eat each day? Do you ever skip a meal? If so, how many times a week? Do you have healthy food options at home or at school? What are they? How many servings of milk or other milk products, such as yogurt or cheese, did you have yesterday? How many servings of other calcium-containing foods did you have yesterday? How many fruits did you eat yesterday? How many vegetables? How often do you drink juice, soda, or sports or energy drinks? Are there any foods you won't eat? If so, which ones? What changes would you like to make in the way you eat?

Ask the Parent

Do you think your child eats healthy foods? What kinds of healthy foods? Do you have any difficulty getting healthy foods for your family? What gets in the way of your family eating healthy foods? Do you have any concerns about your child's eating behaviors (eg, not drinking milk, drinking soda or energy drinks, or skipping meals)? How often are you able to eat meals together as a family?

Anticipatory Guidance

For the Youth

- Eat in ways that help your body be as healthy as possible.
  - Respond to your body's signals. Eat when you are hungry. Stop eating when you feel satisfied.
  - Eat 3 healthy meals a day. Breakfast is an especially important meal.
  - Eat meals with your family as often as you can.
- Choose healthy, nutrient-dense food and drinks for meals and snacks.
  - Eat a lot of vegetables and fruits.
  - Choose whole grains, like whole-wheatbread, brown rice, and oats, not refined grains, like white bread.
  - Get enough protein from foods like chicken, fish, lean meat, eggs, legumes, nuts, and seeds.
  - Keep your bones strong by having 20 to 24 oz of low-fat or fat-free milk every day, plus an additional serving of yogurt, or cheese. If you don't drink milk or eat cheese or yogurt, choose other foods that contain calcium and foods and drinks that are fortified with calcium and vitamin D, like some orange juices and cereals.
- Limit foods and drinks that are high in calories, saturated fat, salt, added sugars, and refined grains, but low in nutrients, like chips, pizza, ice cream, and cupcakes.
- Drink water throughout the day. Choose water or low-fat or fat-free milk instead of juice, fruit drinks, soda, vitamin waters, sports and energy drinks, and caffeine drinks.

For the Parent

- Support positive nutrition habits by keeping a variety of healthy foods at home and encouraging your child to make healthy food choices.
- Be a role model by making healthy nutrition choices yourself.
- Make family meals a priority. Eat together as a family as often as possible and make mealtimes pleasant and encourage conversation. Avoid having the television (TV) on or using phones during meals. Make sure your child has breakfast before going off to school.
- Support your child's choices by providing healthy food and drink options at home, such as vegetables, fruits, whole grains, lean protein, and low-fat or fat-free dairy products. Limit the availability of high-calorie, low-nutrient foods and drinks.
- Calcium and vitamin D are important for healthy bones, so help your child get 20 to 24 oz of low-fat or fat-free milk each day, plus an additional serving of low-fat yogurt and cheese. If your child doesn't drink milk or consume other dairy products, then let's talk about alternatives. These can include foods that naturally contain calcium as well as foods and beverages that are fortified with calcium and vitamin D, like some orange juices and cereals.
- When your child is hungry between meals, offer healthy snacks, like vegetables, fruits, yogurt, and cheese and whole-grain crackers.

Physical Activity and Sleep

Adolescents should engage in 60 minutes or more of physical activity daily. Early adolescents can be physically active through play, games, physical education, recreational activities, and sports at school or in the community. It is important for adolescents to participate in physical activities that are appropriate for their age, that are enjoyable, and that offer variety. Youth with special health care needs should be encouraged to participate in physical activities that are appropriate for their ability and medical diagnosis. Attention to balancing physical activity and inactivity is needed because computers or portable digital devices present numerous opportunities for physical inactivity. Using computers and portable digital devices is often an important recreational outlet for many adolescents; therefore, guidance in limiting screen time is usually needed.

Getting enough sleep is also important to mental and physical health, school performance, and safety.

Sample Questions
Ask the Youth
What do you do to be physically active, such as walking, biking, hiking, skating, swimming, or running? Which physical activities do you participate in? How often? For how long each time? What do you think you can do to be more active? How much time each day do you spend watching TV or playing video games? How many hours a day do you use a computer or Internet-connected device? How much sleep do you get on weeknights?

Ask the Parent

Does your child participate in physical activity daily? Are there opportunities for safe recreation in your neighborhood? How can you help him become more physically active? Do you and your child participate in physical activities together? If so, which ones? How often? How much time does your child spend on recreational screen time each day? Does your child have a TV or digital device in his bedroom? Do you have guidelines or rules about screen time for your child? What are they? How are they working for you and your child? Does your child have a regular bedtime?

Anticipatory Guidance

For the Youth

- Be physically active as part of play, games, physical education, planned physical activities, recreation, and organized sports. Try to be physically active for 60 minutes or more every day. You don't have to do it all at once. You can break it up into shorter times of activity throughout the day. Doing a mix of physical activities you enjoy is a great way to reach the 60-minute-a-day goal.

- To prevent injuries, use appropriate safety equipment, such as a helmet, a mouth guard, eye protection, wrist guards, and elbow and knee pads (**for boys:** also an athletic supporter with cup), when participating in physical activity.

- Drink plenty of water to maintain hydration lost during physical activity to prevent heat-related illnesses, such as heat cramps, exhaustion, and heatstroke.

- It's important to get enough sleep at night. Having a regular bedtime helps. The use of digital devices just before bedtime can negatively affect sleep. If sleep is a problem for you, please talk to me about it.

For the Parent

- Motivate and promote your child's physical activity by encouraging and offering indoor and outdoor choices for physical activity, and by providing games and equipment that encourage physical activity. Identify community resources, like recreation centers and schools, that offer programs.

- Be a role model by being physically active yourself. Create special family times that involve physical activities.

- Do not allow your child to sleep with any electronic device in his bedroom, including phones or tablets.

- In order to balance your child's needs for physical activity, sleep, school activities, and unplugged time, consider making a family media use plan to balance these important health behaviors and media use time in your child's day. The family media use plan is an online tool that you and your child can fill out together. The tool prompts you and your child to enter daily health priorities such as an hour for physical activity, 8 to 11 hours of sleep, time for homework and school activities, and unplugged time each day for time with family and independently. You and your child can then view the time left over and decide on rules around daily screen time for your child. The AAP has information on making a plan at **www.HealthyChildren.org/MediaUsePlan.**

- Take into account not only the quantity but the quality and location of media use. Consider TVs, phones, tablets and computers. Rules should be followed by parents as well as children. Construct it so that it suits your families' media needs, but also helps you preserve face-to-face time during family routines such as meals, playtime, and bedtime. Create guidelines around times or locations in the house that are media free so that devices, such as tablets or smartphones, are not used. Having a TV or Internet-connected device in the bedroom has been associated with increased risks of obesity and poor sleep.
- Review safety issues with your child. Talk with him about ensuring privacy in what he posts online, such as on social networking sites. Stress that there are times in which it is inappropriate or dangerous to use smartphones or handheld devices, such as while walking.
- Encourage your children to get enough sleep. It can be important to their mental and physical health, their safety, and their school performance. Having a regular bedtime and limiting caffeine and the late-night use of tablets and smartphones may be helpful.

Priority

Emotional Well-being
Mood regulation and mental health, sexuality

Mood Regulation and Mental Health

Many adolescents may not present with classic adult symptoms of depression. Irritability or pervasive boredom may be symptoms of depression in this age group. Because parents often do not know that their adolescent has been having suicidal thoughts or has made attempts, it is important to question the adolescent directly if there is any concern about depression or other mental health problems. Bright Futures recommends the administration of a standardized depression screen, such as the *Patient Health Questionnaire (PHQ)*,[22] at every health supervision visit, beginning at the 12 Year Visit.

Anxiety falls along a spectrum of intensity, and symptoms may cause significant distress and affect the early adolescent's functioning at school, at home, or with friends.

Post-traumatic stress disorder is frequently overlooked and can present with symptoms of depression and anxiety. Past traumatic events can include being in a motor vehicle crash, experiencing physical or sexual abuse or other major life events, witnessing violence, or experiencing a natural disaster.

Fighting and bullying behaviors can indicate the presence of a conduct disorder and may co-occur with problems with substance use, depression, or anxiety. *(For more information on this topic, see the Bullying section of the Promoting Mental Health theme.)*

Worsening or poor academic achievement may be a sign of depression, anxiety, attention or learning problems, or alcohol or drug use.

Not adhering to parental rules and requests can indicate problems with the parent-youth relationship or with other authority figures. Disagreements over cultural values can lead to distress and high levels of conflict in the family and can affect the child's functioning and developing identity and may increase the risk of alcohol or drug use.

Any youth with a substance use disorder also may be struggling with a mental health problem. These youth need to be evaluated for both substance use and mental health problems because they occur more often together in adolescents than they do in adults.

Sample Questions

Ask the Youth

Have you been feeling bored all the time? Do you feel sad? Have you had difficulty sleeping or do you often feel annoyed? Do you ever feel so upset that you wished you were not alive or that you wanted to die? Do you find yourself continuing to remember or think about an unpleasant experience that happened in the past? Do you find that you and your parents are often arguing about what your culture expects of you and what your friends are doing?

Ask the Parent

Is your child frequently irritable? Have you noticed any changes in your child's weight or sleep habits? Does your child have recurring thoughts or memories about an unpleasant event in the past, such as a motor vehicle crash or being hurt by someone? Do you and your child have frequent conflict about what your culture expects of her behavior and how her friends behave? Do you have any concerns about your child's emotional health? Has anyone in the family had mental health problems (eg, anxiety or depression) or attempted or died by suicide?

Anticipatory Guidance

For the Youth

- Everyone has difficult times and disappointments, but these usually are temporary and you can keep on track with school, family, friends, and a generally positive attitude toward life.
- Sometimes, though, people your age may feel like they're too sad, depressed, hopeless, nervous, or angry to be able to do these things. If you feel that way now, I'd like to talk with you about it. If you ever feel that way, it is important for you to seek help. Turn to your parents, me, or another adult you trust when you feel sad, down, or alone.

For the Parent

- As your child's health care professional, I am just as interested in her emotional well-being and mental health as I am in her physical health. If you are concerned about your child's behavior, moods, mental health, or substance use, please talk with me.

Sexuality

Concerns about puberty often preoccupy early adolescents, and these concerns can be a frequent topic of discussion during the visit. Health care professionals are uniquely positioned to discuss the young person's individual pubertal developmental trajectory. This can be especially helpful for early-maturing and late-maturing adolescents. For example, it is helpful to reassure parents that most breast development in boys is normal and temporary, and that asymmetrical breast development in females is normal. Because of its importance at this developmental stage, health care professionals should educate young girls and their parents about menarche and subsequent cycle length as well as issues related to hygiene, dysmenorrhea, and irregular bleeding.

During early adolescence, youth also may have questions about gender identity, sexual attraction, and relationships. It is important for health care professionals to provide a safe place for youth to get accurate information and discuss these issues. *(For a detailed discussion of these issues, see the Promoting Healthy Sexual Development and Sexuality theme.)*

In general, it is helpful to advise parents to be open to listening about and discussing sexuality with their children. Being sensitive to cultural issues related to sexuality, gender identity, and sexual attraction while paying close attention to understanding parents' views can help the health care professional be perceived as a credible resource. Consider partnering with members of the family's community to identify strategies to support adolescents who are not following the traditions of their family. Some families will perceive it to be inappropriate for a health care professional to talk to youth about this topic, so it is useful to provide them with information and sources of support in their community.

Sample Questions

Ask the Youth

For boys and girls: *What do you know about how your body changes during puberty?*

For girls: *Have you had your first period? If you have menstruated, tell me more about your periods, such as how often they are and how heavy.*

For boys and girls: *Have you talked with your parents about dating and sex? What have they shared with you?*

Other options for questions: *Do you know or wonder about who you might be romantically or sexually attracted to?* **Alternative questions, if desired:** *Are you interested in boys? Girls? Both? Not sure? Do you know any kids who are gay or lesbian? What would it be like for you if one of your friends told you he or she was gay or lesbian?*

Ask the Parent

Have you and your child discussed the physical changes that occur during puberty? Would you like more information about puberty and the emotional changes that occur? What are your house rules about curfews, dating, and friends?

Anticipatory Guidance

For the Youth

- **For boys and girls:** Youth go through the physical changes of puberty at different times, so if you have any questions about these changes, please ask me.
- **For girls:** I want to make sure you understand about your periods (your menstrual cycles). Please ask me if you have any questions.
- Around your age, youth start to think about romantic and sexual attractions toward others. Middle schoolers are figuring out their sexual attractions. You may have times when you have strong feelings for someone of the opposite or the same sex.
- I am available to discuss these issues with you.

For the Parent

- Youth go through the physical changes of puberty at different times, so if you or your adolescent has any questions about her particular developmental path and developing sexuality, please ask me.
- During adolescence, youth typically start to think about romantic and sexual attractions toward others. Middle schoolers are often figuring out sexual attractions and may go through times of attraction to the same or opposite sex. If you have any questions about adolescent sexual development, or would like more information about adolescent sexual development, sexual orientation, or gender identity, please ask me.

Priority

Risk Reduction

Pregnancy and sexually transmitted infections; tobacco, e-cigarettes, alcohol, prescription or street drugs; acoustic trauma

Pregnancy and Sexually Transmitted Infections

Abstinence for those who have not had sex, and as an option for those who are sexually experienced, is the safest protection from pregnancy and sexually transmitted infections (STIs). Knowing how to protect oneself and one's partner from pregnancy and STIs is critical for those who are sexually active. The majority of youth aged 11 to 14 years have not had sex. According to data from the 2013 Youth Risk Behavior Survey, the percentage of adolescents, both boys and girls, who have had sexual intercourse (including nonconsensual sex) before age 13 years was 5.6% in 2013. A higher percentage of boys (8.3%) are sexually active before age 13 years as compared to girls (3.1%). Among survey participants, 30% reported having had sexual intercourse by the spring semester of grade 9, typically age 14 or 15 years.[23] The youth who are having or have had sex may have risks related to sexual abuse, pregnancy, and STIs that need to be identified.

For older youth, it may be helpful to preface your questions with an explanation of why they are being asked.

- Most youth this age are not involved in a sexual relationship even though some may be in romantic relationships.
- Some youth may not have all the information they need to make healthy decisions.
- Some youth may be in situations where they are being forced or pressured, often by someone older. This can be confusing even though it's not their fault, so it's important that they tell someone.
- Different kinds of physical closeness that count as sex can spread disease (including oral sex).

Sample Questions

Ask the Youth

Have you ever been in a romantic relationship? Have you always felt safe and respected? Have any of your relationships been sexual relationships? What are your thoughts about having sex? Have you ever been touched in a way that made you feel uncomfortable? Have you ever been forced or pressured to do something sexual that you haven't wanted to do?

If the youth is sexually active, the following questions may be helpful: *Were your partners male or female, or have you had both male and female partners? Were your partners younger, older, or your age? Have you had oral sex? Vaginal sex? Anal sex? Did you use other birth control instead of, or along with, a condom? How often do you use condoms? Are you aware of emergency contraception? If you are having sex, are you making good choices to avoid emotional hurt for you and your partner? How are you protecting yourself against STIs and pregnancy?*

Ask the Parent

Have you talked to your child about sex? How do you plan to help him deal with pressures to have sex? How does your culture help you do this?

Anticipatory Guidance

For the Youth

- Not having sexual intercourse, including oral sex, is the safest way to prevent pregnancy and STIs.
- Figure out ways to make sure you can carry through on your decisions regarding your sexual behaviors. Plan how to avoid risky places and relationships. For example, don't use drugs or alcohol, because these can raise the risk of unwanted sex and other risky behaviors.
- If you are sexually active, protect yourself and your partners from STIs and pregnancy.

For the Parent

- Encourage abstinence from sexual activity or a return to abstinence.
- Help your child make a plan to resist pressures to use substances or have sex. Be there for him when he needs support or help.
- Support safe activities at school, with community and faith organizations, and with volunteer groups to encourage personal and social development.
- If you feel you can't talk with your child because you don't know enough about teen development, sexual pressures, teen pregnancy, and STIs, learn more through reliable resources.
- Talk about relationships and sex when issues arise on TV, at school, or with friends. Be open and nonjudgmental, but honest, about your personal views.

Tobacco, E-cigarettes, Alcohol, Prescription or Street Drugs

Provide information or role-play on how to resist peer pressure to smoke or use e-cigarettes, drink alcohol, misuse prescription drugs, or use street drugs.[24] If screening questions about tobacco, e-cigarettes, alcohol, or drug use have not already been asked in a Previsit Questionnaire, Bright Futures recommends they be included during anticipatory guidance. Many youth incorrectly consider e-cigarettes safer than traditional cigarettes. It is important to specifically ask about e-cigarette use, known by many youth as vaping.

Sample Questions

Ask the Youth

What are your thoughts about smoking, vaping, drinking, and using drugs? Have you ever been offered any drugs? Have you ever taken prescription drugs that were not given to you for a specific medical condition? If no: How would you handle that? If yes: How did you handle that?

Ask the Parent

Does anyone in your home smoke or use e-cigarettes? Has your child come to you with questions about alcohol or drugs? What have you discussed about the topic? Do you know your child's friends? Do you know where your child is and what he does after school and on the weekends? What are the expected consequences or disciplinary actions that you would take (or have taken) if you discovered that your child was using tobacco, e-cigarettes, alcohol, or other drugs? To your knowledge, has your child ever used alcohol or drugs? If so, how do you know? How did you react to the situation? Did your child say he would stop? Has he?

Anticipatory Guidance

For the Youth

- Don't smoke, use tobacco or vape, drink alcohol, or use drugs, inhalants, anabolic steroids, or diet pills. Smoking marijuana, vaping, and smoking hookah and other drugs can hurt your lungs. Alcohol and other drugs are bad for your brain's development.

- Prescription drugs can kill when used inappropriately. Do not share medications with friends or take anyone else's medications. Take your own medications only as prescribed.

- Avoid situations in which drugs or alcohol are readily available. If you can't avoid situations with drugs or alcohol, have a plan for how you are going to avoid using. I can help you make your plan.

- Support friends who choose not to use tobacco, e-cigarettes, alcohol, drugs, steroids, or diet pills. Choose friends who support your decision not to use tobacco, e-cigarettes, alcohol, or drugs.

- If you ever have questions about alcohol or drugs, please ask me. If you smoke, vape, misuse prescription drugs, use street drugs, or drink alcohol, let's talk about it. We can work out a way to help you quit or cut down on your use.

- If you are worried about any family members' drug or alcohol use, you can talk with me.

For the Parent

- Know where and with whom your child is spending leisure time.

- Clearly discuss rules and expectations for acceptable behavior.

- Praise your child for not using tobacco, e-cigarettes, alcohol, or other drugs. Reinforce this decision through positive and open conversations about these issues.

- Lock or monitor your liquor cabinet and prescription medications. Do NOT save leftover prescription medicines. Dispose of these medications properly, using a method that is recommended in your community.

Acoustic Trauma

The Occupational Safety Health Administration has rules for noise exposure in the workplace to prevent a temporary threshold shift in hearing (a change of at least 10 dB from a previous test) that can become a permanent hearing loss.[25] No similar recommendation exists for noise from personal devices. Mild hearing loss (ie, >25 dB) was found in 3.5% of adolescents aged 12 to 19 years in the National Health and Nutrition Examination Survey (NHANES) III 1988–1994 and 5.3% in NHANES 2005–2006.[26]

To protect hearing, the CDC recommends avoiding or limiting exposure to excessively loud sounds, turning down the volume of music systems, moving away from the source of loud sounds when possible, and using hearing protection devices when it is not feasible to avoid exposure to loud sounds, or reduce them to a safe level.[27,28]

Sample Questions

Ask the Adolescent

Are you aware that loud noise can cause both temporary and permanent hearing loss? How loud do you usually have your music?

Ask the Parent

Are you concerned about how loudly your adolescent plays his music?

Anticipatory Guidance

For the Adolescent

- Wear hearing protection when you are exposed to loud noise, such as music, at concerts, or in loud working conditions, such as running lawn, garden, or snow removal machinery.
- When you use earbuds, make sure the volume on your device isn't too high.

For the Parent

- Encourage hearing protection when your adolescent is exposed to loud noise, such as when he listens to music, is at concerts, or is in loud working conditions.
- Encourage your adolescent to keep the volume at a reasonable level when he uses a device with earbuds.

Priority

Safety

Seat belt and helmet use, sun protection, substance use and riding in a vehicle, firearm safety

Seat Belt and Helmet Use

Everyone should wear seat belts when riding in a car, and helmets or other protective gear when participating in activities such as biking, skating, or water sports. Smaller adolescents may still need to use a belt-positioning booster seat in the car to help the seat belt fit properly; a low-profile backless booster seat may be less noticeable and more acceptable to the adolescent than a high-back booster.

If parents and peers wear seat belts and bicycle helmets, the early adolescent is more likely to do so.

Children and adolescents younger than 16 years should not ride an all-terrain vehicle (ATV).

Sample Questions

Ask the Youth

How do you feel about wearing a seat belt and helmet? Do you always wear a seat belt? Do you always wear a helmet or other protective gear when you bike, play team sports, or do water sports? What would make it easier for you to wear a seat belt and helmet all of the time?

Ask the Parent

Do you always wear a seat belt and bicycle helmet? Do you insist that your child wear a seat belt when in a car? Do you insist that your child use appropriate safety equipment when she participates in physical activities, such as biking, team sports, or water sports?

Anticipatory Guidance

For the Youth

- Always wear a seat belt in a vehicle.
- Always wear a helmet and other protective gear when you are biking, skateboarding, or skating.
- Always wear protective gear when engaged in team sports.
- Always wear an appropriately fitting US Coast Guard–approved life jacket when engaged in water sports.

For the Parent

- It's important that you and everyone else always wear a seat belt in the car and helmet on your bicycle.

For information about how to keep your child safe in and around cars, visit www.safercar.gov/parents.

Toll-free Auto Safety Hotline: 888-327-4236

Sun Protection

Sun protection is now of increasing importance because of climate change and the thinning of the atmospheric ozone layer. Sun protection is accomplished through limiting sun exposure, using sunscreen, and wearing protective clothing. About one-fourth of a person's exposure to the sun occurs before age 18 years. Early exposure to ultraviolet radiation (UVR) increases skin cancer risk. Youth may visit tanning parlors, which also raises their skin cancer risk.

Sample Questions

Ask the Youth

Do you always use sunscreen? Do you limit outside time during the middle of the day, when the sun is at its strongest? Do you visit tanning parlors?

Ask the Parent

Is your child protected from excessive sun exposure? Does she use sunscreen?

Anticipatory Guidance

For the Youth

- Protect yourself from the sun by covering up with clothing and hats. Whenever possible, time your activities so you're not outside from 11:00 am to 3:00 pm, when the sun is strongest.
- Use sunscreen and reapply frequently.
- Wear sunglasses.

For the Parent

- Encourage your adolescent to protect herself from overexposure to the sun and to avoid tanning parlors.
- Encourage her to use sunscreen with an SPF of 15 or higher and to wear a hat.

Substance Use and Riding in a Vehicle

The use of alcohol and other drugs has been associated with car crash deaths in adolescents. Sometimes, young adolescents don't have control over the substance use of people with whom they ride (eg, rides home from an adult after babysitting or rides with older friends and siblings). Counsel parents to develop strategies with their adolescent on how to avoid these situations.

Sample Questions

Ask the Youth

Have you ever ridden in a vehicle with someone who has been drinking or using drugs? Whom can you call for a ride if you feel unsafe riding with someone?

Ask the Parent

Have you discussed with your child how she should get home safely if she is with someone who has been using drugs or alcohol? What plans have you made with your child to get her home safely?

Anticipatory Guidance

For the Youth

- Do not ride in a vehicle with someone who has been using drugs or alcohol. Call your parents or another trusted adult and get help.

For the Parent

- Help your child make a plan for what to do in case she ever feels unsafe riding in a vehicle because the driver has been drinking or using drugs, or if any situation is out of hand.

Firearm Safety

The AAP recommends that homes be free of firearms and that if it is necessary to keep a firearm, it should be stored unloaded and locked, with the ammunition locked separately from the firearm.

Firearms should be removed from the homes of adolescents who have a history of aggressive or violent behaviors, suicide attempts, or depression. The presence of a firearm in the home increases the risk of suicide and homicide.

Sample Questions

Ask the Youth

Do you ever carry a firearm or knife (even for self-protection)? **If yes:** *When have you carried a firearm or knife? If there is a firearm in your home, do you know how to get hold of it?*

Ask the Parent

Is there a firearm in your house? Is it locked, and is the ammunition locked and stored separately? Is there a firearm in the homes where you and your child visit, such as the homes of grandparents, other relatives, or friends? Have you talked to your child about firearm safety?

Anticipatory Guidance

For the Youth

- Fighting and carrying weapons can be dangerous. Would you like to discuss how to avoid these situations?

For the Parent

- The best way to keep your child safe from injury or death from firearms is to never have a firearm in the home. If it is necessary to keep a firearm in your home, it should be stored unloaded and locked, with the ammunition locked separately from the firearm. Keep the key where your child cannot have access.

Middle Adolescence
15 Through 17 Year Visits

Context

The middle adolescent continues to rapidly develop in many directions simultaneously—physically, cognitively, emotionally, and socially. High school and its associated activities, such as academics, sports, clubs, and the arts, become the central focus of life for most middle adolescents. Many youth also begin working after school or on weekends. Youth with special health care needs are often mainstreamed and, therefore, able to take advantage of the educational opportunities of large schools. Some youth with cognitive challenges also may be eligible for extended educational opportunities in high school until they reach age 21 years.[29] All the experiences that become available to a middle adolescent provide wonderful opportunities for her to solidify life skills and positive habits that will serve her well as she encounters new experiences and makes decisions about whether to experiment with risk behaviors. By now, the adolescent should have a good opinion of herself and a feeling of competency. The ability to bounce back from stressors is evolving into the important quality of resiliency.

As much as high school is a positive formative experience for many middle adolescents, others have a different experience. In 2012, 6.6% of youth and young adults aged 16 to 24 years had not completed high school and were not enrolled.[30] Health care professionals should learn the dropout rates in their area and which youth may be at highest risk.

Appearance is an especially important issue during middle adolescence. Health care professionals should be sensitive to a patient's concerns about body image and the continued problem of disordered eating, from anorexia to obesity. Evaluating the level of body satisfaction and practices that the adolescent uses to maintain body weight (eg, dieting or binge eating and physical activity patterns) will help the health care professional recognize early symptoms of disordered eating or patterns that promote unhealthy body weight and behaviors.

By middle adolescence, peers are an important source of health information to adolescents and are a key reference group. Peers frame behaviors that adolescents feel are appropriate and may offer insight into practices that pose a health risk. For example, the adolescent who engages in competitive sports, such as gymnastics or wrestling, may be vulnerable to misinformation about unhealthy or even unsafe nutrition choices and behaviors (eg, chewing gum to reduce food craving and eating less or drinking excessive amounts of water to maintain a low body weight). An adolescent patient should be directly involved in identifying priority areas for behavior change.

Beginning at age 14 years, the adolescent is entering the developmental period of highest risk for mental health problems.[31] The most common mental health concerns for adolescents are mood disorders (depression and anxiety), learning disorders and attention-deficit disorders, and conduct disturbances. Emotional well-being is related to the adolescent's biophysical development. As she moves into high school, skills used successfully in junior high may be insufficient or ineffective for the increased rigor of the high school curriculum. Support is critical for the adolescent and family with school concerns or behavioral issues that emerge with this new academic environment and developmental stage. Health care professionals must be aware of this and refer their adolescent patients for neuropsychological assessment or behavioral counseling as needed.

Many middle adolescents experiment with risk behaviors, such as drug use or unsafe sexual behavior. Adolescents who have a chronic illness may question whether medications they have used during middle childhood are still needed. Many middle adolescents receive a driver's permit or license, which allows them increased freedom and unsupervised time. By the end of this developmental period, the health care professional should have discussed topics such as tobacco use, alcohol and illicit drug experimentation, healthy sexual development, abstinence, and the importance of responsible and safe driving. Discussions also may include ways in which the youth's culture, religion, and family can be viewed as supports in making healthy behavior choices.

During this developmental stage, the adolescent's interpersonal relationships evolve, and interest in dating, sexual intimacy, and related behaviors increases. These issues can be particularly complex for lesbian, gay, bisexual, transgender, or questioning youth. The health care professional should create a clinical environment where clear messages that are sensitive to personal issues, including sexual orientation and gender identity, can be given whenever the adolescent feels ready to discuss them. Experimentation with sexual behaviors, including oral sex and vaginal or anal intercourse, can occur at this age. Frank and supportive conversations about these issues and behavior within the context of the youth's cultural perspective are important.

The legal age of majority is 18 years of age, but the circumstances in which minors can consent to their own health care varies according to state law. Some minor adolescents may be deemed emancipated (eg, those who are married or divorced, a member of the armed forces, or those living separate from parents and managing their own financial affairs). Others may be considered a mature minor and thus able to consent to their own care under certain conditions (eg, pregnancy-related services, reportable diseases and STIs, mental health, and substance use). Patient-provider confidentiality related to such care is a delicate issue, especially when supporting parental involvement. If an adolescent patient is entitled to confidential care (either because she is legally at the age of majority or she has been deemed an emancipated or a mature minor), a health care professional generally needs the adolescent's permission to discuss her case with her parents. Health care professionals should be aware of their state and local laws, community standards, and public health regulations.[32]

The adolescent patient and her parents should be informed of the practice's terms of confidentiality, as well as any exceptions, such as patient safety. Ultimately, clinical judgment, ethical principles, and moral certitude guide decisions about individual cases. (For more information on this topic, see the introduction to the visits.)

Early consideration may be given to supporting an adolescent in developing decisional capacity to take on the responsibility for his own health care. Developing a transition plan to adult health care and discussing issues such as confidentiality, informed consent, and the adolescent's preference about the presence of parents during part of the visit are steps toward medical autonomy.[33,34]

Priorities for the 15 Through 17 Year Visits

The first priority is to address the concerns of the adolescent and the parents.

In addition, the Bright Futures Adolescence Expert Panel has given priority to the following additional topics for discussion in the 3 Middle Adolescence Visits.

The goal of these discussions is to determine the health care needs of the youth and family that should be addressed by the health care professional. The following priorities are consistent in all the Middle Adolescence Visits. However, the questions used to effectively obtain information and the anticipatory guidance provided to the adolescent and family can vary.

Although each of these issues is viewed as important, they may be prioritized by the individual needs of each patient and family. The goal should be to address issues important to this age group over the course of multiple visits. The issues are

▶ Social determinants of health[a] (risks [interpersonal violence, food security and living situation, family substance use], strengths and protective factors [connectedness with family and peers, connectedness with community, school performance, coping with stress and decision-making])

▶ Physical growth and development (oral health, body image, healthy eating, physical activity and sleep)

▶ Emotional well-being (mood regulation and mental health, sexuality)

▶ Risk reduction (pregnancy and sexually transmitted infections; tobacco, e-cigarettes, alcohol, prescription or street drugs; acoustic trauma)

▶ Safety (seat belt and helmet use, driving, sun protection, firearm safety)

---

[a] Social determinants of health is a new priority in the fourth edition of the *Bright Futures Guidelines*. For more information, see the *Promoting Lifelong Health for Families and Communities theme*.

Health Supervision

The *Bright Futures Tool and Resource Kit* contains Previsit Questionnaires to assist the health care professional in taking a history, conducting developmental surveillance, and performing medical screening.

History

Interval history, including a review of systems, can be obtained according to the health care professional's preference or style of practice. In most cases, the adolescent will be alone at the visit. In some situations, especially if the adolescent has a special health care need, she may be accompanied by a parent, guardian, partner, spouse, or friend. Some clinicians use the HEEADSSS or SSHADESS mnemonics to help organize the questions for their young adult patients.[17,18] The following questions may encourage in-depth discussion to determine changes in health status that would warrant further physical or emotional assessment:

General Questions for the Adolescent

- Since your last visit here, how have you been? What health problems, concerns, or questions have you had?
- How are things going with your family, friends, school, and work?
- Do you have a question or worry about anything that you would like to talk about today?

General Questions for the Parent

- What questions do you have about your adolescent's physical well-being or growth?
- What questions or concerns do you have about your adolescent's emotional well-being, feelings, behavior, or learning?
- What have you and your adolescent discussed about feelings and behaviors that are contributing to her emotional well-being and a healthy lifestyle?
- What have you and your adolescent discussed about avoiding risk behaviors? What adolescent behaviors are you concerned about?

Past Medical History

- Has your adolescent received any specialty or emergency care since the last visit?

Family History

- Has your child or anyone in the family, such as parents, brothers, sisters, grandparents, aunts, uncles, or cousins, developed a new health condition or died? **If the answer is Yes:** Ascertain who in the family has or had the condition, and ask about the age of onset and diagnosis. If the person is no longer living, ask about the age at the time of death.

Social History

- See the Social Determinants of Health priority in Anticipatory Guidance for social history questions.

Surveillance of Development

The developmental tasks of middle adolescence can be addressed by asking questions, through information obtained in the medical examination, by observation, and through general discussion. The following areas can be assessed to better understand the developmental health of the adolescent. A goal of this assessment is to determine whether the adolescent is developing in an appropriate fashion and, if not, to provide information for assistance or intervention. In the assessment, determine whether the adolescent is making progress on the following developmental tasks[19]:

- Forms caring and supportive relationships with family members, other adults, and peers
- Engages in a positive way with the life of the community
- Engages in behaviors that optimize wellness and contribute to a healthy lifestyle
  - Engages in healthy nutrition and physical activity behaviors
  - Chooses safety (wearing bike helmets, using seat belts, avoiding alcohol and drugs)
- Demonstrates physical, cognitive, emotional, social, and moral competencies (including self-regulation)
- Exhibits compassion and empathy
- Exhibits resiliency when confronted with life stressors
- Uses independent decision-making skills (including problem-solving skills)
- Displays a sense of self-confidence, hopefulness, and well-being

Review of Systems

The Bright Futures Adolescence Expert Panel recommends a complete review of systems as a part of every health supervision visit. This review can be done through the following questions:

Do you have any problems with

- Regular or frequent headaches or dizziness
- Fainting or passing out
- Eyes or vision
- Ears or hearing
- Nose or throat
- Breathing problems or chest pains
- Belly aches or pains, throwing up, problems with bowel movements
- Painful urination or other urine problems
- Rashes, moles, sunburn
- Muscle aches, injury, or other problems
- Fatigue

For Girls

- Have you had your first period?
  - If so, when was your last period?
  - Do you have any problems with your periods?
  - Do you have any itching, burning, or discharge in your vaginal area?

Observation of Parent-Adolescent Interaction

Much of each visit with a middle adolescent will be spent with the adolescent alone, but the health care professional still has opportunities to observe parent-adolescent interactions, including

- Do parents encourage self-management and independent decision-making about health?
- How comfortably do the adolescent and parent interact, both verbally and nonverbally?
- Who asks and answers most of the questions?
- Does the adolescent express an interest in self-management of health issues, including adolescents who have special health care needs?

Cultural norms and values shape parent-adolescent interactions. To accurately interpret observations, the health care professional should learn about the norms and expectations of the populations served. Different cultures have different norms about how adolescents and adults interact and whether adolescents speak directly to adults or offer their own opinions in front of adults.

Physical Examination

A complete physical examination is included as part of every health supervision visit.

When performing a physical examination, the practitioner's attention is directed to the following components of the examination that are important for adolescents aged 15 through 17 years. Use of a chaperone is advised, especially when performing sensitive parts of the examination.[20]

- **Measure and compare with norms for age, sex, and height**
  - Blood pressure
- **Measure and plot on appropriate CDC Growth Chart**
  - Height
  - Weight
- **Calculate and plot on appropriate CDC Growth Chart**
  - BMI
- **Skin**
  - Inspect for acne, acanthosis nigricans, atypical nevi, piercings, and signs of abuse or self-inflicted injury.
- **Spine**
  - Examine the back and spine for deformities, including scoliosis and kyphosis.
- **Breast**
  FEMALE
  - Perform visual inspection for sexual maturity rating.
  MALE
  - Observe for gynecomastia.

- **Genitalia**

  FEMALE
  - Perform visual inspection for sexual maturity rating.

  MALE
  - Perform visual inspection and palpate testicles for sexual maturity rating.
  - Examine testicles for hydrocele, hernias, varicocele, or masses.

Screening

Universal Screening	Action	
Depression: Adolescent	Depression screen[a]	
Dyslipidemia (once between 17 Year and 21 Year Visits)	Lipid profile	
Hearing (once between 15 Year and 17 Year Visits)	Audiometry, including 6,000 and 8,000 Hz high frequencies	
HIV (once between 15 Year and 18 Year Visits)	HIV test[b]	
Tobacco, Alcohol, or Drug Use	Tobacco, alcohol, or drug use screen	
Vision (15 Year Visit)	Objective measure with age-appropriate visual-acuity measurement using HOTV or LEA symbols, Sloan letters, or Snellen letters	

Selective Screening	Risk Assessment[c]	Action if Risk Assessment Positive (+)
Anemia	+ on risk screening questions	Hematocrit or hemoglobin
Dyslipidemia (if not universally screened at this visit)	+ on risk screening questions and not previously screened with normal results	Lipid profile
HIV (if not universally screened at this visit)	+ on risk screening questions	HIV test[b]
Oral Health (through 16 Year Visit)	Primary water source is deficient in fluoride.	Oral fluoride supplementation
STIs		
▸ Chlamydia	Sexually active girls	Chlamydia test
	Sexually active boys + on risk screening questions	
▸ Gonorrhea	Sexually active girls	Gonorrhea test
	Sexually active boys + on risk screening questions	
▸ Syphilis	Sexually active and + on risk screening questions	Syphilis test
Tuberculosis	+ on risk screening questions	Tuberculin skin test

continued

Screening *(continued)*

Selective Screening	Risk Assessment[c]	Action if Risk Assessment Positive (+)
Vision (16 and 17 Year Visits)	+ on risk screening questions	Objective measure with age-appropriate visual-acuity measurement using HOTV or LEA symbols, Sloan letters, or Snellen letters

Abbreviations: AAP, American Academy of Pediatrics; HIV, human immunodeficiency virus; STI, sexually transmitted infection; USPSTF, US Preventive Services Task Force.

[a] If depression screen is positive, further evaluation should be considered during the Bright Futures Visit. Suicide risk and the presence of firearms in the home must be considered. Disorders of mood are further discussed in the *Anticipatory Guidance section* of this visit.

[b] Adolescents should be screened for STIs per recommendations in the current edition of the AAP *Red Book: Report of the Committee on Infectious Diseases*. Additionally, all adolescents should be screened for HIV according to the USPSTF recommendations (**www.uspreventiveservicestaskforce.org/uspstf/uspshivi.htm**) once between the ages of 15 and 18, making every effort to preserve confidentiality of the adolescent. Those at increased risk of HIV infection should be tested for HIV and reassessed annually.

[c] See *Evidence and Rationale chapter* for the criteria on which risk screening questions are based.

Immunizations

Consult the CDC/ACIP or AAP Web sites for the current immunization schedule.

CDC National Immunization Program: **www.cdc.gov/vaccines**

AAP *Red Book:* **http://redbook.solutions.aap.org**

Anticipatory Guidance

The following sample questions, which address the Bright Futures Adolescent Expert Panel's Anticipatory Guidance Priorities for this visit, are intended to be used selectively to invite discussion, gather information, address the needs and concerns of the family, and build partnerships. Use of the questions may vary from visit to visit. Not all questions need to be asked at every visit. Questions can be modified to match the health care professional's communication style. Any anticipatory guidance for the family should be geared to questions, issues, or concerns for that particular adolescent and family.

During the Middle Adolescence Visits, a primary focus of discussion should be with the adolescent, without dismissing the concerns or questions of the parent. The discussion and guidance is first directed to the adolescent. Discussion and guidance can include the parent later, as needed. Tools and handouts to support anticipatory guidance can be found in the *Bright Futures Tool and Resource Kit. (For more information on this topic, see the introduction to the visits.)*

Priority

Social Determinants of Health

Risks: Interpersonal violence (fighting, bullying), food security and living situation, family substance use (tobacco, e-cigarettes, alcohol, drugs)

Strengths and protective factors: Connectedness with family and peers, connectedness with community, school performance, coping with stress and decision-making

---

Risks: Interpersonal Violence (Fighting, Bullying)

Adolescents in families that are affected by intimate partner violence, or in schools or neighborhoods with high levels of violence, are dealing with a level of stress that affects their current and future health. The health care professional can identify these issues in a supportive and non-blaming way and help the adolescent (and his parents, if appropriate) formulate steps toward solutions, and make referrals to appropriate community services.

Interpersonal violence at home, in school, or in the neighborhood and gang involvement are key issues in this age group. The adolescent engaging in fighting or bullying behaviors can indicate the presence of conduct disorders or may co-occur with problems of substance use, depression, or anxiety.[35,36] *(For more information on this topic, see the Bullying section of the Promoting Mental Health theme.)*

Bullying, including cyberbullying, is still a concern. Youth who identify as lesbian, gay, bisexual, transgender, or questioning experience high rates of bullying.[37] Discuss youth involvement with negotiating anger or conflict with peers and adults to avoid physical fights in school, at home, or in the neighborhood and ways to avoid dating violence.

Bright Futures Guidelines for Health Supervision of Infants, Children, and Adolescents

Sample Questions

Ask the Adolescent

Do you feel safe at home? In your neighborhood? At school? Getting back and forth to school? Do you feel you have been bullied in person, on the Internet, or through social media? What do you do when someone tries to pick a fight with you? What do you do when you are angry? Have you been in a fight in the past 12 months? Do you carry a weapon? Have you carried a weapon to school? If so, why? Do you know anyone in a gang? Do you belong to a gang? Has your girlfriend or boyfriend ever hit, slapped, or physically hurt you? Have you ever been touched in a sexual way against your wish or without your consent? Have you ever been forced to have sexual intercourse? Are you in a relationship with a person who threatens you physically or hurts you?

Ask the Parent

Are there frequent reports of violence in your community or school? Is your adolescent involved in it? Has he ever been threatened with a firearm or knife or some other physical harm, or been injured in a fight? Has your adolescent bullied others? Has he been suspended from school because of fighting or bullying or carrying a weapon? Do you know your adolescent's friends and the activities they participate in or attend? Does your adolescent have a boyfriend or girlfriend and, if so, is their relationship respectful toward each other? Would your adolescent feel comfortable enough to inform you whether anyone has ever attempted to force sex with him?

Anticipatory Guidance

For the Adolescent

- Learn to manage conflict nonviolently. Walk away if necessary.
- Avoid risky situations. Avoid violent people. Call for help if things get dangerous.
- Confide in your parents or guardians; health care professionals, including me; or other trusted adults, such as teachers, if anyone bullies, stalks, or abuses you or threatens your safety in person, on the Internet, or through social media.
- Be thoughtful about the possible hurtful effects on others in your e-mail, social media, and texting communications. Consider how to be true to your values of respect and kindness in all of these postings. If you see another person being bullied, tell an adult.
- Healthy dating relationships are built on respect, concern, and doing things both of you like to do.
- Leave a relationship when you see signs of violence. If you are scared to do this alone, talk with your parent or other trusted adult for help and support.
- In dating situations, remember that, "No," means NO. Saying, "No," is OK, even if you have said, "Yes," in the past.

For the Parent

- Teach nonviolent conflict resolution.
- Talk to your adolescent about Internet safety and avoiding cyberbullying.
- Talk to your adolescent about safe dating practices.

MIDDLE ADOLESCENCE
15 THROUGH 17 YEAR VISITS

776

Risks: Food Security and Living Situation

Families in difficult living situations or with limited resources may have concerns about their ability to acquire sufficient food. Questions on this topic, especially those directed to the youth, can be sensitive. If the family has housing difficulties, refer the family to community housing and nutrition resources.

Increased caloric needs during the adolescent growth spurt make food security a critical issue in middle adolescence. If the family is having difficulty obtaining nutritious food, provide information about SNAP, the Commodity Supplemental Food Program, local food shelves, and local community food programs.

Sample Questions

Ask the Adolescent

In the past 12 months, have you had trouble having enough food to eat or have concerns that you might not have enough?

Ask the Parent

Tell me about your living situation. Within the past 12 months, did you worry if your food would run out before you got money to buy more? Within the past 12 months, did the food you bought just not last and you did not have money to buy more?

Anticipatory Guidance

For the Adolescent

- Community resources are available to help you and your family. You also may be eligible for food and nutrition assistance programs.

For the Parent

- The people at community agencies have expertise in housing issues and can get you the help you need. Would you like me to help you get in touch with them?
- Community food and nutrition programs and resources, like food banks, food pantries, and community food programs, are available to help you and your family. You may be eligible for the Commodity Supplemental Food Program and SNAP, the program formerly known as Food Stamps.

Risks: Family Substance Use (Tobacco, E-cigarettes, Alcohol, Drugs)

Exposure to tobacco smoke remains an important environmental risk. Although the long-term health effects of e-cigarettes have not yet been established, exposure to secondhand vapor from them likely carries health risks. Adolescents with family members and peers who use e-cigarettes (also called vaping) are more likely to begin using these devices themselves, and adolescents who use e-cigarettes are more likely to start using conventional cigarettes.

Worrying about a family member with a substance use or mental health problem may be a source of significant stress.

Sample Questions

Ask the Adolescent

Does anyone in your house or other places where you spend a lot of time smoke cigarettes or vape with e-cigarettes? Are you worried about a family member's use of alcohol, tobacco, e-cigarettes, or prescription or street drugs?

Ask the Parent

Is there anyone in your adolescent's life whose alcohol or drug use concerns you?

Anticipatory Guidance

- It's not always possible, but, when you can, avoid spending time indoors or in cars where people are smoking cigarettes or vaping with e-cigarettes.
- If someone in your family uses nicotine from either cigarettes or e-cigarettes, he or she has probably tried to stop many times. Nicotine is one of the most addicting drugs we know, and that's why it's so hard for people to stop. That's also why your family and I don't want you to start using cigarettes or e-cigarettes.
- If you are worried about any family member's drug or alcohol use problems, you can talk with me.

Strengths and Protective Factors: Connectedness With Family and Peers

In concert with identifying risks, providing anticipatory guidance about protective factors and strengths is a critical component of surveillance of adolescent developmental tasks. Identifying strengths and providing feedback to adolescents (and families, when appropriate) about what they are doing well helps provide a comprehensive and balanced view of the young person's health and well-being. Often, adolescents and parents can build on these strengths when they make plans about how to deal with the challenges of chronic health conditions or a needed behavior change, such as better nutrition or more physical activity. For adolescents and families living in difficult circumstances, such strengths may help protect the adolescent from, or reduce the degree of, negative health outcomes. The more developmental assets or strengths adolescents have, the less likely they are to engage in risky health behaviors. All adolescents and parents need to know that they can positively influence healthy development no matter what difficulties or problems exist. This anticipatory guidance provides parents with ideas about opportunities they can give their adolescent, such as the chance to become good at things, begin to make independent decisions, have social connections, and do things for others.

Young people are more likely to make healthy choices if they stay connected with family members and if clear rules and limits are set. Many family rules relate to safety and common courtesy. Following these rules will continue to be important in their relationships with friends and family when they become adults.

Friends continue to be very important in this period, and adolescents tend to have a small group of friends who share similar interests and activities, including dress, hairstyle, music, and behaviors. Peer pressure can work in a positive as well as a negative direction at this time. At the older end of this age group, adolescents also take pride in their uniqueness, so they can be encouraged to develop their own sense of identity and take on challenges that increase their skills and self-confidence. Asking parents whether they understand their adolescent's world and daily life is particularly important for families who have immigrated to the United States.

Sample Questions

Ask the Adolescent

How do you get along with your family? What do you like to do together? Do you follow your family rules and limits? What happens if you break the rules?

How closely do you feel connected to your family's cultural and religious life? How do you like school? How do you get along with others at school? How do you get along with your friends? Would you like to discuss any concerns about this?

Ask the Parent

How are you getting along as a family? What do you do together? What is your adolescent's world and daily life? What rules and expectations do you set for your adolescent?

Anticipatory Guidance

For the Adolescent

- In most situations, it's important to stay connected with your family as you get older. Work with your family to solve problems, especially around difficult situations or topics.
- How to make friends and keep them is an important life skill. Evaluating whether a friendship is no longer good for you is also important.
- Spend time with family members. Help out at home.
- Take responsibility for getting your schoolwork done and being at school on time.
- Follow your family rules, such as for curfews and driving.
- Ask for help when you need it.

For the Parent

- Have a positive relationship with your adolescent. Show affection. Praise his efforts and achievements.
- Model the positive behaviors you want your adolescent to have.
- Monitor and be aware. Know where your adolescent is and who his friends are.
- Reach agreement about limits, consequences, and independent decision-making.
- Provide opportunities for your adolescent to develop independent decision-making skills.

Strengths and Protective Factors: Connectectedness With Community

Adolescents who take part in activities they enjoy are more confident, manage their time better, and do better in school than adolescents who do not. These activities can nurture the strengths and assets that will help a middle adolescent navigate these formative years.

Sample Questions

Ask the Adolescent

What are your interests outside of your school classes? What activities are you good at or are you most proud of?

Ask the Parent

What does your adolescent like to do after school? What interests does he have? What activities is he good at? What are you proud of about your adolescent?

Anticipatory Guidance

For the Adolescent

- This is a good time to start figuring out what interests you have. How about art, drama, mentoring, volunteering, construction, and individual and organized sports? Consider learning new skills that can be helpful to your friends, family, or community, such as lifesaving CPR, or peer mentoring.
- Consider getting involved in your community about an issue that is important to you.

For the Parent

- Provide opportunities for your adolescent to find activities, other than academics, that truly interest him, especially if he is struggling academically.
- Help your adolescent see things from another person's point of view, becoming more aware of other peoples' situations in your community.

Strengths and Protective Factors: School Performance

Success in school is associated with reduction in risky behaviors and an increase in positive social relationships.

Worsening or poor academic achievement can be a sign of depression, anxiety, drug or alcohol use, or attention or learning problems. School attendance continues to be an important issue.

Adolescents should be planning for college or beginning to think about potential career options. Having no plan may indicate a lack of connectedness to school and community.

Sample Questions

Ask the Adolescent

Are you attending school? Are you going every day or have you been missing more than a couple of days a month.? How are you doing in school? What classes give you trouble in school? How are your grades? What do you plan to do after high school? Do you have a job?

Ask the Parent

Is your adolescent getting to school on time? Is he attending school almost every day? How is your adolescent doing in school? How do you support him in getting his homework done, for example, by expressing interest in his schoolwork or making sure he has dedicated time and space at home for homework? How are his grades? What do you see your adolescent doing after he completes high school?

Anticipatory Guidance

For the Adolescent

- Take responsibility for getting your homework done and getting to school on time.
- This is a good time to discuss college or work plans and goals with your family and other appropriate adults.

For the Parent

- Emphasize the importance of school.
- Praise positive efforts.
- Recognize success and achievements.
- Encourage your adolescent to take responsibility for school-related issues, but continue to be ready to help out with organizational issues or new activities, such as applying for jobs and college.
- Encourage him to read for pleasure and relaxation.
- Encourage him to keep up with the daily news.

Strengths and Protective Factors: Coping With Stress and Decision-making

Strategies for coping effectively with stress are an important aspect of emotional well-being and developing resiliency. Time-management skills, problem-solving skills, and refusal skills have all been identified as helpful. Some adolescents use their social support network, exercise, journaling, or meditation to help them manage.

Sample Questions

Ask the Adolescent

How do you cope with stress? Are you feeling really stressed out all the time? What causes you to feel stressed?

Ask the Parent

How are you helping your adolescent become a good decision-maker? Cope with stress?

Anticipatory Guidance

For the Adolescent

- Most people your age experience ups and downs as they transition from adolescence to adulthood. They have great days and not-so-great days, and successes and failures. Everyone has stress in their lives. It's important for you to figure out how to deal with stress in the ways that work best for you. If you would like some help with this, I would be happy to give you some ideas.

For the Parent

- Involve your adolescent in family decision-making, as appropriate, to give him experience with solving problems and making decisions.
- Encourage your adolescent to think through solutions rather than giving him all the answers.

Priority

Physical Growth and Development

Oral health, body image, healthy eating, physical activity and sleep

---

Oral Health

The value of brushing the teeth with fluoridated toothpaste extends to all ages. Fluoride is beneficial because it remineralizes tooth enamel and inhibits bacterial growth, thereby preventing caries. Daily flossing also is important to prevent gum disease. To maximize topical benefit through the adolescent caries-risk period, a fluoride supplement should be prescribed up to the age of 16 years if the fluoride level in community water supplies (at home and at school) is low. Adolescents should have regularly scheduled visits with their dentist at least twice each year.

Sample Questions

Ask the Adolescent

Do you brush your teeth every day? Do you floss your teeth every day? When did you last see a dentist? How frequently do you snack? Do you drink soda and other sweetened beverages or energy drinks? Do you chew gum or tobacco? Do you wear a mouth guard when you play contact sports?

Ask the Parent

Does your adolescent see a dentist regularly? Do you have trouble accessing dental care?

Anticipatory Guidance

For the Adolescent

- Brush your teeth twice a day with fluoridated toothpaste and floss every day also. See a dentist twice a year and discuss ways to keep your teeth healthy.
- Use a mouth guard for all contact sports.
- Limit soda and other sweetened beverages, sport drinks, and energy drinks.
- Limit the frequency of between-meal snacks.
- If you chew gum, make sure that it is sugarless gum.
- Don't use chewing tobacco. It causes mouth cancer.

For the Parent

- Continue dental appointments according to the individual schedule that is set for your adolescent within her dental home.
- Help your adolescent establish a daily oral health routine that includes brushing with a fluoride-containing toothpaste twice a day and flossing once a day.
- Give your adolescent fluoride supplements as recommended by your dentist.
- Monitor and limit her consumption of sweetened beverages and sports and energy drinks.
- Tell your adolescent to not use chewing tobacco because it causes mouth cancer.
- Advise your adolescent to limit the frequency of snacking and establish a regular pattern of 3 meals a day.

Body Image

An adolescent's body image is influenced by many emotional and physical factors that are associated with the changes of puberty. In middle adolescence, these issues can gain prominence when the normal weight gain and body shape changes associated with puberty combine with influences of media, advertising, and peers.

Sample Questions

Ask the Adolescent

How do you feel about the way you look? Do you feel that you weigh too little? Too much? Just right? How much would you like to weigh? Are you doing anything to change your weight? Are you teased about your weight?

Ask the Parent

What questions or concerns do you have about your adolescent's weight, eating, or physical activity behaviors? Does she talk about getting fat or dieting to lose weight?

Anticipatory Guidance

For the Adolescent

- This is a good time to start figuring out what combination of healthy eating and physical activity works to keep your body strong and healthy.

For the Parent

- Support a healthy weight for your adolescent by emphasizing eating healthy foods and being physically active.
- Support your adolescent's evolving self-image by commenting on the positive things she does or has learned rather than on her physical appearance only.

Healthy Eating

Adolescents spend a good deal of time away from home, and many consume foods that are convenient, but often high in calories, saturated fat, and added sugars. It is common for adolescents to skip meals and snack frequently. As the middle adolescent takes increasing responsibility for what she eats, parents can support this decision by providing healthy foods at home and opportunities for the adolescent to learn about selecting, purchasing, and preparing foods. This can help the adolescent choose healthy foods (eg, vegetables, fruits, whole grains, and foods lower in saturated fat and added sugars). Advocating for healthy food in school cafeterias, vending machines, snack bars, school stores, and other venues that offer food and beverages to students also can be an important strategy.

Adequate calcium intake continues to be an important concern during middle adolescence. Educate adolescents and parents on ways to ensure adolescents receive sufficient calcium intake through daily choices of milk and milk products, such as low-fat or fat-free milk, yogurt, and cheese. Supplementation can be considered for youth who cannot consume calcium-containing foods. Fortified orange juice typically has calcium and vitamin D. Soy milk generally has both, but families should be encouraged to check the package label. Not all yogurt has vitamin D. Vegetarian or vegan diets require careful attention to ensure adequate intakes of protein and nutrients.

Sample Questions

Ask the Adolescent

Which meals do you usually eat each day? Do you ever skip a meal? Do you have healthy food options at home or at school? What are they? How many servings of milk did you have yesterday? How many servings of other milk products, such as yogurt or cheese? How many servings of other calcium-containing foods did you have yesterday? How many vegetables did you eat yesterday? How many fruits? How often do you drink soft drinks? Juice? Are there any foods you won't eat? If so, which ones? What changes would you like to make in the way you eat? How often do you eat meals together as a family?

Ask the Parent

Do you think your adolescent eats healthy foods? What kinds of healthy foods? Do you have any difficulty getting healthy foods for your family? What gets in the way of your family eating healthy foods? Do you have any concerns about your adolescent's eating behaviors, such as not drinking milk, drinking soda or sports or energy drinks, or skipping meals? How often do you eat meals together as a family?

Anticipatory Guidance

For the Adolescent

- Eat in ways that help your body be as healthy as possible.
  - Respond to your body's signals. Eat when you are hungry. Stop eating when you feel satisfied.
  - Eat 3 healthy meals a day. Breakfast is an especially important meal.
  - Eat meals with your family as often as you can.
  - Pick a healthy lunch from the school cafeteria or other food venues, or pack a healthy lunch.

- Choose healthy, nutrient-dense food and drinks for meals and snacks.
  - Eat a lot of vegetables and fruits.
  - Choose whole grains, like whole-wheat bread, brown rice, and oats, not refined grains, like white bread.
  - Get enough protein from foods like chicken, fish, lean meat, eggs, legumes, nuts, and seeds.
  - Keep your bones strong by having 20 to 24 oz of low-fat or fat-free milk every day, plus an additional serving of yogurt or cheese. If you don't drink milk or eat cheese or yogurt, choose other foods that contain calcium and foods and drinks that are fortified with calcium and vitamin D, like some orange juices and cereals.
- Limit foods and drinks that are high in calories, saturated fat, salt, added sugars, and refined grains, but low in nutrients, like chips, pizza, ice cream, and cupcakes.
  - Drink water throughout the day. Choose water or low-fat or fat-free milk instead of juice, fruit drinks, soda, vitamin waters, sports and energy drinks, and caffeine drinks.
  - Don't drink too many caffeinated beverages, such as soda, coffee, and sports and energy drinks.

For the Parent
- Support positive nutrition habits by keeping a variety of healthy foods at home and encouraging your adolescent to make healthy food choices.
- Be a role model by making healthy nutrition choices yourself.
- Make family meals a priority. Eat together as a family as often as possible and make mealtimes pleasant and encourage conversation. Avoid having the TV on during meals. Make sure your adolescent has breakfast before going off to school.
- Support your adolescent's choices by providing healthy food and drink options at home, such as vegetables, fruits, whole grains, lean protein, and low-fat or fat-free dairy products. Limit the availability of high-calorie, low-nutrient foods and drinks.
- Calcium and vitamin D are important for healthy bones, so help your adolescent get 20 to 24 oz of low-fat or fat-free milk each day, plus an additional serving of low-fat yogurt and cheese. If your adolescent doesn't drink milk or eat yogurt or cheese, have her consider other foods that contain calcium as well as foods and beverages that are fortified with calcium and vitamin D, like some orange juices and cereals.
- When your adolescent is hungry in between meals, offer healthy snacks, like vegetables, fruits, yogurt, and cheese and whole-grain crackers.

Physical Activity and Sleep

Current recommendations state that adolescents should engage in 60 minutes or more of physical activity daily. The middle adolescent may need help in maintaining adequate daily physical activity. School physical education programs are often phased out by the second year of high school, sports teams begin limiting their membership to highly successful players, and participation in other clubs and school activities, as well as an increasing academic load, can limit the time available for physical activity. Depending on the safety and resources of the community, this can pose a challenge to adolescents and families. Problem-solving and helping adolescents identify activities that they can pursue may be an important part of these visits.

Attention to balancing physical activity and inactivity is needed because computers or portable devices present numerous opportunities for physical inactivity. Using computers and portable digital devices are often an important recreational outlet for many adolescents; therefore, guidance in limiting screen time is usually needed.

Sleep hygiene is important for the adolescent, yet a sleep deficit is common during these years. A phase delay in circadian rhythm that begins in early puberty makes it easiest for many adolescents to go to bed at 11:00 pm and wake up at 8:00 am, even though the junior high and senior high school classes start early.[14,16] In addition, the use of both traditional and new media delay the adolescent going to sleep.

Sample Questions

Ask the Adolescent

What do you do to be physically active, such as walking, biking, hiking, skating, swimming, or running? How often? For how long each time? How many hours a day do you use a computer? Do you do any physical activities with your family or friends? Do you participate in sports activities or dancing? How much time do you spend each day watching TV, playing video games, or using a computer or other digital device? Do you have a regular bedtime? Do you have trouble waking up in the morning? How much sleep do you get on school nights?

Ask the Parent

Does your adolescent participate in regular daily physical activity for at least 60 minutes? Do you have opportunities for safe recreation in your neighborhood? What are some ways you can support your adolescent in becoming more physically active? Do you and your adolescent participate in physical activities together? If so, which ones? How often? Does she participate in sports activities? How much time does your adolescent spend on recreational screen time each day? Does she have a TV in her bedroom? Do you have guidelines or rules about screen time? Does your adolescent have a regular bedtime? Do you think your adolescent gets enough sleep?

Anticipatory Guidance

For the Adolescent

- Be physically active as part of play, games, physical education, planned physical activities, recreation activities, and organized sports. Try to be active for 60 minutes or more every day. You don't have to do it all at once. You can break it up into shorter times of activity throughout the day. Doing a mix of physical activities you enjoy is a great way to reach the 60-minutes-a-day goal.
- To prevent injuries, use appropriate safety equipment, such as a helmet, a mouth guard, eye protection, wrist guards, and elbow and knee pads (**for boys:** also an athletic supporter with cup), when participating in physical activity.
- Drink plenty of water to maintain hydration lost during physical activity to prevent heat-related illnesses, such as heat cramps, exhaustion, and heatstroke.
- It's important to get enough sleep at night. Having a regular bedtime helps, as does limiting caffeine and the use of digital devices just before bedtime. If sleep is a problem for you, please talk to me about it.

For the Parent

- Motivate and promote your adolescent's physical activity by encouraging and offering her indoor and safe outdoor choices for physical activity, and by providing games and equipment that encourage physical activity. Identify community resources, like recreation centers, that offer programs.
- Be a role model by being physically active yourself. Create special family times that involve physical activities.
- Help your adolescent limit screen time other than for homework, by setting rules and providing alternatives.
- If your adolescent has special health care needs, encourage her to be physically active, within the limits of her medical or physical conditions. Adaptive physical education can be helpful, and a physical therapist can help you identify appropriate activities.
- Encourage your adolescent to get enough sleep. It can be important to her mental and physical health, school performance, and safety, especially if she has started driving. Having a regular bedtime and limiting caffeine and late-night use of digital devices may help.

Priority

Emotional Well-being

Mood regulation and mental health, sexuality

Mood Regulation and Mental Health

Many adolescents may not present with classic adult symptoms of depression. Pervasive boredom or irritability may be symptoms of depression in this age group. Because parents often do not know that their adolescent has been having suicidal thoughts or has made attempts, it is important to question them directly if there is any concern about depression or other mental health problems. Bright Futures recommends the administration of a standardized depression screen, such as the *PHQ*,[22] at every health supervision visit.

Anxiety falls along a spectrum of intensity, and symptoms may cause significant distress and affect the adolescent's functioning at school, at home, or with friends.

Post-traumatic stress disorder is frequently overlooked and can present with symptoms of depression and anxiety. Past traumatic events can include being in a motor vehicle crash, experiencing physical or sexual abuse or other major life events, witnessing violence, or experiencing a natural disaster.

Fighting and bullying behaviors can indicate the presence of a conduct disorder and may co-occur with problems with substance use, depression, or anxiety. *(For more information on this topic, see the Bullying section of the Promoting Mental Health theme.)*

Worsening or poor academic achievement or job performance may be a sign of depression, anxiety, attention or learning problems, or a substance misuse problem.

Not adhering to parental rules and requests can indicate problems with the parent-youth relationship or significant problems with other authority figures.

Any adolescent with substance use disorders also may be struggling with a mental health problem. These adolescents need to be evaluated for both substance misuse and mental health problems because they occur more often together in adolescents than they do in adults.

Sample Questions

Ask the Adolescent

Have you been feeling sad, had difficulty sleeping, or frequently feel irritable? Do you ever feel so upset that you wish you were not alive or that you want to die? Do you worry a lot or feel overly stressed out? Do you find yourself continuing to remember or think about an unpleasant experience that happened in the past? Who do you go to for advice and help when you have these feelings? Do you ever use any substances to make you feel better? Do you harm yourself, such as by cutting, hitting, or pinching yourself?

Ask the Parent

Have you noticed any changes in your adolescent's weight, sleep habits, or behaviors, such as becoming more isolated from his peers? Is your adolescent frequently irritable? Do you have any concerns about his emotional health? Do you think your adolescent worries too much or appears overly anxious? Does he have recurring thoughts or worries about a past unpleasant event, such as a motor vehicle crash or being hurt by someone? What helps your adolescent manage his feelings? Has anyone in the family had mental health problems or attempted or died by suicide?

Anticipatory Guidance

For the Adolescent

- Even with the ups and downs of everyday life, most people can figure out how to find and do the things they enjoy in life, such as doing their job or schoolwork; having good relationships with friends, family, and other adults; making decisions, often after talking with trusted friends and family members; having goals for the future; and adhering to their values.
- Sometimes, though, people your age may feel like they're too sad, depressed, bored, hopeless, nervous, or angry to do these things. If you feel that way now, I'd like to talk about it with you. If you ever feel that way, it is important for you to ask for help.

For the Parent

- As your adolescent's health care professional, I am just as interested in his emotional well-being and mental health as I am in his physical health. If you are concerned about your adolescent's behavior, moods, mental health, or substance use, please talk with me.

Sexuality

The physical changes of puberty are still in process for youth, especially for later maturing boys. Questions for girls often focus on menstrual issues. Sexuality and relationships are an important issue in middle adolescence. Parents and adolescents need accurate information and support to help them communicate with each other. Adolescents can develop sexual feelings and attraction for others of the opposite sex, the same sex, or both. Adolescents may have questions about gender identity, sexual attraction, and relationships in general. They will benefit from parental and health care professional support. It is helpful to advise parents to be open to listening and discussing sexuality with their children. *(For a detailed discussion of these issues, see the Promoting Healthy Sexual Development and Sexuality theme.)*

Sample Questions

Ask the Adolescent

Have you talked with your parents about dating and relationships, and about sex? **Other options for questions:** *In terms of your sexual attraction, are you attracted to anyone now? Boys? Girls? Both? Not sure? Do you have any questions or concerns about your gender identity, meaning your identity as a male or female?*

Ask the Parent

Have you talked with your adolescent about relationships, dating, and sex? About his sexuality? Have you shared your hopes, expectations, and values about relationships and sex with your adolescent? Have you established house rules about curfews, parties, dating, and friends? Do you spend time getting to know your adolescent's friends and know where they are and what they're doing? Does he have any special relationships or someone he dates steadily?

Anticipatory Guidance

For the Adolescent

- It's important for you to have accurate information about sexuality, your physical development, your gender identity, and your sexual attraction and feelings. Please ask me if you have any questions.

For the Parent

- Communicate frequently and share expectations clearly.
- Support from parents can make a positive difference for all adolescents as they go through the pubertal changes and the development of their sexual identity. If you have any questions about adolescent sexual development, or would like more information about adolescent sexual development, sexual orientation, or gender identity, please ask me.

Priority

Risk Reduction

Pregnancy and sexually transmitted infections; tobacco, e-cigarettes, alcohol, prescription or street drugs; acoustic trauma

Pregnancy and Sexually Transmitted Infections

Abstinence for those who have not had sex, and as an option to those who are sexually experienced, is the safest protection from pregnancy and STIs. In the 2013 Youth Risk Behavior Survey, 41% of 10th graders, 54% of 11th graders, and 64% of 12th graders reported that they have ever had sexual intercourse.[23] Knowing how to protect oneself and one's partner from pregnancy and STIs is critical for those who are sexually active. It may be helpful to preface your questions with an explanation of why they are being asked.

- Adolescents your age may be involved in romantic relationships. Some may be involved in a sexual relationship.
- Some adolescents may not have all the information they need to make healthy decisions.
- Some adolescents may be in situations where they are being forced or pressured, often by someone older. This can be confusing even though it's not their fault, so it's important that they tell someone.
- Different kinds of physical closeness that count as sex can spread disease (including oral sex).

Sample Questions

Ask the Adolescent

Initial options: *Are you now in a romantic relationship? Have you always felt safe and respected? Have any of your relationships been sexual relationships? Are you currently having sex, including oral sex, with anyone? In the past have you had sex? Have you ever been touched in a way that made you feel uncomfortable? Have you ever been forced or pressured to do something sexual that you haven't wanted to do?*

If the adolescent is sexually active currently or was in the past: *How many people have you had sex with in the past year? Were your partners male or female, or have you had both male and female partners? Were your partners younger, older, or your age? Have you had oral sex? Vaginal sex? Anal sex? Did you use other birth control instead of, or along with, a condom? How often do you use condoms? Are you aware of emergency contraception? If you are having sex, are you making good choices to avoid emotional hurt for you and your partner? How are you protecting yourself against STIs and pregnancy?*

Ask the Parent

Are you worried about sexual pressures on your adolescent? How do you plan to help her deal with these issues? How does your culture help you do this? What are your thoughts about your adolescent using birth control?

Anticipatory Guidance

For the Adolescent

- Abstaining from sexual intercourse is the safest way to prevent pregnancy and STIs. Many people don't know that STIs can be transmitted by oral and anal sex.
- Plan how to avoid risky places and relationships.
- If you are sexually active, protect yourself and your partners from STIs and pregnancy by correctly and consistently using a long-acting reversible contraceptive, such as an intrauterine device (IUD) or contraceptive implant, or birth control pills. Use one of these methods along with a condom. Consider having emergency contraception available. Make sure you understand what protection contraceptives do and don't offer.
- Know where to get condoms in your community and how to properly use them.

For the Parent

- Help your child make a plan to resist pressures to have sex. Be there for her when she needs support or assistance.
- Have discussions with your adolescent to help her accept responsibility for her decisions and relationships.
- Help your adolescent make healthy decisions about sex, including consistent use of birth control if she is sexually active.

Tobacco, E-cigarettes, Alcohol, Prescription or Street Drugs

Provide information on how to resist peer pressure to smoke, use e-cigarettes, drink alcohol, misuse prescription drugs, use street drugs, or have sex.

If screening questions about alcohol or drug use have not already been asked in a Previsit Questionnaire, Bright Futures recommends they be included during anticipatory guidance. Many adolescents incorrectly consider e-cigarettes safer than traditional cigarettes. It is important to specifically ask about e-cigarette use, known by many youth as vaping.

Sample Questions

Ask the Adolescent

What are your thoughts about smoking, vaping, drinking, and using drugs? Have you ever been offered any drugs? **If no:** *How would you handle that?* **If yes:** *How did you handle that?*

Have you ever taken prescription drugs that were not given to you for a specific medical condition?

Ask the Parent

Does anyone in your home smoke or use e-cigarettes? Are you worried about any family members and how much they smoke, drink, or use drugs? Has your adolescent come to you with questions about alcohol or drugs? What have you discussed about the topic? Do you know where your adolescent is and what she does after school and on the weekend? To your knowledge, has your adolescent ever used alcohol or drugs? If so, how do you know? How did you react to the situation? Did your adolescent say she would stop? Has she?

Anticipatory Guidance

For the Adolescent

- Do not smoke, use tobacco or vape with e-cigarettes, drink alcohol, or use drugs, inhalants, anabolic steroids, or diet pills. Smoking marijuana, vaping, and smoking hookah and other drugs can hurt your lungs. Alcohol and other drugs are bad for your brain's development.
- Prescription drugs can kill when used inappropriately. Do not share medications with friends or take anyone else's medications. Take your own medications only as prescribed.
- Avoid situations in which drugs or alcohol are readily available.
- Support friends who choose not to use tobacco, e-cigarettes, alcohol, drugs, steroids, or diet pills. Choose friends who support your decision not to use tobacco, e-cigarettes, alcohol, or drugs.
- If you smoke, vape, misuse prescription drugs, use street drugs, or drink alcohol, let's talk about it. We can work on a plan together to help you quit or cut down on your use.
- If you are worried about any family member's drug or alcohol use, you can talk to me.

For the Parent

- Be involved in your adolescent's life. Know where and with whom she is spending leisure time.
- Clearly discuss rules and expectations for acceptable behavior.
- Praise your adolescent for not using tobacco, e-cigarettes, alcohol, or other drugs. Encourage her to stick to this decision.
- Help your adolescent plan for situations when she will be offered alcohol, tobacco, e-cigarettes, or other drugs.
- Set a good example for your adolescent through your own responsible use of alcohol and other substances.
- Lock your liquor cabinet. Put your prescription medicines in a place where your adolescent and her friends cannot get them, preferably also in a locked place. Medications at the homes of relatives and friends should be locked as well. If you are concerned that your medications are being misused, count the pills. Do NOT save leftover prescription medicines. Dispose of these medications properly, using a method that is recommended in your community.

Acoustic Trauma

The Occupational Safety Health Administration has rules for noise exposure in the workplace to prevent a temporary threshold shift in hearing (a change of at least 10 dB from a previous test) that can become a permanent hearing loss.[25] No similar recommendation exists for noise from personal devices. Mild hearing loss (ie, >25 dB) was found in 3.5% of adolescents aged 12 to 19 years in NHANES III 1988–1994 and 5.3% in NHANES 2005–2006.[26]

To protect hearing, the CDC recommends avoiding or limiting exposure to excessively loud sounds, turning down the volume of music systems, moving away from the source of loud sounds when possible, and using hearing protection devices when it is not feasible to avoid exposure to loud sounds, or reduce them to a safe level.[27,28]

Sample Questions

Ask the Adolescent

Are you aware that loud noise can cause both temporary and permanent hearing loss? How loud do you usually have your music?

Ask the Parent

Are you concerned about how loudly your adolescent plays her music?

Anticipatory Guidance

For the Adolescent

- Wear hearing protection when you are exposed to loud noise, such as music, at concerts, or in loud working conditions, such as running lawn, garden, or snow removal machinery.
- When you use earbuds, make sure the volume on your device isn't too high.

For the Parent

- Encourage hearing protection when your adolescent is exposed to loud noise, such as when she listens to music, is at concerts, or is in loud working conditions.
- Encourage your adolescent to keep the volume at a reasonable level when she uses a device with earbuds.

Priority

Safety

Seat belt and helmet use, driving; sun protection; firearm safety

Seat Belt and Helmet Use, Driving

Everyone should wear seat belts when riding in a vehicle, and helmets when riding a bicycle, a motorcycle, or an ATV, and other protective gear when participating in activities such as biking, skating, or water sports. Graduated driver requirements have been shown to be effective, and it is important for parents to enforce them and for adolescents to understand their importance. However, no state's graduated driver licensing law includes all the rules and restrictions that are known to reduce crash risk, so parents should be advised that they can and should set rules and limits of their own in addition to those set by the state.

Learning to drive is a rite of passage for many adolescents and a reflection of their growing independence and maturity. Health care professionals should encourage parents to be closely involved with their adolescent's driver's education by doing practice driving sessions together and by establishing rules that foster safe, responsible driving behaviors. Parents should familiarize themselves with the provisions of the Graduated Driver License law in their state and continue to monitor their adolescent's driving skills and habits to ensure that safe behaviors persist.

Sample Questions

Ask the Adolescent

Do you always wear a seat belt? Do you always wear a helmet or protective gear when biking, playing team sports, or doing water sports? Have you started to learn how to drive? Do you follow the driving regulations for young drivers? Do you have someone you can call for a ride if you feel unsafe driving yourself or riding with someone else?

Ask the Parent

Do you always wear a seat belt and bicycle or motorcycle helmet? Do you insist that your adolescent wear them? What kinds of rules and restrictions have you set regarding his driving?

Anticipatory Guidance

For the Adolescent

- Always wear a seat belt in a vehicle, and a helmet when riding a bike, a motorcycle, or an ATV, or when skateboarding.
- Always wear an appropriately fitting US Coast Guard–approved life jacket when you do water sports.
- Always wear protective gear when you play in team sports.
- Distracted driving is dangerous. Your brain cannot pay attention to your driving and a mobile device at the same time. Do not talk, text, or manipulate a mobile device while the keys are in the ignition. Turn off your cell phone and put it in the trunk of the car so you are not tempted to use it while you are driving.
- Do not ride in a vehicle with a driver who has been using drugs or alcohol.
- Limit night driving and driving with other teen passengers.
- If you feel unsafe driving yourself or riding with someone else, call someone to drive you.

For the Parent

- If you wear seat belts and helmets, your adolescent is more likely to do so also. Insist that everyone in the vehicle wear a seat belt.
- Be involved with your adolescent's life. Know where he is and who his friends are.
- Be a good role model and reinforce that distracted driving is dangerous. Do not talk, text, or use a mobile device while the keys are in the ignition. Turn off your cell phone and put it in the trunk of the car so you aren't tempted to use it while driving.
- Set limits and expectations for your adolescent about driving, such as number of passengers, the amount of night driving allowed, how to minimize distracted driving, and how to avoid high-risk situations. Consider using a written parent-teen driving agreement to document that you and your adolescent understand the rules and the consequences for breaking them, and when the rules will be relaxed if he demonstrates safe and responsible driving behavior.
- Be involved in your adolescent's driving, because parents who are involved are successful at imposing limits.
- Make a plan with your adolescent for situations when he feels unsafe driving or riding with someone.

For information about how to keep your youth safe in and around cars, visit www.safercar.gov/parents.

Toll-free Auto Safety Hotline: 888-327-4236

Sun Protection

Sun protection is now of increasing importance because of climate change and the thinning of the atmospheric ozone layer. Sun protection is accomplished through limiting sun exposure, using sunscreen, and wearing protective clothing. About one-fourth of a person's exposure to the sun occurs before age 18 years. Early exposure to UVR increases skin cancer risk. Adolescents may visit tanning parlors, which also raises their skin cancer risk.

Sample Questions

Ask the Adolescent

Do you always use sunscreen? Do you limit outside time during the middle of the day, when the sun is strongest? Do you visit tanning parlors?

Ask the Parent

Is your adolescent protected from excessive sun exposure? Does he use sunscreen?

Anticipatory Guidance

For the Adolescent

- Protect yourself from the sun by covering up with clothing and hats. Whenever possible, time your activities so you're not outside from 11:00 am to 3:00 pm, when the sun is strongest.
- Use sunscreen SPF 15 or higher and reapply frequently.
- Wear sunglasses.
- Don't go to tanning parlors.

For the Parent

- Encourage your adolescent to protect himself from overexposure to the sun and to avoid tanning parlors.
- Encourage him to use sunscreen of SPF 15 or higher and wear a hat.

Firearm Safety

The AAP recommends that homes be free of firearms and that if it is necessary to keep a firearm, it should be stored unloaded and locked, with the ammunition locked separately from the firearm.

Firearms should be removed from the homes of adolescents who have a history of aggressive or violent behaviors, suicide attempts, or depression. The presence of a firearm in the home increases the risk of suicide and homicide, even in those without a mental health diagnosis.

Sample Questions

Ask the Adolescent

Do you ever carry a firearm? Can you get a firearm if you want to? Is there a firearm at home? If so, do you know how to get hold of it? Have you ever carried a firearm for protection?

Ask the Parent

Is there a firearm in your house? Is it locked and is the ammunition locked and stored separately? Is there a firearm in the homes where you and your adolescent visit, such as the homes of grandparents, other relatives, or friends? Have you talked with your adolescent about firearm safety?

Anticipatory Guidance

For the Adolescent

- Fighting and carrying weapons can be dangerous. Let's talk about some ways to avoid these situations.

For the Parent

- The best way to keep your adolescent safe from injury or death from firearms is to never have a firearm in the home. If it is necessary to keep a firearm in your home, it should be stored unloaded and locked, with the ammunition locked separately from the firearm. Keep the key where your adolescent cannot have access.

Late Adolescence
18 Through 21 Year Visits

Context

The late adolescent stands at a transforming moment in life. He has progressed through a huge developmental trajectory that began 18 years ago. The accumulated physical, cognitive, emotional, and social experiences of infancy, early childhood, middle childhood, and the earlier phases of adolescence have prepared him for the final transition to adulthood. This transition is the work of late adolescence.

Physical development is generally complete by late adolescence. By this point, the young adult also typically has developed a sense of self-identity and a rational and realistic conscience, and he has refined his moral, religious, and sexual values. He is able to compromise, set limits, and think through issues to make decisions. Cognitively, the young adult is still developing, and new research evidence suggests that this process may continue into the third decade of life.[38] Society, however, regards him as a legal adult in many ways.

The experiences of late adolescence vary greatly and depend on the adolescent's resources, previous academic performance, life choices, opportunities, motivations, and cultural expectations about independence. It is important for young adults to either finish high school and obtain a high school diploma or, for those who drop out of high school, to obtain a high school equivalency certificate (the GED, or General Educational Development). The late adolescent may enter college, enter a trade or start a job, participate in Job Corps, or join the military. A growing minority of high school graduates delay college matriculation for a "gap year."

Living situations vary widely among young adults. They may live at home or college, on their own, with a roommate or partner, or in a group setting. They may be getting married and starting their own family. A young adult with special health care needs may be in high school or at work and still living at home. In some cultures, young adults are expected to live at home until they are married.

It is argued that "emerging adulthood is neither adolescence nor young adulthood, but is theoretically and empirically distinct from them both."[1] Compared to earlier times contemporary young adults experience a longer and less structured transition period from their late teens through their mid-20s, including more years of education and training and later ages of entering marriage and parenthood. Attending college typically delays moving into the work force full-time and entails paying historically high tuition rates. This expensive lengthening of the education process makes it difficult for young people to become financially independent, even though a college education often ultimately results in a higher-paying job.

All these transitional experiences expose the young adult to new relationships, lifestyles, driving habits, dietary patterns, and exercise habits. He may start new sexual relationships and define his sexual identity. Parental and other adult supervision decreases and autonomy increases. Responsibilities and life stresses also increase, as does access to alcohol and drugs. Personal health behaviors may change. The nutrition and physical activity habits of this age group may change, too, as their food and physical activity choices are no longer supervised. For some young adults, the transition to independent living creates opportunities to improve their nutrition and physical activity patterns. For others, nutritious foods may be perceived as unaffordable or inconvenient. Access to formal exercise programs or team participation also may be limited.

The health care needs of the young adult vary greatly on the basis of his situation; thus, the young adult should have medical preventive visits annually to assess any new positive and negative influences that may be affecting his health. Inquiring about these issues can often lead to topics that merit further exploration and assistance. Unfortunately, young adults' participation in health supervision visits tends to decrease. Many in this age group are no longer legally considered "dependents" of their parents. However, currently a young adult can remain on his parent's commercial health plan until he turns 26 years of age if the plan covers dependent children. Other sources of health supervision exist for young adults, depending on their life choices. For example, college and university health care centers can play an important role in addressing the health conditions and risky behaviors (eg, episodic heavy drinking/binge drinking, drinking and driving, cigarette smoking, and overweight) of young adults.[39] The military provides health care to active duty personnel, and many workplaces sponsor wellness and health-promotion activities.

Optimal health care for the young adult includes a formal plan for the transition to an adult health care professional. Successful transition involves the early engagement and participation of the young adult and his family with the pediatric and adult health care teams in developing a formal plan.[33,34] *(For more information on this topic, see the Promoting Health for Children and Youth With Special Health Care Needs theme.)* As a legal adult after age 18 years, young adults now consent for their own health care. A health care professional must obtain permission to discuss the young adult's care with the parents without the young adult's permission. All the anticipatory guidance information should be directed toward the young adult patient.

The *Bright Futures Tool and Resource Kit* contains Previsit Questionnaires to assist the health care professional in taking a history, conducting developmental surveillance, and performing medical screening.

Priorities for the 18 Through 21 Year Visits

The first priority is to address any specific concerns that the young adult may have.

In addition, the Bright Futures Adolescence Expert Panel has given priority to the following topics for discussion in the 4 Late Adolescence Visits.

The goal of these discussions is to determine the health care needs of the young adult that should be addressed by the health care professional. The following priorities are consistent in all the Late Adolescence Visits. However, the questions used to effectively obtain information and the anticipatory guidance provided to the young adult can vary.

Although each of these issues is viewed as important, they may be prioritized by the individual needs of each patient. The goal should be to address issues important to this age group over the course of multiple visits. The issues are

▶ Social determinants of health[a] (risks [interpersonal violence, living situation and food security, family substance use], strengths and protective factors [connectedness with family and peers, connectedness with community, school performance, coping with stress and decision-making])

▶ Physical health and health promotion (oral health, body image, healthy eating, physical activity and sleep, transition to adult health care)

▶ Emotional well-being (mood regulation and mental health, sexuality)

▶ Risk reduction (pregnancy and sexually transmitted infections; tobacco, e-cigarettes, alcohol, prescription or street drugs; acoustic trauma)

▶ Safety (seat belt and helmet use, driving and substance use; sun protection; firearm safety)

---

[a] Social determinants of health is a new priority in the fourth edition of the *Bright Futures Guidelines*. For more information, see the *Promoting Lifelong Health for Families and Communities theme.*

Health Supervision

History

Interval history, including a review of systems, can be obtained according to the health care professional's preference or style of practice. In most cases, the young adult will be alone at the visit. In some situations, especially if the young adult has a special health care need, he may be accompanied by a parent, guardian, partner, spouse, or friend. Some clinicians use the HEEADSSS or SSHADESS mnemonics to help organize the questions for their young adult patients.[17,18] The following questions may encourage in-depth discussion to determine changes in health status that would warrant further physical or emotional assessment:

General Questions for the Young Adult

- Have you been in good health since your last visit here? Do you have any medical questions, problems, or concerns? What questions or worries do you have that you want to cover today?
- How are things going with your family, your friends, your job, in school?
- What are your future plans for employment, further education, or relationships?

Past Medical History

- Have you received any specialty or emergency care since the last visit?

Family History

- Has your child or anyone in the family, such as parents, brothers, sisters, grandparents, aunts, uncles, or cousins, developed a new health condition or died? **If the answer is Yes:** Ascertain who in the family has or had the condition, and ask about the age of onset and diagnosis. If they are no longer living, ask about their age at the time of death.

Social History

- See the Social Determinants of Health priority in Anticipatory Guidance for social history questions.

Surveillance of Development

The developmental tasks of late adolescence can be addressed by asking specific questions, through information obtained in the medical examination, by observation, and through general discussion. The following areas can be assessed to better understand the developmental health of the young adult. A goal of this assessment is to determine whether the young adult is developing in an appropriate fashion and, if not, to provide information for assistance or intervention. In the assessment, determine whether the young adult is making progress on the following developmental tasks[19]:

- Forms caring and supportive relationships with family members, other adults, and peers
- Engages in a positive way with the life of the community
- Engages in behaviors that optimize wellness and contribute to a healthy lifestyle
  - Engages in healthy nutrition and physical activity behaviors
  - Chooses safety (wearing bike helmets, using seat belts, avoiding alcohol and drugs)

- Demonstrates physical, cognitive, emotional, social, and moral competencies (including self-regulation)
- Exhibits compassion and empathy
- Exhibits resiliency when confronted with life stressors
- Uses independent decision-making skills (including problem-solving skills)
- Displays a sense of self-confidence, hopefulness, and well-being

Review of Systems

The Bright Futures Adolescent Expert Panel recommends a complete review of systems as a part of every health supervision visit. This review can be done through the following questions:

Do you have any problems with

- Regular or frequent headaches or dizziness
- Fainting or passing out
- Eyes or vision
- Ears or hearing
- Nose or throat
- Breathing problems or chest pains
- Belly aches or pains, throwing up, problems with bowel movements
- Painful urination or other urine problems
- Rashes, moles, sunburn
- Muscle aches, injury, or other problems
- Fatigue

For Young Women

- When was your last period?
- Do you have any problems with your periods?
- Do you have any itching, burning, or discharge in your vaginal area?

Observation of Parent–Young Adult Interaction

Most of the Late Adolescence Visits will be with the young adult alone, without a parent, unless the young adult requests differently. However, if parents are present, the health care professional can observe the interactions between the parent and young adult, including

- How comfortably do the young adult and parent interact, both verbally and nonverbally?

For all young adults who have a parent, guardian, partner, or spouse accompanying them to the visit, and especially for those with special health care needs, these visits provide an excellent opportunity to see whether the young adults are being appropriately encouraged toward managing and making independent decisions about their own health.[35,36]

Physical Examination

A complete physical examination is included as part of every health supervision visit.

When performing a physical examination, the health care professional's attention is directed to the following components of the examination that are important for young adults aged 18 to 21 years:

- **Measure and compare with norms for age, sex, and height**
  - Blood pressure

- **Measure and plot on appropriate CDC Growth Chart**
  - Height
  - Weight

- **Calculate and plot on appropriate CDC Growth Chart**
  - BMI

- **Skin**
  - Inspect for acne, acanthosis nigricans, atypical nevi, piercings, hirsutism, and signs of abuse or self-inflicted injuries.

- **Breast**

  MALE
  - Observe for gynecomastia.

- **Genitalia**

  FEMALE
  - Perform examination as indicated by patient or practitioner concerns.

  MALE
  - Perform visual inspection and examine testicles for sexual maturity rating.
  - Examine testicles for hydrocele, hernias, varicocele, or masses.

Screening

Universal Screening	Action
Cervical Dysplasia (all young women at the 21 Year Visit)	Pap smear
Depression: Adolescent	Depression screen[a]
Dyslipidemia (once between 17 Year and 21 Year Visits)	Lipid profile
Hearing (once between 18 Year and 21 Years Visits)	Audiometry including 6,000 and 8,000 Hz high frequencies
HIV (once between 15 Year and 18 Year Visits)	HIV test[b]
Tobacco, Alcohol, or Drug Use	Tobacco, alcohol, or drug use screen

continued

Screening *(continued)*

Selective Screening	Risk Assessment[c]	Action if Risk Assessment Positive (+)
Anemia	+ on risk screening questions	Hematocrit or hemoglobin
Dyslipidemia (if not universally screened at this visit)	+ on risk screening questions and not previously screened with normal results	Lipid profile
HIV (if not universally screened at this visit[b])	+ on risk screening questions	HIV test[b]
STIs		
▶ **Chlamydia**	All sexually active young women Sexually active young men + on risk screening questions	Chlamydia test
▶ **Gonorrhea**	All sexually active young women Sexually active young men + on risk screening questions	Gonorrhea test
▶ **Syphilis**	Sexually active and + on risk screening questions	Syphilis test
Tuberculosis	+ on risk screening questions	Tuberculin skin test
Vision	+ on risk screening questions	Objective measure with age-appropriate visual-acuity measurement using HOTV or LEA symbols, Sloan letters, or Snellen letters

Abbreviations: AAP, American Academy of Pediatrics; HIV, human immunodeficiency virus; STI, sexually transmitted infection; USPSTF, US Preventive Services Task Force.

[a] If depression screen is positive, further evaluation should be considered during the Bright Futures Health Supervision Visit. Suicide risk and the presence of firearms in the home must be considered. Disorders of mood are further discussed in the *Anticipatory Guidance section* of this visit.

[b] Adolescents should be screened for STIs per recommendations in the current edition of the AAP *Red Book: Report of the Committee on Infectious Diseases.* Additionally, all adolescents should be screened for HIV according to the USPSTF recommendations (**www.uspreventiveservicestaskforce.org/uspstf/uspshivi.htm**) once between the ages of 15 and 18, making every effort to preserve confidentiality of the adolescent. Those at increased risk of HIV infection should be tested for HIV and reassessed annually.

[c] See *Evidence and Rationale chapter* for the criteria on which risk screening questions are based.

Immunizations

Consult the CDC/ACIP or AAP Web sites for the current immunization schedule.

CDC National Immunization Program: **www.cdc.gov/vaccines**

AAP *Red Book:* **http://redbook.solutions.aap.org**

Anticipatory Guidance

The following sample questions, which address the Bright Futures Adolescent Expert Panel's Anticipatory Guidance Priorities for this visit, are intended to be used selectively to invite discussion, gather information, address the needs and concerns of the young adult, and build partnerships. Use of the questions may vary from visit to visit. It will not be feasible to ask all the questions at every visit. Questions should be modified to match the health care professional's communication style and the local culture. Any anticipatory guidance for the young adult should be geared to questions, issues, or concerns for that particular young adult. Tools and handouts to support anticipatory guidance can be found in the *Bright Futures Tool and Resource Kit*.

Priority

Social Determinants of Health

Risks: Interpersonal violence, living situation and food security, family substance use (tobacco, e-cigarettes, alcohol, drugs)

Strengths and protective factors: Connectedness with family and peers, connectedness with community, school performance, coping with stress and decision-making

Risks: Interpersonal Violence

Whether young adults are living on their own, with friends, with their parents, or with their own families, poverty, intimate partner violence, or neighborhood violence create a level of stress that affects the young adults' current and future health. The health care professional can identify these issues in a supportive and non-blaming way and help the young adult formulate steps toward solutions, and make referrals to appropriate community services.

Fighting behaviors can indicate the presence of conduct disorders or may co-occur with problems of substance use, depression, or anxiety. Many young adults are unaware of the prevalence of dating violence and would benefit from understanding the warning signs and actions to take.

Sample Questions

Can you tell me about your living situation? In general, how does everybody get along? Do you feel safe at home? What do you do when you get angry? Do you often get into fights? Physical or verbal? Have you been in a fight in the past 12 months? Do you know anyone in a gang? Do you belong to a gang? Have you ever been hit, slapped, or physically hurt while on a date? Have you ever been touched sexually against your wish or without your consent? Have you ever been forced to have sexual intercourse? Are you in a relationship with a person who threatens you physically or hurts you? Do you feel threatened by anyone? Are you worried that you might ever hurt someone else?

Anticipatory Guidance

- Learn to manage conflict nonviolently. Walk away if necessary.
- Avoid risky situations. Avoid violent people. Call for help if things get dangerous.
- Leave a relationship if there are any signs of violence.
- Confide in your parents or guardians; health care professionals, including me; or other trusted adults (such as teachers) if anyone bullies, stalks, or abuses you or threatens your safety.
- You can also call the toll-free **National Domestic Violence Hotline** at **800-799-SAFE (7233).**
- When dating, remember that, "No," means NO. Saying, "No," is OK, even if you have said, "Yes," in the past.
- Healthy dating relationships are built on respect, concern, and doing things both of you like to do.

Risks: Living Situation and Food Security

Difficult living situations or limited resources may cause concerns about the ability to acquire adequate housing and sufficient food. If the young adult or her family does not have enough money to buy food, refer them to resources, such as food bank and pantries, SNAP, or other federal nutrition assistance programs. Food security is still a critical issue in late adolescence, particularly because young adults may be newly responsible for providing for themselves financially and may be at higher risk than younger adolescents for income insecurity and food insecurity. Homelessness or inadequate housing also may affect the families of young adults or individual young adults who are emancipated, who have run away, or who have been excluded from the family home.

Sample Questions

Who are you living with? How long do you anticipate living in that situation? Do you feel safe? If not, have you tried to get help with this issue? In the past 12 months, did you worry that your food would run out before you got money to buy more? In the past 12 months, did the food you bought not last and you did not have money to buy more?

Anticipatory Guidance

- The people at community agencies have expertise in housing issues and can get you the help you need. Would you like me to help you get in touch with them?
- Programs and resources are available to help you and your family. You may be eligible for food and nutrition programs. The Commodity Supplemental Food Program and SNAP, the program formerly known as Food Stamps, can help you. Food banks, food pantries, and community food programs also can help.

Risks: Family Substance Use (Tobacco, E-cigarettes, Alcohol, Drugs)

Exposure to tobacco smoke remains an important environmental risk. Although the long-term health effects of e-cigarettes have not yet been established, exposure to secondhand vapor from them likely carries health risks. Adolescents with family members and peers who use e-cigarettes (also called vaping) are more likely to begin using these devices themselves, and adolescents who use e-cigarettes are more likely to start using conventional cigarettes.

A young adult's worries about a substance use or mental health problem of a family member or other person they live with may be a source of significant stress.

Sample Questions

Does anyone in your house or other places where you spend a lot of time smoke cigarettes or vape with e-cigarettes? Is there anyone in your life whose alcohol or drug use concerns you?

Anticipatory Guidance

- It's not always possible, but, when you can, avoid spending time indoors or in cars where people are smoking cigarettes or vaping with e-cigarettes.
- Nicotine from cigarettes and e-cigarettes is one of the most addicting drugs we know. That's why it's so hard for people to stop. That's also why I don't want you to products that contain it.
- If you are worried about the drug or alcohol use of anyone in your family or the people you live with, you can talk with me.

Strengths and Protective Factors: Connectedness With Family and Peers

In concert with identifying risks, providing anticipatory guidance about protective factors and strengths is a critical component of surveillance of the developmental tasks of late adolescence and early adulthood. Identifying strengths and providing feedback about what the young adult is doing well helps provide a comprehensive and balanced view of the young person's health and well-being. Often, young adults can build on these strengths when they make plans about how to deal with the challenges of chronic health conditions or a needed behavior change, such as better nutrition or more physical activity. For young adults living in difficult circumstances, such strengths may help protect them from, or reduce the degree of, negative health outcomes. All young adults need to know that they can positively influence healthy development no matter what difficulties or problems exist. *(For more information on this topic, see the Promoting Lifelong Health for Families and Communities theme.)*

Peer relationships can positively or negatively affect a young adult's outlook and choice of behaviors. Even though young adults spend increasing amounts of time with peers, it is still important for them to have the support of their families when they need help.

Sample Questions

Do you have a close friend? If not, what stands in the way? How do you get along with members of your family? What interests do you have outside of school and work?

Anticipatory Guidance

- It's still important to stay connected with your family as you grow to adulthood. Talk with your family to solve problems, especially around difficult situations or topics.
- Making friends and keeping them is an important life skill. Evaluating whether a friendship is no longer good for you also is important.
- If you're in a new situation and making new friends, consider choosing people who share your interests and approach to life. You can look for them in organizations, groups, faith communities, or volunteer situations.
- As you leave high school and begin a new life with new interests, you may find that you drift away from some of your old friends. That's a normal part of growing up and becoming an adult.

Strengths and Protective Factors: Connectedness With Community

Young adults who take part in a range of activities that interest them are more confident and manage their time better than those who do not. These activities can nurture strengths and assets that will help young adults successfully navigate this developmental stage. Living in a community or neighborhood that is safe, with positive community norms and opportunities for engagement and participation, also is a protective factor, especially for youth who may have significant risk factors.

Sample Questions

What are your interests outside of school or work? What do you like to do after school or work or on weekends? Do you have a chance to help others out at home or at school or in your community?

Anticipatory Guidance

- This is a good time to get involved in activities that interest you. Art, drama, mentoring, volunteering, construction, gardening, and individual and organized sports are only a few possibilities. Consider learning new skills that can be helpful to your friends, family, or community, such as lifesaving CPR or peer mentoring.

Strengths and Protective Factors: School Performance

Students who complete high school are more successful in supporting themselves and living independently than adolescents who do not. Poor academic achievement can be a sign of depression, anxiety, or attention or learning problems.

Sample Questions

Have you graduated from high school? If not, have you considered getting a GED? What are your plans for work or school? How can I or your parents help you reach your goal?

Anticipatory Guidance

- Take responsibility for being organized enough to get yourself to school or work on time.
- As you head to college, the military, or your first full-time job, consider getting involved in your community on an issue that is important to you.

Strengths and Protective Factors: Coping With Stress and Decision-making

Strategies for coping effectively with stress are an important aspect of emotional well-being and developing resiliency. Time-management skills, problem-solving skills, and refusal skills have all been identified as helpful. Some young adults have found that their social support network, exercise, journaling, or meditation help them manage.

The ability to solve problems, make good decisions, and cope with stress is an important skill for young adults. Parents, health care professionals, and other trusted adults can be a valuable resource in helping young adults set priorities, manage stress, and make progress toward goals.

Sample Questions

How do you cope with stress? Are you feeling really stressed out all the time? What causes you to feel stressed? What do you do to reduce or relieve your stress?

Anticipatory Guidance

- Most people your age experience ups and downs as they make the transition from adolescence to adulthood. They have great days and not so great days, and successes and failures. Everyone has stress in their lives. It's important for you to figure out how to deal with stress in ways that work well for you. If you would like some help with this, I would be happy to give you some ideas.

Priority

Physical Health and Health Promotion

Oral health, body image, healthy eating, physical activity and sleep, transition to adult health care

Oral Health

The value of brushing the teeth with a fluoridated toothpaste extends to all ages. Fluoride is beneficial because it remineralizes tooth enamel and inhibits bacterial growth, thereby preventing caries. Flossing daily is important to prevent gum disease. Young adults should have regularly scheduled visits with their dentist twice each year. Of note, wisdom teeth (2 sets of third molars), usually appear between the ages of 17 and 25 years.

Sample Questions

Do you brush twice a day? Do you floss once a day? When was the last time you saw a dentist? Do you have trouble accessing dental care?

Anticipatory Guidance

- Brush your teeth twice daily with fluoridated toothpaste and floss once a day. See a dentist twice a year and discuss ways to keep your teeth healthy.
- Don't use chewing tobacco. It causes mouth cancer.

Body Image

As young adults move away from home to college, the military, or their own apartments, they must take responsibility for establishing a healthy balance of physical activity and nutrition. Eating disorders are still a significant risk for young people in this age group, especially women.

Sample Questions

How do you feel about the way you look? How much would you like to weigh? Are you doing anything to change your weight? If so, what are you doing?

Anticipatory Guidance

- It's important for you to begin to figure out the right balance for you between your eating and physical activity so you can maintain a weight that is healthy for you.

Healthy Eating

Many young adults aged 18 through 21 years are making most food decisions on their own. They may be living on their own, eating college cafeteria food, and eating out often. Even if they are still living at home, their schedules often do not foster participation in family meals. Vegetarian or vegan diets require careful attention to ensure adequate intakes of protein and nutrients.

Sample Questions

Which meals do you usually eat each day? Do you ever skip a meal? If so, how many times a week? How many servings of milk or milk products, such as yogurt or cheese, did you have yesterday? How many fruits did you eat yesterday? How many vegetables? How often do you drink soda or sports or energy drinks? Are there any foods you won't eat? If so, which ones? What changes would you like to make in the way you eat? Do you have difficulty getting healthy foods?

Anticipatory Guidance

- Eat in ways that help your body be as healthy as possible.
  - Respond to your body's signals. Eat when you are hungry. Stop eating when you feel satisfied.
  - Eat 3 healthy meals a day. Breakfast is an especially important meal.
  - Pick a healthy lunch from the school or work cafeteria or other food venues, or pack a healthy lunch.
- Choose healthy, nutrient-dense food and drinks for meals and snacks.
  - Eat a lot of vegetables and fruits.
  - Choose whole grains, like whole-wheat bread, brown rice, and oats, not refined grains, like white bread.
  - Get enough protein from foods like chicken, fish, lean meat, eggs, legumes, nuts, and seeds.
  - Keep your bones strong by having 20 to 24 oz of low-fat or fat-free milk every day, plus an additional serving of yogurt, or cheese. If you don't drink milk or eat cheese or yogurt, have other foods that contain calcium as well as foods and drinks that are fortified with calcium and vitamin D, like some orange juices and cereals.
- Limit foods and drinks that are high in calories, saturated fat, salt, added sugars, and refined grains, but low in nutrients, like chips, pizza, ice cream, and cupcakes.
- Drink water throughout the day. Choose water or low-fat or fat-free milk instead of juice, fruit drinks, soda, vitamin waters, sports or energy drinks, and caffeine drinks.
- If you're concerned about having enough money to buy healthy foods for your family, please talk with me. I can tell you about food and nutrition assistance programs and local community resources that can help you.

For Young Women

- It's a good idea for you to consume foods rich in folate, like dark green leafy vegetables, foods fortified with folic acid, or a folic acid supplement, because, if you should become pregnant, having enough folate will reduce the risk that your baby might develop a birth defect, such as a neural tube defect.
- Be sure to avoid alcohol, tobacco, and drugs if you are considering becoming pregnant. Alcohol can seriously and permanently harm a baby.

Physical Activity and Sleep

Current recommendations state that young adults should engage in at least 150 minutes of moderate-intensity physical activity, or 75 minutes of vigorous-intensity physical activity, or a combination of both, per week. Physical activity is one cornerstone of a healthy adult life and is essential to maintaining a healthy weight. Young adults who have transitioned from their usual high school activities to different living and working situations may benefit the most from encouragement, advice, and problem-solving tailored to their individual situation.

Attention to balancing physical activity and inactivity is needed because mobile devices, computers, movies, and social media present numerous opportunities for physical inactivity. Using computers and digital devices are an important recreational outlet for many young adults. Therefore, guidance about limiting screen time is usually needed.

Sleep hygiene also is important for the young adult—8 to 10 hours of sleep are recommended for those on the younger side of this age spectrum, and 7 to 9 hours are recommended for older young adults.

Sample Questions

What do you do to be physically active, such as walking, biking, hiking, skating, swimming, or running? How often? For how long each time? What do you think you can do to be more active? Do you participate in any physical activities with your family or friends, such as biking, hiking, skating, swimming, or running? How much time do you spend on recreational screen time each day? Do you have a regular bedtime? Do you have trouble getting to sleep or waking up in the morning?

Anticipatory Guidance

- Be physically active as part of physical education, planned physical activities, recreation activities, and organized sports. Try to do 150 minutes or more every week of moderate-intensity physical activity, or 75 minutes a week or more of vigorous-intensity activity.
- You can be physically active throughout the week by walking to class and climbing stairs rather than using elevators. You can break it up into shorter times of activity throughout the week. Or, you can do a mixture of moderate- and vigorous-intensity activities. Doing a mix of physical activities you enjoy is a great way to reach the 150-minutes-a-week goal.
- To prevent injuries, use appropriate safety equipment, such as a helmet, a mouth guard, eye protection, wrist guards, and elbow and knee pads (**for young men:** also an athletic supporter, with cup), when participating in physical activity.
- Drink plenty of water to maintain hydration lost during physical activity lasting longer than 1 hour to prevent heat-related illnesses, such as heat cramps, exhaustion, and heatstroke.
- If the safety of the environment or neighborhood is a concern, find other places to participate in physical activity.
- Getting enough sleep may be difficult, but it is important for your physical and emotional health. Having a regular bedtime helps, as does limiting caffeine and the use of digital devices just before bedtime. If sleep is a problem for you, please talk to me about it.

For Young Adults With Special Health Care Needs

- Engage in physical activity for cardiovascular fitness within the limits of your medical or physical condition. Adaptive physical education can be helpful, and a physical therapist can help you identify appropriate activities.

Transition to Adult Health Care

It is important to assess the young adult's readiness for taking on his own health care. Over the course of the Late Adolescence Visits, the health care professional can work with the young adult to continue developing a transition plan.[34] Depending on the young adult's individual situation and whether he has a special health care need, these discussions can include explanations about legal changes that occur at age 18 years, especially issues related to confidentiality, informed consent, the presence of parents or others at the visit, and access to medical information by others.

Review the office policy about transition with the young adult, including what the office will offer during the next several years to make the transition to an adult provider successful.

Sample Questions

How confident do you feel about your ability to begin seeing an adult doctor? Tell me about your preferences for an adult doctor. Do you know about your health insurance coverage, and whether you can keep it over the next several years? Can you explain your medical conditions and medications, your allergies, your family history, and your emergency care plan?

Anticipatory Guidance

- When you were younger, your parents were the managers for your health care. As you grew up, that gradually changed and now you're ready to take on more of that responsibility. Let's talk about what you need to know and what skills you need to have to manage your health care as an adult.
- It's a big change to start seeing a new doctor for your adult health care. Let me tell you how our office can help you make the transition a success.

Priority

Emotional Well-being
Mood regulation and mental health, sexuality

Mood Regulation and Mental Health

- Many young adults may not present with classic adult symptoms of depression. Pervasive boredom or irritability still may be symptoms of depression in this age group, as can self-injuring behaviors. It is important to question them directly about suicidal thoughts or attempts if there is any concern about depression or other mental health problems. Bright Futures recommends the administration of a standardized depression screen, such as the *PHQ,*[22] at every health supervision visit.
- Anxiety falls along a spectrum of intensity, and symptoms can cause significant distress and affect the young adult's functioning at school, at home, or with friends.
- Post-traumatic stress disorder is frequently overlooked and can present with symptoms of depression and anxiety. Past traumatic events can include being in a motor vehicle crash, experiencing physical or sexual abuse or other major life events, witnessing violence, or experiencing a natural disaster.
- Fighting behaviors can indicate the presence of conduct disorder and may co-occur with problems with substance use, depression, or anxiety. Consistently not adhering to rules and requests from parents, teachers, or employers can indicate problems with the relationship or significant problems with other authority figures.
- Worsening or poor academic achievement or job performance may be a sign of depression, anxiety, attention or learning problems, or a substance misuse problem.
- Any young adult with substance use disorders also may be struggling with a mental health problem. These young adults need to be evaluated for both substance misuse and mental health.

Sample Questions
Do you often feel sad, feel irritable, or have difficulty sleeping? Did you ever feel so upset that you wished you were not alive or that you wanted to die? Do you find yourself continuing to remember or think about an unpleasant experience that happened in the past? Do you harm yourself, such as by cutting, hitting, or pinching yourself? Has anyone in your family had mental health problems or attempted or died by suicide?

Anticipatory Guidance

- Even with life's ups and downs, most people can figure out how to find and do the things they enjoy, such as doing their job or schoolwork; having good relationships with friends, family, and other adults; making decisions, often after talking with trusted friends and family members; having goals for the future; and sticking to their values.
- Sometimes, though, people your age may feel like they're too sad, depressed, hopeless, nervous, or angry to do these things. If you feel that way now, I'd like to talk about it with you. If you ever feel that way, it is important for you to ask for help.
- When people feel severely depressed, suicide may feel like the only option, but there are always more options. Please seek help as soon as possible by talking with me, seeking out a trusted friend or family member, calling 911, going to the closest emergency department, or calling the **National Suicide Prevention Lifeline** at **800-273-8255.**

Sexuality

For the young adult, the issue of sexuality is central. Some young adults may have questions or concerns about their sexual orientation, gender identity, or sexual maturity. For some, the decision to have an intimate relationship and become sexually active may be relevant. For others, thoughts about the emotional intensity of romantic relationships or protection from STIs and pregnancy may be uppermost in their minds. *(For a detailed discussion of these issues, see the Promoting Healthy Sexual Development and Sexuality theme.)*

Sample Questions

What are your values about dating and relationships? In terms of sexual attraction, are you attracted to males, females, or both? Do you have any questions or concerns about your gender identity, meaning your identity as a male or female? What are your plans and values about relationships, sex, and future family or marriage?

Anticipatory Guidance

- Sexuality is an important part of your normal development as a young adult.
- If you have any questions or concerns about sexuality, your sexual orientation, or your gender identity, I hope you will consider me one of the people you can discuss these issues with. I am available as a confidential resource for you. Please ask me if you have any questions.

Priority

Risk Reduction

Pregnancy and sexually transmitted infections; tobacco, e-cigarettes, alcohol, prescription or street drugs; acoustic trauma

Pregnancy and Sexually Transmitted Infections

It is important for all young adults to understand how to avoid pregnancy and STIs. By understanding both the physical and emotional health aspects of a young adult's sexual decision-making, the health care professional can ensure that the young adult has all the accurate information necessary to foster healthy decisions. This health focus also conveys that the health care professional is not making judgments about the young adults' worth as a person, but providing guidance and support for healthy behaviors. *(For a detailed discussion of these issues, see the Promoting Healthy Sexual Development and Sexuality theme.)*

Sample Questions

Initial options: *Are you now in a romantic relationship? Have you always felt safe and respected? Have any of your relationships been sexual relationships? Are you currently having sex with anyone? Oral sex? Vaginal sex? Anal sex? In the past, have you had sex? Have you ever been touched in a way that made you feel uncomfortable? Have you ever been forced or pressured to do something sexual that you haven't wanted to do?*

If the young adult is sexually active currently or was in the past: *How many people have you had sex with in the past year? Were your partners male or female, or have you had both male and female partners? Were your partners younger, older, or your age? Have you had oral sex? Vaginal sex? Anal sex? Did you use other birth control instead of, or along with, a condom? How often do you use condoms? Are you aware of emergency contraception? If you are having sex, are you making good choices to avoid emotional hurt for you and your partner? How are you protecting yourself against STIs and pregnancy?*

Anticipatory Guidance

- If you are sexually active, it's important to protect you and your partner or partners from an unwanted pregnancy and STIs by correctly and consistently using a long-acting reversible contraceptive, such as an IUD or contraceptive implant, or birth control pills. Use one of these methods along with a condom.
- Consider having emergency contraception available.
- One important issue is that any sexual activity should be something you want. No one should ever force you or try to convince to do something you do not want to do.
- It can be helpful to think through ahead of time how to make sure you can carry out your decisions about sex. Two things that have helped other young adults are to be careful with alcohol and drug use and to avoid risky places and relationships.

Tobacco, E-cigarettes, Alcohol, Prescription or Street Drugs

The use of tobacco, alcohol, and other drugs has adverse health effects on young adults and their still-developing brain. This focus on the health effects is often the most helpful approach and may help some young adults with quitting or cutting back on substance use. Others may be concerned about problems with substance use by their friends or family members. If screening questions about tobacco, e-cigarettes, alcohol, or drug use have not already been asked in a Previsit Questionnaire, Bright Futures recommends they be included during anticipatory guidance. Many young adults incorrectly consider e-cigarettes safer than traditional cigarettes. It is important to specifically ask about e-cigarette use, known by many youth as vaping.

Sample Questions

Do you or your friends smoke? Chew tobacco or use other tobacco products, like e-cigarettes, hookah, or snus? Does anyone in your home use tobacco products or e-cigarettes? Drink alcohol? Tell me about any experiences you've had with alcohol, marijuana, or other drugs.

Anticipatory Guidance

- Do not smoke, use tobacco or e-cigarettes, drink alcohol, or use drugs, anabolic steroids, or diet pills. Avoid situations in which drugs or alcohol are readily available. Smoking marijuana and other drugs can hurt your lungs. Alcohol and other drugs are bad for brain development.
- Alcohol poisoning is a serious and sometimes deadly consequence of binge drinking large amounts of alcohol in a short period of time. This can affect your breathing, heart rate, body temperature, and gag reflex. If you think someone has alcohol poisoning, call for emergency medical help.
- Support friends who choose not to use tobacco, e-cigarettes, alcohol, drugs, steroids, or diet pills. Choose friends who support you in your decision to not use tobacco, e-cigarettes, alcohol, or drugs.
- If you use alcohol, street drugs, or prescription drugs that weren't prescribed for you, talk to me about it. I can help you with quitting or cutting down on your use. To be safe, do not drink alcohol or use drugs when driving, swimming, boating, riding a bike or motorcycle, or operating farm equipment, since, in these situations, even small amounts of alcohol or drugs can be dangerous.
- If you or your friends drink or use drugs, plan to ride with a designated driver or call for a ride.

Acoustic Trauma

The Occupational Safety Health Administration has rules for noise exposure in the workplace to prevent a temporary threshold shift in hearing (a change of at least 10 dB from a previous test) that can become a permanent hearing loss.[26] No similar recommendation exists for noise from personal devices. Mild hearing loss (ie, >25 dB) was found in 3.5% of adolescents aged 12 to 19 years in NHANES III 1988–1994 and 5.3% in NHANES 2005–2006.[26]

To protect hearing, the CDC recommends avoiding or limiting exposure to excessively loud sounds, turning down the volume of music systems, moving away from the source of loud sounds when possible, and using hearing protection devices when it is not feasible to avoid exposure to loud sounds, or reduce them to a safe level.[27,28]

Sample Questions

Are you aware that loud noise can cause both temporary and permanent hearing loss? How loud do you usually have your music?

Anticipatory Guidance

- Wear hearing protection when you are exposed to loud noise, such as music, at concerts, or in loud working conditions, such as running lawn, garden, or snow removal machinery.
- When you use earbuds, make sure the volume on your device isn't too high.

Priority

Safety

Seat belt and helmet use, driving and substance use; sun protection; firearm safety

Seat Belt and Helmet Use, Sun Protection, Driving and Substance Use

Everyone should wear seat belts when riding in a vehicle and wear helmets when riding a bicycle, a motorcycle, or an ATV. Crashes are the leading cause of morbidity and mortality for young adults. Substance use by the driver can be a factor in many of these crashes. An arrest for driving while under the influence of a substance can have significant negative effect on a young adult's educational plans and insurance and employment prospects.

Sample Questions

Do you always wear a seat belt? Do you always wear a helmet when you are riding a bike, a motorcycle, or an ATV? Do you ever use your wireless mobile device while driving, even when at stop signs? Have you and your parents discussed what to do if you feel unsafe riding with someone who is driving?

Anticipatory Guidance

- Always wear a seat belt in a vehicle and wear a helmet when biking or riding a motorcycle or an ATV.
- Do not drive after using alcohol or drugs.
- Do not ride in a vehicle with someone who has been using drugs or alcohol.
- If you feel unsafe driving yourself or riding with someone else, call someone to drive you.
- Do not talk, text, or use a mobile device while the keys are in the ignition. Turn off your cell phone. If it feels impossible to drive without your device in your hand, put it in the trunk of the car.

Sun Protection

Sun protection is now of increasing importance because of climate change and the thinning of the atmospheric ozone layer. Sun protection is accomplished through limiting sun exposure, using sunscreen, and wearing protective clothing. About one-fourth of a person's exposure to the sun occurs before age 18 years. Early exposure to UVR increases skin cancer risk. Young adults may visit tanning parlors, which also raises their skin cancer risk.

Sample Questions

Do you always use sunscreen? Do you limit outside time during the middle of the day, when the sun is strongest? Do you visit tanning parlors?

Anticipatory Guidance

- Protect yourself from the sun by covering up with clothing and hats. Whenever possible, time your activities so you're not outside from 11:00 am to 3:00 pm, when the sun is strongest.
- Use sunscreen of SPF 15 or higher and reapply frequently.
- Wear sunglasses.
- Don't go to tanning parlors.

Firearm Safety

The AAP recommends that homes be free of firearms and that if it is necessary to keep a firearm, it should be stored unloaded and locked, with the ammunition locked separately from the firearm.

It is particularly important that firearms be removed from the homes of young adults who have a history of aggressive or violent behaviors, suicide attempts, or depression. The presence of a firearm in the home raises the risk of suicide and homicide, even in those without a mental health diagnosis.

Sample Questions

Do you know anyone with a weapon? Do you have access to firearms? Do you carry a weapon? Is there a firearm at home? If so, do you know how to get hold of it? Have you carried a weapon to school or work? Do any of your friends carry a weapon? If so, why?

Anticipatory Guidance

- Fighting and carrying weapons can be dangerous. Would you like to discuss how to avoid these situations?
- The best way to keep you, your family, and your friends safe from injury or death from firearms is to never have a firearm in the home. If it is necessary to keep a firearm in your home, it should be stored unloaded and locked, with the ammunition locked separately from the firearm. If children live with you, you must be sure that they cannot get to the key.

References

1. Bordini B, Rosenfield RL. Normal pubertal development: part II; clinical aspects of puberty. *Pediatr Rev.* 2011;32(7):281-292
2. American Academy of Pediatrics Committee on Adolescence; American College of Obstetricians and Gynecologists Committee on Adolescent Health. Menstruation in girls and adolescents: using the menstrual cycle as a vital sign. *Pediatrics.* 2006;118(5):2245-2250
3. Murphy NA, Elias ER. Sexuality of children and adolescents with developmental disabilities. *Pediatrics.* 2006;118(1):398-403
4. Euling SY, Selevan SG, Pescovitz OH, Skakkebaek NE. Role of environmental factors in the timing of puberty. *Pediatrics.* 2008;121 (suppl 3):S167-S171
5. Herman-Giddens ME, Steffes J, Harris D, et al. Secondary sexual characteristics in boys: data from the Pediatric Research in Office Settings Network. *Pediatrics.* 2012;130(5):e1058-e1068
6. Herman-Giddens ME, Slora EJ, Wasserman RC, et al. Secondary sexual characteristics and menses in young girls seen in office practice: a study from the Pediatric Research in Office Settings Network. *Pediatrics.* 1997;99(4):505-512
7. Weinberger DR, Elvevag B, Giedd JN. *The Adolescent Brain: A Work in Progress.* Washington, DC: The National Campiagn to Prevent Teen Pregnancy; 2005. http://web.calstatela.edu/faculty/dherz/Teenagebrain.workinprogress.pdf. Accessed November 16, 2016
8. The Teen Brain: Still Under Construction. National Institute of Mental Health Web site. www.nimh.nih.gov/health/publications/the-teen-brain-still-under-construction/index.shtml. Accessed August 9, 2016
9. Smith AR, Chein J, Steinberg L. Impact of socio-emotional context, brain development, and pubertal maturation on adolescent risk-taking. *Horm Behav.* 2013;64(2):323-332
10. Nelson LJ, Padilla-Walker LM, Christensen KJ, Evans CA, Carroll JS. Parenting in emerging adulthood: an examination of parenting clusters and correlates. *J Youth Adolesc.* 2011;40(6):730-743
11. Harper Browne C. *Youth Thrive: Advancing Healthy Adolescent Development and Well-Being.* Washington, DC: Center for the Study of Social Policy; 2014. http://www.cssp.org/reform/child-welfare/youth-thrive/2014/Youth-Thrive_Advancing-Healthy-Adolescent-Development-and-Well-Being.pdf. Accessed August 9, 2016.

12. Eisenberg ME, Resnick MD. Suicidality among gay, lesbian and bisexual youth: the role of protective factors. *J Adolesc Health*. 2006;39(5):662-668

13. Snapp SD, Watson RJ, Russell ST, Diaz RM, Ryan C. Social support networks for LGBT young adults: low cost strategies for positive adjustment. *Fam Relat*. 2015;64(3):420-430

14. Hirshkowitz M, Whiton K, Albert SM, et al. National Sleep Foundation's updated sleep duration recommendations: final report. *Sleep Health*. 2015;1(4):233-243

15. National Sleep Foundation. *Summary of Findings: 2006 Sleep in America Poll*. Washington, DC: National Sleep Foundation; 2006. https://sleepfoundation.org/sites/default/files/2006_summary_of_findings.pdf. Accessed August 9, 2016

16. American Academy of Pediatrics Adolescent Sleep Working Group, Committee on Adolescence, Council on School Health. School start times for adolescents. *Pediatrics*. 2014;134(3):642-649

17. Ginsburg KR, Kinsman SB. *Reaching Teens: Strength-Based Communication Strategies to Build Resilience and Support Healthy Adolescent Development*. Elk Grove Village, IL: American Academy of Pediatrics; 2014

18. Klein DA, Goldenring JM, Adelman WP. HEEADSSS 3.0: the psychosocial interview for adolescents updated for a new century fueled by media. *Contemp Pediatr*. 2014. http://contemporarypediatrics.modernmedicine.com/contemporary-pediatrics/content/tags/adolescent-medicine/heeadsss-30-psychosocial-interview-adolesce?page=full. Accessed August 9, 2016

19. Fine A, Large R. *A Conceptual Framework for Adolescent Health*. Washington, DC: Association of Maternal and Child Health Programs, National Network of State Adolescent Health Coordinators; 2005. http://www.amchp.org/programsandtopics/AdolescentHealth/Documents/conc-framework.pdf. Accessed August 9, 2016

20. American Academy of Pediatrics Committee on Practice and Ambulatory Medicine. Use of chaperones during the physical examination of the pediatric patient. *Pediatrics*. 2011;127(5):991-993

21. Attendance Works: Advancing Student Success By Reducing Chronic Absence Web site. http://www.attendanceworks.org. Accessed August 9, 2016

22. Richardson LP, Rockhill C, Russo JE, et al. Evaluation of the PHQ-2 as a brief screen for detecting major depression among adolescents. *Pediatrics*. 2010;125(5):e1097-e1103

23. Kann L, Kinchen S, Shanklin SL, et al. Youth risk behavior surveillance—United States, 2013 [published correction appears in *Morb Mortal Wkly Rep Surveill Summ*. 2014;63(26):576]. *Morb Mortal Wkly Rep Surveill Summ*. 2014;63(4):1-168

24. Sims TH; American Academy of Pediatrics Committee on Substance Abuse. Technical report—tobacco as a substance of abuse. *Pediatrics*. 2009;124(5):e1045-e1053

25. Noise. In: *OSHA Technical Manual*. Washington, DC: Occupational Safety and Health Administration; 2013. https://www.osha.gov/dts/osta/otm/new_noise/index.html. Accessed August 9, 2016

26. Shargorodsky J, Curhan SG, Curhan GC, Eavey R. Change in prevalence of hearing loss in US adolescents. *JAMA*. 2010;304(7):772-778

27. Franks JR, Stephenson MR, Merry CJ, eds. *Preventing Occupational Hearing Loss: A Practical Guide*. Washington, DC: US Department of Health and Human Services, Public Health Service, Centers for Disease Control and Prevention, National Institute for Occupational Safety and Health, Division of Biomedical and Behavioral Science, Physical Agents Effects Branch; 1996. DHHS (NIOSH) publication 96-110. http://www.cdc.gov/niosh/docs/96-110. Accessed August 9, 2016

28. Vasconcellos AP, Kyle ME, Gilani S, Shin JJ. Personally modifiable risk factors associated with pediatric hearing loss: a systematic review. *Otolaryngol Head Neck Surg*. 2014;151(1):14-28

29. Individuals with Disabilities Education Improvement Act (IDEA) of 2004. National Center for Homeless Education Web site. http://center.serve.org/nche/legis/idea.php. Accessed August 9, 2016

30. Stark P, Noel AM, McFarland J. *Trends in High School Dropout and Completion Rates in the United States: 1972-2012: Compendium Report*. Washington, DC: National Center for Education Statistics; Institute of Education Sciences; 2015. http://nces.ed.gov/pubs2015/2015015.pdf. Accessed August 9, 2016

31. Mental Illness Facts and Numbers fact sheet. National Alliance on Mental Illness Web site. http://www.nami.org/Learn-More/Mental-Health-By-the-Numbers. Accessed September 21, 2016

32. English A, Bass L, Boyle AD, Eshragh F. *State Minor Consent Laws: A Summary*. 3rd ed. Chapel Hill, NC: Center for Adolescent Health & the Law; 2010

33. American Academy of Pediatrics; American Academy of Family Physicians; American College of Physicians; Transitions Clinical Report Authoring Group. Supporting the health care transition from adolescence to adulthood in the medical home. *Pediatrics*. 2011;128(1):182-200

34. The National Alliance to Advance Adolescent Health. Got Transition Web site. http://www.gottransition.org. Accessed August 9, 2016

35. Institute of Medicine, National Research Council. *Building Capacity to Reduce Bullying: Workshop Summary*. Washington, DC: National Academies Press; 2014

36. Espelage DL, Low S, Rao MA, Hong JS, Little TD. Family violence, bullying, fighting, and substance use among adolescents: a longitudinal mediational model. *J Res Adolesc*. 2014;24(2):337-349

37. Kosciw JG, Greytak EA, Bartkiewicz MJ, Boesen MJ, Palmer NA. *The 2011 National School Climate Survey: The Experiences of Lesbian, Gay, Bisexual and Transgender Youth in Our Nation's Schools*. New York, NY: Gay, Lesbian & Straight Education Network; 2012

38. Weinberger DR, Elvevag B, Giedd JN. *The Adolescent Brain: A Work in Progress*. Washington, DC: The National Campaign to Prevent Teen and Unplanned Pregnancy; 2005. http://web.calstatela.edu/faculty/dherz/Teenagebrain.workinprogress.pdf. Accessed August 9, 2016

39. American College Health Association. *American College Health Association-National College Health Assessment II: Reference Group Executive Summary Spring 2015*. Hanover, MD: American College Health Association; 2015. http://www.acha-ncha.org/reports_ACHA-NCHAII.html. Accessed August 9, 2016

Appendix A
World Health Organization
Growth Charts

Birth to 24 months: Boys
Length-for-age and Weight-for-age percentiles

NAME

RECORD #

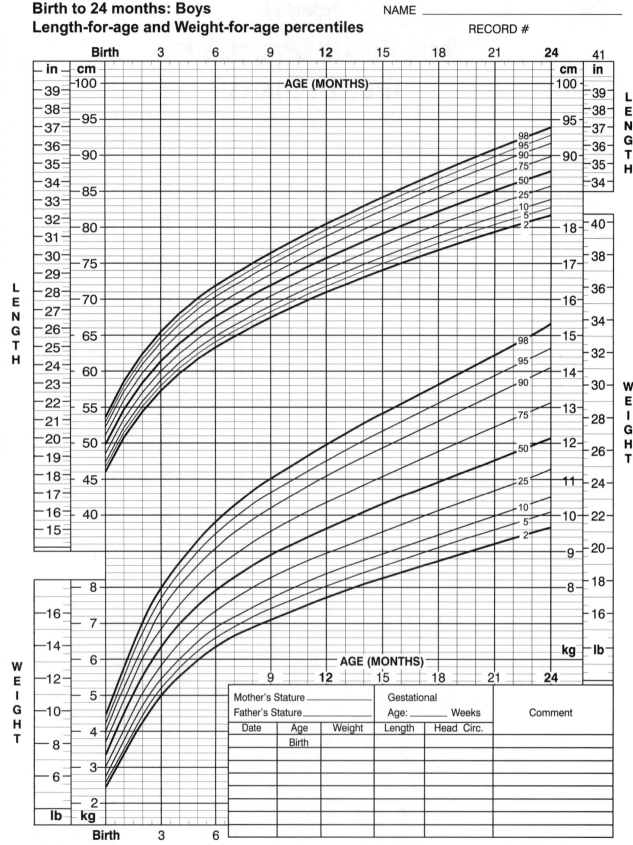

Published by the Centers for Disease Control and Prevention, November 1, 2009
SOURCE: WHO Child Growth Standards (http://www.who.int/childgrowth/en)

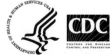

SAFER · HEALTHIER · PEOPLE™

Birth to 24 months: Girls
Length-for-age and Weight-for-age percentiles

NAME _____

RECORD # _____

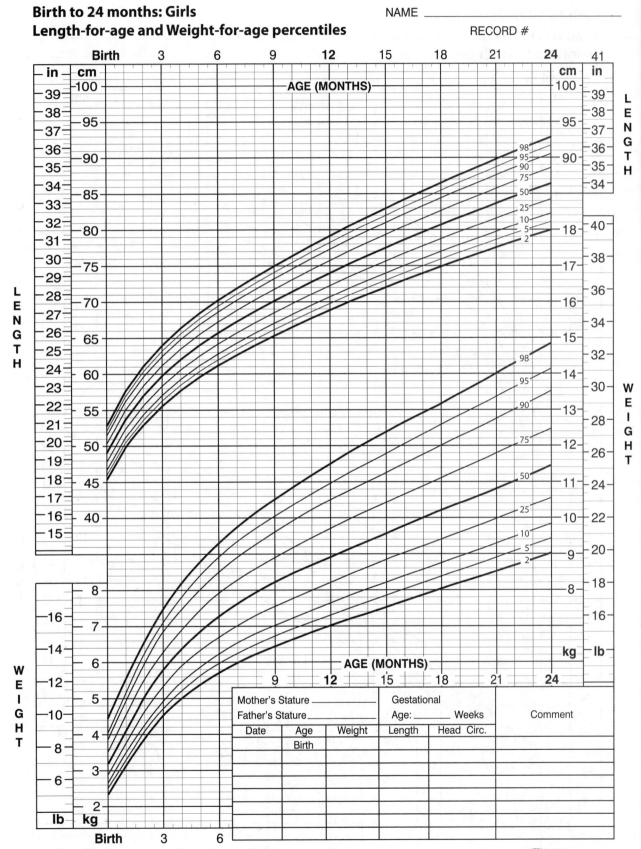

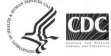

WORLD HEALTH ORGANIZATION
GROWTH CHARTS

Birth to 24 months: Boys
Head circumference-for-age and
Weight-for-length percentiles

NAME _____

RECORD # _____

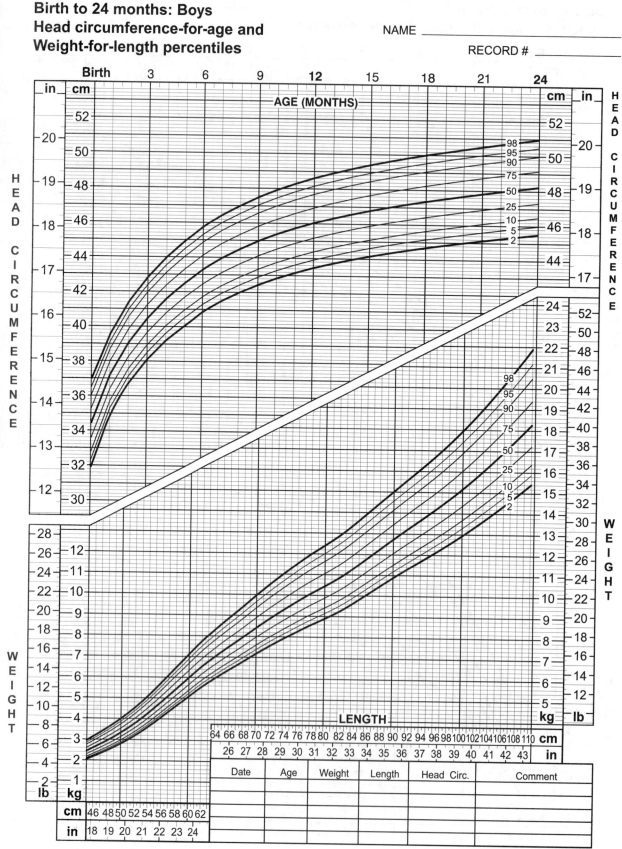

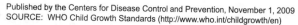

Date	Age	Weight	Length	Head Circ.	Comment

Published by the Centers for Disease Control and Prevention, November 1, 2009
SOURCE: WHO Child Growth Standards (http://www.who.int/childgrowth/en)

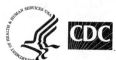

Birth to 24 months : Girls
Head circumference-for-age and
Weight-for-length percentiles

NAME _____

RECORD # _____

WORLD HEALTH ORGANIZATION
GROWTH CHARTS

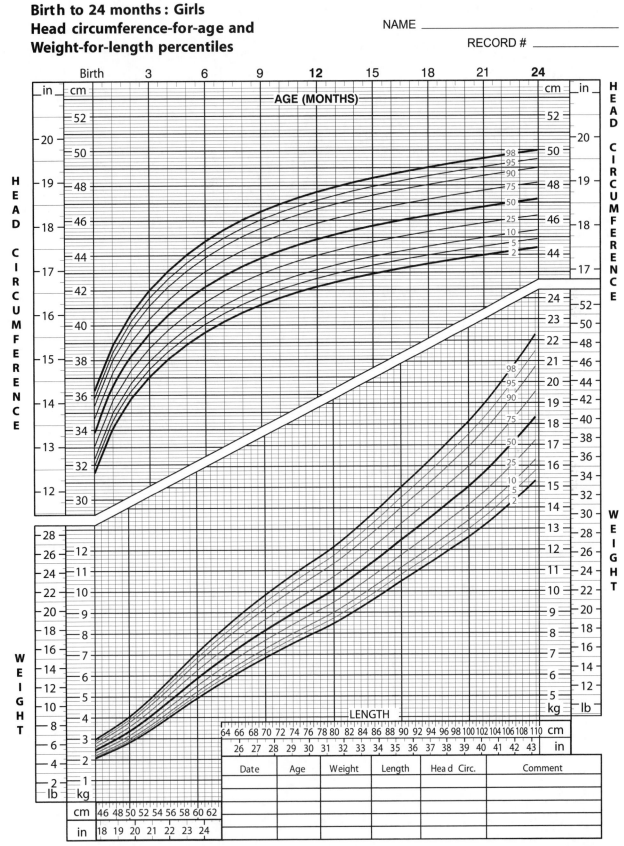

Published by the Centers for Disease Control and Prevention, November 1, 2009
SOURCE: WHO Child Growth Standards (http://www.who.int/childgrowth/en)

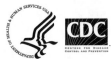

Centers for Disease Control and Prevention Growth Charts

2 to 20 years: Boys
Stature-for-age and Weight-for-age percentiles

NAME _____

RECORD # _____

Mother's Stature _____ Father's Stature _____

Date	Age	Weight	Stature	BMI*

*To Calculate BMI: Weight (kg) ÷ Stature (cm) ÷ Stature (cm) x 10,000
or Weight (lb) ÷ Stature (in) ÷ Stature (in) x 703

AGE (YEARS)

STATURE

WEIGHT

AGE (YEARS)

Published May 30, 2000 (modified 11/21/00).
SOURCE: Developed by the National Center for Health Statistics in collaboration with
the National Center for Chronic Disease Prevention and Health Promotion (2000).
http://www.cdc.gov/growthcharts

830

SAFER·HEALTHIER·PEOPLE™

2 to 20 years: Girls
Stature-for-age and Weight-for-age percentiles

NAME _____

RECORD # _____

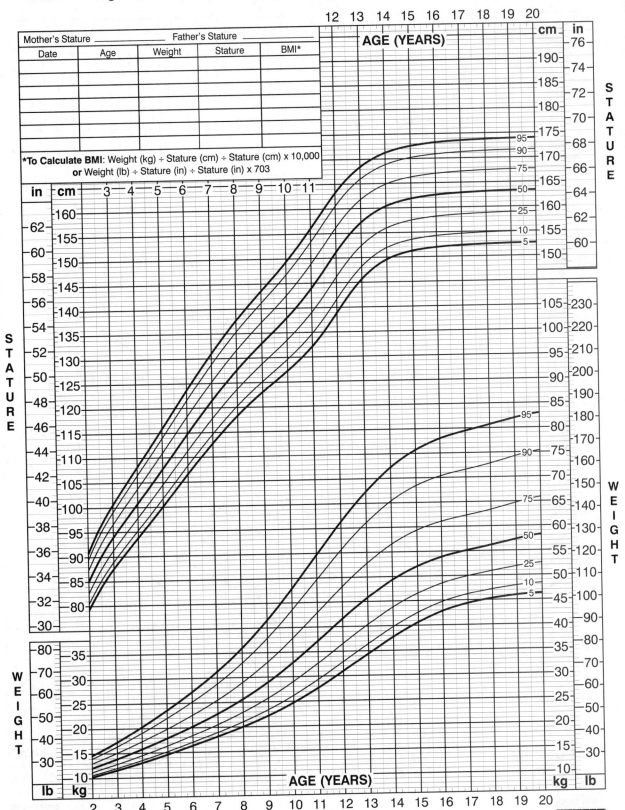

*To Calculate BMI: Weight (kg) ÷ Stature (cm) ÷ Stature (cm) x 10,000
or Weight (lb) ÷ Stature (in) ÷ Stature (in) x 703

Published May 30, 2000 (modified 11/21/00).
SOURCE: Developed by the National Center for Health Statistics in collaboration with
the National Center for Chronic Disease Prevention and Health Promotion (2000).
http://www.cdc.gov/growthcharts

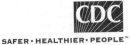

SAFER · HEALTHIER · PEOPLE™

CENTERS FOR DISEASE CONTROL AND
PREVENTION GROWTH CHARTS

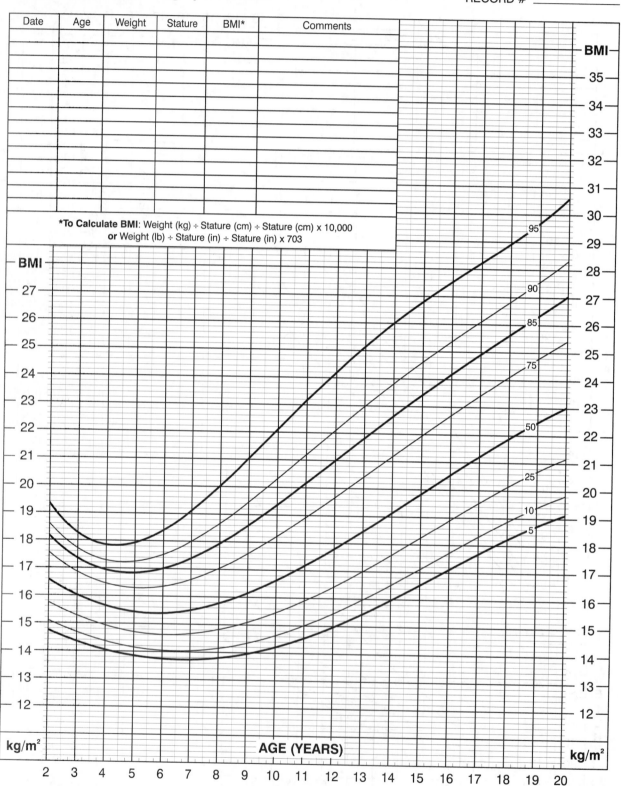

Bright Futures Guidelines for Health Supervision of Infants, Children, and Adolescents

2 to 20 years: Boys
Body mass index-for-age percentiles

NAME _____

RECORD # _____

Date	Age	Weight	Stature	BMI*	Comments

*To Calculate BMI: Weight (kg) ÷ Stature (cm) ÷ Stature (cm) x 10,000
or Weight (lb) ÷ Stature (in) ÷ Stature (in) x 703

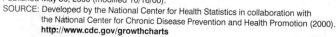

Published May 30, 2000 (modified 10/16/00).
SOURCE: Developed by the National Center for Health Statistics in collaboration with
the National Center for Chronic Disease Prevention and Health Promotion (2000).
http://www.cdc.gov/growthcharts

SAFER · HEALTHIER · PEOPLE™

2 to 20 years: Girls
Body mass index-for-age percentiles

NAME _____

RECORD # _____

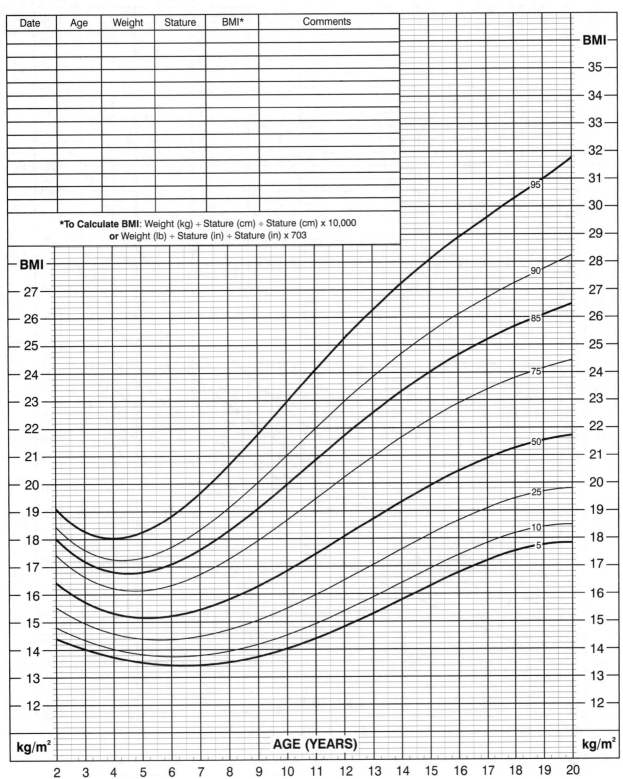

Date	Age	Weight	Stature	BMI*	Comments

*To Calculate BMI: Weight (kg) ÷ Stature (cm) ÷ Stature (cm) x 10,000
or Weight (lb) ÷ Stature (in) ÷ Stature (in) x 703

AGE (YEARS)

Published May 30, 2000 (modified 10/16/00).
SOURCE: Developed by the National Center for Health Statistics in collaboration with
the National Center for Chronic Disease Prevention and Health Promotion (2000).
http://www.cdc.gov/growthcharts

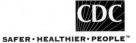

CENTERS FOR DISEASE CONTROL AND PREVENTION GROWTH CHARTS

Weight-for-stature percentiles: Boys

NAME _____

RECORD # _____

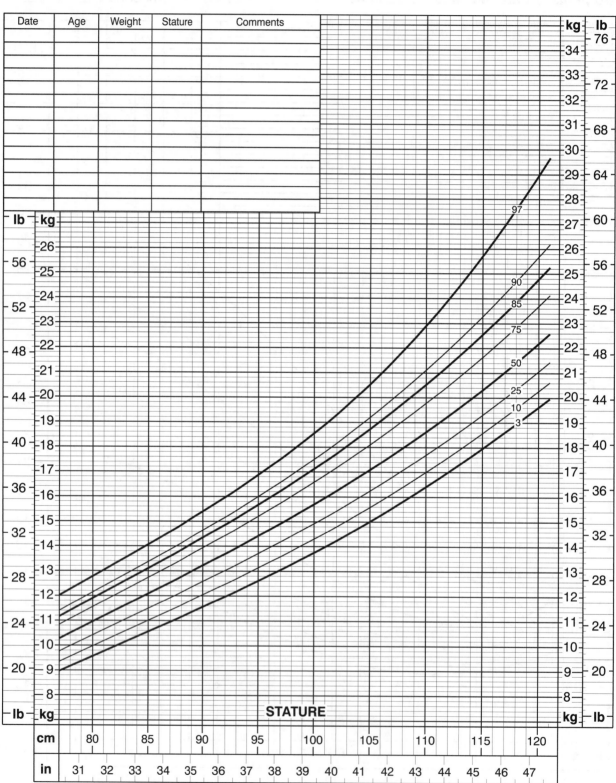

Date	Age	Weight	Stature	Comments

STATURE

Published May 30, 2000 (modified 10/16/00).
SOURCE: Developed by the National Center for Health Statistics in collaboration with
the National Center for Chronic Disease Prevention and Health Promotion (2000).
http://www.cdc.gov/growthcharts

SAFER · HEALTHIER · PEOPLE™

NAME _____

Weight-for-stature percentiles: Girls

RECORD # _____

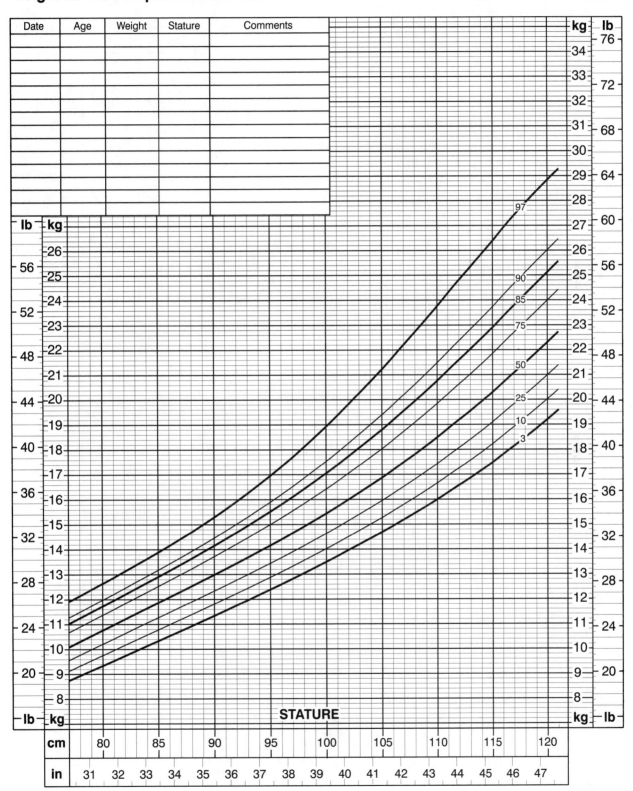

Date	Age	Weight	Stature	Comments

STATURE

Published May 30, 2000 (modified 10/16/00).

SOURCE: Developed by the National Center for Health Statistics in collaboration with
the National Center for Chronic Disease Prevention and Health Promotion (2000).
http://www.cdc.gov/growthcharts

SAFER · HEALTHIER · PEOPLE™

Appendix C

BRIGHT FUTURES/AMERICAN ACADEMY OF PEDIATRICS

Recommendations for Preventive Pediatric Health Care
(Periodicity Schedule)

Available at

www.aap.org/periodicityschedule

Index

Page numbers followed by an *f* or a *t* or *b* denote a figure, table, or box, respectively.

A

Abuse. *See* Family violence; Intimate partner violence; Maltreatment and neglect; Sexual abuse
Abusive head trauma (AHT), 121–122
ACE Study. *See* Adverse Childhood Experiences (ACE) Study
Acoustic trauma
    11 through 14 Year Visits, 761–762
    15 through 17 Year Visits, 793–794
    18 through 21 Year Visits, 819
ADHD. *See* Attention-deficit/hyperactivity disorder (ADHD)
Adolescence
    acoustic trauma in
        11 through 14 Year Visits, 761–762
        15 through 17 Year Visits, 793–794
        18 through 21 Year Visits, 819
    alcohol use/exposure in
        11 through 14 Year Visits, 745–746, 760–761
        15 through 17 Year Visits, 777–778, 792–793
        18 through 21 Year Visits, 808, 818
    anxiety disorders in, 138–139
    asset models for, 110, 110*t*
    attachment patterns in, 138
    attention deficits in, 139
    behavioral concerns/problems in, 140
    bisexual, youth who identify as, 224–225
    body image in, 189–190
        11 through 14 Year Visits, 751
        15 through 17 Year Visits, 783
        18 through 21 Year Visits, 811
    brushing teeth in, 214
    bullying in
        11 through 14 Year Visits, 743–744
        15 through 17 Year Visits, 775–776
        18 through 21 Year Visits, 805–806
    calcium in, 183*b*, 188*b*
    cheerleading safety, 252
    cognitive development/skills in, 108
        cognitive deficits, 139
    communication skills in, 108
    community connectedness/engagement in
        11 through 14 Year Visits, 747–748
        15 through 17 Year Visits, 779–780
        18 through 21 Year Visits, 809
    concussions from sports, 251
    conduct disturbances in, 140
    connectedness in, 138
        social connections/skills, 108–109
    contraception in, 222
    coping with stress in
        11 through 14 Year Visits, 749
        15 through 17 Year Visits, 781
        18 through 21 Year Visits, 810

    decision-making skills in
        11 through 14 Year Visits, 749
        15 through 17 Year Visits, 781
        18 through 21 Year Visits, 810
    deficit models for, 110*t*
    depression in, 138–139
        screening for, 283
    development/developmental surveillance in, 78–79
        11 through 14 Year Visits, 739
        15 through 17 Year Visits, 771
        18 through 21 Year Visits, 802–803
        cognitive deficits, 139
        cognitive development/skills, 108
        developmental domains, 107*t*, 108–109
        developmental highlights/milestones, 110
        growth, nutrition for, 187–189
        healthy development, promotion of, 106–110
        sexual development and sexuality, 221–225
    diet and nutrition in, 187–190
        dietary reference intakes, 183*b*, 188*b*
        growth, nutrition for, 187–189
        oral health promotion, 213–214
    driving safely in, 248–249
        15 through 17 Year Visits, 795–796
        18 through 21 Year Visits, 820
    eating disorders in, 189–190
    eating habits in, 189–190
        11 through 14 Year Visits, 751–753
        15 through 17 Year Visits, 784–785
        18 through 21 Year Visits, 812
        eating disorders, 189–190
    e-cigarette use/exposure in
        11 through 14 Year Visits, 745–746, 760–761
        15 through 17 Year Visits, 777–778, 792–793
        18 through 21 Year Visits, 808, 818
    emotional development/well-being in, 108–109, 137, 137*t*
    family dynamic/relationships in
        11 through 14 Year Visits, 746–747
        15 through 17 Year Visits, 778–779
        18 through 21 Year Visits, 808–809
    family support in, 60–61
    fighting in
        11 through 14 Year Visits, 743–744
        15 through 17 Year Visits, 775–776
        18 through 21 Year Visits, 805–806
    firearm safety in
        11 through 14 Year Visits, 765
        15 through 17 Year Visits, 797
        18 through 21 Year Visits, 821
    fluoride in, 213–214